Brief Contents

evolve

ELSEVIER

YOU'VE JUST PURCHASED
MORE THAN
A TEXTBOOK!

Evolve Student Resources for *Sorrentino & Remmert: Mosby's Essentials for Nursing Assistants, 6th edition*, include the following:

- Video Clips
- Audio Glossary
- Spanish Vocabulary and Phrases Audio Glossary
- Procedure Checklists
- Chapter Review Questions
- Scenarios in Practice Questions
- Body Spectrum Coloring Book

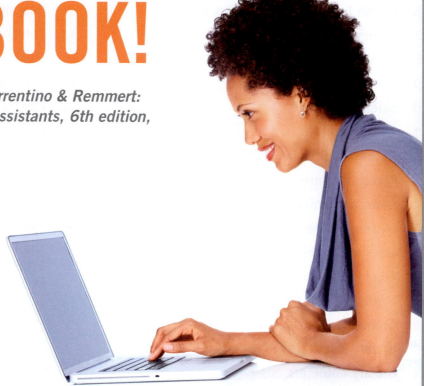

Activate the complete learning experience that comes with each textbook purchase by registering at

http://evolve.elsevier.com/Sorrentino/essentials/

REGISTER TODAY!

2015v1.0

EDITION **6**

Mosby's ESSENTIALS
FOR Nursing Assistants

SHEILA A. SORRENTINO, PhD, RN
Delegation Consultant
Anthem, Arizona

LEIGHANN N. REMMERT, MS, RN
Nursing Assistant Instructor
Mt. Pulaski, Illinois

ELSEVIER

ELSEVIER

3251 Riverport Lane
St. Louis, Missouri 63043

MOSBY'S ESSENTIALS FOR NURSING ASSISTANTS, SIXTH EDITION

ISBN: 978-0-323-52392-9

Notices

Practitioners and researchers must always rely on their own experience and knowledge in evaluating and using any information, methods, compounds or experiments described herein. Because of rapid advances in the medical sciences, in particular, independent verification of diagnoses and drug dosages should be made. To the fullest extent of the law, no responsibility is assumed by Elsevier, authors, editors or contributors for any injury and/or damage to persons or property as a matter of products liability, negligence or otherwise, or from any use or operation of any methods, products, instructions, or ideas contained in the material herein.

Previous editions copyrighted 2014, 2010, 2006, 2001, and 1997.

Library of Congress Cataloging-in-Publication Data

Names: Sorrentino, Sheila A., author. | Remmert, Leighann N., author.
Title: Mosby's essentials for nursing assistants / Sheila A. Sorrentino, Leighann N. Remmert.
Other titles: Essentials for nursing assistants
Description: Sixth edition. | St. Louis, Missouri : Elsevier, [2018] | Includes bibliographical references and index.
Identifiers: LCCN 2017049764 | ISBN 9780323523929 (pbk. : alk. paper)
Subjects: | MESH: Nurses' Aides | Nursing Care–methods
Classification: LCC RT84 | NLM WY 193 | DDC 610.7306/98–dc23 LC record available at https://lccn.loc.gov/2017049764

Senior Content Strategist: Nancy O'Brien
Senior Content Development Manager: Luke Held
Content Development Specialist: Kelly Skelton
Publishing Services Manager: Jeff Patterson
Book Production Specialist: Carol O'Connell
Design Direction: Renee Duenow

Printed in Canada

Last digit is the print number: 9 8 7 6 5 4 3

Working together to grow libraries in developing countries

www.elsevier.com • www.bookaid.org

Dedication

To my brother, Tony

and

My sister, Sandra

Because we are family

Love you both,

Sheila

To Shane

*For 20 years together
and the hope of
many, many more*

I love you,

Leighann

About the Authors

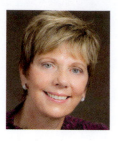

Sheila A. Sorrentino was instrumental in the development and approval of CNA-PN-ADN career-ladder programs in the Illinois community college system and has taught at various levels of nursing education—nursing assistant, practical nursing, associate degree nursing, and baccalaureate and higher degree programs. Her career includes experiences in nursing practice and higher education—nursing assistant, staff nurse, charge and head nurse, nursing faculty, program director, assistant dean, and dean.

A Mosby author and co-author of several nursing assistant titles since 1982, Dr. Sorrentino's titles include:
- *Mosby's Textbook for Nursing Assistants* (ed 1–9)
- *Mosby's Essentials for Nursing Assistants* (ed 1–6)
- *Mosby's Textbook for Long-Term Care Nursing Assistants* (ed 1–6)
- *Mosby's Textbook for Nursing Assistive Personnel* (ed 1–2)
- *Mosby's Basic Skills for Nursing Assistants*
- *Mosby's Textbook for Medication Assistants*

She was also involved in the development of an early version of *Mosby's Nursing Assistant Video Skills* and *Mosby's Nursing Video Skills*, winner of the 2003 AJN Book of the Year Award (electronic media). An earlier version of nursing assistant video skills won an International Films Award on caregiving.

Dr. Sorrentino has a Bachelor of Science degree in nursing, a Master of Arts degree in education, a Master of Science degree in nursing, and a PhD in higher education administration. She is a member of Sigma Theta Tau International, the Honor Society of Nursing. Her past community activities include the Rotary Club of Anthem (Anthem, Arizona), the Provena Senior Services Board of Directors (Mokena, Illinois), the Central Illinois Higher Education Health Care Task Force, the Iowa-Illinois Safety Council Board of Directors, and the Board of Directors of Our Lady of Victory Nursing Center (Bourbonnais, Illinois).

She received an alumni achievement award from Lewis University for outstanding leadership and dedication in nursing education. She is also a member of the Illinois State University College of Education Hall of Fame.

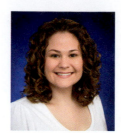

Leighann N. Remmert is a nursing assistant instructor in central Illinois. Teaching in vocational and high school programs, she guides students in acquiring the skills and knowledge needed to succeed as nursing assistants.

Leighann has a Bachelor of Science degree in nursing from Bradley University (Peoria, Illinois) and a Master of Science degree in nursing education from Southern Illinois University Edwardsville (Edwardsville, Illinois). She is a member of Sigma Theta Tau International, the Honor Society of Nursing, and the Certified Nursing Assistant Educator's Association (Illinois, Central Region).

Leighann's background includes diverse clinical and teaching experiences in acute care and long-term care settings. She began her nursing career as a nursing assistant/tech and nurse extern at St. John's Hospital (Springfield, Illinois). As an RN, Leighann concentrated in the area of emergency nursing at Memorial Medical Center (Springfield, Illinois). There, her career included the roles of staff nurse, charge nurse, trauma nurse specialist, and nurse preceptor. Recognizing her passion for teaching, Leighann began working as a clinical nursing instructor at Capital Area School of Practical Nursing (Springfield, Illinois) and teaching community Basic Life Support courses.

Leighann provides nursing assistant instruction for Lincolnland Technical Education Center (Lincoln, Illinois) and Fishes & Loaves Vocational and Literacy Center (Springfield, Illinois). Her teaching emphasizes the importance of professionalism and work ethics, safety, teamwork, communication, and accountability. Valuing the role of the nursing assistant and treating the person with dignity, care, and respect are integral to her instruction.

Leighann is co-author of *Mosby's Textbook for Nursing Assistants* (ed 8–9), *Mosby's Essentials for Nursing Assistants* (ed 4–6), and *Mosby's Textbook for Medication Assistants*. She was a consultant on *Mosby's Textbook for Long-Term Care Nursing Assistants* (ed 6) and served as a content adviser for *Mosby's Nursing Assistant Video Skills* (version 4.0).

Leighann and her husband, Shane, have 2 daughters, Olivia and Ava. Leighann and Shane are active in various ministry areas at Elkhart Christian Church (Elkhart, Illinois).

Acknowledgments

Many individuals help us develop an accurate, up-to-date, and timely publication. Therefore we extend a "thank you" and appreciation to:

- The staff of the Christian Village and Abraham Lincoln Memorial Hospital in Lincoln, Illinois. Many of the new photos were shot at these locations.
- The artists at Graphic World (St. Louis, Missouri) for their talented work and patience with revisions.
- Jordan Rick, RN (Peru, Illinois) for his insight and contributions.
- Artist Jeanne Robertson (Apex, North Carolina) for her prompt and detailed figure revisions.
- The reviewers who made comments and offered suggestions to improve our textbook. See "Reviewers" list below.
- Susan Broadhurst (New Orleans, Louisiana) for her role as copy editor. She accommodates our style well.
- Heather Faucher for her proofreading efforts. The task requires attention to detail.
- And finally the Elsevier/Mosby staff involved:
  - Nancy O'Brien, Senior Content Strategist
  - Kelly Skelton, Content Development Specialist
  - Carol O'Connell, Book Production Specialist
  - Suzanne Fannin, Project Manager
  - Renee Duenow, Designer

To all individuals who contributed to this effort in any way, we are sincerely grateful.

Sheila A. Sorrentino and Leighann N. Remmert

CONTRIBUTOR

Jordan Rick, RN, BSN
Registered Nurse II
Illinois Veteran's Home
LaSalle, Illinois

REVIEWERS

Beverly Banks, RN, BSN, MSN
Faculty
Alpena Community College
Alpena, Michigan

Tricia Berry, PhD, MATL, OTR/L
Associate Dean and Director of Clinical and Practicum Programs
Medical Assisting Program Chair
Kaplan University
Chicago, Illinois

Sherie Courchaine, RN, BSN
Nurse Aide Instructor
Dickinson-Iron Technical Education Center, Bay College
Kingsford, Michigan

Sylvia J. Crews, RN, MSN-L
Registered Nurse
Matrix Medical Network
Scottsdale, Arizona

MeLynnda Paulette Dunn, LPN
Certified Nurse Assistant Instructor
PRN Medical Services
Fort Smith, Arkansas

Jamie Hale, BSN, RN
Registered Nurse
PRN Medical Services
Springdale, Arkansas

Tiffany Jakubowski, BSN, RN, ONC, CMSRN
Adjunct Faculty
Front Range Community College
Clinical Nurse III
Longmont United Hospital
Longmont, Colorado

Stephanie Johnson, RN, ADN, BA
Staff Development, IPC, QAPI
SCVGS
St. Croix Falls, Wisconsin

Janis Longfield McMillan, MSN, RN, CNE
Assistant Professor of Nursing
Northern Arizona University
Flagstaff, Arizona

Dusty Marie Milne-Jones, LPN
CNA Instructor/Licensed Practical Nurse
PRN Medical Services
Springdale Arkansas

Mary Beth Riggins, RN, BA, MS
Mason Co ATC, Meadowview Regional Medical Center
Maysville, Kentucky

The sixth edition of *Mosby's Essentials for Nursing Assistants* serves several purposes.

- Prepares students to function as nursing assistants in nursing centers and hospitals.
- Assists faculty in meeting educational goals.
- Serves as a resource to prepare for the competency evaluation.
- Serves as a resource to review or learn new information for safe care.

The following foundational principles are presented in specific chapters while values, objectives, and organizational strategies are integrated in content and key features throughout the book. (See "Student Preface," p. xii for key features.)

- Patients and residents are *persons* with dignity having a past, a present, and a future. They are physical, social, psychological, and spiritual beings with basic needs and protected rights.
- Nursing assistant roles, functions, and limitations are described in federal and state laws with dependence on effective delegation and good work ethics.
- Body structure and function, body mechanics, preventing infection, and safety and comfort measures form an essential knowledge base.
- Communication skills enhance relationships with the nursing and health teams, patients and residents, and families and visitors.
- The nursing assistant has a key role in the nursing process.

CONTENT ISSUES

Content decisions are based on changes in laws or in guidelines and standards issued by federal and state governments, accrediting agencies, and national organizations. So are changes to state curricula and competency evaluations.

Student learning needs and abilities, instructor desires, work-related issues, course/program and book length, and student cost also are among the many factors considered.

New Content
Chapter 1: Introduction to Health Care
- *Patient Protection and Affordable Care Act* of 2010

Chapter 2: The Person's Rights
- Box 2-1 Resident Rights

Chapter 3: The Nursing Assistant
- Working in Another State
- PROMOTING SAFETY AND COMFORT: Who Can Delegate
- DELEGATION GUIDELINES: Step 2—Communication

Chapter 4: Ethics and Laws *(new!)*
- Box 4-3 Boundary Signs
- PROMOTING SAFETY AND COMFORT: Intentional Torts (Defamation)
- Wrongful Use of Electronic Communications
- Box 4-5 Electronic Communications
- FOCUS ON COMMUNICATION: Wrongful Use of Electronic Communications
- PROMOTING SAFETY AND COMFORT: Intimate Partner Violence

Chapter 5: Student and Work Ethics
- Bullying
- Unethical Student Behavior

Chapter 6: Health Team Communications
- Table 6-1 Defining Medical Terms

Chapter 10: Safety Needs
- FOCUS ON OLDER PERSONS: Preventing Burns
- PROMOTING SAFETY AND COMFORT: Preventing Poisoning

Chapter 11: Preventing Falls
- FOCUS ON OLDER PERSONS: Causes and Risk Factors for Falls
- Bed and Chair Alarms
- PROMOTING SAFETY AND COMFORT: The Falling Person

Chapter 12: Restraint Alternatives and Restraints
- PROMOTING SAFETY AND COMFORT: Risks From Restraint Use

Chapter 13: Preventing Infection
- Donning and Removing PPE
- PROMOTING SAFETY AND COMFORT: Donning and Removing PPE
- Surgical Asepsis

Chapter 14: Body Mechanics
- Back Injuries
- PROMOTING SAFETY AND COMFORT: Back Injuries
- Preventing MSDs
- PROMOTING SAFETY AND COMFORT: Preventing MSDs
- FOCUS ON MATH: Fowler's Positions

Chapter 15: Moving the Person *(new!)*
- Box 15-1 Guidelines for Moving Persons in Bed

Chapter 16: Transferring the Person *(new!)*

New Key Terms

- Psychosis (Chapter 34)
- Pulse oximetry (Chapter 30)
- Reasonable accommodation (Chapter 38)
- Reciprocity (Chapter 3)
- Resuscitate (Chapter 36)
- Straight catheter (Chapter 21)
- Surveyor (Chapter 1)
- Tinnitus (Chapter 32)
- Vertigo (Chapter 32)

New Procedures

- Transferring the Person Using a Stand-Assist Mechanical Lift (Chapter 16)
- Caring for Eyeglasses (Chapter 32)

New Figures

- Figure 1-1 A hospital room.
- Figure 1-2 Nursing care patterns.
- Figure 2-3 A nursing assistant is helping residents with an activity.
- Figure 2-4 This resident's personal items include an electronic device.
- Figure 3-1 Nursing assistant training program. An instructor demonstrates a skill to her students.
- Figure 3-3 The nurse considers the person's needs, the task, and the staff member's abilities when making delegation decisions.
- Figure 4-3 Some physical signs of elder abuse.
- Figure 6-5 Electronic charting sample.
- Figure 6-6 The nursing assistant uses an electronic device to record.
- Figure 9-3 A nursing center is as home-like as possible.
- Figure 11-3 Bed alarm.
- Figure 12-19 Charting sample.
- Figure 13-3 Cross-contamination.
- Figure 13-10 Hands are dried starting at the fingertips and working up to the forearms.
- Figure 13-16, **C** Method 2: Removing PPE.
- Figure 15-11 Re-positioning the person in a reclining chair.
- Figure 16-12, **A** Parts of a stand-assist lift.
- Figure 16-13, **A–E** Using a stand-assist lift.
- Figure 17-9, **A–B** Bariatric bed.
- Figure 18-22 A shower cabinet.
- Figure 18-26, **A–C** Cleaning the perineum.
- Figure 18-29, **B** Cleaning the penis. Clean the shaft with downward strokes.
- Figure 19-1, **A–B** Grooming aids.
- Figure 19-22, **A–B** Applying pullover garments.
- Figure 21-2 Parts of an indwelling catheter and urine drainage system.

- Figure 21-3 Urine drainage bag secured to the bed frame.
- Figure 21-4, **C** The catheter is secured to the man's thigh with a leg band.
- Figure 21-5, **B** Start at the meatus and clean downward at least 4 inches.
- Figure 22-1 Color chart for stools.
- Figure 22-2 Stool shapes and consistencies.
- Figure 22-5 A stoma on the surface of the body.
- Figure 23-3 Percent of food eaten.
- Figure 23-4 Percents measure parts of a whole.
- Figure 24-2 A graduate is on a flat surface. The amount is read at eye level.
- Figure 24-3 Calculating unlabeled measurements.
- Figure 25-10 Values used to read thermometers.
- Figure 25-11 Reading thermometers.
- Figure 25-20 Parts of an aneroid sphygmomanometer.
- Figure 25-21 Reading the manometer.
- Figure 26-7 A blood glucose test.
- Figure 27-25 Walker tennis balls on the rear legs of a walker.
- Figure 27-27 Ankle-foot orthosis (AFO).
- Figure 28-4, **I** Fungal infection of the toenail.
- Figure 29-5 Blanchable and non-blanchable skin.
- Figure 29-6 Stage 1 Pressure Injury. **B**, Dark skin.
- Figure 29-14 Unstageable Pressure Injury. **A**, Dark eschar. **B**, Slough and eschar.
- Figure 29-15 **A**, Unstageable Pressure Injury with eschar. **B**, Unstageable Pressure Injury with slough.
- Figure 33-4 Knee replacement prosthesis.
- Figure 33-22 Fluid in the membrane lining the abdominal cavity (ascites).
- Figure 33-25 Urine is poured through a strainer to collect stones.
- Figure 35-1 A large clock can help persons who are confused.
- Figure 35-2 Nerve cell death and tissue loss shrink the brain in the person with AD.
- Figure 38-3 Sample thank-you note written after a job interview.

FEATURES AND DESIGN

For features and design elements, see "Student Preface," p. xii.

May this book serve you and your students well. We aim to provide current information for teaching and learning safe and effective care during a time of dynamic change in health care.

Sheila A. Sorrentino, BSN, MA, MSN, PhD, RN
Leighann N. Remmert, BSN, MS, RN

Student Preface

This book with special features (p. xiii) was designed to help you learn. This preface gives study guidelines to help you use the book. To study effectively, use a study system with these steps.

- Survey or preview
- Question
- Read and record
- Recite and review

SURVEY OR PREVIEW

Preview or survey the reading assignment for a few minutes. This gives an idea of what the assignment covers. It also helps you to recall what you know about the subject. Carefully look over the assignment. Preview the chapter title, objectives, key terms and abbreviations, headings, subheadings, and key ideas in italics. Also survey the boxes and chapter review questions.

QUESTION

Questioning sets a purpose for reading. Form questions to answer while reading. Questions should relate to how the information applies to care or possible test questions. Use the headings and subheadings to form questions. What, why, or how questions are helpful. Avoid questions with 1-word answers. If a question does not help you study, change the question.

READ AND RECORD

You read to:

- Gain new information.
- Connect new information to what you already know.
- Find answers to your questions.

Break the assignment into small parts. Then answer your questions as you read each part. Underline or highlight important information. This reminds you of what you need to learn. Review the marked parts later. Make notes by writing down important information in the margins or in a notebook. Use words and statements to prompt your memory about the material.

To remember what you read, organize information into a study guide. Create diagrams or charts to show relationships or steps in a process. Note taking in an outline also is very useful. For example:

1 Main heading
  A Second level
  B Second level
    (1) Third level
    (2) Third level

RECITE AND REVIEW

Finally, recite and review. Use your notes and study guides. Answer your questions and others from reading and answering chapter "Review Questions." Answer all questions out loud (recite).

Reviewing is more about *when* to study rather than *what* to study. You decided *what* to study during your preview, question, and reading steps. It is best to review right after the first study session, 1 week later, and before a quiz or test.

We hope you enjoy learning and your work. You and your work are important. You and the care you give make a difference in the person's life!

Sheila A. Sorrentino
Leighann N. Remmert

SPECIAL FEATURES

CHAPTER 14 — Body Mechanics

OBJECTIVES

- Define the key terms and key abbreviations in this chapter.
- Explain the purpose and rules of body mechanics.
- Identify the risk factors for work-related injuries.
- Identify the signs, symptoms, and activities associated with back injuries.
- Explain how to prevent work-related injuries.
- Position persons in the basic bed positions and in a chair.
- Explain how to promote PRIDE in the person, the family, and yourself.

KEY TERMS

base of support The area on which an object rests
body alignment The way the head, trunk, arms, and legs are aligned with one another; posture
body mechanics Using the body in an efficient and careful way
dorsal recumbent position The back-lying or supine position
ergonomics The science of designing a job to fit the worker; *ergo* means *work, nomos* means *law*
Fowler's position A semi-sitting position; the head of the bed is raised between 45 and 60 degrees
lateral position The person lies on 1 side or the other; side-lying position

musculo-skeletal disorders (MSDs) Injuries and disorders of the muscles, tendons, ligaments, joints, and cartilage
posture See "body alignment"
prone position The person lies on the abdomen with the head turned to 1 side
semi-prone side position See "Sims' position"
side-lying position See "lateral position"
Sims' position A left side-lying position in which the upper leg (right leg) is sharply flexed so it is not on the lower leg (left leg) and the lower arm (left arm) is behind the person; semi-prone side position
supine position The back-lying or dorsal recumbent position

KEY ABBREVIATIONS

MSD	Musculo-skeletal disorder	**OSHA**	Occupational Safety and Health Administration

Body mechanics *means using the body in an efficient and careful way.* It involves good posture, balance, and using your strongest and largest muscles for work. Fatigue, muscle strain, and injury can result from the incorrect use and positioning of the body during activity or rest.

PRINCIPLES OF BODY MECHANICS

Body alignment (posture) is the way the head, trunk, arms, and legs are aligned with one another. Good alignment lets the body move and function with strength and efficiency. Standing, sitting, and lying down require good alignment.

Base of support is the area on which an object rests. A good base of support is needed for balance (Fig. 14-1). When standing, your feet are your base of support. Stand with your feet apart for a wider base of support and more balance.

Your strongest and largest muscles are in your shoulders, upper arms, hips, and thighs. Use these muscles to handle and move persons and heavy objects. Otherwise, you place strain and exertion on the smaller and weaker muscles. This causes fatigue and injury. *Back injuries are a major risk.* For good body mechanics:

- Bend your knees and squat to lift a heavy object (Fig. 14-2). Do not bend from your waist. Bending from the waist places strain on small back muscles.
- Hold items close to your body and base of support (see Fig. 14-2). This involves upper arm and shoulder muscles. Holding objects away from the body places strain on small muscles in the lower arms.

All activities require good body mechanics. Follow the rules in Box 14-1.

174

The skin defends the body against disease. Intact skin prevents microbes from entering the body and causing an infection. Likewise, mucous membranes of the mouth, genital area, and anus must be clean and intact. Besides cleansing, hygiene measures prevent body and breath odors. They also are relaxing and increase circulation.

Culture and personal choice affect hygiene. (See *Caring About Culture: Personal Hygiene.*) The person's care preferences are part of the care plan.

See *Focus on Communication: Hygiene Needs,* p. 248.
See *Focus on Older Persons: Hygiene Needs,* p. 248.
See *Promoting Safety and Comfort: Hygiene Needs,* p. 248.

CARING ABOUT CULTURE

Personal Hygiene

Personal hygiene is very important to *East Indian Hindus.* For religious duty, at least 1 bath a day is required. Some believe bathing after a meal is harmful. Another belief is that a cold bath prevents a blood disease. Some believe that eye injuries can occur if bath water is too hot. Hot water can be added to cold water. However, cold water is not added to hot water for a bath. After bathing, the body is carefully dried with a towel.

(*NOTE: Each person is unique. A person may not follow all of the beliefs and practices of his or her culture. Follow the care plan.*)

Modified from Giger JN: *Transcultural nursing: assessment and intervention,* ed 6, St Louis, 2013, Mosby.

247

Objectives—what is presented in the chapter.

Key Terms—important words and phrases in the chapter with definitions. The key terms introduce chapter content and are a useful study guide.

Key Abbreviations—important abbreviations used in the chapter.

Magenta bolded type and magenta italics—key terms and definitions in the text.

Caring About Culture—describes some cultural practices.

Focus on Communication—suggest what to say and questions to ask when interacting with patients, residents, visitors, and the nursing team.

Color illustrations and photographs—visually present key ideas, concepts, and procedure steps.

Heading icons—alert to associated procedures. Procedure boxes have the same icon.

Callouts in blue font—callouts for boxes, tables, illustrations and photographs, procedures, and special boxes (*Focus on Commmunication, Delegation Guidelines, Promoting Safety and Comfort,* and so on) are in blue font.

Boxes and tables—rules, principles, guidelines, signs and symptoms, nursing measures, and other information. They are useful study guides.

Focus on Math *(NEW!)*—math involved in various care measures and procedures.

---

284   MOSBY'S ESSENTIALS FOR NURSING ASSISTANTS

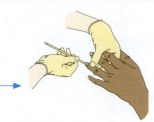

FIGURE 19-12 Push the cuticle back with an orangewood stick.

CHANGING GARMENTS

Hospital patients wear patient gowns or other sleepwear. Nursing center residents wear street clothes during the day and sleepwear at bedtime. Garments are changed:
- After bathing
- When wet or soiled
- On admission and discharge

Dressing and Undressing

Some persons dress and undress themselves. Others need help. Personal choice is a resident right. Let the person choose what to wear. To assist with dressing and undressing, follow the rules in Box 19-2.

See *Focus on Communication: Dressing and Undressing.*
See *Focus on Older Persons: Dressing and Undressing.*
See *Delegation Guidelines: Dressing and Undressing.*
See *Promoting Safety and Comfort: Dressing and Undressing.*
See procedure: *Undressing the Person.*
See procedure: *Dressing the Person,* p. 287.

Text continued on p. 289.

FOCUS ON COMMUNICATION

Dressing and Undressing

Promote personal choice and independence when assisting with dressing and undressing. You can ask:
- "What would you like to wear today?"
- "There's a concert today. Do you want to wear something special?"
- "Can I help you with those buttons?"
- "Do you need help with that zipper?"

FOCUS ON OLDER PERSONS

Dressing and Undressing

Persons with dementia may not want to change clothes. Or they may not know how. For example, a person tries to put slacks over his or her head. Or summer shorts are worn in the winter. The Alzheimer's Disease Education and Referral Center (ADEAR) suggests the following.
- Try to assist with dressing at the same time each day. Dressing becomes part of the daily routine.
- Let the person dress to the extent possible. Allow extra time. Do not rush the person.
- Let the person choose from 2 or 3 outfits. The family may buy several of the same outfit. Dressing is easier if the person insists on wearing the same thing.
- Choose comfortable, easy to get on and off clothes. Garments with elastic waistbands and Velcro closures are examples. There are no zippers, buttons, hooks, snaps, or other closures.
- Stack clothes in the order they are put on. The person sees 1 item at a time. For example, an under-garment is put on first. The item is on top of the stack.
- Give clear, simple, and step-by-step directions.

DELEGATION GUIDELINES

Dressing and Undressing

To assist with dressing and undressing, you need this information from the nurse and the care plan.
- How much help the person needs
- Which side is the person's strong side
- If certain garments are needed
- What observations to report and record:
  - How much help was given
  - How the person tolerated the procedure
  - Complaints by the person
  - Changes in the person's behavior
- When to report observations
- What patient or resident concerns to report at once

PROMOTING SAFETY AND COMFORT

Dressing and Undressing

Safety

To assist with dressing and undressing, you turn the person from side to side. If the person uses bed rails, raise the far bed rail. If bed rails are not used, ask a co-worker to help turn and position the person. This protects the person from falling.

BOX 19-2	Rules for Dressing and Undressing

- Provide for privacy. Do not expose the person.
- Encourage the person to do as much as possible.
- Let the person choose what to wear. Have the person choose the right under-garments.
- Make sure garments and footwear are the correct size.
- Remove clothing from the strong or "good" side first. This is often called the *unaffected side.*
- Put clothing on the weak side first. This is often called the *affected side.*
- Support the arm or leg to remove or put on a garment.
- Move and handle the body gently. Do not force a joint beyond its range of motion or to the point of pain. See Chapter 27.

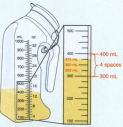

FIGURE 24-2 A graduate is on a flat surface. The amount is read at eye level.

FOCUS ON MATH

Measuring Intake and Output

To measure I&O, you must accurately read measurements. You may have to do some math.

Measuring Intake

To measure intake, subtract the amount left in each liquid served from the full serving amount. Add the intake amounts from each liquid together.

Intake is measured in mL (milliliters). Some containers show the serving amount in oz (ounces). You need to convert (change) the serving amount from oz to mL. One oz equals 30 mL (1 oz = 30 mL). To convert, multiply the number of oz by 30. For example:

A coffee cup holds 8 oz. Multiply 8 oz by 30 (the number of mL in each oz). The full serving amount is 240 mL.

$$8 \text{ oz} \times 30 \text{ mL/oz} = 240 \text{ mL}$$

(mL/oz is read as "milliliters per ounce")

You measure 90 mL left in the cup. Subtract 90 mL (amount left) from 240 mL (serving amount). The person drank 150 mL.

$$240 \text{ mL (full serving)} - 90 \text{ mL (amount left)} = 150 \text{ mL intake}$$

Measuring Output

Measuring containers are marked in oz and mL. Urinals and specimen pans used to measure output may not have all lines labeled. To calculate unlabeled measurements (Fig. 24-3):

1 Choose the labeled line above the fluid level and the labeled line below it.

$$400 \text{ mL and } 300 \text{ mL}$$

2 Subtract these 2 numbers. The result is called the *difference.*

$$400 \text{ mL} - 300 \text{ mL} = 100 \text{ mL}$$

3 Count the number of spaces between the 2 labeled lines in step 1.

$$4 \text{ spaces}$$

4 Divide the difference in step 2 by the number of spaces.

$$100 \text{ mL} \div 4 \text{ spaces} = 25 \text{ mL}$$
Each line increases by 25 mL.

Totaling Intake and Output

Intake and output amounts are each totaled at the end of the shift and 24-hour day. See Figure 24-1. Add the amounts for intake and the amounts for output. For example:
- Total 24-hour intake amount: *A person had 125 mL during the first shift, 1100 mL during the second shift, and 600 mL during the third shift. The total 24-hour day intake amount is 1825 mL.*

$$125 \text{ mL} + 1100 \text{ mL} + 600 \text{ mL} = 1825 \text{ mL}$$

- Total shift output amount: *A person voided 3 times during your shift—200 mL, 250 mL, and 100 mL. The total output for your shift is 550 mL.*

$$200 \text{ mL} + 250 \text{ mL} + 100 \text{ mL} = 550 \text{ mL}$$

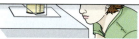

$$400 \text{ mL} - 300 \text{ mL} = 100 \text{ mL}$$
$$100 \text{ mL} \div 4 = 25 \text{ mL}$$
Each line increases by 25 mL.

FIGURE 24-3 Calculating unlabeled measurements. Divide the difference between 2 labeled lines by the number of spaces between the 2 lines. For example, each line on the urinal increases by 25 mL. The measurements between 300 mL and 400 mL are 325 mL, 350 mL, and 375 mL.

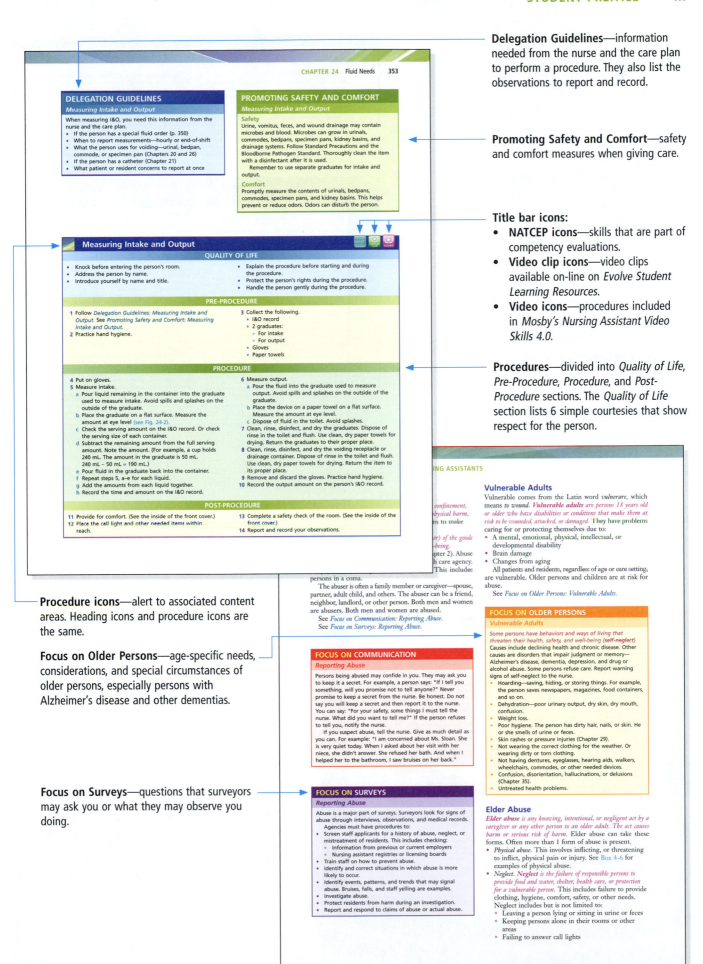

Delegation Guidelines—information needed from the nurse and the care plan to perform a procedure. They also list the observations to report and record.

Promoting Safety and Comfort—safety and comfort measures when giving care.

Title bar icons:
- **NATCEP icons**—skills that are part of competency evaluations.
- **Video clip icons**—video clips available on-line on *Evolve Student Learning Resources.*
- **Video icons**—procedures included in *Mosby's Nursing Assistant Video Skills 4.0.*

Procedures—divided into *Quality of Life, Pre-Procedure, Procedure,* and *Post-Procedure* sections. The *Quality of Life* section lists 6 simple courtesies that show respect for the person.

Procedure icons—alert to associated content areas. Heading icons and procedure icons are the same.

Focus on Older Persons—age-specific needs, considerations, and special circumstances of older persons, especially persons with Alzheimer's disease and other dementias.

Focus on Surveys—questions that surveyors may ask you or what they may observe you doing.

CHAPTER 24 Fluid Needs   353

DELEGATION GUIDELINES
Measuring Intake and Output

When measuring I&O, you need this information from the nurse and the care plan.
- If the person has a special fluid order (p. 350)
- When to report measurements—hourly or end-of-shift
- What the person uses for voiding—urinal, bedpan, commode, or specimen pan (Chapters 20 and 26)
- If the person has a catheter (Chapter 21)
- What patient or resident concerns to report at once

PROMOTING SAFETY AND COMFORT
Measuring Intake and Output

Safety
Urine, vomitus, feces, and wound drainage may contain microbes and blood. Microbes can grow in urinals, commodes, bedpans, specimen pans, kidney basins, and drainage systems. Follow Standard Precautions and the Bloodborne Pathogen Standard. Thoroughly clean the item with a disinfectant after it is used.
   Remember to use separate graduates for intake and output.

Comfort
Promptly measure the contents of urinals, bedpans, commodes, specimen pans, and kidney basins. This helps prevent or reduce odors. Odors can disturb the person.

Measuring Intake and Output

QUALITY OF LIFE
- Knock before entering the person's room.
- Address the person by name.
- Introduce yourself by name and title.
- Explain the procedure before starting and during the procedure.
- Protect the person's rights during the procedure.
- Handle the person gently during the procedure.

PRE-PROCEDURE
1. Follow *Delegation Guidelines: Measuring Intake and Output.* See *Promoting Safety and Comfort: Measuring Intake and Output.*
2. Practice hand hygiene.
3. Collect the following.
   - I&O record
   - 2 graduates:
     - For intake
     - For output
   - Gloves
   - Paper towels

PROCEDURE
4. Put on gloves.
5. Measure intake.
   a. Pour liquid remaining in the container into the graduate used to measure intake. Avoid spills and splashes on the outside of the graduate.
   b. Place the graduate on a flat surface. Measure the amount at eye level (see Fig. 24-2).
   c. Check the serving amount on the I&O record. Or check the serving size of each container.
   d. Subtract the remaining amount from the full serving amount. Note the amount. (For example, a cup holds 240 mL. The amount in the graduate is 50 mL. 240 mL − 50 mL = 190 mL.)
   e. Pour fluid in the graduate back into the container.
   f. Repeat steps 5, a–e for each liquid.
   g. Add the amounts from each liquid together.
   h. Record the time and amount on the person's I&O record.
6. Measure output.
   a. Pour the fluid into the graduate used to measure output. Avoid spills and splashes on the outside of the graduate.
   b. Place the device on a paper towel on a flat surface. Measure the amount at eye level.
   c. Dispose of fluid in the toilet. Avoid splashes.
7. Clean, rinse, disinfect, and dry the graduates. Dispose of rinse in the toilet and flush. Use clean, dry paper towels for drying. Return the graduates to their proper place.
8. Clean, rinse, disinfect, and dry the voiding receptacle or drainage container. Dispose of rinse in the toilet and flush. Use clean, dry paper towels for drying. Return the item to its proper place.
9. Remove and discard the gloves. Practice hand hygiene.
10. Record the output amount on the person's I&O record.

POST-PROCEDURE
11. Provide for comfort. (See the inside of the front cover.)
12. Place the call light and other needed items within reach.
13. Complete a safety check of the room. (See the inside of the front cover.)
14. Report and record your observations.

ING ASSISTANTS

... confinement, ... physical harm, ... ns to make

... er) of the goods ...-being.

... pter 2). Abuse ... h care agency. ... This includes persons in a coma.
   The abuser is often a family member or caregiver—spouse, partner, adult child, and others. The abuser can be a friend, neighbor, landlord, or other person. Both men and women are abusers. Both men and women are abused.
   See *Focus on Communication: Reporting Abuse.*
   See *Focus on Surveys: Reporting Abuse.*

Vulnerable Adults
Vulnerable comes from the Latin word *vulnerare,* which means *to wound.* *Vulnerable adults are persons 18 years old or older who have disabilities or conditions that make them at risk to be wounded, attacked, or damaged.* They have problems caring for or protecting themselves due to:
- A mental, emotional, physical, intellectual, or developmental disability
- Brain damage
- Changes from aging
   All patients and residents, regardless of age or care setting, are vulnerable. Older persons and children are at risk for abuse.
   See *Focus on Older Persons: Vulnerable Adults.*

FOCUS ON COMMUNICATION
Reporting Abuse

Persons being abused may confide in you. They may ask you to keep it a secret. For example, a person says: "If I tell you something, will you promise not to tell anyone?" Never promise to keep a secret from the nurse. Be honest. Do not say you will keep a secret and then report it to the nurse. You can say: "For your safety, some things I must tell the nurse. What did you want to tell me?" If the person refuses to tell you, notify the nurse.
   If you suspect abuse, tell the nurse. Give as much detail as you can. For example: "I am concerned about Ms. Sloan. She is very quiet today. When I asked about her visit with her niece, she didn't answer. She refused her bath. And when I helped her to the bathroom, I saw bruises on her back."

FOCUS ON OLDER PERSONS
Vulnerable Adults

Some persons have behaviors and ways of living that threaten their health, safety, and well-being (self-neglect). Causes include declining health and chronic disease. Other causes are disorders that impair judgment or memory—Alzheimer's disease, dementia, depression, and drug or alcohol abuse. Some persons refuse care. Report warning signs of self-neglect to the nurse.
- Hoarding—saving, hiding, or storing things. For example, the person saves newspapers, magazines, food containers, and so on.
- Dehydration—poor urinary output, dry skin, dry mouth, confusion.
- Weight loss.
- Poor hygiene. The person has dirty hair, nails, or skin. He or she smells of urine or feces.
- Skin rashes or pressure injuries (Chapter 29).
- Not wearing the correct clothing for the weather. Or wearing dirty or torn clothing.
- Not having dentures, eyeglasses, hearing aids, walkers, wheelchairs, commodes, or other needed devices.
- Confusion, disorientation, hallucinations, or delusions (Chapter 35).
- Untreated health problems.

FOCUS ON SURVEYS
Reporting Abuse

Abuse is a major part of surveys. Surveyors look for signs of abuse through interviews, observations, and medical records. Agencies must have procedures to:
- Screen staff applicants for a history of abuse, neglect, or mistreatment of residents. This includes checking:
  - Information from previous or current employers
  - Nursing assistant registries or licensing boards
- Train staff on how to prevent abuse.
- Identify and correct situations in which abuse is more likely to occur.
- Identify events, patterns, and trends that may signal abuse. Bruises, falls, and staff yelling are examples.
- Investigate abuse.
- Protect residents from harm during an investigation.
- Report and respond to claims of abuse or actual abuse.

Elder Abuse
Elder abuse is any knowing, intentional, or negligent act by a caregiver or any other person to an older adult. The act causes harm or serious risk of harm. Elder abuse can take these forms. Often more than 1 form of abuse is present.
- *Physical abuse.* This involves inflicting, or threatening to inflict, physical pain or injury. See Box 4-6 for examples of physical abuse.
- *Neglect.* **Neglect** is the failure of responsible persons to provide food and water, shelter, health care, or protection for a vulnerable person. This includes failure to provide clothing, hygiene, comfort, safety, or other needs. Neglect includes but is not limited to:
  - Leaving a person lying or sitting in urine or feces
  - Keeping persons alone in their rooms or other areas
  - Failing to answer call lights

Focus on PRIDE: The Person, Family, and Yourself—build on chapter content to help you promote *pride* in the person, the family, and yourself. The first letter of each section spells *PRIDE*.

- **P**ersonal and Professional Responsibility—how to have pride in yourself through personal and professional behaviors and development.

- **R**ights and Respect—how to promote the person's rights and respect him or her as a person with dignity and value.

- **I**ndependence and Social Interaction—ways to help the person remain or attain independence and interact socially with others.

- **D**elegation and Teamwork—how to work efficiently with and help nursing team members.

- **E**thics and Laws—laws affecting nursing care and doing the right thing when dealing with patients, residents, and co-workers.

Focus on PRIDE: Application *(NEW!)*—how to apply information in Focus on PRIDE. Questions are intended for personal thought or classroom discussion.

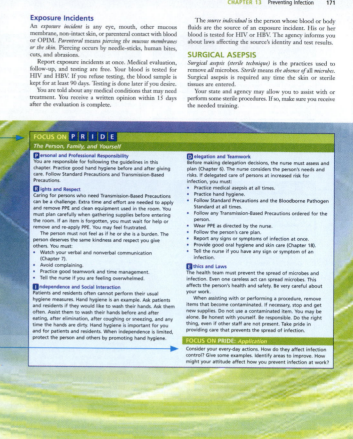

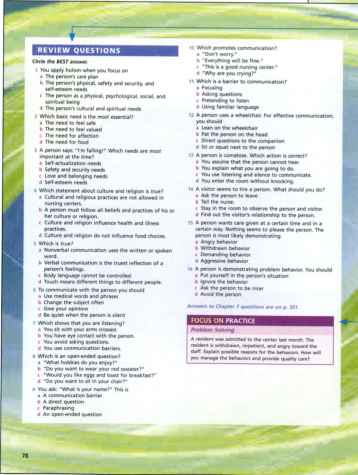

Review Questions—study guides to review what you have learned. Use them to study for a test or for the competency evaluation. Answers are at the back of the book. See p. 551.

Focus on Practice: Problem Solving—follow the Review Questions. A situation is presented that you may encounter as a student or in the work setting. For classroom discussion or self-study, questions relate to what you should do, how you should act, or how you can improve the situation.

Contents

Introduction to Health Care

OBJECTIVES

- Define the key terms and key abbreviations in this chapter.
- Describe hospitals and long-term care centers.
- Describe the persons cared for in long-term care centers.
- Describe the members of the health team and nursing team.
- Describe 5 nursing care patterns.

- Describe the programs that pay for health care.
- Explain your role in meeting standards.
- Explain how to promote PRIDE in the person, the family, and yourself.

KEY TERMS

acute illness A sudden illness from which the person is expected to recover

assisted living residence (ALR) Provides housing, personal care, support services, health care, and social activities in a home-like setting to persons needing help with daily activities

chronic illness An on-going illness that is slow or gradual in onset; it has no known cure; it can be controlled and complications prevented with proper treatment

health team The many health care workers whose skills and knowledge focus on the person's total care; interdisciplinary health care team

hospice A health care agency or program for persons who are dying

licensed practical nurse (LPN) A nurse who has completed a practical nursing program and has passed a licensing test; called licensed vocational nurse (LVN) in California and Texas

licensed vocational nurse (LVN) See "licensed practical nurse (LPN)"

nursing assistant A person who has passed a nursing assistant training and competency evaluation program (NATCEP); performs delegated nursing tasks under the supervision of a licensed nurse

nursing team Those who provide nursing care—RNs, LPNs/LVNs, and nursing assistants

registered nurse (RN) A nurse who has completed a 2-, 3-, or 4-year nursing program and has passed a licensing test

surveyor A person who collects information by observing and asking questions

terminal illness An illness or injury from which the person will not likely recover

KEY ABBREVIATIONS

ALR	Assisted living residence	**LVN**	Licensed vocational nurse
DON	Director of nursing	**RN**	Registered nurse
LPN	Licensed practical nurse	**SNF**	Skilled nursing facility

Health care is needed by persons of all ages. The *person* is always the focus of care.

Health care agencies are owned by individuals, groups, and corporations. Some are owned by city, county, or state health departments. The U.S. Department of Veterans Affairs operates health care agencies across the country.

HOSPITALS

Hospitals provide emergency care, surgery, nursing care, x-ray procedures and treatments, and laboratory testing. They also provide respiratory, physical, occupational, speech, and other therapies. Hospital care is either in-patient or out-patient. *In-patient care* is health care a person receives when admitted to an agency such as a hospital or skilled nursing facility. See Figure 1-1. *Out-patient (ambulatory) care* includes medical or surgical care received when a person is not admitted to an agency.

People of all ages need hospital care. They have babies, surgery, physical and mental health disorders, and broken bones. Some are dying.

Hospital patients have acute, chronic, or terminal illnesses.

- *Acute illness is a sudden illness from which the person is expected to recover.* A heart attack is an example.
- *Chronic illness is an on-going illness that is slow or gradual in onset. There is no known cure. The illness can be controlled and complications prevented with proper treatment.* Diabetes is an example.
- *Terminal illness is an illness or injury from which the person will not likely recover.* The person will die (Chapter 37). Cancers not responding to treatment are examples.

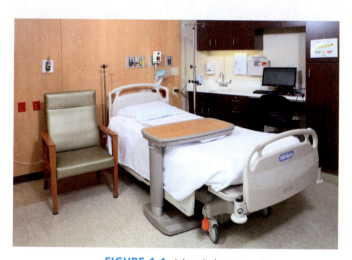

FIGURE 1-1 A hospital room.

LONG-TERM CARE CENTERS

Some persons cannot care for themselves at home but do not need hospital care. Long-term care centers are designed to meet their needs. Care needs range from simple to complex. Medical, nursing, dietary, recreation, rehabilitation, and social services are provided.

Persons in long-term care centers are called *residents.* They are not *patients.* The center is their short- or long-term home.

Most residents are older. Many have chronic diseases, poor nutrition, memory problems, or poor health. Not all residents are old. Some are disabled from birth defects, accidents, or disease. Hospital patients are often discharged while still recovering from illness or surgery. Some need home care. Others need long-term care until able to go home. Others need care until death.

See *Focus on Older Persons: Long-Term Care Centers.*

Board and Care Homes

Board and care homes (group homes) provide a room, meals, laundry, and supervision. Some homes are for older persons. Others are for people with certain problems. Dementia, mental health disorders, and developmental disabilities are examples.

Homes house 4 to 10 people or more. Residents share common living areas and eat together. A safe setting is provided but not 24-hour nursing care. Residents can usually dress and meet grooming and elimination needs with little help.

Assisted Living Residences

An *assisted living residence (ALR) provides housing, personal care, support services, health care, and social activities in a home-like setting to persons needing help with daily activities.* Some ALRs are part of nursing centers or retirement communities.

FOCUS ON OLDER PERSONS

Long-Term Care Centers

Most residents are older. Their problems and care needs vary.

- *Alert, oriented persons.* They know who they are and where they are. They have physical problems. The amount of care required depends on their needs.
- *Confused and disoriented persons.* These persons are mildly to severely confused and disoriented. The problem may be temporary. For others, confusion and disorientation are permanent and become worse (Chapter 35).
- *Persons needing complete care.* They are very disabled, confused, or disoriented. They cannot meet their own needs. Some cannot say what they need or want.
- *Short-term residents.* These people are recovering from fractures, acute illness or surgery, and other injuries. Often they are younger than most residents. Some may need tube feedings, wound care, or other treatments. They usually recover and return home.

- *Persons needing respite care.* Some people living at home go to nursing centers for short stays. This is *respite care. Respite* means *rest* or *relief.* The caregiver can take a trip, tend to business, or simply rest.
- *Life-long residents.* Birth defects and childhood injuries and diseases can cause disabilities. Disabilities may be physical impairments, intellectual impairments, or both. The person needs life-long assistance, support, and special devices.
- *Residents with mental health disorders.* Behavior and function are affected. In severe cases, self-care and independent living are impaired. Some persons have both physical and mental health disorders.
- *Terminally ill residents.* Terminally ill persons are dying. The goal is to provide quality end-of-life care (Chapter 37).

ALR residents may need help with 1 or more of the following.

- Personal care—bathing, dressing, grooming, elimination
- Meals—cooking, eating
- Taking drugs
- Housekeeping
- Personal safety
- Transportation

Mobility is often a requirement. The person walks or uses a wheelchair or motor scooter. The person can leave the building in an emergency. The person has stable health or needs limited health care or treatment.

The person has a room, an apartment, or cottage. Three meals a day and 24-hour supervision are provided. So are housekeeping, laundry, social, recreational, transportation, and some health care services.

Nursing Centers

A *nursing center (nursing facility, nursing home)* provides medical, nursing, dietary, recreation, rehabilitation, and social services. Licensed nurses are required.

Skilled nursing facilities (SNFs) provide complex care for severe health problems. They are part of hospitals or nursing centers. SNF residents need time to recover or rehabilitation. Others never go home.

Some nursing centers and hospitals provide sub-acute care. *Sub-acute care* is complex medical care or rehabilitation when hospital care is no longer needed. Often called *patients*, they may have nervous system problems, bone or joint surgeries or injuries, or wounds that are not healing. Short stays are common.

The *Omnibus Budget Reconciliation Act of 1987 (OBRA)* and "Resident Rights" are discussed in Chapter 2.

Memory Care Units.
A memory care unit is designed for persons with Alzheimer's disease and other dementias (Chapter 35). Such persons suffer increasing memory loss and confusion. Over time, they cannot tend to simple personal needs. Often they wander and may become agitated and combative. The unit is usually closed off from other parts of the center. The closed unit provides a safe setting where residents can wander freely.

Hospices

A *hospice is a health care agency or program for persons who are dying.* Such persons no longer respond to treatments aimed at cures. Usually they have less than 6 months to live.

The physical, emotional, social, and spiritual needs of the person and family are met. The focus is on comfort, not cure.

Hospice care is provided by hospitals, nursing centers, and home care and hospice agencies.

ORGANIZATION

An agency has a governing body called the *board of trustees* or *board of directors*. The board makes policies. It makes sure that safe care is given at the lowest possible cost. Local, state, and federal laws are followed.

An administrator manages the agency. He or she reports directly to the board. Directors or department heads manage certain areas (Fig. 1-2).

Nursing centers are usually owned by an individual or a corporation. Some are owned by county or state health departments. The U.S. Department of Veterans Affairs (Veterans Administration; VA) also has nursing centers.

Nursing centers have nursing, therapy, and food service departments. They also have housekeeping, maintenance, laundry, social service, activity, and other departments. Department directors report to the administrator.

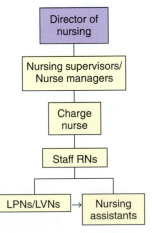

FIGURE 1-2 Sample organizational chart of the nursing department. (*LPN*—Licensed practical nurse; *LVN*—licensed vocational nurse; *RN*—registered nurse.)

TABLE 1-1	Health Team Members
Title	**Description**
Activities director/recreational therapist	Assesses, plans, and implements recreational needs.
Audiologist	Tests hearing; prescribes hearing aids; works with persons who are hard-of-hearing.
Cleric (clergyman; clergywoman)	Assists with spiritual needs.
Clinical nurse specialist	Advanced practice RN who consults in a specialty. Geriatrics, critical care, diabetes, rehabilitation, and wound care are examples.
Dietitian and nutritionist	Assesses and plans for nutritional needs. Teaches about diet and healthy eating.
Licensed practical/vocational nurse (LPN/LVN)	Provides nursing care and gives drugs under an RN's direction.
Medical or clinical laboratory technician	Collects specimens. Performs laboratory tests on blood, urine, and other body fluids, secretions, and excretions.
Medication assistant-certified (MA-C)	Gives drugs as allowed by state law under the supervision of a licensed nurse.
Nurse practitioner (NP)	Advanced practice RN in a nursing specialty. Does physical exams, diagnoses common health problems, and prescribes some drugs and treatments.
Nursing assistant	Assists nurses and gives care. Supervised by a licensed nurse.
Occupational therapist registered (OTR)	Assists persons to learn or retain skills needed for daily living.
Pharmacist	Fills drug orders; monitors and evaluates drug interactions; consults with doctors and nurses about drug actions and interactions.
Physical therapist (PT)	Assists ill and injured persons with movement and pain management.
Physician (doctor)	Diagnoses and treats diseases and injuries.
Podiatrist	Prevents, diagnoses, and treats foot disorders.
Radiographer/radiologic technologist	Takes images using x-rays and other equipment.
Registered nurse (RN)	Assesses, makes nursing diagnoses, plans, implements, and evaluates nursing care. Supervises LPNs/LVNs and nursing assistants.
Respiratory therapist (RT)	Assists in treating lung and heart disorders; gives respiratory treatments and therapies.
Social worker	Deals with social, emotional, and environmental issues affecting illness and recovery. Coordinates community agencies to assist the person and family.
Speech-language pathologist/speech therapist	Diagnoses and treats communication and swallowing disorders.

Modified from Bureau of Labor Statistics, U.S. Department of Labor: Occupational outlook handbook, October 24, 2017.

The Health Team

The *health team* (interdisciplinary health care team) involves the many health care workers whose skills and knowledge focus on the person's total care (Table 1-1). The goal is to provide quality care. The person is the focus of care.

Many team members are involved in the care of each person. Coordinated care is needed. A registered nurse (RN) leads this team.

See *Focus on Communication: The Health Team.*

FOCUS ON COMMUNICATION

The Health Team

Many staff members work together to provide care. Each member has different roles. Health team members communicate often. You may have questions or concerns about a person and his or her care. Tell the team leader. The leader will communicate with other health team members.

Nursing Service

Nursing service is a large department (see Fig. 1-2). The director of nursing (DON) is an RN. (*Director of nursing services, vice president of nursing,* and *vice president of patient services* are some other titles.) Usually a bachelor's or higher degree is required. The DON is responsible for the entire nursing staff and the nursing care given.

Nursing supervisors and nurse managers over-see a work shift, nursing unit, or certain function. Nurse supervisors or managers are responsible for all nursing care and the actions of nursing staff in their areas.

Nursing units usually have charge nurses for each shift. Usually RNs, LPNs/LVNs can be charge nurses in some states. The charge nurse is responsible for all nursing care and nursing staff actions during that shift. Staff RNs report to the charge nurse. LPNs/LVNs report to staff RNs or to the charge nurse. You report to the nurse supervising your work.

Nursing education (staff development) is part of nursing service. Nursing education staff:

- Plan and present educational programs (in-service programs). This includes programs that meet federal and state educational requirements.
- Provide new and changing information.
- Show how to use new equipment and supplies.
- Review policies and procedures on a regular basis.
- Educate and train nursing assistants.
- Conduct new employee orientation programs.

THE NURSING TEAM

The *nursing team involves those who provide nursing care— RNs, LPNs/LVNs, and nursing assistants.* All focus on the physical, social, emotional, and spiritual needs of the person and family.

Registered Nurses

A *registered nurse (RN) has completed a 2-, 3-, or 4-year nursing program and has passed a licensing test.*

- Community college programs—2 years
- Hospital-based diploma programs—2 or 3 years
- College or university programs—4 years

Graduates take a licensing test offered by their state board of nursing. They receive a license and become *registered* after passing the test. RNs must have a license recognized by the state in which they work.

RNs assess, make nursing diagnoses, plan, implement, and evaluate nursing care (Chapter 6). They provide care and delegate (Chapter 3) nursing care and tasks to the nursing team. They evaluate how nursing care affects each person. RNs teach the person and family how to improve health and independence.

RNs follow the doctor's orders. They may delegate them to other nursing team members. RNs do not prescribe treatments or drugs. However, RNs can become *clinical nurse specialists* or *nurse practitioners*. These RNs have limited diagnosing and prescribing functions.

Licensed Practical Nurses and Licensed Vocational Nurses

A *licensed practical nurse (LPN) has completed a practical nursing program and has passed a licensing test.* Hospitals, community colleges, vocational schools, and technical schools offer programs. Programs are 10, 12, or 18 months long. Some high schools offer 2-year programs.

Graduates take a licensing test for practical nursing. After passing the test, they have a license to practice and the title of *licensed practical nurse. Licensed vocational nurse (LVN) is used in California and Texas.* LPNs/LVNs must have a license recognized by the state where they work.

LPNs/LVNs are supervised by RNs, licensed doctors, and licensed dentists. They have fewer responsibilities and functions than RNs do. They need little supervision when the person's condition is stable and care is simple. They assist RNs with acutely ill persons and complex procedures.

Nursing Assistants

A *nursing assistant has passed a nursing assistant training and competency evaluation program (NATCEP).* Nursing assistants *perform delegated nursing tasks under the supervision of a licensed nurse.* Nursing assistants are discussed in Chapter 3.

NURSING CARE PATTERNS

The nursing care pattern used depends on how many persons need care, the staff, and the cost. See Figure 1-3, p. 6.

- *Functional nursing* focuses on tasks and jobs. Each nursing team member has certain tasks and jobs to do. For example, 1 nurse gives all drugs. Another gives all treatments. Nursing assistants give baths, make beds, and serve meals.
- *Team nursing* involves a team of nursing staff led by an RN. Called the "team leader," he or she delegates the care of certain persons to other nurses and nursing assistants. Delegation (Chapter 3) is based on the person's needs and team member abilities. Team members report observations and the care given to the team leader.
- *Primary nursing* involves total care. The primary nurse (an RN) is responsible for the person's total care. The nursing team assists as needed. The RN gives nursing care and makes discharge plans. The RN teaches and counsels the person and family.
- *Case management.* A nursing case manager coordinates the care of specific groups of patients from admission through discharge and into the home or long-term care setting. He or she communicates with doctors and the health team. Communication also is with insurance companies and community agencies. Case managers work with certain doctors, certain age-groups, or persons with certain health problems. Heart disease, diabetes, and cancer are examples.
- *Patient-focused care* is when services are moved from departments to the bedside. Besides nursing care, the nursing team performs basic skills usually done by other health team members. For example, an RN draws a blood sample. This reduces the number of staff involved and the care costs.

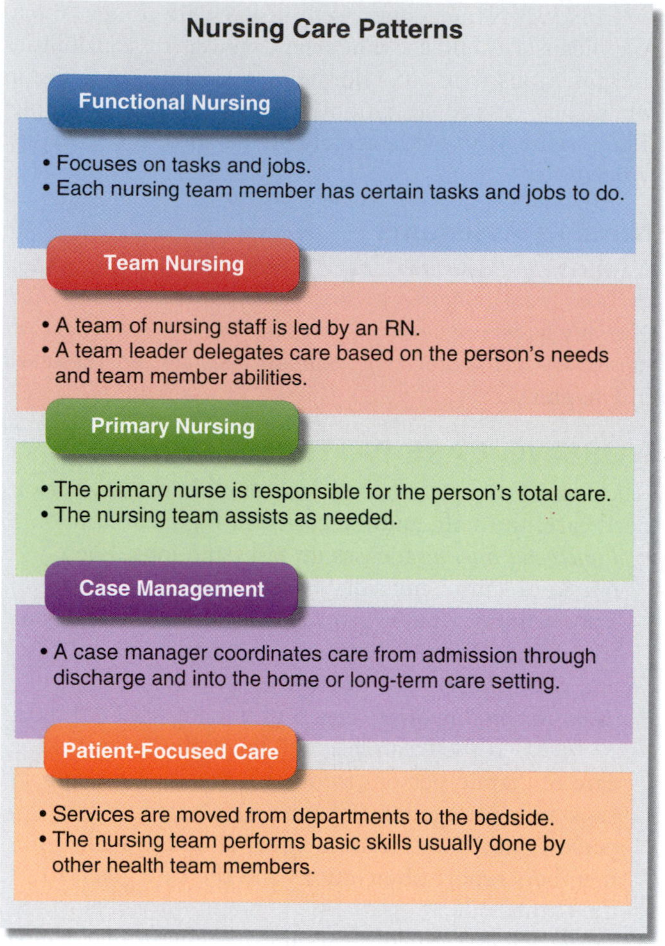

Nursing Care Patterns

Functional Nursing

- Focuses on tasks and jobs.
- Each nursing team member has certain tasks and jobs to do.

Team Nursing

- A team of nursing staff is led by an RN.
- A team leader delegates care based on the person's needs and team member abilities.

Primary Nursing

- The primary nurse is responsible for the person's total care.
- The nursing team assists as needed.

Case Management

- A case manager coordinates care from admission through discharge and into the home or long-term care setting.

Patient-Focused Care

- Services are moved from departments to the bedside.
- The nursing team performs basic skills usually done by other health team members.

FIGURE 1-3 Nursing care patterns.

PAYING FOR HEALTH CARE

Health care is costly. Some people avoid health care because they cannot pay. Others pay doctor bills but go without food or drugs. Health insurance covers some costs. Rarely are all costs covered.

These programs help pay for health care.

- *Private insurance* is bought by individuals and families.
- *Group insurance* is bought by groups or organizations for individuals. This is often an employee benefit.
- *Medicare* is a federal program for persons 65 years of age or older. Some younger people with certain disabilities qualify. Part A covers hospital, SNF, nursing home, hospice, and home care costs. Part B covers doctor visits, ambulance services, medical equipment, mental health care, and some drugs. Part B is voluntary. The person pays a monthly premium.
- *Medicaid* is jointly funded by the federal government and the states. People and families with low incomes usually qualify. It covers children and older, blind, and disabled persons.

See *Promoting Safety and Comfort: Paying for Health Care.*

PROMOTING SAFETY AND COMFORT
Paying for Health Care

Safety
Some conditions can be prevented with proper care. Medicare pays a lower rate for such conditions if they are acquired during a hospital stay. Pressure injuries (Chapter 29) and certain types of falls, trauma, and infections are examples. You must help prevent such conditions.

Patient Protection and Affordable Care Act of 2010

In 2010 the *Patient Protection and Affordable Care Act* became law. Commonly called "Obamacare" after President Barack Obama who signed the law, it is sometimes called the *Affordable Care Act (ACA)*.

Some people do not qualify for Medicare or Medicaid. They can buy insurance through health insurance exchanges. These are market-places for buying health insurance. Exchanges are run by the federal government, by states, or both.

Currently the law provides for the following.

- Up to age 26, children can be part of their parents' insurance plans.
- If a person becomes ill, the insurance company cannot limit coverage or cancel the plan.
- An insurance company cannot deny coverage for children who are chronically ill.
- Insurance companies must provide some essential benefits. Preventive and wellness care and management of chronic diseases are examples.

Efforts have been made to repeal and replace the law or to make some changes. Follow your preferred news sources and government websites to remain current and up-to-date about the law.

Prospective Payment Systems

Prospective payment systems limit the amount paid by insurers, Medicare, and Medicaid. *Prospective* means *before*. The amount paid for services is determined before giving care. If costs are less than the amount paid, the agency keeps the extra money. If costs are greater, the agency takes the loss.

MEETING STANDARDS

Health care agencies must meet standards set by federal and state governments and accrediting agencies. Standards relate to policies, procedures, and quality of care. An agency must meet standards for:

- *Licensure.* A state license is required to operate and provide care.
- *Certification.* This is required to receive Medicare and Medicaid funds.
- *Accreditation.* This is voluntary. It signals quality and excellence.

The Survey Process

Surveys are done to see if standards are met. A survey team will:

- Review policies, procedures, and medical records.
- Interview staff, patients and residents, and families.
- Observe how care is given.
- Observe if dignity and privacy are promoted.
- Check for cleanliness and safety.
- Make sure staff meet state requirements. (Are doctors and nurses licensed? Are nursing assistants on the state registry?)

If standards are met, the agency receives a license, certification, or accreditation. Sometimes problems (*deficiencies*) are found. The agency usually has 60 days or less to correct the problem. The agency can be fined for uncorrected or serious deficiencies. Or it can lose its license, certification, or accreditation.

Your Role

You have an important role in meeting standards and in the survey process. You must:

- Provide quality care.
- Protect the person's rights.
- Provide for the person's and your own safety.
- Help keep the agency clean and safe.
- Act in a professional manner.
- Have good work ethics.
- Follow agency policies and procedures.
- Answer questions honestly and completely. See *Focus on Surveys: Your Role.*

FOCUS ON SURVEYS

Your Role

Survey teams are made up of surveyors. A *surveyor is a person who collects information by observing and asking questions.*

A surveyor may ask you questions. If so, be polite. Answer questions honestly and completely. If you do not understand a question, ask the surveyor to re-phrase it. Do not guess. Tell the surveyor where you can find the answer. You can say: "I'm not sure, but I would ask the nurse."

For example, a surveyor approaches you.

Surveyor: "May I ask you a few questions?"
You: "Yes. I am happy to answer your questions."
Surveyor: "Thank you. First, when should you practice hand hygiene?"
You: "I wash my hands before and after contact with a patient. I also wash my hands when they are dirty and after I take off gloves."

Surveyor: "Thank you. Next, what are 2 appropriate patient identifiers?"
You: "I don't understand the question. Can you re-phrase it?"
Surveyor: "Yes. Name 2 things you can use to identify a patient."
You: "Okay. Thank you. I can use the patient's full name and date of birth. I cannot use the room number."
Surveyor: "I have 1 last question. In a disaster, where would you find the Emergency Preparedness Plan?"
You: "Well, I'm not sure. I will ask the charge nurse where to find it."

The Person, Family, and Yourself

P ersonal and Professional Responsibility

Working in health care is rewarding. You provide care for a *person.* Your work affects the person's quality of care. Value the work that you do.

Focus on PRIDE helps you promote pride in the person, his or her family, and yourself. Building on chapter content, it focuses on:

- *Personal and Professional Responsibility*—how personal and professional behaviors and development affect yourself and others.
- *Rights and Respect*—how to promote others' rights and respect them as persons with dignity and value.
- *Independence and Social Interaction*—ways to promote independence and positive interactions.
- *Delegation and Teamwork*—how to practice safe delegation (Chapter 3) and work well with and help other team members.
- *Ethics and Laws*—how to do the right thing when dealing with patients, residents, and co-workers. Laws affecting nursing care are also presented.

For discussion purposes, each chapter ends with a *Focus on PRIDE: Application* section. The questions challenge you to think about your role and how you will value the person, family, or yourself.

R ights and Respect

Why do you want to work in health care? Maybe you want to help people. Maybe a health team member inspired you. Or you may have a job opportunity or career goal in mind. Think about your reasons.

Consider what type of agency would suit you. One person may prefer working in long-term care while another prefers a hospital setting. Careful career planning shows respect for employers, patients and residents, and yourself.

I ndependence and Social Interaction

You will interact with many people. Patients and residents, nursing staff, health team members, surveyors, and visitors are examples. Good work ethics and communication skills are important. See Chapters 5 and 6. How you interact with others affects quality of care and job satisfaction.

D elegation and Teamwork

Health team members must work together to provide quality care. Offer to help others when you can. Helping others shows you are dependable and value teamwork.

E thics and Laws

RNs, LPNs/LVNs, and nursing assistants have different roles. Federal and state laws determine the legal limits of these roles. See Chapter 3 for your role limits. Functions may also vary among agencies. A job description (Chapter 3) states the agency's expectations. To protect yourself and others, know the limits of your role in your state and agency.

FOCUS ON PRIDE: *Application*

Health care offers many opportunities. Why do you want to work in health care? Where do you want to work? What are your career goals?

REVIEW QUESTIONS

Circle the BEST answer.

1 A person is admitted to a hospital. Which is *true*?
   a The person is called a resident.
   b Chronic illnesses are not treated.
   c The person cannot leave.
   d The person receives in-patient care.

2 A health care program for dying persons is a
   a Hospice
   b Board and care home
   c Skilled nursing facility
   d Hospital

3 You work in an assisted living residence. You
   a Give care in the person's home
   b Care for patients recovering from surgery
   c Help persons with their daily activities
   d Care for persons with acute illnesses

4 Who controls policy in a health care agency?
   a The survey team
   b The board of directors
   c The health team
   d Medicare and Medicaid

5 Who is responsible for the entire nursing staff and safe nursing care?
   a The case manager
   b The director of nursing
   c The charge nurse
   d The RN

6 You are a member of
   a The health team and the nursing team
   b The health team and the medical team
   c The nursing team and the medical team
   d The board of trustees

7 The nursing team includes
   a Doctors
   b Pharmacists
   c Physical and occupational therapists
   d RNs, LPNs/LVNs, and nursing assistants

8 Nursing assistants are supervised by
   a Licensed nurses
   b Other nursing assistants
   c The health team
   d The medical director

9 The nursing assistant's role is to
   a Meet Medicare and Medicaid standards
   b Perform delegated tasks
   c Follow the doctor's orders
   d Manage care

10 Nursing tasks are delegated according to a person's needs and staff member abilities. This nursing care pattern is called
   a Team nursing
   b Functional nursing
   c Case management
   d Primary nursing

11 Medicare is for persons who
   a Are 65 years of age or older
   b Need nursing center care
   c Have group insurance
   d Have low incomes

12 Which is required for an agency to operate and provide care?
   a Accreditation
   b Certification
   c A license
   d A survey

13 Which is voluntary for health care agencies?
   a Licensure
   b Certification
   c Accreditation
   d Surveys

14 Surveys are done to
   a Reduce health care costs
   b See if agencies meet set standards
   c Educate the nursing team
   d Determine the amount paid by insurers

15 A surveyor asks you some questions. You should
   a Refer all questions to the nurse
   b Answer as the DON tells you to
   c Give as little information as possible
   d Give honest and complete answers

Answers to Chapter 1 questions are on p. 551.

FOCUS ON PRACTICE

Problem Solving

The nurse supervising you has not returned from a meal break. You have a question about a patient's care. Your nursing department is organized as shown in **Figure 1-2.** What will you do?

OBJECTIVES

- Define the key terms and key abbreviation in this chapter.
- Explain the purpose of *The Patient Care Partnership: Understanding Expectations, Rights, and Responsibilities.*
- Describe the purposes and requirements of the *Omnibus Budget Reconciliation Act of 1987 (OBRA).*
- Identify the person's rights under OBRA.
- Explain how to protect the person's rights.
- Explain the ombudsman role.
- Explain how to promote PRIDE in the person, the family, and yourself.

KEY TERMS

involuntary seclusion Separating the person from others against his or her will, keeping the person to a certain area, or keeping the person away from his or her room without consent
ombudsman Someone who supports or promotes the needs and interests of another person

representative A person with the legal right to act on the patient's or resident's behalf when he or she cannot do so for himself or herself
treatment The care provided to maintain or restore health, improve function, or relieve symptoms

KEY ABBREVIATION

OBRA Omnibus Budget Reconciliation Act of 1987

People want to know about their health problems and treatment. They want to understand and take part in treatment decisions. As patients and residents, they have certain rights.

PATIENT RIGHTS

The Patient Care Partnership: Understanding Expectations, Rights, and Responsibilities is from the American Hospital Association. The document explains the person's rights and expectations during hospital stays. The relationship between the doctor, health team, and patient is stressed. See Appendix A, p. 553.

RESIDENT RIGHTS

The *Omnibus Budget Reconciliation Act of 1987 (OBRA)* is a federal law. It applies to all 50 states.

OBRA requires that nursing centers provide care in a manner and in a setting that maintains or improves each person's quality of life, health, and safety. Resident rights are a major part of OBRA.

Residents have rights as United States citizens. They also have rights relating to their every-day lives and care in a nursing center. Some residents cannot exercise their rights. A representative (spouse, partner, adult child, court-appointed guardian) does so for them. A *representative is a person with the legal right to act on the patient's or resident's behalf when he or she cannot do so for himself or herself.*

Nursing centers must inform residents of their rights. Residents are informed orally and in writing before or during admission to the center. Resident rights and other information are given in the language the person uses and understands. An interpreter is used if the person speaks and understands a foreign language or communicates by sign language.

Resident rights (Box 2-1) also are posted throughout the center. Those affecting your role are described in this chapter.

See *Focus on Surveys: Resident Rights.*

BOX 2-1	Resident Rights

- To be treated with dignity and respect. And to receive quality care.
- To exercise his or her rights as a center resident and as a United States citizen.
- To be informed orally and in writing of rights and center rules. This is done in a language the person understands.
- To access all his or her records, including current clinical records.
- To obtain copies of his or her records. This is at the resident's expense.
- To refuse treatment.
- To refuse to take part in experimental research. This is the development and testing of new treatments and drugs.
- To make advance directives (Chapter 37).
- To be informed of Medicare benefits and services. This includes costs and charges covered and not covered.
- To file complaints with the appropriate state agency about abuse, neglect, and the mis-use of his or her property.
- To be informed of center services and service charges.
- To choose his or her doctor.
- To know the doctor's name, specialty, and contact information.
- To be fully informed of his or her total health status and medical condition.
- To be informed of:
  - Any accident or injury that may need medical attention
  - A change in physical, mental, or psycho-social status
  - The need to stop, change, or add a treatment
  - A decision to transfer or discharge the person
  - A change in the person's room or roommate
  - A change in rights under federal or state law
- To manage personal and financial affairs.
- To be fully informed in advance about care and treatment. This includes changes in care and treatment.
- To privacy and confidentiality:
  - Of personal and medical records
  - Of treatment and care
  - Of written and phone communications
  - During visits with family and friends
  - When meeting with resident groups

- To voice grievances and have them solved promptly.
- To see the results of federal and state surveys and plans to correct problems or areas of weakness.
- To perform services for the center or to refuse to perform services.
- To send and receive un-opened mail. To buy supplies to send mail.
- To receive information about protecting persons with intellectual and developmental disabilities and mental health disorders.
- To have and use personal items and clothing.
- To take his or her drugs without help if able.
- To refuse to change to a different room.
- To be free from restraints (Chapter 12).
- To be free from abuse (verbal, sexual, physical), bodily punishment, involuntary seclusion, and other abuse or mistreatment (p. 13 and Chapter 4).
- To be cared for in a manner and setting that maintains or enhances quality of life.
- To choose activities, schedules, and health care that meet his or her interests and needs.
- To interact with community members inside and outside the center.
- To make choices about his or her life in the center.
- To organize and take part in resident groups.
- To take part in social, religious, and community activities.
- To a setting and services that consider his or her needs and choices.
- To be informed of his or her health and medical condition in a language that he or she understands. That language is used when taking part in care planning.
- To a clean, comfortable, and home-like setting. This includes temperature, lighting, and sound levels.
- To attain or maintain his or her highest level of function.
- To closet space.
- To visit with his or her spouse or partner, family, and friends at any reasonable hour.

FOCUS ON SURVEYS

Resident Rights

Resident rights are a major focus of surveys. Surveyors observe staff behaviors and actions. They listen to staff comments and remarks. You may not know they are doing so. What you say and do must promote the person's quality of life, health, and safety. For example, a surveyor may observe:

- How you prevent exposure of the person's body
- How you help a person dress for the season and time of day
- How you label clothing
- If you knock on a person's door before entering the room
- If you change a person's music or TV without permission
- If you move a person's personal items without permission
- How you address and speak to a person

You will learn how to protect the person's rights as you study this and other chapters. Always act and speak in a professional manner.

Information

The *right to information* means access to all records about the person. They include the medical record, contracts, incident reports, and financial records. The request can be oral or written.

The person has the right to be fully informed of his or her health condition. The person must also have information about his or her doctor. This includes the doctor's name, specialty, and how to contact the doctor.

Report any request for information to the nurse. *You do not give the information described above to the person or family* (Chapter 3).

See *Focus on Communication: Information.*

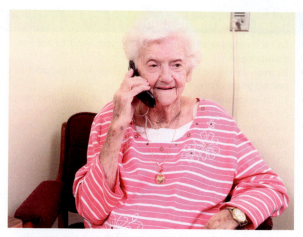

FIGURE 2-1 A resident is talking privately on her phone.

FOCUS ON COMMUNICATION

Information

You may be asked about a person's care. You must not give out information. This is the nurse's responsibility. You can say: "I am sorry. I am not allowed to give that information. I will report your request to the nurse."

Communicate the request promptly. You can tell the person: "I told the nurse about your question. The nurse will speak with you soon."

Refusing Treatment

The person has the *right to refuse treatment. Treatment means the care provided to maintain or restore health, improve function, or relieve symptoms.* A person who does not give consent (Chapter 4) or refuses treatment cannot be treated against his or her wishes. The center must find out what the person is refusing and why. The center must:

- Find out the reason for the refusal.
- Explain the problems that can result from the refusal.
- Offer other treatment options.
- Continue to provide all other services.

Advance directives are part of the right to refuse treatment (Chapter 37). They include living wills and instructions about life support. *Advance directives* are written instructions about health care when the person is not able to make such decisions.

Report any treatment refusal to the nurse. The nurse may change the person's care plan (Chapter 6).

Privacy and Confidentiality

Residents have the *right to personal privacy.* Staff must maintain privacy of the person's body. Expose the person's body only as necessary. Only staff directly involved in care and treatment are present. Consent is needed for others to be present.

Privacy is maintained for all personal care measures. Bathing, dressing, and elimination are examples. To protect privacy:

- Close privacy curtains, doors, and window coverings.
- Remove residents from public view.
- Provide clothes or drape the person to prevent unnecessary exposure of body parts.
- Practice the measures listed in Chapter 4.

Residents have the right to visit with others in private—where others cannot see or hear them. This includes phone calls (Fig. 2-1). Centers provide phones or phone jacks. Phones are at the correct height for use by persons in wheelchairs. Phones for hard-of-hearing persons are also available. Some residents have wireless phones.

The right to privacy also involves mail. No one can open mail the person sends or receives without his or her consent.

Information about the person's care, treatment, and condition is kept confidential. So are medical and financial records.

Privacy and confidentiality are discussed in Chapters 4 and 5.

Personal Choice

Residents have the *right to make their own choices.* This includes:

- Choosing doctors
- Choosing friends and visitors
- Helping to plan care and treatment
- Choosing preferred activities, schedules, and care:
  - When to go to bed and when to get up
  - What to wear (Fig. 2-2)
  - How to spend time
  - What to eat

Personal choice promotes quality of life, dignity, and self-respect. Allow personal choice whenever safely possible.

Grievances

Residents have the *right to voice concerns, questions, and complaints about treatment and care.* The problem may involve another person. It may be about care that was given or not given. The center must promptly try to correct the matter. No one can punish the person in any way for voicing the grievance.

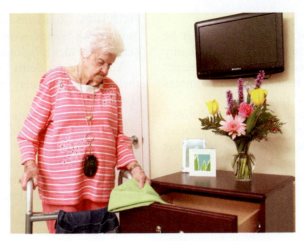

FIGURE 2-2 A resident is choosing what clothing to wear.

Work

The person does not work for care, care items or other things, or privileges. The person is not required to perform services for the center.

However, the person has the *right to work or perform services if he or she wants to do so.* Some people like to garden, repair or build things, clean, sew, mend, or cook. Other persons need work for rehabilitation or activity reasons. The care plan reflects the person's desire or need to work. Residents volunteer or are paid for their services.

Resident Groups

The person has the *right to form and take part in resident groups.* Families can meet with other families. These groups can plan activities, discuss concerns, and suggest center improvements. They can support and comfort group members.

Residents have the right to take part in social, cultural, religious, and community events. They have the right to help in getting to and from events of their choice.

Personal Items

Residents have the *right to keep and use personal items.* Treat the person's property with care and respect. The items may lack value to you but have meaning to the person. They also relate to personal choice, dignity, a home-like setting, and quality of life.

The person's property is protected. Items are labeled with the person's name. The center must investigate reports of lost, stolen, or damaged items. Sometimes the police help.

Protect yourself and the center from being accused of stealing. Do not go through a person's closet, drawers, purse, or other space without the person's knowledge and consent. A nurse may ask you to inspect closets and drawers. Center policy should require that a co-worker and the person or legal representative be present. They witness your actions.

Freedom From Abuse, Mistreatment, and Neglect

Residents have the *right to be free from verbal, sexual, physical, and mental abuse* (Chapter 4). They also have the right to be free from ***involuntary seclusion.***

- *Separating the person from others against his or her will*
- *Keeping the person to a certain area*
- *Keeping the person away from his or her room without consent*

No one can abuse, neglect, or mistreat a resident. This includes center staff, volunteers, and staff from other agencies or groups. It also includes other residents, family members, visitors, and legal representatives. Centers must investigate suspected or reported cases of abuse. They cannot employ persons who:

- Were found guilty of abusing, neglecting, or mistreating others by a court of law.
- Have a finding entered into the state's nursing assistant registry (Chapter 3) about abuse, neglect, mistreatment, or wrongful acts involving the person's money or property. A *finding* means that a state determined that the employee abused, neglected, mistreated, or wrongfully used the person's money or property.

Freedom From Restraint

Residents have the *right not to have body movements restricted.* Restraints and certain drugs can restrict body movements (Chapter 12). Some drugs are restraints because they affect mood, behavior, and mental function. Sometimes residents are restrained to protect them from harming themselves or others. A doctor's order is needed for restraint use. Restraints are not used for staff convenience or to discipline a person.

Quality of Life

Residents have the *right to quality of life*. They must be cared for in a manner and in a setting that promotes dignity and respect for self. Care must promote physical, mental, and social well-being. Protecting resident rights promotes quality of life. It shows respect for the person.

Speak to the person in a polite and courteous manner. Good, honest, and thoughtful care enhances the person's quality of life. Box 2-2 lists OBRA-required actions that promote dignity and privacy.

See *Focus on Communication: Quality of Life.*

Activities. Residents have the *right to activities that enhance each person's physical, mental, and psycho-social well-being.* The center provides religious services for spiritual health.

You assist residents to and from activity programs of their choice. You may need to help them with activities (Fig. 2-3).

See *Focus on Communication: Activities.*
See *Focus on Surveys: Activities.*

Environment. Residents have the *right to a safe, clean, comfortable, and home-like setting.* The person is allowed to have and use personal items (Fig. 2-4). Doing so promotes personal choice and a home-like setting.

BOX 2-2	OBRA-Required Actions to Promote Dignity and Privacy

Courteous and Dignified Interactions
- Use the right tone of voice.
- Use good eye contact.
- Stand or sit close enough as needed.
- Use the person's proper name and title. For example: "Mrs. Crane." Or use the name the person prefers.
- Gain the person's attention before interacting with him or her.
- Use touch if the person approves.
- Respect the person's social status.
- Listen with interest to what the person is saying.
- Do not yell at, scold, or embarrass the person.

Privacy and Self-Determination
- Drape properly during care and procedures to avoid exposure and embarrassment.
- Use privacy curtains or screens during care and procedures.
- Close the room door during care and procedures as the person desires. Also close window coverings.
- Knock on the door before entering. Wait to be asked in.
- Close the bathroom door when the person uses the bathroom.
- Drape properly in a chair.

Personal Choice and Independence
- Person smokes in allowed areas.
- Person takes part in activities of his or her interest.
- Person takes part in scheduling activities and care.
- Person gives input into the care plan about preferences and independence.
- Person is involved in a room or roommate change.
- The person's items are moved or inspected only with the person's consent.

Courteous and Dignified Care
- Groom hair, beards, and nails as the person wishes.
- Assist with dressing in the right clothing for time of day and personal choice.
- Promote independence and dignity in dining.
- Respect private space and property. For example, change music or TV stations only with the person's consent.
- Assist with walking and transfers. Do not interfere with independence.
- Assist with hygiene and grooming preferences. Do not interfere with independence.
  - Appearance is neat and clean.
  - The person is clean shaven or has a groomed beard and mustache.
  - Nails are trimmed and clean.
  - Dentures, hearing aids, eyeglasses, and other devices are used correctly.
  - Clothing is clean.
  - Clothing fits and is properly fastened.
  - Shoes, hose, and socks are on properly and fastened.
  - Extra clothing is worn for warmth as needed. Sweaters and lap blankets are examples.

FOCUS ON COMMUNICATION
Quality of Life

Every person deserves to be addressed in a manner that shows dignity and respect. Address the person by his or her title and last name. For example: Mr. Baker, Mrs. Harty, or Dr. Collins. Do not use a person's first name or another name unless the person requests it. Avoid using terms like *Sweetheart, Honey, Grandpa,* and *Dear.*

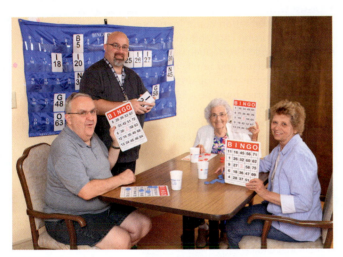

FIGURE 2-3 A nursing assistant is helping residents with an activity.

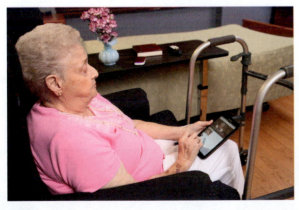

FIGURE 2-4 This resident's personal items include an electronic device.

FOCUS ON COMMUNICATION
Activities

You may need help assisting residents to and from activity programs. Politely ask a co-worker to help you. Share the following with your co-worker.

- What time you need help.
- How much of the co-worker's time you need.
- The residents you need help with.
- If the person walks or uses a wheelchair.
- What assistive (adaptive) devices are used. Eyeglasses, hearing aids, canes, and walkers are examples.

Always say "please" when asking for help. And thank the person for helping you. For example:

Jane, can you please help me assist 2 residents to the concert? It starts at 2:00, so I'll need your help at 1:45. Mr. Harris needs his glasses and hearing aid. He'll use a walker. Mrs. Janz uses a wheelchair. She needs her glasses and a blanket for her lap. The blanket is in her wheelchair. The concert is over at 3:00. Can you help me then, too? Thanks so much for helping me.

FOCUS ON SURVEYS
Activities

Surveyors may ask you about:
- Your role in helping residents get ready for a group activity.
  - How do you make sure the person is out of bed, dressed, and ready for an activity?
  - How do you provide needed transportation?
- Your role in helping with activities of daily living during an activity. For example, does the person need to use the bathroom? Does the person need help eating?
- Your role in helping a person with an individual activity. For example, you play cards with a person. Do you have needed supplies? Is the person properly positioned? Do you provide good lighting?
- How are activities provided when the activities staff members are not available?

P ersonal and Professional Responsibility

OBRA is concerned with quality of life, health, and safety. All care must maintain or improve each person's quality of life. You are responsible for the care you give. To provide quality care:

- Protect the person's rights.
- Provide for safety (Chapter 10) and prevent falls (Chapter 11).
- Help keep the agency clean and safe.
- Act in a professional manner.
- Have good work ethics (Chapter 5).
- Follow agency policies and procedures.

Take pride in your work. Your care helps improve each person's quality of life, health, and safety.

R ights and Respect

The person has the right to refuse treatment. This does not mean that all treatment stops. The health team offers other treatment options. For example, the doctor suggests short-term placement in a nursing center. The person refuses. The family agrees to help the person at home. A social worker helps the person and family arrange for home care and respite care. *Respite care* relieves caregivers of daily care for a short time.

I ndependence and Social Interaction

Many patients and residents feel a loss of independence and social interaction. To promote independence, have the person choose food, clothing, activities, and schedules.

For social interaction, tell the person about activities and offer help to and from activities. Also respect the person's right to privacy during visits with others and phone calls. These actions promote independence, self-worth, and quality of life.

D elegation and Teamwork

Health care agencies must meet the person's needs and preferences. Schedules, care assignments, and room arrangements may need to change to meet the person's needs. Flexibility, good teamwork, and communication are required to provide quality care.

For example, a person likes to bathe at night. However, the day shift gives baths. You share the person's preference with the nurse. The day-time and evening staffs work together so the person can bathe at night.

E thics and Laws

The *Older Americans Act* is a federal law. It requires a long-term care ombudsman program in every state. An ***ombudsman*** *is someone who supports or promotes the needs and interests of another person.*

Ombudsmen act on behalf of persons receiving health care. They protect a person's health, safety, welfare, and rights. They:

- Investigate and resolve complaints.
- Provide services to assist the person.
- Assist with hospital access or discharge concerns.
- Provide information about long-term care services.
- Monitor nursing care and conditions.
- Provide support to resident and family groups.
- Help the person and family resolve family conflicts.
- Help the center manage difficult problems.

Nursing centers must post contact information for local and state ombudsmen. A resident or family may share a concern with you. Follow center policies and procedures for contacting an ombudsman. Ombudsman services are useful when:

- There is concern about a person's care or treatment.
- Someone interferes with a person's rights, health, safety, or welfare.

FOCUS ON PRIDE: *Application*

You have an important role in protecting the person's rights. Identify 3 ways you can promote the person's right to:

- Personal choice
- Privacy and confidentiality
- A safe, clean, and comfortable setting

REVIEW QUESTIONS

*Circle **T** if the statement is TRUE or **F** if it is FALSE.*

1 T F OBRA applies to all 50 states.

2 T F Nursing center residents have rights as U.S. citizens.

3 T F Residents are informed of their rights only in writing.

4 T F Residents have the right to choose their own doctors.

5 T F You should open the person's mail within 24 hours of delivery to the center.

6 T F A resident complains about the food. The center must try to provide desired foods.

7 T F Residents must provide some type of work for the center.

8 T F Resident groups can discuss ideas for activity programs.

9 T F An employee was found guilty of abusing a resident. The center can continue to employ the person.

10 T F You can restrain a resident to provide care.

Circle the BEST answer.

11 *The Patient Care Partnership: Understanding Expectations, Rights, and Responsibilities* is concerned with
 a Hospital care
 b Home care
 c Long-term care
 d All health care agencies and settings

12 A son has the legal right to act on his mother's behalf. The son is his mother's legal
 a Ombudsman
 b Representative
 c Caregiver
 d Health care provider

13 A daughter wants to read her father's medical record. What should you do?
 a Give her the medical record.
 b Ask the resident if she can read the record.
 c Tell the nurse.
 d Tell her that she cannot do so.

14 A resident refuses to have a shower. What should you do?
 a Tell him or her that a shower cannot be refused.
 b Tell the family.
 c Comply, but say that he or she must shower tomorrow.
 d Tell the nurse.

15 Which violates the person's right to privacy?
 a Closing the bathroom door when the person uses the bathroom
 b Opening window blinds when assisting with bathing
 c Covering the person for personal care
 d Asking the person's permission to observe a treatment

16 A resident has a phone and wants to make a call. What should you do?
 a Leave the room.
 b Tell the nurse.
 c Ask the person to use the phone at the nurses' station.
 d Close the privacy curtain so you can finish your tasks in the room.

17 Who decides how to style a person's hair?
 a The person
 b The nurse
 c You
 d The ombudsman

18 Residents have the right to
 a Bring weapons into the center
 b Mistreat other residents
 c Use other residents' personal items
 d Voice complaints about care

19 Residents have the right to be free from
 a Disease
 b Grievances
 c Involuntary seclusion
 d Rules

20 Who selects activities for a resident?
 a The nurse
 b You
 c The person's representative
 d The person

21 A nursing center must provide
 a A safe, clean, and comfortable setting
 b An indoor smoking area
 c A bed near a window
 d A noise-free setting

22 Which is the correct way to address a person?
 a "Hello, sweetie."
 b "Hello."
 c "Hello, Mrs. Smith."
 d "Hello, Grandpa."

23 Which promotes privacy?
 a Entering a person's room without knocking
 b Closing the privacy curtain for a procedure
 c Leaving the door open during personal care
 d Looking through the person's belongings

24 A long-term care ombudsman
 a Is employed by the nursing center
 b Investigates resident complaints
 c Grants a nursing center a license or certification
 d Can prevent a resident from leaving the center

Answers to Chapter 2 questions are on p. 551.

FOCUS ON PRACTICE

Problem Solving

A resident refuses to eat. What will you do? Does the resident have the right to refuse to eat? What is the nursing center's responsibility?

The Nursing Assistant

OBJECTIVES

- Define the key terms and key abbreviations in this chapter.
- Describe the training and competency evaluation requirements for nursing assistants.
- Identify the information in the nursing assistant registry.
- List the reasons for denying, suspending, or revoking a nursing assistant's certification, license, or registration.
- Explain how to obtain certification, a license, or registration in another state.

- Describe what nursing assistants can do and their role limits.
- Describe the standards for nursing assistants developed by the National Council of State Boards of Nursing.
- Explain why a job description is important.
- Describe the delegation process and your role.
- Explain how to accept or refuse a delegated task.
- Explain how to promote PRIDE in the person, the family, and yourself.

KEY TERMS

certification Official recognition by a state that standards or requirements have been met

delegate To authorize another person to perform a nursing task in a certain situation

endorsement A state recognizes the certificate, license, or registration issued by another state; reciprocity or equivalency

equivalency See "endorsement"

job description A document that describes what the agency expects you to do

nursing task Nursing care or a nursing function, procedure, activity, or work that can be delegated to nursing assistants when it does not require a nurse's professional knowledge or judgment

reciprocity See "endorsement"

KEY ABBREVIATIONS

LPN	Licensed practical nurse
LVN	Licensed vocational nurse
NATCEP	Nursing assistant training and competency evaluation program

NCSBN	National Council of State Boards of Nursing
OBRA	Omnibus Budget Reconciliation Act of 1987
RN	Registered nurse

Federal and state laws and agency policies combine to define your roles and functions. To protect patients and residents from harm, you need to know:
- What you can and cannot do
- Rules and standards of conduct affecting your work
- Your role limits

Laws, job descriptions, and the person's condition shape your work. So does the amount of supervision you need.

NURSE PRACTICE ACTS

Each state has a nurse practice act. A nurse practice act:
- Defines RN (registered nurse) and LPN/LVN (licensed practical nurse/licensed vocational nurse) and their scope of practice.
- Describes RN and LPN/LVN education and licensing requirements.
- Protects the public from persons practicing nursing without a license. Persons who do not meet the state's requirements cannot perform nursing functions.

The law allows for denying, revoking, or suspending a nursing license. The intent is to protect the public from unsafe nurses. Reasons include:

- Selling or distributing drugs
- Using a person's drugs for oneself
- Placing a person in danger from the over-use of alcohol or drugs
- Being convicted of abusing or neglecting children or older persons
- Demonstrating incompetent behaviors
- Prescribing drugs and treatments

Nursing Assistants

Nurse practice acts are used to decide what nursing assistants can do. Some also regulate nursing assistant roles, functions, education, and certification requirements. Other states have separate laws for nursing assistants.

If you do something beyond the legal limits of your role, you could be practicing nursing without a license. This means serious legal problems for you, your supervisor, and your employer. Like nurses, you can have your certification (license, registration) denied, revoked, or suspended. (See "Certification," p. 20.)

THE OMNIBUS BUDGET RECONCILIATION ACT OF 1987

The *Omnibus Budget Reconciliation Act of 1987 (OBRA)* is a federal law. It applies to all 50 states.

OBRA sets minimum requirements for nursing assistant training and evaluation. Each state must have a nursing assistant training and competency evaluation program (NATCEP). A nursing assistant must successfully complete a NATCEP to work in a nursing center, hospital long-term care unit, or home care agency receiving Medicare funds.

The Training Program

OBRA requires at least 75 hours of instruction. Some states require more hours. Classroom and at least 16 hours of supervised practical training are required (Fig. 3-1). Practical training (clinical practicum or clinical experience) occurs in a laboratory or clinical setting. Students perform nursing tasks on another person. A nurse supervises this training.

See *Focus on Communication: The Training Program.*

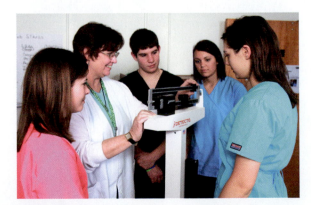

FIGURE 3-1 Nursing assistant training program. An instructor demonstrates a skill to her students.

FOCUS ON COMMUNICATION

The Training Program

Student clinical experiences involve giving care to patients or residents. The patient or resident has the right to know who you are. Introduce yourself. Tell the person you are a student. For example: "Hello. My name is Jenna Smith. I am a nursing assistant student. I will be working with your nurse today."

Competency Evaluation

The competency evaluation has a written test and a skills test (Appendix B, p. 554).

- The written test has multiple-choice questions. Each has 4 choices. Only 1 answer is correct.
- For the skills test you perform certain skills learned in your training program.

You take the competency evaluation after your training program. Your instructor knows the testing service used in your state and when and where the tests are given. You complete the application in writing or on-line. The evaluation has a fee. If working in a nursing center, the employer pays the fee. Otherwise you pay the fee.

If you listen, study hard, and practice safe care, you should do well. If the first attempt was not successful, you can re-test. OBRA allows at least 3 attempts to successfully complete the evaluation.

Each testing service has a candidate handbook. Review the handbook carefully as you prepare for the competency evaluation.

Nursing Assistant Registry

OBRA requires a nursing assistant registry in each state. It is the official record or listing of persons who have successfully completed that state's approved NATCEP. The registry has information about each nursing assistant.

- Full name, including maiden name and any married names.
- Last known home address.
- Registry number and the date it expires.
- Date of birth.
- Last known employer, date hired, and date employment ended.
- Date the competency evaluation was passed.
- Information about findings of abuse, neglect, or dishonest use of property. It includes the nature of the offense and supporting evidence. If a hearing was held, the date and its outcome are included. The person has the right to include a statement disputing the finding. All information stays in the registry for at least 5 years.

Any health care agency can access registry information. You also receive a copy of your registry information. The copy is sent when the first entry is made and when information is changed or added. You can correct wrong information.

BOX 3-1	Losing Certification, a License, or Registration

The National Council of State Boards of Nursing (NCSBN) lists these reasons for doing so.

- Substance abuse or dependency.
- Abandoning, abusing, or neglecting a person.
- Fraud or deceit. Examples are:
  - Filing false personal information
  - Providing false information when applying for initial certification, re-instatement, or renewal
- Violating professional boundaries (Chapter 4).
- Giving unsafe care.
- Performing acts beyond the nursing assistant role.
- Misappropriation (stealing, theft) or mis-using property.
- Obtaining money or property from a patient or resident. This can be done through fraud, falsely representing oneself, or by force.
- Being convicted of a crime. Examples include murder, assault, kidnapping, rape or sexual assault, robbery, sexual crimes involving children, criminal mistreatment of children or a vulnerable person (Chapter 4), drug trafficking, embezzlement (to take a person's property for one's own use), theft, and arson (starting fires).
- Failing to conform to the standards of nursing assistants (p. 22).
- Putting patients or residents at risk for harm.
- Violating a person's privacy.
- Failing to maintain the confidentiality of patient or resident information.

PROMOTING SAFETY AND COMFORT
Certification

Safety

OBRA and other federal and state laws require background screenings on individuals with direct patient or resident contact in long-term care agencies. The background screening may include FBI (Federal Bureau of Investigation) fingerprint checks. Long-term care agencies include:

- Nursing centers and skilled nursing facilities
- Home care agencies
- Hospices
- Long-term care hospitals
- Assisted living residences
- Adult day-care centers
- Centers for persons with intellectual disabilities

Findings of abuse, neglect, mistreatment, or misappropriation of property (Chapter 4) may affect your certification (license, registration) status. Also, OBRA does not allow persons convicted of such crimes to be employed in long-term care agencies.

Your NATCEP may require a background screening before enrolling in the program or before clinical experiences begin. This is because clinical sites have the right to deny student participation depending on his or her criminal record. Satisfactory completion of clinical is a NATCEP requirement. Follow your NATCEP's guidelines.

Certification

Certification is the official recognition by a state that standards or requirements have been met. After successfully completing your state's NATCEP, you have the title used in your state. Titles include:

- Certified nursing assistant (CNA) or certified nurse aide (CNA). CNA is used in most states.
- Licensed nursing assistant (LNA).
- Registered nurse aide (RNA).
- State registered nurse aide (SRNA).
- State tested nurse aide (STNA).

Nursing assistants can have their certification (licenses, registration) denied, revoked, or suspended. See Box 3-1 for the reasons listed by the National Council of State Boards of Nursing (NCSBN).

See *Promoting Safety and Comfort: Certification.*

Maintaining Competence

Re-training and a new competency evaluation are required for nursing assistants who have not worked for 24 months. It does not matter how long you worked as a nursing assistant before. What matters is how long you did *not* work. States can require:

- A new competency evaluation
- Both re-training and a new competency evaluation

Agencies must provide 12 hours of education to nursing assistants every year. Performance reviews also are required. That is, your work is evaluated. These requirements help ensure that you have the current knowledge and skills to give safe, effective care.

See *Focus on Surveys: Maintaining Competence.*

WORKING IN ANOTHER STATE

To work in another state, you must meet that state's NATCEP requirements. First, contact the state agency responsible for NATCEPs and the nursing assistant registry. To find that agency, do 1 of the following.

- Contact your current nursing assistant registry.
- Search on-line to locate the state agency.

Then apply to the state agency for endorsement (reciprocity, equivalency) as a CNA (LNA, RNA, SRNA, STNA). *Endorsement (reciprocity, equivalency) means that a state recognizes the certificate, license, or registration issued by another state.* This means that your application is reviewed to see if you meet the state's requirements.

The application review results in 1 or more of the following.

- Being granted or denied certification (a license, registration).
- Having to take a NATCEP competency test. This may be the written test, the skills test, or both.
- Having to take the entire NATCEP in that state (training program and competency test).

ROLES AND RESPONSIBILITIES

Nurse practice acts, OBRA, state laws, and legal and advisory opinions direct what you can do. To protect persons from harm, you must understand what you can do, what you cannot do, and the legal limits of your role. This is called *scope of practice* or *range of functions.*

Licensed nurses supervise your work. You perform nursing tasks related to the person's care. A ***nursing task*** *is the nursing care or a nursing function, procedure, activity, or work that can be delegated to nursing assistants when it does not require a nurse's professional knowledge or judgment.* Often you function without a nurse in the room. At other times you help nurses give care. The rules in Box 3-2 will help you understand your role.

The range of functions for nursing assistants varies among states and agencies. Before performing a nursing task make sure that:

- Your state allows nursing assistants to do so.
- It is in your job description.
- You have the education and training to do so.
- A nurse is available to answer questions and to supervise you.

You perform nursing tasks to meet the person's hygiene, safety, comfort, nutrition, exercise, and elimination needs. You move and transfer persons and make observations. You measure temperatures, pulses, respirations, and blood pressures. And you help promote the person's mental comfort.

Box 3-3 (p. 22) describes the limits of your role—tasks that you should never do. State laws differ. Know what you can do in the state in which you are working.

State laws and rules limit nursing assistant functions. Your job description reflects those laws and rules. An agency can further limit what you can do. So can a nurse based on the person's needs. However, no agency or nurse can expand your range of functions beyond what your state's laws and rules allow.

BOX 3-3	Role Limits

- *Never give drugs.* Nurses give drugs. Many states allow nursing assistants to give some drugs after completing a state-approved medication assistant training program.
- *Never insert tubes or objects into body openings. Do not remove them from the body.* Exceptions to this rule are the procedures you will study during your training. Giving enemas is an example.
- *Never take oral or phone orders from doctors.* Politely give your name and title, and ask the doctor to wait for a nurse. Promptly find a nurse to speak with the doctor.
- *Never perform procedures that require sterile technique.* With sterile technique, all objects in contact with the person are free of microorganisms (Chapter 13). You can assist a nurse with a sterile procedure. However, you will not perform the procedure yourself.
- *Never tell the person or family the person's diagnosis or medical or surgical treatment plans.* This is the doctor's responsibility. Nurses may clarify what the doctor has said.
- *Never diagnose or prescribe treatments or drugs for anyone.* Doctors and some advanced practice nurses diagnose and prescribe. Nurse practitioners and clinical nurse specialists are advanced practice nurses.
- *Never supervise others including other nursing assistants.* This is a nurse's responsibility. You will not be trained to supervise others. Supervising others can have serious legal problems.
- *Never ignore an order or request to do something.* This includes nursing tasks that you can do, those you cannot do, and those beyond your legal limits. Promptly and politely explain to the nurse why you cannot carry out the order or request. The nurse assumes you are doing what you were told to do unless you explain otherwise. You cannot neglect the person's care.

BOX 3-4	Nursing Assistant Standards

The nursing assistant:
- Performs nursing tasks within the range of functions allowed by the state's nurse practice act and its rules.
- Is honest and shows integrity. (*Integrity* involves following a code of ethics. See Chapter 4.)
- Bases nursing tasks on education, training, and the nurse's directions.
- Is accountable for his or her behavior and actions.
- Performs delegated aspects of the person's care.
- Assists the nurse in observing patients and residents. Also assists in identifying their needs.
- Communicates:
  - Progress toward completing nursing tasks
  - Problems in completing nursing tasks
  - Changes in the person's status
- Asks the nurse to clarify what is expected when unsure.
- Uses educational and training opportunities as available.
- Practices safety measures to protect the person, others, and self.
- Respects the person's rights, concerns, decisions, and dignity.
- Functions as a member of the health team. Helps implement the care plan (Chapter 6).
- Respects the person's property and the property of others.
- Protects confidential information unless required by law to share the information.

Modified from National Council of State Boards of Nursing, Inc.: *NCSBN model rules,* Chicago, 2017, Author.

Nursing Assistant Standards

OBRA defines the basic range of functions for nursing assistants. All NATCEPs include those functions. Some states allow other functions. NATCEPs also prepare nursing assistants to meet the standards listed in Box 3-4.

Job Description

The *job description is a document that describes what the agency expects you to do* (Fig. 3-2). It also states educational requirements and your job title.

Always obtain a written job description when you apply for a job. Ask questions about it during your job interview (Chapter 38). Before accepting a job, tell the employer about:

- Functions you did not learn
- Functions you cannot do for moral or religious reasons

Clearly understand what is expected before taking a job. Do not take a job that requires you to:

- Act beyond the legal limits of your role.
- Function beyond your training limits.
- Perform acts that are against your morals or religion.

No one can force you to do something beyond the legal limits of your role. Sometimes jobs are threatened for refusing to follow a nurse's orders. Often staff obey out of fear. That is why you must understand:

- Your roles and responsibilities
- What you can safely do
- The things you should never do
- Your job description
- The ethical and legal aspects of your role
  See *Focus on Communication: Job Description.*

FOCUS ON COMMUNICATION

Job Description

Your training prepares you for certain nursing tasks. The agency may not let you do everything you learned. Other agencies may want you to do things not learned. Use your job description to discuss these issues with the nurse.

For example, a hospital job description includes changing a dressing (Chapter 28). You did not learn this skill in your training program. You can say: "I see changing dressings in the job description. I did not learn to do that. Will I be trained to perform this skill?"

Carefully review your job description. Know what you can and cannot do. Ask if you have questions.

POSITION DESCRIPTION/PERFORMANCE EVALUATION

Job Title: LTC Certified Nursing Assistant (CNA) Supervised by: CNA Coordinator, Charge Nurse

Prepared by: _____ Approved by: _____

Date: _____ Date: _____

Job Summary: Provides direct and indirect resident care activities under the direction of an RN or LPN/LVN. Assists residents with activities of daily living, provides for personal care and comfort, and assists in the maintenance of a safe and clean environment for an assigned group of residents.

DUTIES AND RESPONSIBILITIES:

3 = Exceeds Performance   2 = Expected Performance   1 = Needs Improvement

<u>**Demonstrates Competency in the Following Areas:**</u>

Assists in the preparation for admission of residents.	3	2	1
Assists in and accompanies residents in the admission, transfer and discharge procedures.	3	2	1
Provides morning care, which may include bed bath, shower or whirlpool, oral hygiene, combing hair, back care, dressing residents, changing bed linen, cleaning overbed table and bedside stand, straightening room and other general care as necessary throughout the day.	3	2	1
Provides evening care which includes hands/face washing as needed, oral hygiene, back rubs, peri-care, freshening linen, cleaning overbed tables, straightening room and other general care as needed.	3	2	1
Notifies appropriate licensed staff when resident complains of pain.	3	2	1
Provides postmortem care and assists in transporting bodies to the morgue.	3	2	1
Assists LPN/LVN in treatment procedures.	3	2	1
Provides general nursing care such as positioning residents, lifting and turning residents, applying/utilizing special equipment, assisting in use of bedpan or commode and ambulating the residents.	3	2	1
Performs all aspects of resident care in an environment that optimizes resident safety and reduces the likelihood of medical/health care errors.	3	2	1
Supports and maintains a culture of safety and quality.	3	2	1
Takes and records temperature, pulse, respiration, weight, blood pressure and intake-output.	3	2	1
Makes rounds with outgoing shift; knows whereabouts of assigned residents.	3	2	1
Makes rounds with oncoming shift to ensure the unit is left in good condition.	3	2	1
Adheres to policies and procedures of the facility and the Nursing Department.	3	2	1
Participates in socialization activities on the unit.	3	2	1
Turns and positions residents as ordered and/or as needed, making sure no rough surfaces are in direct contact with the body. Lifts and turns with proper and safe body mechanics and with available resources.	3	2	1
Checks for reddened areas or skin breakdown and reports to RN or LPN/LVN.	3	2	1
Ensures residents are dressed properly and assists, as necessary. Ensures that used clothing is properly stored in bedside stand or on hangers in closet. Ensures that all residents are clean and dry at all times.	3	2	1
Checks unit for adequate linen. Folds neatly and arranges linen in linen closet. Cleans linen cart. Provides clean linen and clothing. Makes beds.	3	2	1
Treats residents and their families with respect and dignity.	3	2	1
Restrains residents properly, when ordered.	3	2	1
Accompanies residents to appointments, as directed.	3	2	1
Provides reality orientation in daily care.	3	2	1
Prepares residents for meals; serves and removes food trays and assists with meals or feeds residents, if necessary.	3	2	1
Distributes drinking water and other nourishments to residents.	3	2	1
Performs general care activities for residents in isolation.	3	2	1
Answers residents' call lights, anticipates residents' needs and makes rounds to assigned residents.	3	2	1
Assists residents with handling and care of clothing and other personal property (including dentures, glasses, contact lenses, hearing aids and prosthetic devices).	3	2	1
Transports residents to and from various departments, as requested.	3	2	1
Reports and, when appropriate, records any changes observed in condition or behavior of residents and unusual incidents.	3	2	1
Participates in and contributes to interdisciplinary care conferences.	3	2	1
Must be able to follow directions, both oral and written, and work cooperatively with other staff members.	3	2	1

FIGURE 3-2 A sample nursing assistant job description. Note that the job description is also a performance evaluation. (Provided by MCN Healthcare, Denver, Colo. www.MCNHealthcare.com. All rights reserved.)

Continued

POSITION DESCRIPTION/PERFORMANCE EVALUATION—cont'd

Must have the ability to acquire knowledge of and develop skills in basic nursing procedures and simple charting.	3	2	1
Establishes and maintains interpersonal relationship with residents, family members and other facility staff while assuring confidentiality of resident information.	3	2	1
Attends inservice education programs, as assigned, to learn new treatments, procedures, developmental skills, etc.	3	2	1
Practices careful, efficient and nonwasteful use of supplies and linen and follows established charge procedure for resident charge items.	3	2	1
Maintains personal health in order to prevent absence from work due to health problems.	3	2	1
Possesses a genuine interest and concern for geriatric and disabled persons.	3	2	1

Professional Requirements:

Adheres to dress code, appearance is neat and clean.	3	2	1
Completes annual education requirements.	3	2	1
Maintains regulatory requirements.	3	2	1
Maintains resident confidentiality at all times.	3	2	1
Reports to work on time and as scheduled, completes work within designated time.	3	2	1
Wears identification while on duty, uses computerized punch time system correctly.	3	2	1
Completes inservices and returns in a timely fashion.	3	2	1
Attends annual review and department inservices, as scheduled.	3	2	1
Attends at least _____ staff meetings annually, reads and returns all monthly staff meeting minutes.	3	2	1
Represents the organization in a positive and professional manner.	3	2	1
Actively participates in performance improvement and continuous quality improvement (CQI) activities.	3	2	1
Complies with all organizational policies regarding ethical business practices.	3	2	1
Communicates the mission, ethics and goals of the facility.	3	2	1

TOTAL POINTS _____   _____   _____

Regulatory Requirements:
- High School graduate or equivalent.
- Current Certified Nursing Assistant (CNA) certification in State of _____ for Long Term Care Facilities.
- Current Basic Cardiac Life Support certification within three (3) months of hire date.

Language Skills:
- Able to communicate effectively in English, both verbally and in writing.
- Additional languages preferred.

Skills:
- Basic computer knowledge.

Physical Demands:
- For physical demands of position, including vision, hearing, repetitive motion and environment, see following description.

  Reasonable accommodations may be made to enable individuals with disabilities to perform the essential functions of the position without compromising patient care.

I have received, read and understand the Position Description/Performance Evaluation above.

_____   _____

Name/Signature   Date Signed

FIGURE 3-2, cont'd

DELEGATION

Delegate means to authorize another person to perform a nursing task in a certain situation. The person must be competent to perform the task in the given situation. *Competent means having the necessary ability, knowledge, or skill to perform a task safely and successfully.* For example, you know how to give a bed bath. However, the nurse wants to assess a new resident's nursing needs. You do not assess. Therefore the nurse gives the bath.

Who Can Delegate

RNs can delegate nursing tasks to LPNs/LVNs and nursing assistants. In some states, LPNs/LVNs can delegate nursing tasks to nursing assistants. A nurse's delegation decisions must protect the person's health and safety.

The nurse must make sure that the task was completed safely and correctly. If the RN or LPN/LVN delegates, he or she is responsible for the delegated task. The RN supervises LPNs/LVNs. Therefore the RN is legally responsible for the tasks that LPNs/LVNs delegate to nursing assistants. The RN is responsible for all nursing care.

Nursing assistants cannot delegate. You cannot delegate any task to other nursing assistants or to any other worker. You can ask someone to help you. But you cannot ask or tell someone to do your work. Also, you cannot re-delegate a task to another nursing assistant or other worker.

See *Promoting Safety and Comfort: Who Can Delegate.*

PROMOTING SAFETY AND COMFORT

Who Can Delegate

Safety

Delegation requires a nurse's knowledge and judgment. Delegated nursing tasks must be:
- Within the nursing assistant range of functions allowed by your state. For example, your state does not allow nursing assistants to cut toenails. The nurse cannot delegate cutting toenails to you. The nurse must know:
  - The range of functions allowed in your state
  - The content and skills learned in your NATCEP
- Listed in your job description. For example, your state allows you to give enemas. The task is not in your job description. The nurse cannot delegate the task to you. The nurse must know the tasks allowed by your job description.

You must know what you can and cannot do. You must refuse a task that you were not trained to do. You also must refuse a delegated task that is:
- Beyond the nursing assistant range of functions allowed by your state
- Not in your job description

See "Refusing a Task" (p. 27).

Delegation Process

To make delegation decisions, the nurse follows a process. The person's needs, the nursing task, and the staff member doing the task must fit (Fig. 3-3). The nurse decides if the task will be delegated to you. The person's needs and the task may require a nurse's knowledge, judgment, and skill. You may be asked to assist.

Delegation decisions must result in the best care for the person. Otherwise the person's health and safety are at risk. The NCSBN has described the delegation process in 4 steps (pp. 26-27).
- Step 1—Assessment and Planning
- Step 2—Communication
- Step 3—Surveillance and Supervision
- Step 4—Evaluation and Feedback

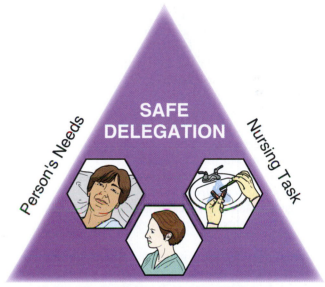

Nursing Team Member
(RN, LPN/LVN, Nursing Assistant)

FIGURE 3-3 The nurse considers the person's needs, the task, and the staff member's abilities when making delegation decisions.

Step 1—Assessment and Planning. The nurse needs to understand the person's needs. And the nurse needs to know your knowledge, skills, and job description.

When assessing the person's needs, the nurse answers these questions.

- What are the person's needs? How complex are they? How can they vary? How urgent are the care needs?
- What are the most important long-term needs? What are the most important short-term needs?
- How much judgment is needed to meet the person's needs and give care?
- How predictable is the person's health status? How does the person respond to health care?
- What problems might arise from the task? How severe might they be?
- What actions are needed if a problem occurs? How complex are the needed actions?
- What emergencies or incidents might arise? How likely might they occur?
- How involved is the person in health care decisions? How involved is the family?
- How will delegating the task help the person? What are the risks to the person?

To assess your knowledge and skills, the nurse answers these questions.

- What knowledge and skills are needed to safely perform the task?
- What is in your job description?
- What are the conditions affecting the task?
- What is expected from the task?
- What problems can arise from the task?
- What problems might the person develop during the task?

The nurse decides if it is safe to delegate the task. It must be safe for the person and you. If unsafe, the nurse stops the delegation process. If safe for the person and you, the nurse moves to step 2.

Step 2—Communication. This step involves the nurse and you. The nurse must give clear and complete directions about:

- How to perform and complete the task
- What observations to report and record
- When to report observations
- What patient or resident concerns to report at once
- Priorities for tasks
- What to do if the person's condition changes or needs change

The nurse must make sure that you understand the directions to give safe care. The nurse asks questions to make sure you understand. You may be asked to explain what you need to do. Do not be insulted by such questions. The intent is to protect the person and you.

Before performing a delegated task, discuss the task with the nurse. Make sure that you:

- Ask questions about the task and what you are expected to do.
- Tell the nurse if you have not done the task before or not often.
- Ask for needed training or supervision.
- Re-state what is expected of you.
- Re-state what patient or resident concerns to report to the nurse.
- Explain how and when you will report progress in completing the task.
- Know how to call the nurse for an emergency.
- Know what to do during an emergency.

After completing a delegated task, report and record the care given. Also report and record your observations. See "Reporting and Recording" in Chapter 6.

See *Delegation Guidelines: Step 2—Communication.*

DELEGATION GUIDELINES

Step 2—Communication

"Delegation Guidelines" boxes accompany the procedures in this book. The guidelines describe information you need from the nurse and care plan before a procedure. They also tell you the observations to report and record.

Review "Delegation Guidelines" boxes carefully. They provide the information you need to perform tasks safely.

Step 3—Surveillance and Supervision. *Surveillance* means *to keep a close watch over someone or something.* *Supervise* means *to over-see, direct, or manage.* In this step, the nurse:

- Observes the care you give.
- Makes sure that you complete the task correctly.
- Observes the person's condition and response to care. Frequency of observations depends on:
  - The person's health status and needs
  - If the person's condition is stable or unstable
  - If the nurse can predict the person's responses and risks to care
  - The setting where the task occurs
  - The resources and support available
  - If the task is simple or complex

The nurse follows up on problems or concerns. For example, the nurse takes action if:

- You did not complete the task in a timely manner.
- The task did not meet expectations.
- There is a change in the person's condition.

The nurse is alert for possible changes in the person's condition. With your help, the nurse can take action before the person's condition changes.

Sometimes problems arise during a task. By supervising you, the nurse can detect and solve problems early. This helps you complete the task safely and on time.

After you complete the task, the nurse may review and discuss what happened with you. This helps you learn. If something similar happens again, you have ideas about how to adjust.

Step 4—Evaluation and Feedback. *Evaluate* means *to judge*. The nurse decides if the delegation was successful. The nurse answers these questions.

- Was the task done correctly?
- Did the person respond as expected?
- Was the outcome (the result) as desired? Was the result good or bad?
- Was communication between you and the nurse timely and effective?
- What went well? What were the problems?
- Does the care plan need to change (Chapter 6)?
- Did the nurse give you feedback? *Feedback* means *to respond*. The nurse tells you what you did correctly and about any errors. Feedback helps you learn and improve the care you give.
- Did the nurse thank you for completing the task?

Your Role in Delegation

You perform delegated tasks for or on *a person*. You must protect the person from harm. You have 2 choices when delegated a task. You either *accept* or *refuse* a task.

The NCSBN describes *Five Rights of Delegation*. Use the *Five Rights of Delegation* in Box 3-5.

Accepting a Task. When you agree to perform a task, you are responsible for your actions. What you do or fail to do can harm the person. *You must complete the task safely.* Ask for help if you are unsure or have questions about a task. Report to the nurse what you did and your observations.

Refusing a Task. You have the right to say "no." Sometimes refusing to follow the nurse's directions is your right and duty. You should refuse to perform a task when:

- The task is beyond the legal limits of your role. That is, the task is beyond the range of functions allowed by your state.
- The task is not in your job description.
- You were not trained to perform the task.
- The task could harm the person.
- The person's condition has changed.
- You do not know how to use the supplies or equipment.
- Directions are not ethical or legal.
- Directions are against agency policies.
- Directions are not clear or complete.
- A nurse is not available for supervision.

Use common sense. This protects you and the person. Ask yourself if what you are doing is safe for the person.

BOX 3-5	The *Five Rights of Delegation* for Nursing Assistants

The Right Task
- Does your state allow you to perform the task?
- Were you trained to do the task?
- Do you have experience performing the task?
- Is the task in your job description?

The Right Circumstance
- Do you have experience with the task given the person's condition and needs?
- Do you understand the purposes of the task for the person?
- Can you perform the task safely under the current circumstances?
- Do you have the equipment and supplies to safely complete the task?
- Do you know how to use the equipment and supplies?

The Right Person
- Are you comfortable performing the task?
- Do you have concerns about performing the task?

The Right Directions and Communication
- Did the nurse give clear directions and instructions?
- Did you review the task with the nurse?
- Do you understand what the nurse expects?

The Right Supervision and Evaluation
- Is a nurse available to answer questions?
- Is a nurse available if the person's condition changes or if problems occur?
- Did the nurse evaluate the outcome?

Modified from National Council of State Boards of Nursing, Inc.: *The five rights of delegation*, as referenced in *National Guidelines for nursing delegation*, April 2016, Chicago, Author.

Never ignore an order or a request to do something. Tell the nurse about your concerns. For tasks within the legal limits of your role and in your job description, the nurse can help increase your comfort. The nurse can:

- Answer your questions.
- Demonstrate the task.
- Show you how to use supplies and equipment.
- Help you as needed.
- Observe you doing the task.
- Check on you often.
- Arrange for needed training.

Do not refuse a task because you do not like it or do not want to do it. You must have sound reasons. Otherwise you place the person at risk for harm. You could lose your job.

See *Focus on Communication: Refusing a Task.*

FOCUS ON COMMUNICATION
Refusing a Task

A nurse may delegate a task that was not part of your training. The task is in your job description. You can say:

I know this task is in my job description, but I did not learn it in school. Can you show me what to do and then observe me doing it? That would really help me.

A nurse may ask you to do something that is not in your job description. With respect, you must firmly refuse the nurse's request. You can say: "I'm sorry, but that task is not in my job description. Can I help you with something else?"

FOCUS ON PRIDE
The Person, Family, and Yourself

P ersonal and Professional Responsibility
Your training program will prepare you with the knowledge and skills to be a nursing assistant. Personal and professional qualities allow you to do your job well. Examples include communication skills, patience, compassion, and teamwork. You will learn about other qualities when you study work ethics in Chapter 5. Continue to develop personal and professional qualities during and after your training.

R ights and Respect
Most NATCEPs involve practice in a clinical setting. Sometimes a patient or resident refuses to have a student. Or the person refuses to allow a student to watch a procedure. The person's right to refuse must be respected.

If this happens to you, you may feel disappointed, rejected, ashamed, or upset. Or you may feel that you did something wrong. Kindly respect the person's request. Tell your instructor. Do not speak badly about the person. The person may have had a bad experience. This had nothing to do with you. Respect the person's right to choose who provides his or her care.

I ndependence and Social Interaction
Staff relationships and interactions affect delegation outcomes. Delegation experiences are positive when staff:

- Communicate openly.
- Trust each other.
- Help and encourage each other.
- Work toward a common goal.

With positive interactions, the person benefits from effective care.

D elegation and Teamwork
Delegation deals with what you are asked to do. To safely assist the nurse, you must know what you can and cannot do. This protects the person and you.

Do not be discouraged by what you *cannot* do. Value what you *can* do. You have a very important role. Your attitude affects the work you do. Take pride in your role.

E thics and Laws
Some nursing assistants work in more than 1 setting. Some are also emergency medical technicians (EMTs). EMTs give emergency care outside of health care settings. State laws and rules for EMTs and nursing assistants differ. For example, you work as an EMT and a nursing assistant. Your state laws allow EMTs to start intravenous (IV) lines. Nursing assistants do not start IVs.

The ability to do something does not give the right to do so in all settings. There are legal limits to your role. Be proud of the advanced skills and training you may have. But when working as a nursing assistant, follow your state's laws and rules for nursing assistants.

FOCUS ON PRIDE: *Application*
What must you consider when deciding to accept or refuse a delegated task? How would you respectfully refuse? Give an example.

*Circle **T** if the statement is TRUE or **F** if it is FALSE.*

1 **T F** OBRA requires a nursing assistant training and competency evaluation program in every state.

2 **T F** You are allowed 1 attempt to pass your state's competency evaluation.

3 **T F** Each state must have a nursing assistant registry.

4 **T F** You have not worked for 3 years. Your certification (license, registration) is still current.

5 **T F** An agency can expand your range of functions beyond what is allowed in your state.

Circle the BEST answer.

6 What state law affects what nursing assistants can do?
   a Standards for nursing assistants
   b Medicaid
   c OBRA
   d Nurse practice act

7 Your nursing assistant certification (license, registration) can be revoked for
   a Refusing a nursing task
   b Asking the nurse questions
   c Performing acts beyond your role
   d Keeping the person's information confidential

8 As a nursing assistant, you
   a Can take verbal or phone orders from doctors
   b Report observations to the nurse
   c Can remove tubes from the person's body
   d Can ignore a nursing task if it is not in your job description

9 Who assigns and supervises your work?
   a A nurse
   b The health team
   c Another nursing assistant
   d You

10 You are responsible for
   a Supervising other nursing assistants
   b Telling the person his or her diagnosis
   c Knowing what you can safely do
   d Deciding what treatments are needed

11 You perform a task not allowed by your state. Which is *true?*
   a If a nurse asked you to do the task, there is no legal problem.
   b You could be practicing nursing without a license.
   c You can perform the task if it is in your job description.
   d If you complete the task safely, there is no legal problem.

12 As a nursing assistant, you
   a Must accept all tasks delegated by the nurse
   b Make decisions about a person's care
   c Must know what tasks are in your job description
   d Give a drug when a nurse tells you to

13 The communication step of the delegation process involves
   a Observing care
   b Determining who should perform a task
   c Deciding if the delegation was successful
   d Asking questions about a task

14 You can refuse to perform a task if
   a The task is within the legal limits of your role
   b The task is in your job description
   c You do not like the task
   d A nurse is not available to supervise you

15 You decide to refuse a task. What should you do?
   a Communicate your concerns to the nurse.
   b Delegate the task to a nursing assistant.
   c Ignore the request.
   d Talk to the director of nursing.

Answers to Chapter 3 questions are on p. 551.

FOCUS ON PRACTICE

Problem Solving

You are training in the clinical setting. A nursing assistant asks you to do a patient's catheter care. You have not learned that skill yet. Can the nursing assistant delegate? How will you respond?

Ethics and Laws

OBJECTIVES

- Define the key terms and key abbreviations in this chapter.
- Describe ethical conduct.
- Describe the rules of conduct for nursing assistants.
- Explain how to maintain professional boundaries.
- Explain how to prevent negligent acts.
- Give examples of unintentional and intentional torts.
- Describe how to protect the right to privacy.

- Explain the correct use of electronic communications.
- Explain the purpose of informed consent.
- Describe elder abuse, child abuse and neglect, and intimate partner violence.
- Explain how to promote PRIDE in the person, the family, and yourself.

KEY TERMS

abuse The willful infliction of injury, unreasonable confinement, intimidation, or punishment that results in physical harm, pain, or mental anguish; depriving the person (or the person's caregiver) of the goods or services needed to attain or maintain well-being

assault Intentionally attempting or threatening to touch a person's body without the person's consent

battery Touching a person's body without his or her consent

boundary crossing A brief act or behavior of being over-involved with the person; the intent of the act or behavior is to meet the person's needs

boundary sign Acts, behaviors, or thoughts that warn of a boundary crossing or boundary violation

boundary violation An act or behavior that meets your needs, not the person's

child abuse and neglect The intentional harm or mistreatment of a child under 18 years old; it involves any recent act or failure to act on the part of a parent or caregiver; it results in death, serious physical or emotional harm, sexual abuse, or exploitation; and it presents a likely or immediate risk for harm

civil law Laws concerned with relationships between people

crime An act that violates a criminal law

criminal law Laws concerned with offenses against the public and society in general

defamation Injuring a person's name and reputation by making false statements to a third person

elder abuse Any knowing, intentional, or negligent act by a caregiver or any other person to an older adult; the act causes harm or serious risk of harm

ethics Knowledge of what is right conduct and wrong conduct

false imprisonment Unlawful restraint or restriction of a person's freedom of movement

fraud Saying or doing something to trick, fool, or deceive a person

informed consent The process by which a person receives and understands information about a treatment or procedure and is able to decide if he or she will receive it

intimate partner violence (IPV) Physical, sexual, or psychological harm by a current or former partner or spouse

invasion of privacy Violating a person's right not to have his or her name, photo, or private affairs exposed or made public without giving consent

law A rule of conduct made by a government body

libel Making false statements in print, in writing (including e-mail and text messages), through pictures or drawings, through broadcast (radio, TV, or video), posted on-line on websites, or through video sites and social media sites

malpractice Negligence by a professional person

neglect The failure of responsible persons to provide food and water, shelter, health care, or protection for a vulnerable person

negligence An unintentional wrong in which a person did not act in a reasonable and careful manner and a person or the person's property was harmed

professional boundary That which separates helpful behaviors from behaviors that are not helpful

professional sexual misconduct An act, behavior, or comment that is sexual in nature

protected health information Identifying information and information about the person's health care that is maintained or sent in any form (paper, electronic, oral)

self-neglect A person's behaviors and way of living that threaten his or her health, safety, and well-being

slander Making false statements through the spoken word, sounds, sign language, or gestures

vulnerable adult A person 18 years old or older who has a disability or condition that makes him or her at risk to be wounded, attacked, or damaged

KEY ABBREVIATIONS

CDC Centers for Disease Control and Prevention
HIPAA Health Insurance Portability and Accountability Act of 1996

IPV Intimate partner violence
OBRA Omnibus Budget Reconciliation Act of 1987

Nurse practice acts, your training and job description, and safe delegation serve to protect patients and residents from harm (Chapter 3). Protecting them from harm also involves ethical and legal aspects of care.

ETHICAL ASPECTS

Ethics is knowledge of what is right conduct and wrong conduct. Ethics also deals with choices or judgments about what should or should not be done. An ethical person behaves and acts in the right way. He or she does not cause another person harm.

Ethical behavior also involves not being prejudiced or biased. To be *prejudiced* or *biased* means *making judgments and having views before knowing the facts.* Judgments and views often are based on one's values and standards. They are based on culture, religion, education, and experiences. The person's situation and yours may be very different. For example:

- Children think their mother needs nursing home care. In your culture, children care for older parents at home.
- An older man does not want life-saving measures. You believe that everything must be done to save a life.

Do not judge the person by your values and standards. Do not avoid persons whose standards and values differ from your own.

Ethical problems involve making choices. You must decide what is the right thing to do.

Codes of Ethics

Professional groups have codes of ethics. A *code of ethics* has rules, or standards of conduct, for group members to follow. The rules of conduct in Box 4-1 can guide your thinking and behavior. See Chapter 5 for student and work ethics.

BOX 4-1	Code of Conduct for Nursing Assistants

- Respect each person as an individual.
- Know the limits of your role and knowledge.
- Perform only the tasks within the legal limits of your role.
- Perform only the tasks that you have been trained to do.
- Perform no act that will harm the person.
- Take drugs only if prescribed and supervised by a doctor.
- Follow the nurse's directions to your best possible ability.
- Follow agency policies and procedures.
- Complete each task safely.
- Be loyal to your employer and co-workers.
- Act as a responsible citizen at all times.
- Keep the person's information confidential.
- Protect the person's privacy.
- Protect the person's property.
- Consider the person's needs to be more important than your own.
- Report errors and incidents honestly and at once.
- Be accountable for your actions.

Professional Boundaries

A *boundary* limits or separates something. A fence forms a boundary. You stay inside or outside of the fenced area. As a nursing assistant, you enter into a helping relationship with patients, residents, and families. The helping relationship has professional boundaries.

Professional boundaries separate helpful behaviors from behaviors that are not helpful (Fig. 4-1). The boundaries create a helpful zone. If your behaviors are outside of the helpful zone, you are over-involved or under-involved with the person.

Professional Boundaries

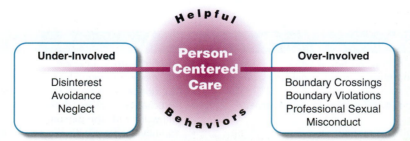

FIGURE 4-1 Professional boundaries guide your behavior. Your focus is on helping the person. Being under-involved or over-involved is not helpful. (Modified from National Council of State Boards of Nursing, Inc.: *A nurse's guide to professional boundaries*, Chicago, 2014, Author.)

If you are *under-involved*, the following can occur.
- Disinterest—you lack interest in the person.
- Avoidance—you avoid the person.
- Neglect—you do not properly care for the person (p. 36).

If you are *over-involved*, the following can occur.
- *Boundary crossing is a brief act or behavior of being over-involved with the person. The intent of the act or behavior is to meet the person's needs.* The act or behavior may be thoughtless or something you did not mean to do. Or it could have purpose if it meets the person's needs. For example, you give a crying patient a hug. The hug meets the person's needs at the time. If the hug meets your needs, the act is wrong. Also, it is wrong to hug the person every time you see him or her.
- *Boundary violation is an act or behavior that meets your needs, not the person's.* The act or behavior is not ethical. It violates the code of conduct in Box 4-1. The person can be harmed. Boundary violations include:
  - Abuse (p. 36).
  - Giving a lot of information about yourself. You tell the person about your personal relationships or problems.
  - Keeping secrets with the person.
- *Professional sexual misconduct is an act, behavior, or comment that is sexual in nature.* It is sexual misconduct even if the person consents or makes the first move.

Some boundary violations and some types of professional sexual misconduct also are crimes. To maintain professional boundaries, follow the rules in Box 4-2. Be alert to boundary signs. *Boundary signs are acts, behaviors, or thoughts that warn of a boundary crossing or boundary violation* (Box 4-3).

See *Focus on Communication: Professional Boundaries.*

BOX 4-2	Maintaining Professional Boundaries

- Follow the code of conduct in Box 4-1. Maintain a professional relationship at all times.
- Talk to the nurse if you sense a boundary sign, crossing, or violation.
- Avoid caring for family, friends, and people you know. This may be hard to do in a small community. Always tell the nurse if you know the person. The nurse may change your assignment.
- Do not make sexual comments or jokes.
- Do not use offensive language.
- Use touch correctly (Chapter 7). Touch or handle sexual and genital areas only for needed care. The areas include the breasts, nipples, perineum, buttocks, and anus.
- Do not visit or spend extra time with someone who is not part of your assignment.
- The following apply to patients, residents, and families.
  - Do not date, flirt with, kiss, or have a sexual relationship with them.
  - Do not discuss your sexual relationships with them.
  - Do not say or write things that could suggest a romantic or sexual relationship with them.
  - Do not accept gifts, loans, money, credit cards, or other valuables from them.
  - Do not give gifts, loans, money, credit cards, or other valuables to them.
  - Do not borrow from them. This includes money, personal items, and transportation.
  - Do not develop a personal relationship or friendship with them.
  - Do not share personal or financial information with them.
  - Do not help with their finances.
  - Do not take a person home with you. This includes for holidays or other events.
- Ask yourself these questions before you date or marry a person whom you cared for. Be aware of the risk for professional sexual misconduct.
  - When were you involved with the person's care?
  - Was the person's care short-term or long-term?
  - What kind and how much information do you have about the person? How will that information affect your relationship with the person?
  - Will the person need more care in the future?
  - Does dating or marrying the person place the person at risk for harm?

BOX 4-3	Boundary Signs

- You think about the person when not at work.
- You visit with the person during breaks, meal times, when off duty, and so on.
- You give more attention to the person at the expense of others.
- The person gives you gifts or money.
- You give the person gifts or money.
- You share information about yourself with the person.
- You flirt with the person.
- You make comments with a sexual message.
- You notice more touch between you and the person.
- You change how you dress or your appearance when you will work with the person.
- You have contact with the person after he or she leaves the agency.

LEGAL ASPECTS

A *law is a rule of conduct made by a government body.* The U.S. Congress and state legislatures make laws. Enforced by the government, laws protect the public welfare.

Criminal laws are concerned with offenses against the public and society in general. An act that violates a criminal law is called a **crime**. A person found guilty of a crime is fined or sent to prison. Murder, robbery, stealing, rape, kidnapping, and abuse (p. 36) are crimes.

Civil laws are concerned with relationships between people. Examples are contracts and nurse practice acts. A person found guilty of breaking a civil law usually has to pay a sum of money to the injured person.

Torts are part of civil law. *Tort* comes from the French word meaning *wrong.* A *tort* is a wrong committed against a person or the person's property. Some torts are *unintentional.* Harm was not intended. Some torts are *intentional.* The act was done on purpose and harm was intended.

Unintentional Torts

Negligence is an unintentional wrong. The negligent person did not act in a reasonable and careful manner. A person or the person's property was harmed. The person causing the harm did not intend or mean to cause harm. The person failed to do what a reasonable and careful person *would have done.* Or he or she did what a reasonable and careful person *would not have done.*

Malpractice is negligence by a professional person. A person has professional status because of education and services provided. Nurses, doctors, dentists, and pharmacists are examples.

What you do or do not do can lead to a lawsuit if you harm a person or the property of another. You are legally responsible (*liable*) for your own actions. The nurse is liable as your supervisor. However, you have personal liability. Sometimes refusing to follow the nurse's directions is your right and duty (Chapter 3).

Intentional Torts

Intentional torts are meant to be harmful.

- *Defamation is injuring a person's name and reputation by making false statements to a third person.*
  - *Libel is making false statements in print, in writing (including e-mail and text messages), through pictures or drawings, through broadcast (radio, TV, or video), posted on-line on websites, or through video sites and social media sites.* See "Wrongful Use of Electronic Communications," p. 34.
  - *Slander is making false statements through the spoken word, sounds, sign language, or gestures.*
- *False imprisonment is the unlawful restraint or restriction of a person's freedom of movement.* It involves:
  - Threatening to restrain a person
  - Restraining a person
  - Preventing a person from leaving the agency
- *Invasion of privacy is violating a person's right not to have his or her name, photo, or private affairs exposed or made public without giving consent.* You must treat the person with respect and ensure privacy. Only staff involved in the person's care should see, handle, or examine his or her body. See Box 4-4 (p. 34) for measures to protect privacy.
- *Fraud is saying or doing something to trick, fool, or deceive a person.* The act is fraud if it does or could harm a person or the person's property. Telling someone that you are a nurse is fraud. So is giving wrong or incomplete information on a job application.
- *Assault is intentionally attempting or threatening to touch a person's body without the person's consent.* The person fears bodily harm. Threatening to "tie down" a person is an example of assault.
- *Battery is touching a person's body without his or her consent.* The person must consent to any procedure, treatment, or other act that involves touching the body. The person has the right to withdraw consent at any time.

See *Focus on Communication: Intentional Torts (Invasion of Privacy)*, p. 34.

See *Promoting Safety and Comfort: Intentional Torts (Defamation)*, p. 34.

BOX 4-4   Protecting the Right to Privacy

- Keep all information about the person confidential.
- Cover the person when in hallways and elevators.
- Ask visitors to leave the room when care is given.
- Screen the person. Close the privacy curtain as in Figure 4-2. Close the room door and window coverings to give care.
- Close the bathroom door for elimination or personal hygiene.
- Expose only the body part involved in a task.
- Do not discuss the person or the person's treatment with anyone except the nurse supervising your work.
- Do not open the person's mail.
- Allow the person to visit with others in private.
- Allow the person to use the phone in private.
- Follow agency policies and procedures required to protect privacy.

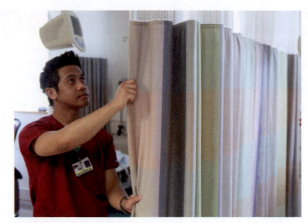

FIGURE 4-2 Pulling the privacy curtain around the bed helps protect the person's privacy.

FOCUS ON COMMUNICATION

Intentional Torts (Invasion of Privacy)

The *Health Insurance Portability and Accountability Act of 1996 (HIPAA)* protects the privacy and security of a person's health information. *Protected health information refers to identifying information and information about the person's health care that is maintained or sent in any form (paper, electronic, oral).* Failure to follow HIPAA rules can result in fines, penalties, and criminal actions including jail time.

To avoid HIPAA violations:

- *Always follow agency policies and procedures.*
- *Never take photos or videos of patients or residents or any person in the health care setting. Sharing photos or videos or posting them on video sites or social media sites is a very serious violation of HIPAA.*
- *Never send an e-mail or text message or post anything on a website, video site, or social media site about a patient, resident, family member, or visitor. Sharing information is a very serious violation of HIPAA.*
- *Never write anything for a newspaper, magazine, or print source about a patient, resident, family member, or visitor.*
- *Never broadcast (through TV, radio, or video) anything about a patient, resident, family member, or visitor.*
- *Only discuss the person's health information with staff directly involved in the person's care.*
- See "Wrongful Use of Electronic Communications."

You may be asked questions about the person or the person's care. Direct any questions about the person or the person's care to the nurse. Also follow the rules for using computers and other electronic devices (Chapter 6).

PROMOTING SAFETY AND COMFORT

Intentional Torts (Defamation)

Safety

To protect yourself from defamation, never make false statements about a patient, resident, family member, visitor, co-worker, or any other person. This includes:

- Through e-mails or text messages
- On websites, video sites, or social media sites
- In newspapers, magazines, or other print sources
- Through broadcasts (TV, radio, or film)
- With words, sounds, signs, gestures, or any form of communication

Wrongful Use of Electronic Communications

Electronic communications include e-mail, text messages, faxes, websites, video sites, and social media sites. Video and social media sites include Facebook, Twitter, YouTube, Instagram, and so on.

Correct use of electronic communications is essential in your personal life and as a nursing assistant. Follow the rules in Box 4-5. Do so whether using a computer, phone, camera, or other electronic device at home, at school, at work, or in any other setting. Wrongful use of electronic communications can result in job loss and loss of your certification (license, registration).

Wrongful use also can result in:

- Civil action resulting in a fine
- Criminal action resulting in a fine or jail time
  See *Focus on Communication: Wrongful Use of Electronic Communications.*

BOX 4-5	Electronic Communications

- Follow agency policies for using electronic communications.
- Remember that:
  - Anything you send or post electronically can be sent or shared with someone other than the intended person.
  - Electronic communications last forever. Deleted content can be retrieved for legal purposes.
  - Private information shared with the intended person still violates the rights to privacy and confidentiality.
  - Referring to a person by nickname, room number, diagnosis, or other means but not by name still violates the rights to privacy and confidentiality.
- Protect privacy and maintain confidentiality at all times.
- Never take photos or videos of the person or any part of the person's body.
- Never send in any way information about the person or images (photos, videos, art) of the person.
- Never share information that can lead to the person being identified.
- Maintain professional boundaries. Avoid on-line contact with patients and residents, former patients and residents, and their family members.
- Do not use electronic communications to share or discuss workplace issues or co-workers.
- Tell the nurse at once if you may have violated the person's right to privacy or confidentiality. If you suspect that a co-worker has done so, also tell the nurse.
- See "Gossip" in Chapter 5.
- See "Unethical Student Behavior" in Chapter 5.
- See "Electronic Devices" in Chapter 6.

Modified from National Council of State Boards of Nursing: *A nurse's guide to the use of social media,* Chicago, 2011, Author.

FOCUS ON COMMUNICATION

Wrongful Use of Electronic Communications

The following are examples of wrongful use of electronic communications.

- Laura is a nursing assistant student. On the last day of clinical, she asks 2 residents if she can take a picture with them. Laura posts the picture on Facebook with this comment: "Done with clinical! I'll miss my residents."
- Justin works on a cancer unit. A patient posts on a blog about a tiring day of treatments. Justin posts: "Chemo can wear you down. Maybe the new medicine will help you rest. Hope you feel better tomorrow. See you then."

What did Laura do wrong? What did Justin do wrong?

Often wrongful use of electronic communications is not intentional. You must be very careful. Your communication must protect privacy and confidentiality at all times.

Informed Consent

Informed consent is the process by which a person receives and understands information about a treatment or procedure and is able to decide if he or she will receive it.

A person has the right to decide what will be done to his or her body and who can touch his or her body. The doctor is responsible for informing the person about all aspects of treatment. Consent is informed when the person clearly understands all aspects of treatment.

Persons under legal age (usually 18 years) cannot give consent. Nor can persons who are mentally incompetent. Such persons are unconscious, sedated, or confused. Or they have certain mental health disorders. Informed consent is given by a responsible party—a wife, husband, parent, daughter, son, guardian, or legal representative.

You are never responsible for obtaining written consent. In some agencies, you can witness the signing of a consent. When a witness, you are present when the person signs the consent.

See *Focus on Communication: Informed Consent.*

FOCUS ON COMMUNICATION

Informed Consent

There are different ways to give consent.

- *Written consent.* The person signs a form agreeing to a treatment or procedure. You are not responsible for obtaining written consent.
- *Verbal consent.* The person says aloud that he or she consents. "Yes" and "okay" are examples.
- *Implied consent.* For example, you ask a person if you can check his or her blood pressure. He or she extends an arm. The movement implies consent.

Before any procedure or task, explain the steps to the person. This is how you obtain verbal or implied consent. Also explain each step. This allows the person to refuse at any time.

REPORTING ABUSE

Abuse is:
- *The willful infliction of injury, unreasonable confinement, intimidation, or punishment that results in physical harm, pain, or mental anguish.* Intimidation means to make afraid with threats of force or violence.
- *Depriving the person (or the person's caregiver) of the goods or services needed to attain or maintain well-being.*

Abuse includes involuntary seclusion (Chapter 2). Abuse is a crime. It can occur at home or in a health care agency. All persons must be protected from abuse. This includes persons in a coma.

The abuser is often a family member or caregiver—spouse, partner, adult child, and others. The abuser can be a friend, neighbor, landlord, or other person. Both men and women are abusers. Both men and women are abused.

See *Focus on Communication: Reporting Abuse.*
See *Focus on Surveys: Reporting Abuse.*

FOCUS ON COMMUNICATION
Reporting Abuse

Persons being abused may confide in you. They may ask you to keep it a secret. For example, a person says: "If I tell you something, will you promise not to tell anyone?" Never promise to keep a secret from the nurse. Be honest. Do not say you will keep a secret and then report it to the nurse. You can say: "For your safety, some things I must tell the nurse. What did you want to tell me?" If the person refuses to tell you, notify the nurse.

If you suspect abuse, tell the nurse. Give as much detail as you can. For example: "I am concerned about Ms. Sloan. She is very quiet today. When I asked about her visit with her niece, she didn't answer. She refused her bath. And when I helped her to the bathroom, I saw bruises on her back."

FOCUS ON SURVEYS
Reporting Abuse

Abuse is a major part of surveys. Surveyors look for signs of abuse through interviews, observations, and medical records.
Agencies must have procedures to:
- Screen staff applicants for a history of abuse, neglect, or mistreatment of residents. This includes checking:
  - Information from previous or current employers
  - Nursing assistant registries or licensing boards
- Train staff on how to prevent abuse.
- Identify and correct situations in which abuse is more likely to occur.
- Identify events, patterns, and trends that may signal abuse. Bruises, falls, and staff yelling are examples.
- Investigate abuse.
- Protect residents from harm during an investigation.
- Report and respond to claims of abuse or actual abuse.

Vulnerable Adults

Vulnerable comes from the Latin word *vulnerare*, which means *to wound*. *Vulnerable adults are persons 18 years old or older who have disabilities or conditions that make them at risk to be wounded, attacked, or damaged.* They have problems caring for or protecting themselves due to:
- A mental, emotional, physical, intellectual, or developmental disability
- Brain damage
- Changes from aging

All patients and residents, regardless of age or care setting, are vulnerable. Older persons and children (p. 38) are at risk for abuse.

See *Focus on Older Persons: Vulnerable Adults.*

FOCUS ON OLDER PERSONS
Vulnerable Adults

Some persons have behaviors and ways of living that threaten their health, safety, and well-being (self-neglect). Causes include declining health and chronic disease. Other causes are disorders that impair judgment or memory—Alzheimer's disease, dementia, depression, and drug or alcohol abuse. Some persons refuse care. Report warning signs of self-neglect to the nurse.
- Hoarding—saving, hiding, or storing things. For example, the person saves newspapers, magazines, food containers, and so on.
- Dehydration—poor urinary output, dry skin, dry mouth, confusion.
- Weight loss.
- Poor hygiene. The person has dirty hair, nails, or skin. He or she smells of urine or feces.
- Skin rashes or pressure injuries (Chapter 29).
- Not wearing the correct clothing for the weather. Or wearing dirty or torn clothing.
- Not having dentures, eyeglasses, hearing aids, walkers, wheelchairs, commodes, or other needed devices.
- Confusion, disorientation, hallucinations, or delusions (Chapter 35).
- Untreated health problems.

Elder Abuse

Elder abuse is any knowing, intentional, or negligent act by a caregiver or any other person to an older adult. The act causes harm or serious risk of harm. Elder abuse can take these forms. Often more than 1 form of abuse is present.
- *Physical abuse.* This involves inflicting, or threatening to inflict, physical pain or injury. See Box 4-6 for examples of physical abuse.
- *Neglect.* **Neglect** *is the failure of responsible persons to provide food and water, shelter, health care, or protection for a vulnerable person.* This includes failure to provide clothing, hygiene, comfort, safety, or other needs. Neglect includes but is not limited to:
  - Leaving a person lying or sitting in urine or feces
  - Keeping persons alone in their rooms or other areas
  - Failing to answer call lights

BOX 4-6	Examples of Physical Abuse

- Burning
- Corporal punishment—punishment inflicted directly on the body (beatings, lashings, whippings, and so on)
- Depriving of a basic need—food, water, shelter, and so on (Chapter 7)
- Force-feeding

- Grabbing, pinching
- Hair-pulling
- Hitting, kicking, punching, slapping
- Physical or chemical restraint (Chapter 12)
- Pushing, shaking, shoving
- Striking with or without an object

- *Verbal abuse.* Verbal abuse is using oral or written words or statements that speak badly of, sneer at, criticize, or condemn the person. It includes unkind gestures, threats of harm, or saying things to frighten the person. For example, a person is told that family members cannot visit anymore.
- *Involuntary seclusion.* The person is kept in a certain area. People have been locked in closets, basements, attics, bathrooms, and other spaces.
- *Financial exploitation or misappropriation.* To *exploit* means *to use unjustly. Misappropriate* means *to dishonestly, unfairly, or wrongly take for one's own use.* The older person's resources (money, property, assets) are mis-used or stolen by another person. Or the resources are used for the other person's profit or benefit. Examples include:
  - Using a person's credit card or debit card without permission.
  - Forging a person's signature on checks or other documents.
- *Emotional or mental abuse.* This involves inflicting mental pain, anguish, or distress through verbal or nonverbal acts. Humiliation, harassment, bullying, insults, and threats of punishment are examples. It includes being deprived of needs such as food, clothing, care, a home, or a place to sleep.
- *Sexual abuse.* This is non-consensual sexual contact of any kind. *Non-consensual* means *not giving consent.* Unwanted touching, forced nudity, and taking photos or videos are forms of sexual abuse. So is harassing the person about sex or attacking the person sexually. The person may be forced to perform sexual acts out of fear of punishment or physical harm.
- *Abandonment. Abandon* means *to leave or desert someone.* The person is deserted by someone who is supposed to provide care. Abandonment involves the following 4 points.
  - You accept an assignment to care for a person or group of persons.
  - You accept the assignment for a certain time period.
  - You remove yourself from the care setting— hospital, nursing center, or other agency.
  - You do not report off to a staff member who will assume responsibility for care.

There are many signs of elder abuse. The abused person may show only some of the signs in Box 4-7. See Figure 4-3, p. 38.

BOX 4-7	Signs of Elder Abuse

- The person reports mistreatment—abuse (physical, verbal, financial, emotional or mental, sexual), neglect, seclusion, abandonment.
- Living conditions are not safe, clean, or adequate.
- Personal hygiene is lacking. The person is not clean. Clothes are dirty. The person has poor oral hygiene.
- Weight loss—signs of poor nutrition and poor fluid intake.
- Assistive (adaptive) devices are missing or broken— eyeglasses, hearing aids, dentures, cane, walker, and so on.
- Medical needs are not met.
- Frequent injuries—injuries are strange or seem impossible.
- Old and new injuries—bruises, welts, scars, fractures, punctures, and so on.
- Complaints of pain or itching in the genital or anal area.
- Bleeding and bruising around the breasts or in the genital or anal area.
- Torn, stained, or bloody under-garments.
- Burns on the feet, hands, buttocks, or other parts of the body. Cigarettes and cigars cause small circle-like burns.
- Pressure injuries (Chapter 29) or contractures (Chapter 27).
- The person seems very quiet or withdrawn.
- Unexplained withdrawal from normal activities.
- The person seems fearful, anxious, or agitated.
- The person does not want to talk or answer questions.
- Sudden changes in alertness.
- Depression.
- Sudden changes in finances.
- The person is restrained. Or the person is locked in a certain area for long periods.
- The person cannot reach toilet facilities, food, water, and other needed items.
- Private conversations are not allowed. The caregiver is present during all conversations.
- Strained or tense relationships with a caregiver.
- Frequent arguments with a caregiver.
- The person seems anxious to please the caregiver.
- Drugs are not taken properly. Drugs are not bought. Or too much or too little of the drug is taken.
- Emergency room visits may be frequent.
- The person may change doctors often. Some people do not have a doctor.

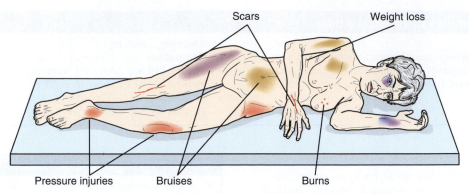

Scars   Weight loss

Pressure injuries   Bruises   Burns

FIGURE 4-3 Some physical signs of elder abuse.

Reporting Elder Abuse. Federal and state laws require the reporting of elder abuse. You may suspect abuse. If so, discuss the matter and your observations with the nurse. Give as many details as possible. The nurse contacts health team members and community agencies as needed. Sometimes the police or courts are involved.

OBRA Requirements. The *Omnibus Budget Reconciliation Act of 1987 (OBRA)* requires these actions if abuse is suspected within the center.

- The matter is reported at once to the administrator. It also is reported at once to other officials as required by federal and state laws.
- All claims of abuse are thoroughly investigated.
- The center must prevent further potential for abuse while the investigation is in progress.
- Investigation results are reported to the center administrator within 5 days of the incident. They also are reported to other officials as required by federal and state laws.
- Corrective actions are taken if the claim is found to be true.

Child Abuse and Neglect

Child abuse and neglect is the intentional harm or mistreatment of a child under 18 years old. It involves the following.
- *Any recent act or failure to act on the part of a parent or caregiver.*
- *The act or failure to act results in death, serious physical or emotional harm, sexual abuse, or exploitation.*
- *The act or failure to act presents a likely or immediate risk for harm.*

Child abuse is complex. You must be alert for signs and symptoms of child abuse. All states require the reporting of suspected child abuse (Box 4-8). If you suspect child abuse, share your concerns with the nurse. Give as much detail as you can. The nurse contacts health team members and child protection agencies as needed.

Intimate Partner Violence

The Centers for Disease Control and Prevention (CDC) defines *intimate partner violence (IPV) as physical, sexual, or psychological harm by a current or former partner or spouse.* Also called domestic abuse, domestic violence, intimate partner abuse, partner abuse, and spousal abuse—IPV occurs in relationships. IPV includes dating violence and teen dating violence. In IPV, 1 partner has power and control over the other through abuse. The abuse may range from 1 hit to chronic, severe battering. Rarely is IPV a 1-time event.

IPV causes fear and harm. Usually more than 1 type of IPV is present.
- *Physical violence*—physical injuries occur. Death is a constant threat.
- *Sexual violence*—unwanted sexual contact.
- *Threats of physical or sexual violence*—words, gestures, or weapons are used to communicate threats of death, disability, injury, or harm.
- *Psychological and emotional violence*—acts, threats of acts, or forceful actions cause trauma to the victim. This includes stalking.

Both males and females can be victims. Patients and residents can suffer from IPV. For example, a husband slaps his wife during a visit. Or a wife uses her husband's money for herself rather than buying her husband's needed medicine. You, yourself, may be a victim of IPV. Warning signs include:
- Unwanted physical or sexual contact
- Threats to you, your children, family members, or pets
- Threats of suicide to get you to do something
- Using or threatening to use a weapon against you
- Keeping or taking your paycheck
- Saying things to put you down or make you feel bad
- Keeping you from seeing family or friends
- Keeping you from going to work

Intimate partner violence is a safety issue. The victim often hides the abuse. He or she may protect the abuser. State laws vary about reporting IPV. However, the health team has an ethical duty to give information about safety and community resources. If you suspect IPV, share your concerns with the nurse. The nurse gathers information to help the person.

See *Promoting Safety and Comfort: Intimate Partner Violence.*

BOX 4-8	Child Abuse and Neglect—Signs and Symptoms

General Behaviors
- Reports bad treatment or abuse by a parent or caregiver.
- Has sudden changes in behavior.
- Has sudden changes in school performance or grades.
- Has health problems that go untreated.
- Lacks adult supervision.
- Is overly agreeable or obedient.
- Is quiet, withdrawn, or uninvolved.
- Arrives early at school or stays late.
- Fears a parent or a certain person; does not want to be around a certain person.

Physical Abuse
- Bruises, fractures, welts, bites, or burns.
- The shape of the object causing the welt may be seen. The shape of a welt may be of a belt, belt buckle, chain, clothes hanger, rope, or other object.
  - Intentional burns leave a pattern from the item causing the burn. Cigarettes and irons are examples.
  - In scalds, the area put in hot liquid is clearly marked. For example, a scald to the hand looks like a glove.

Neglect
- Fails to gain weight.
- Wants to eat large amounts of food.
- Begs or steals food or money.
- Is dirty or has a severe body odor.
- Lacks the correct clothing for the weather.
- Abuses alcohol or drugs.
- States that no one is at home to provide care.
- Is often absent from school.
- Lacks medical or dental care. Does not have needed eyeglasses.

Sexual Abuse
- Bleeding, cuts, or bruises of the genitalia, anus, breasts, or mouth. Stains or blood on under-garments.
- Trouble walking or sitting.
- Bedwetting.
- Sudden change in appetite.
- Signs and symptoms of urinary tract infection (Chapter 33).
- Vaginal discharge.
- Genital odor or pain.
- Pregnancy.
- Sexual knowledge or behavior that does not fit with one's age.

Emotional Abuse
- Headaches.
- Stomach aches.
- Abnormal fears.
- Nightmares.
- Attempts to run away.
- Extremes in behavior—overly agreeable or demanding; quiet and withdrawn or aggressive.
- Depression.
- Avoids certain situations—going to school, riding the school bus.
- Has attempted suicide.
- Rocks oneself or bangs head.

Modified from Child Welfare Information Gateway: *What is child abuse and neglect: recognizing the symptoms,* Washington, DC, July 2013, Children's Bureau.

PROMOTING SAFETY AND COMFORT

Intimate Partner Violence

Safety

Intimate partner violence occurs in relationships. Partners may be:
- Married
- Not married but living together
- Dating
- Divorced or separated
- Female and male; male and male; female and female

If you are a victim of abuse, call 911 or the police. Tell the police everything that happened—the abuser, what happened, marks on your body, and so on. Answer their questions honestly and completely. The police can help you and your children to a safe place. They can give you information about IPV, IPV programs and shelters, and how to develop a personal safety plan.

OTHER LAWS

See "Ethics and Laws" in the *Focus on PRIDE: The Person, Family, and Yourself* boxes at the end of each chapter. They describe other laws affecting your work as a nursing assistant.

Personal and Professional Responsibility

States have laws about who must report abuse and neglect. Such persons are called *mandatory reporters. Mandatory* means *required.* For example, most states require that health care providers report suspected abuse or neglect of children, vulnerable adults, and elders. Tell the nurse if you suspect abuse or neglect.

Rights and Respect

The person has the right to be free from abuse, mistreatment, and neglect. Abuse can take many forms. For example:

- A person constantly crying out for help is left alone with the door closed.
- A person is told to be nice or care will not be given.
- A person is turned in a rough and hurried manner.
- A person lies in a wet and soiled bed all night.
- A person uses the call light a lot. It is removed from the room.
- A person is told that family does not visit because the person is mean.

Independence and Social Interaction

You will interact closely with patients, residents, and families. You may begin to know them well. Social and professional relationships differ. To maintain professional boundaries:

- Follow the "Code of Conduct for Nursing Assistants" in Box 4-1.
- See "Maintaining Professional Boundaries" and "Boundary Signs" in Boxes 4-2 and 4-3.
- Ask the nurse if you have a question about an interaction.

Use good judgment when interacting with patients, residents, and families. Take pride in being professional.

Delegation and Teamwork

Working within the limits of your role protects persons from harm. You must understand your roles and responsibilities to know when a task is outside these limits.

Laws, job descriptions, and agency policies and procedures direct what you do.

- Policies are guides for staff conduct.
- Procedures explain how to perform certain tasks or skills.

You must know what you can and cannot do and how to safely perform procedures. Sometimes refusing a delegated task is your right and duty.

Ethics and Laws

Without intending it, harm can occur. The following actions can lead to charges of negligence.

- You fail to test the water temperature for a shower. The water is too hot. The person is burned.
- You do not answer a call light promptly. The person gets up without help. The person falls and breaks an arm.
- You do not follow the manufacturer's instructions for a mechanical lift. The person slips out of the lift and falls. The person fractures a hip.
- You do not identify the person before a procedure. You perform the procedure on the wrong person. Both residents are harmed. One had a procedure that was not ordered. The other did not have a needed procedure.

Your training helps you develop the skills and judgment needed to give safe care. Take pride in protecting persons from harm.

FOCUS ON PRIDE: *Application*

A code of conduct guides your thinking and behavior. Write a personal code of conduct stating what you expect of yourself as a nursing assistant.

Circle the BEST answer.

1 Which is ethical behavior?
   a Sharing information about a person with a friend
   b Accepting gifts from a resident's family
   c Reporting errors
   d Calling your family before answering a call light

2 On your days off, you call the agency to check on a patient. This is a
   a Professional boundary
   b Tort
   c Boundary violation
   d Boundary sign

3 To maintain professional boundaries, focus on
   a Helping the person
   b Meeting your needs
   c Being biased
   d Showing that you care

4 You help with a friend's hospital care. This is a
   a Professional boundary
   b Boundary crossing
   c Tort
   d Crime

5 Which is a crime?
   a Abuse
   b Slander
   c Negligence
   d Fraud

6 These statements are about negligence. Which is *true?*
   a It is an intentional tort.
   b The negligent person acted in a reasonable manner.
   c The person or the person's property was harmed.
   d A prison term is likely.

7 You do not tell the nurse about a patient's chest pain. The patient dies from a heart attack. You
   a Did nothing wrong
   b Could face negligence charges
   c Are not legally responsible
   d Are guilty of fraud

8 Threatening to touch the person's body without the person's consent is
   a Assault
   b Battery
   c Defamation
   d False imprisonment

9 Restraining a person's freedom of movement is
   a Neglect
   b Invasion of privacy
   c Defamation
   d False imprisonment

10 Sharing a resident's photo on a social media site is
   a Fraud
   b Allowed with the family's consent
   c A violation of HIPAA
   d Allowed if you obtain informed consent

11 You tell others that you are nurse. This is
   a Negligence
   b Fraud
   c Libel
   d Slander

12 Informed consent is when the person
   a Fully understands all aspects of treatment
   b Signs a consent form
   c Is admitted to the agency
   d Agrees to a procedure

13 Self-neglect is when
   a A caregiver harms a person
   b The person's behaviors put him or her at risk for harm
   c A person is deprived of food, clothing, hygiene, and shelter
   d The person does not receive attention or affection

14 You scold an older person for not eating lunch. This is
   a Physical abuse
   b Neglect
   c Battery
   d Verbal abuse

15 Which is a sign of elder abuse?
   a Stiff joints and joint pain
   b Weight gain
   c Poor personal hygiene
   d Forgetfulness

16 Depriving a child of food, clothing, and shelter is
   a Physical abuse
   b Neglect
   c Abandonment
   d Emotional abuse

17 An older adult has a black eye and bruises on the face. These are signs of
   a Physical abuse
   b Sexual abuse
   c Neglect
   d Substance abuse

18 Blood stains on a child's underpants are a sign of
   a Physical abuse
   b Sexual abuse
   c Neglect
   d Substance abuse

19 These statements are about intimate partner violence. Which is *true?*
   a It always involves physical harm.
   b It is usually a 1-time event.
   c One partner has control over the other partner.
   d Only 1 type of abuse is usually present.

20 You suspect a resident was abused. You should
   a Tell the nurse
   b Call the police
   c Tell the family
   d Ask the person about the abuse

Answers to Chapter 4 questions are on p. 551.

FOCUS ON PRACTICE

Problem Solving

A resident in your nursing center asks you to bring your children to visit. How will you respond? How do professional boundaries protect the person?

Student and Work Ethics

OBJECTIVES

- Define the key terms and key abbreviation in this chapter.
- Describe the qualities and traits of a successful nursing assistant.
- Describe good health and hygiene practices.
- Explain how to look professional.
- Explain how to plan for childcare and transportation.
- Describe ethical behavior on the job.
- Explain how to manage stress.
- Explain how to problem solve and deal with conflict.

- Explain the aspects of harassment.
- Explain how to resign from a job.
- Identify the common reasons for losing a job.
- Explain the reasons for drug testing.
- Describe unethical student behavior and possible consequences.
- Explain how to promote PRIDE in the person, the family, and yourself.

KEY TERMS

bullying Repeated attacks or threats of fear, distress, or harm by a bully toward a victim

confidentiality Trusting others with personal and private information

gossip To spread rumors or talk about the private matters of others

harassment To trouble, torment, offend, or worry a person by one's behavior or comments

priority The most important thing at the time

professionalism Following laws, being ethical, having good work ethics, and having the skills to do your work

stress The response or change in the body caused by any emotional, physical, social, or economic factor

teamwork Staff members work together as a group; each person does his or her part to give safe and effective care

work ethics Behavior in the workplace

KEY ABBREVIATION

NATCEP Nursing assistant training and competency evaluation program

As a student and a nursing assistant, you must act and function in a professional manner. *Professionalism involves following laws, being ethical, having good work ethics, and having the skills to do your work.* Certain behaviors (conduct), choices, and judgments are expected. *Work ethics deals with behavior in the workplace.* Your conduct reflects your choices and judgments. Work ethics involves:

- How you look
- What you say
- How you behave
- How you treat and work with others
- The qualities and traits described in Box 5-1

In this chapter, *work ethics* also applies to you as a student. To be a successful student, practice good work ethics in the classroom and clinical setting and with instructors and fellow students.

BOX 5-1	Qualities and Traits for Good Work Ethics

- *Being caring.* Have concern for the person. Help make the person's life happier, easier, or less painful.
- *Being dependable.* Report to work on time and as scheduled. Perform delegated tasks. Keep obligations and promises.
- *Being considerate.* Respect the person's physical and emotional feelings. Be gentle and kind toward patients, residents, families, and co-workers.
- *Being cheerful.* Greet and talk to people in a pleasant manner. Do not be moody, bad-tempered, or unhappy while at work.
- *Having empathy.* Empathy is seeing things from the person's point of view—putting yourself in the person's place. How would you feel if you had the person's problems?
- *Being trustworthy.* Patients, residents, families, and staff have confidence in you. They believe you will keep information confidential. They trust you not to gossip about them.
- *Being respectful.* Patients and residents have rights, values, beliefs, and feelings. They may differ from yours. Do not judge or condemn the person. Treat the person with respect and dignity at all times. The person has the right to respectful treatment. Also show respect for the health and nursing teams.
- *Being courteous.* Be polite and courteous to patients, residents, families, visitors, and co-workers. See p. 46 for common courtesies in the workplace.
- *Being conscientious.* Be careful, alert, and exact in following instructions. Give thorough care. Do not lose or damage the person's property.
- *Being honest.* Accurately report the care given, your observations, and any errors.
- *Being cooperative.* Willingly help and work with others. Take that "extra step" during busy and stressful times.
- *Having enthusiasm.* Be eager, interested, and excited about your work. Your work is important.
- *Being self-aware.* Know your feelings, strengths, and weaknesses. Understand yourself so you can understand patients and residents.
- *Having patience.* Tolerate problems and delays without getting upset, annoyed, or angry. Stay calm. Do not hurry or rush the person or a co-worker.

HEALTH, HYGIENE, AND APPEARANCE

Patients, residents, families, and visitors expect you to look, act, and be healthy. For example, a person must stop smoking. Yet because you smoke, you and your clothes smell of smoke. If you do not look or smell clean, people wonder if you give good care. Your health, hygiene, and appearance need careful attention.

Your Health

In order to learn and to give safe and effective care, you must be physically and mentally healthy.

- *Diet.* You need a balanced diet for good nutrition (Chapter 23).
- *Sleep and rest.* Most adults need 7 to 8 hours of sleep daily.
- *Body mechanics.* You will bend, carry heavy objects, and move and turn persons. Use your muscles correctly (Chapter 14).
- *Exercise.* Exercise promotes muscle tone, circulation, and weight loss.
- *Your eyes.* You will read instructions and take measurements. Wrong readings and measurements can harm the person. Have your eyes checked. Wear needed eyeglasses or contact lenses. Have good lighting for reading and fine work.
- *Smoking.* Smoke odors stay on your breath, hands, clothing, and hair. Hand-washing and good hygiene are needed.
- *Drugs.* Some drugs affect thinking, feeling, behavior, and function. Working under the influence of drugs affects the person's safety and yours. Take only those drugs ordered by your doctor.
- *Alcohol.* Alcohol is a drug that affects thinking, balance, coordination, and alertness. Never go to work under the influence of alcohol. Do not drink alcohol while working.

Your Hygiene

Your hygiene needs careful attention. Bathe daily. Use a deodorant or antiperspirant to prevent body odors. Brush your teeth often—upon awakening, before and after meals, and at bedtime. Use mouthwash to prevent breath odors.

Menstrual hygiene is important. Change tampons or sanitary pads often, especially for heavy flow. Wash your genital area with soap and water at least once a day. Also practice good hand-washing.

Foot care prevents odors and infection. Wash your feet daily. Dry thoroughly between the toes. Cut toenails straight across after bathing or soaking them.

Your Appearance

How you look affects the way people think about you and the agency. When staff or students are clean and neat, people think the agency is clean and neat.

Follow the practices in Box 5-2, p. 44. They help you look clean, neat, and professional (Fig. 5-1, p. 44).

BOX 5-2	Professional Appearance

- Practice good hygiene.
- Follow your training program's or the agency's dress code. The dress code tells about uniform style and color, shoes, make-up, jewelry, hair-style, and so on.
- Do not wear home or social attire at work or as a student in the clinical setting.
  - Do not wear jeans, halter tops, short skirts, or low-cut tops or pants.
  - Wear clothing that fits well. Clothing must not be tight, revealing, or sexual.
    - Women—do not show cleavage, tops of breasts, or upper thighs.
    - Men—avoid tight pants and exposing your chest. Open only the top button of your shirt.
- Wear uniforms that fit well. They are modest in length and style. Follow the dress code.
- Keep uniforms clean, pressed, and mended. Sew on buttons. Repair zippers, tears, and hems.
- Wear a clean uniform daily.
- Wear your name badge or photo ID (identification) at all times when on duty. Make sure it can be seen. Wear it according to agency policy. It is best to wear it above your waist. Agencies may use first names only or first and last names. For security, some agencies only use first names. Your student ID will have the school's name.
- Wear under-garments that are clean and fit properly. Change them daily.
- Wear under-garments in the best color for your skin tone. Do not wear colored (red, pink, blue, and so on) ones. They can be seen through white and light-colored uniforms.
- Cover tattoos (body art). They may offend others.

- Follow the dress code for jewelry. Wedding and engagement rings may be allowed. Rings and bracelets can scratch a person. Confused or combative persons and young children might pull on jewelry (necklaces, dangling earrings).
- Do not wear jewelry in pierced eyebrows, nose, lips, cheek, tongue, or other visible sites while on duty.
- Follow the dress code for earrings. Usually 1 set of small, simple earrings is allowed.
- Wear a wristwatch with a second (sweep) hand.
- Wear clean stockings and socks that fit well. Change them daily.
- Wear shoes that fit, are comfortable, give needed support, and have non-skid soles. Do not wear sandals or open-toed shoes.
- Wear clean shoes. Wash or replace shoes and laces as needed.
- Keep fingernails clean, short, and smoothly and neatly shaped. Long or jagged nails can scratch a person. Nails must be natural, not artificial.
- Do not wear nail polish. Chipped nail polish may provide a place for microbes to grow.
- Have a simple, attractive hair-style. Hair is off your collar and away from your face. Use simple pins, combs, barrettes, and bands to keep long hair up and in place.
- Keep beards and mustaches clean and trimmed.
- Use make-up that is modest in amount and moderate in color. Avoid a painted and severe look.
- Do not wear perfume, cologne, or after-shave lotion. The scents may offend, nauseate, or cause breathing problems in patients and residents.

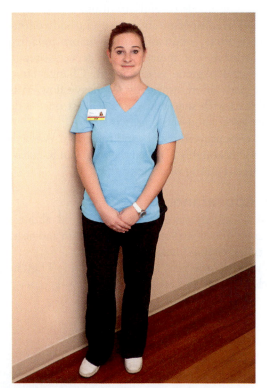

FIGURE 5-1 The nursing assistant is well groomed. Her uniform and shoes are clean. Her hair has a simple style—away from her face and off of her collar. She does not wear jewelry.

PREPARING FOR SCHOOL OR WORK

Being dependable is important as a student and in the workplace. To show you are dependable as a student:

- Be on time for class and clinical experiences. Arrive early to store your things, use the restroom, and gather needed items for class or clinical. Be ready for class or clinical to start.
- Complete and turn in assignments on time.
- Pay attention and follow directions.
- Stay for the entire class or clinical experience.

Absences and tardiness (being late) can affect your success in school. Your state's nursing assistant training and competency evaluation program (NATCEP) requires a certain number of hours. To pass the course, you must complete the required number of hours.

Absences and tardiness are also common reasons for losing a job. Childcare and transportation issues often interfere with getting to school and work. You need to plan carefully. See "Attendance."

Childcare

Someone needs to care for your children when you leave for school or work, while you are at school or work, and before you get home. Also plan for emergencies.

- Your childcare provider is ill or cannot care for your children that day.
- A child becomes ill or injured while you are at school or work.
- You will be late getting home from school or work.

Transportation

Plan for getting to and from school or work. If you drive, keep your car in good working order. Keep enough gas in the car. Or leave early to get gas.

Carpooling is an option. Carpoolers depend on each other. If the driver is late leaving, everyone is late for school or work. If 1 person is not ready when the driver arrives, everyone is late for school or work. Carpool with people you trust to be ready on time. Be on time as a driver and as a passenger.

Know bus or train schedules. Know what bus or train to take if delays occur. Always carry enough money for fares to and from school or work.

Have a back-up plan for getting to school or work. Your car may not start, the carpool driver may not be going that day, or public transportation may not run.

TEAMWORK

Teamwork means that staff members work together as a group. Each person does his or her part to give safe and effective care. Teamwork involves:

- Working when scheduled
- Being cheerful and friendly
- Completing delegated tasks
- Helping others willingly
- Being kind to others

You are an important member of the health and nursing teams. Quality of care is affected by how you work with others and how you feel about your job.

Attendance

Report to work when scheduled and on time. The entire unit is affected when just 1 person is late. Call the agency if you will be late or cannot go to work. Follow the attendance policy in your employee handbook. Poor attendance can cause you to lose your job.

Be *ready to work* when your shift starts.

- Store your things before your shift starts.
- Use the restroom when you arrive at the agency.
- Arrive on your nursing unit a few minutes early. Greet others and settle yourself.

You must stay the entire shift. Watching the clock for your shift to end gives a bad image. You may need to work over-time. Prepare to stay longer if necessary. When it is time to leave, report off duty to the nurse.

See *Focus on Communication: Attendance.*

Your Attitude

You need a good attitude. Show that you enjoy your work. Listen to others. Be willing to learn. Stay busy and use your time well.

Always think before you speak. These statements signal a bad attitude.

- "That's not my resident (patient)."
- "I can't. I'm too busy."
- "I didn't do it."
- "I don't feel like it."
- "It's not my fault."
- "Don't blame me."
- "It's not my turn. I did it yesterday."
- "Nobody told me."
- "That's not my job."
- "You didn't say that you needed it right away."
- "I did more than she (he) did."
- "I work harder than anyone else."
- "No one appreciates what I do."
- "I'm tired of this place."
- "Is it time to leave yet?"
- "Good luck. I had a horrible day."

FOCUS ON COMMUNICATION

Attendance

You may have days that you cannot go to class or clinical or to work. Illness, a family death, and other emergencies are reasons. You must tell your instructor or the agency about your absence. Otherwise you could have an unexcused absence from your NATCEP. If working, you could lose your job. To report an absence:

- *Call well before class, clinical, or your shift begins.* See the attendance policy in your student or employee handbook for when to call. Calling at least 2 hours before the start time is common.

- *Know who to call.* As a student, call your instructor. A charge nurse, nurse manager, or supervisor handles absences in the work setting. You may need your call transferred. For example: "Hello. This is Erin Jones. Please transfer me to the charge nurse." You must give information to the right person.

- *Give the reason for your absence.* Be honest. You can say: "I am sorry. I will be absent from work (class, clinical) today. I have a fever and a cough."

- *Give the length of your absence.* People often miss 1 or 2 days for illness or a family emergency. Longer absences require more communication.

Gossip

To *gossip means to spread rumors or talk about the private matters of others.* Gossiping is unprofessional and hurtful. To avoid being a part of gossip:

- Remove yourself from where people are gossiping.
- Do not make or repeat any comment that can hurt a person, family member, visitor, co-worker, fellow student, instructor, or the school or agency.
- Do not make or repeat any comment that you do not know is true. Making or writing false statements about another person is defamation (Chapter 4).
- Do not talk about patients, residents, family members, visitors, co-workers, fellow students, instructors, or the school or agency at home or in social settings.
- Do not send messages or post comments about others or the school or agency by e-mail, instant messaging, text messaging, video sites, or social media. This is especially true of hurtful, false, or private comments. See "Wrongful Use of Electronic Communications" in Chapter 4.

Confidentiality

The person's information is private and personal. *Confidentiality means trusting others with personal and private information.* The person's information is shared only among staff involved in his or her care. The person has the right to privacy and confidentiality. Agency, family, and co-worker information also is confidential. So is student information.

Share information only with the nurse or your instructor. Avoid talking about patients, residents, families, the agency, or co-workers when others are present. Do not talk about them in hallways, elevators, dining areas, or outside the agency. Others may over-hear you. Do not eavesdrop. To *eavesdrop means to listen in or over-hear what others are saying.* It invades a person's privacy.

Many agencies have intercom systems. They allow for communication between the bedside and the nurses' station (Chapter 17). Be careful what you say. The intercom is like a loud speaker. Others nearby can hear what you are saying.

See *Focus on Communication: Confidentiality.*

FOCUS ON COMMUNICATION

Confidentiality

Your family and friends may ask about patients, residents, families, or staff. For example, your mother says: "I heard my neighbor is in your nurisng home. Do you know what's wrong?"

Do not share any information with your family and friends. Doing so violates the person's right to privacy and confidentiality (Chapters 2 and 4). You can say:

I'm sorry, but I can't tell you about anyone in the center. It is unprofessional and against center policies. And it violates the person's right to privacy and confidentiality. Please don't ask me about anyone in the center.

Speech and Language

Your speech and language must be professional. Words used in home and social settings are not proper in class, the clinical setting, and at work. Such words may offend patients, residents, families, visitors, and co-workers. Remember:

- Do not swear or use foul, vulgar, slang, or abusive language.
- Speak softly and gently.
- Speak clearly. Hearing problems are common.
- Do not shout or yell.
- Do not fight or argue with a person, family member, visitor, co-worker, your instructor, or a fellow student.

Courtesies

A *courtesy* is a polite, considerate, or helpful comment or act. Courtesies take little time or energy. Even the smallest kind act can brighten someone's day.

- Address others by Miss, Mrs., Ms., Mr., or Doctor. Or use the name the person prefers. Do not call your instructor by his or her first name.
- Say "please." Begin or end each request with "please."
- Say "thank you" when someone does something for you or helps you.
- Apologize. Say "I'm sorry" when you make a mistake or hurt someone. Even little things—like bumping someone in the hallway—need an apology.
- Wish the person and family well when they leave the agency. "Stay well" and "stay healthy" are examples.
- Hold doors and elevator doors open for others. If you are at the door first, open the door and let others pass through.
- Let patients, residents, families, and visitors enter elevators first.
- Stand to greet families and visitors.
- Help others willingly when asked.
- Give praise. If you see a co-worker or student do or say something that impresses you, tell that person. Also tell your co-workers or other students.
- Do not take credit for another person's deeds. Give the person credit for the action.

Personal Matters

Personal matters must not interfere with your job. Otherwise care is neglected. You could lose your job. To keep personal matters out of the workplace:

- Make phone calls during meals and breaks.
- Do not let family and friends visit you on the unit. If they must see you, meet them during a meal or break.
- Make appointments (doctor, dentist, lawyer, and others) for your days off.
- Do not use agency computers, printers, fax machines, copiers, or other equipment for your personal use.
- Do not take the agency's supplies (pens, paper, and others) for your personal use.
- Do not discuss personal problems.

- Control your emotions. If you need to cry or express anger, do so in private. Get yourself together quickly and return to your work.
- Do not borrow money from or lend it to co-workers or fellow students.
- Do not sell things or engage in fund-raising.
- Turn off phones.
- Do not send or check e-mail or text messages.

Meals and Breaks

Meal breaks are usually 30 minutes. Other breaks are usually 15 minutes. Meals and break times are scheduled so that some staff are always on the unit. Staff remaining on the unit cover for the staff on break.

Staff members depend on each other. Leave for and return from breaks on time. That way other staff can have their turn. Do not take longer than allowed. Tell the nurse when you leave and return to the unit.

Job Safety

You must protect patients, residents, families, visitors, co-workers, and yourself from harm. Everyone is responsible for safety. Negligent acts affect the safety of others (Chapter 4). Safety practices are presented throughout this book. These guidelines apply to everything you do.

- Understand the roles, functions, and responsibilities in your job description.
- Follow agency rules, policies, and procedures.
- Know what is right and wrong conduct.
- Know what you can and cannot do.
- Develop the desired qualities and traits in Box 5-1.
- Follow the nurse's directions and instructions.
- Question unclear directions and things you do not understand.
- Help others willingly when asked.
- Ask for any training you might need.
- Report accurately—measurements, observations, the care given, the person's complaints, and any errors (Chapters 6 and 10).
- Be responsible for your actions. Admit when you are wrong or make mistakes. Do not blame others. Do not make excuses. Learn what you did wrong and why. Try to learn from your mistakes.
- Handle the person's property carefully and prevent damage.
- Follow the safety measures in Chapter 10 and throughout this book. Also see the *Promoting Safety and Comfort* boxes throughout this book.

Planning Your Work

You will give care and perform routine nursing unit tasks. Some tasks are done at certain times. Others are done at the end of the shift. Deciding what to do and when (Chapter 6) is called *priority setting.* A **priority** *is the most important thing at the time.* Setting priorities involves deciding:

- Who has the greatest or most life-threatening needs.
- What task the nurse or person needs done first.
- What tasks need to be done at a certain time.
- How long it takes to complete a task.
- How much help you need to complete a task.
- Who can help you and when.

Priorities change as the person's needs change. A person's condition can improve or worsen. New patients and residents are admitted. Others are transferred to other nursing units or discharged. These and many other factors can change priorities.

Setting priorities becomes easier with experience. Ask your instructor or the nurse to help you set priorities. Plan your work to give safe, thorough care and to use your time well (Box 5-3).

BOX 5-3	Planning Your Work

- Discuss priorities with the nurse.
- Know the routine of your shift and nursing unit.
- Follow unit policies for shift reports. In an *end-of-shift report,* the nurse gives a report to the on-coming shift. See Chapter 6.
- List tasks that are on a schedule. For example, some persons are turned or offered the bedpan every 2 hours.
- Judge how much time you need for each person and task.
- Identify tasks to do while patients and residents are eating, visiting, or involved with activities or therapies.
- Plan care around meal times, visiting hours, and therapies. Also consider recreation and social activities.
- Identify when you will need help from a co-worker. Ask a co-worker to help you. Give the time when you will need help and for how long.
- Schedule equipment or rooms for the person's use. The shower room is an example.
- Review delegated tasks. Gather needed supplies ahead of time.
- Do not waste time. Stay focused on your work.
- Leave a clean work area. Make sure rooms are neat and orderly. Also clean utility areas.
- Be a self-starter. Have initiative. Ask others if they need help. Follow unit routines, stock supply areas, and clean utility rooms. Stay busy.

MANAGING STRESS

Stress is the response or change in the body caused by any emotional, physical, social, or economic factor. Stress is normal. It occurs every minute of every day in everything you do. No matter the cause—pleasant or unpleasant—stress affects the whole person.

- *Physically*—sweating, increased heart rate, faster and deeper breathing, increased blood pressure, dry mouth, and so on
- *Mentally*—anxiety, fear, anger, dread, apprehension, and using defense mechanisms (Chapter 34)
- *Socially*—changes in relationships, avoiding others, needing others, blaming others, and so on
- *Spiritually*—changes in beliefs and values and strengthening or questioning one's beliefs in God or a higher power

Prolonged or frequent stress threatens physical and mental health. Some problems are often minor—headaches, stomach upset, sleep problems, muscle tension, and so on. Others are life-threatening—high blood pressure, heart attack, stroke, ulcers, and so on.

School and job stresses affect your family and friends. Personal stress affects your studies or work. Stress affects you, the care you give, the person's quality of life, and how you relate to co-workers.

To reduce or cope with stress:

- Exercise regularly.
- Get enough rest and sleep.
- Eat healthy.
- Plan personal and quiet time for you.
- Use common sense about what you can and cannot do. Do not try to do everything that others ask you to do.
- Do 1 thing at a time. Set priorities.
- Do not judge yourself harshly. Do not try to be perfect or expect too much from yourself.
- Give yourself praise. You do good and wonderful things every day.
- Have a sense of humor. Laugh at yourself. Laugh with others. Spend time with those who make you laugh.
- Have a social life that does not include co-workers.
- Talk to the nurse if your work or a person is causing too much stress. The nurse can help you deal with the matter.

Dealing With Conflict

People bring their values, attitudes, opinions, experiences, and expectations to school and work settings. Differences often lead to conflict. *Conflict is a clash between opposing interests or ideas.* People disagree and argue. There are misunderstandings and unrest.

Conflicts arise over issues or events. Work schedules, absences, and the amount and quality of work are examples. The problems must be worked out. Otherwise, unkind words or actions may occur. The learning or work setting becomes unpleasant. Care is affected.

Resolving Conflict.   To resolve conflict, identify the real problem. This is part of *problem solving.*

- Step 1: Define the problem. *A nurse ignores me.*
- Step 2: Collect information about the problem. Do not include unrelated information. *The nurse does not look at me. The nurse does not talk to me. The nurse does not respond when I ask for help. The nurse does not ask me to help with tasks that require 2 people. The nurse talks to other staff members.*
- Step 3: Identify possible solutions. *Ignore the nurse. Talk to my supervisor. Talk to co-workers about the problem. Change jobs.*
- Step 4: Select the best solution. *Talk to my supervisor.*
- Step 5: Carry out the solution. *See below.*
- Step 6: Evaluate the results. *See below.*

Communication and good work ethics help prevent and resolve conflicts. Identify and solve problems before they become major issues. To deal with conflict:

- Ask your instructor or supervisor for time to talk privately. Explain the problem. Give facts and specific examples. Ask for advice to solve the problem.
- Approach the person with whom you have the conflict. Ask to talk privately. Be polite and professional.
- Agree on a time and place to talk.
- Talk in a private setting. No one should hear you or the other person.
- Explain the problem and what is bothering you. Give facts and specific behaviors. Focus on the problem. Do not focus on the person.
- Listen to the person. Do not interrupt.
- Identify ways to solve the problem. Offer your thoughts. Ask for the other person's ideas.
- Set a date and time to review the matter.
- Thank the person for meeting with you.
- Carry out the solution.
- Review the matter as scheduled.
  See *Focus on Communication: Resolving Conflict.*

FOCUS ON COMMUNICATION
Resolving Conflict

You may find it hard to talk to someone with whom you have a conflict. This is hard for many people. However, letting the problem continue will make the matter worse. The following may help you start talking to the person. Always ask the person involved if you can talk privately.

- "You say 'no' when I ask you to help me. I help you when asked. This bothers me. Can we talk privately for a few minutes?"
- "I heard you tell John that I was sitting in a resident's room. You seemed angry when you said it. Can we talk privately? I want to explain why I was sitting and find out why that bothers you."
- "The new schedule shows me working every weekend this month. Please tell me why. The employee handbook says that we work every other weekend."
- "We were late for class 2 times this week when you drove. How can I help so that we are not late?"

HARASSMENT

Harassment means to trouble, torment, offend, or worry a person by one's behavior or comments. Harassment can be sexual. Or it can involve age, race, ethnic background, religion, or disability. Respect others. Do not offend others by your gestures, remarks, use of touch, or through electronic communications. Do not offend others with jokes, photos, or other pictures (drawings, cartoons, and so on). Harassment is not legal.

You have the right not to be harassed as a student. No student should be allowed to harass or bully you. The same applies to your instructor, other school instructors or staff, and clinical staff. If you believe that you are being harassed or bullied, talk to your instructor or school counselor. Follow the steps in "Resolving Conflict."

See *Focus on Communication: Harassment.*

FOCUS ON COMMUNICATION
Harassment

You have the right to feel safe and not threatened. If comments make you uncomfortable, you can say: "Please don't say things like that. It's unprofessional." If someone's actions make you uneasy, you can say: "Please don't do that. It's unprofessional." Leave the area. Report the person's statements or actions to the nurse or your instructor.

Sexual Harassment

Sexual harassment involves unwanted sexual behaviors by another. The behavior may be a sexual advance or a request for a sexual favor. Some remarks, comments, and touch are sexual. The behavior affects work and comfort. In extreme cases, a job (or grade) is threatened if sexual favors are not granted.

Sexual harassment can take the form of sexting. *Sexting* combines the words *sex* and *texting*. Sexting involves creating, sending, and posting sexual text messages, photos, or videos of oneself or others. Phones and other electronic devices are used.

Victims of sexual harassment may be men or women. Men harass women or men. Women harass men or women. If you feel harassed, report the matter to the nurse and the human resources officer. As a student, tell your instructor and school counselor.

Be careful about what you say or do. Even innocent remarks and behaviors can be viewed as harassment. You might not be sure about your own or another person's remarks or behaviors. If so, talk to your instructor or the nurse. You cannot be too careful.

Bullying

Bullying is repeated attacks or threats of fear, distress, or harm by a bully toward a victim. Bullying can be physical (hitting, tripping), verbal (name calling, teasing), or social (rumors, leaving the person out of a group). Property damage and forcing a person to do something against his or her will are other forms of bullying.

Bullying can occur in work, classroom, clinical, or social settings. Cyber-bullying occurs through electronic means (including phones)—phone calls and voice messages, e-mail, chat rooms, instant messaging, text messaging, videos, photos, and social media sites.

According to the Centers for Disease Control and Prevention (CDC), bullying can result in injury, emotional distress, and even death. Victims of bullying are at risk for depression, anxiety, sleep problems, and poor school or work performance. Those who bully are at risk for substance abuse, school or work problems, and violence.

Talk to your instructor or supervisor if you are being bullied. He or she will try to help you with the situation.

RESIGNING FROM A JOB

Whatever your reason for resigning, tell your employer. Do 1 of the following.
- Give a written notice.
- Write a resignation letter.
- Complete a form in the human resources office.

A 2-week notice is a good practice. Do not leave without notice. Include the following in your notice.
- Reason for leaving
- The last date you will work
- Comments thanking the employer for the opportunity to work in the agency

LOSING A JOB

You must perform your job well and protect patients and residents from harm. No pay raise or losing your job results from poor performance. Failing to follow agency policy is often grounds for termination. So is failure to get along with others. Box 5-4 lists the many reasons why you can lose your job. To protect your job, function at your best. Always practice good work ethics.

DRUG TESTING

Drug and alcohol use affect patient, resident, and staff safety. Quality of care suffers. Those who use drugs or alcohol are late to work or absent more often than staff who do not use such substances. Therefore drug testing policies are common. Review your agency's policy for when and how you might be tested.

UNETHICAL STUDENT BEHAVIOR

Your NATCEP and school will likely have a code of conduct. Violating the code of conduct is unethical behavior. Many of the reasons listed in Box 5-4 are violations of your school's and NATCEP's code of conduct. As a result, your school and NATCEP may take 1 or more of the following actions.

- Dismiss you from the school or NATCEP
- Issue a failing grade
- Not recommend that you take the competency evaluation (written and skills tests)

Act in an ethical manner at all times. Always try to do the right thing. If you do, you will be a successful nursing assistant.

BOX 5-4	Common Reasons for Losing a Job

- Poor attendance—not going to work or excessive tardiness (being late).
- Abandonment—leaving the job during your shift.
- Falsifying a record—job application or a person's record.
- Violent behavior in the workplace.
- Weapons in the workplace—guns, knives, explosives, or other dangerous items.
- Having, using, or distributing alcohol or drugs in the work setting. This excludes having or using drugs ordered by your doctor.
- Taking a person's drugs for your own use or giving them to others.
- Harassment.
- Offensive speech and language.
- Stealing or destroying the agency's or a person's property.
- Disrespect to patients, residents, families, visitors, co-workers, or supervisors.
- Abusing or neglecting a person.
- Invading a person's privacy.
- Failing to maintain patient, resident, family, agency, or co-worker confidentiality. This includes access to computer and other electronic information.
- Wrongful use of electronic communications (Chapter 4).
- Using the agency's supplies and equipment for your own use.
- Defamation—see Chapter 4 and "Gossip" (p. 46).
- Abusing meal breaks and break time.
- Sleeping on the job.
- Violating the agency's dress code.
- Violating any agency policy or care procedure.
- Tending to personal matters while on duty.

FOCUS ON P R I D E

The Person, Family, and Yourself

Personal and Professional Responsibility

Your job as a nursing assistant is important. You can help persons feel safe, secure, and cared for. Through good work ethics, you can make others' lives happier, easier, and less painful. Take pride in your work ethics. Your work affects quality of life.

Rights and Respect

Conflict with other students and co-workers will arise. Dealing with conflict can be hard. But it must be addressed. Deal with conflict in a respectful and mature way. Do not gossip, put others down, or talk about people behind their backs. These behaviors are disrespectful and not professional.

Independence and Social Interaction

Social interaction is part of your job. Smile and greet patients and residents by name. Politely introduce yourself. Do not appear hurried. Display a caring and friendly manner all the time. Remain calm and helpful in stressful situations. These actions promote good relationships and reflect well on you and the agency.

Delegation and Teamwork

Your work ethics affect the team. Greet co-workers pleasantly. Help others willingly. After completing tasks, ask if you can help with anything else.

Be available. Stay where you can be found easily. If you will be in 1 area for a while, tell the nurse. Return from breaks on time. Be someone others enjoy working with.

Ethics and Laws

As a student and nursing assistant, you are responsible for following the ethical guidelines in this chapter. Patients, residents, families, visitors, and co-workers depend on you for safe and effective care. You must:

- Attend clinical and work when scheduled.
- Arrive at clinical and work on time.
- Stay the entire clinical time or work shift.
- Complete your assignments.
- Work safely.
- Be pleasant and courteous.

FOCUS ON PRIDE: Application

Think of a person you enjoy working with. What qualities do you value in a co-worker? How will you apply these qualities in your work?

REVIEW QUESTIONS

Circle **T** *if the statement is TRUE and* **F** *if it is FALSE.*

1 **T F** You wear needed eyeglasses. This helps protect the person's safety.

2 **T F** Childcare requires planning before going to school.

3 **T F** Being on time for work means arriving at the agency when your shift starts.

4 **T F** You share confidential information with a friend. You could lose your job.

5 **T F** You do not follow the agency's dress code. You could lose your job.

6 **T F** You can use your phone to send text messages during clinical.

7 **T F** You must follow the agency's attendance policy.

8 **T F** Harassment is legal in the workplace.

Circle the BEST answer.

9 You show honesty when you
   a Help others complete tasks
   b Report mistakes
   c Remain calm
   d Are polite

10 Which will help you do your job well?
   a Sleeping 3 to 4 hours daily
   b Avoiding exercise
   c Using drugs and alcohol
   d Having good nutrition

11 Which is a good hygiene practice?
   a Bathing weekly
   b Wearing strongly scented perfume or cologne
   c Brushing teeth after meals
   d Having long and polished fingernails

12 You are getting ready for clinical. Which is a good practice?
   a Styling hair up and off your collar
   b Wearing jewelry
   c Wearing your name badge at waist level
   d Having tattoos exposed

13 Which statement reflects a good attitude?
   a "It's not my fault."
   b "I'm sorry. I didn't know."
   c "That's not my job."
   d "I did it yesterday. It's your turn."

14 A co-worker tells you that a doctor and nurse are dating. This is
   a Gossip
   b Eavesdropping
   c Confidential information
   d Sexual harassment

15 Which is professional speech and language?
   a Using vulgar words
   b Shouting
   c Arguing
   d Speaking clearly

16 Which is a courteous act?
   a Telling co-workers they did a good job
   b Calling a resident "Honey"
   c Taking credit for a co-worker's work
   d Closing an elevator door as a person approaches

17 You are on a meal break. Which is *true*?
   a You cannot make personal phone calls.
   b Family members cannot meet you.
   c The nurse needs to know that you are off the unit.
   d You can take a few extra minutes if needed.

18 When planning your work
   a Discuss priorities with the nurse
   b Delegate tasks you will not have time to do
   c Do not ask co-workers for help
   d Plan care so that you can watch the person's TV

19 These statements are about stress. Which is *true*?
   a Personal stress does not affect work.
   b Stress affects the whole person.
   c All stress is unpleasant.
   d Stress is abnormal.

20 You have extra work because a co-worker is often late for work. To resolve the conflict
   a Explain the problem to your supervisor
   b Refuse to work with the person
   c Ignore the problem
   d Complain about the person to co-workers

21 Which statement is *true*?
   a Giving a resident a compliment is harassment.
   b Joking about a person's religion is not harassment.
   c Harassment can occur through text messages.
   d Only women are victims of harassment.

22 You are often late for work. Which is *true*?
   a Tardiness is excused if you give the reason.
   b You may be fined.
   c You can make up the time by skipping your break.
   d You can lose your job.

Answers to Chapter 5 questions are on p. 551.

FOCUS ON PRACTICE

Problem Solving

A co-worker did not show up for work. You and the other staff members have extra work. How do you respond? How will you plan, prioritize, and manage the extra work?

Health Team Communications

OBJECTIVES

- Define the key terms and key abbreviations in this chapter.
- Describe the rules for good communication.
- Describe the legal and ethical aspects of medical records.
- Identify common parts of the medical record.
- Explain your role in the nursing process.
- List the information you need to report to the nurse.
- List the rules for recording.
- Explain how electronic devices are used in health care.

- Explain how to protect the right to privacy when using electronic devices.
- Describe how to answer phones.
- Use the 24-hour clock, medical terminology, and medical abbreviations.
- Explain how to promote PRIDE in the person, the family, and yourself.

KEY TERMS

chart See "medical record"

communication The exchange of information—a message sent is received and correctly interpreted by the intended person

electronic health record (EHR) An electronic version of a person's medical record; electronic medical record

electronic medical record (EMR) See "electronic health record"

end-of-shift report A report that the nurse gives at the end of the shift to the on-coming shift; change-of-shift report

medical record The legal account of a person's condition and response to treatment and care; chart

nursing care plan A written guide about the person's nursing care; care plan

nursing diagnosis A health problem that can be treated by nursing measures

nursing process The method nurses use to plan and deliver nursing care; its 5 steps are assessment, nursing diagnosis, planning, implementation, and evaluation

objective data Information that is seen, heard, felt, or smelled by an observer; signs

observation Using the senses of sight, hearing, touch, and smell to collect information

planning Setting priorities and goals

recording The written account of care and observations; charting

reporting The oral account of care and observations

signs See "objective data"

subjective data Things a person tells you about that you cannot observe through your senses; symptoms

symptoms See "subjective data"

KEY ABBREVIATIONS

ADL	Activities of daily living
BMs	Bowel movements
EHR	Electronic health record
EMR	Electronic medical record

EPHI; ePHI	Electronic protected health information
MDS	Minimum Data Set
PHI	Protected health information

Health team communication is needed for coordinated and effective care. Team members share information about:

- What was done for the person
- What needs to be done for the person
- The person's response to treatment

COMMUNICATION

Communication is the exchange of information—a message sent is received and correctly interpreted by the intended person. For good communication:

- Use words that mean the same thing to you and the message receiver. Avoid words with more than 1 meaning. What does "far" mean—50 feet or 100 feet?
- Use familiar words. Avoid terms that the person and family do not understand.
- Be brief and concise. Do not add unrelated or unnecessary information. Stay on the subject. Do not wander in thought or get wordy.
- Give information in a logical and orderly way. Organize your thoughts. Present them step-by-step.
- Give facts and be specific. Reporting a pulse rate of 110 is more specific than the "pulse is fast."

THE MEDICAL RECORD

The *medical record (chart) is the legal account of a person's condition and response to treatment and care.* Medical records are written on paper forms or electronically with computers or other electronic devices. An *electronic health record (EHR) or electronic medical record (EMR) is an electronic version of a person's medical record.*

The health team uses the medical record to share information about the person. The record is a permanent legal document. It can be used in court as legal evidence of the person's problems, treatment, and care.

Agencies have policies about medical records and who can see them. Policies address:

- Who records
- When to record
- Ink color (paper charting)
- Abbreviations
- How to make and sign entries
- How to correct errors

Some agencies allow nursing assistants to record observations and care. Others do not. Follow your agency's policies.

Professional staff involved in a person's care can review charts. You have an ethical and legal duty to keep information confidential. If not involved in the person's care, you have no right to read the person's chart. Doing so is an invasion of privacy.

Common parts of the record include:

- *Admission information*—is gathered when the person is admitted to the agency. It includes the person's identifying information.
- *Health history*—is completed by the nurse. The nurse asks about current and past illnesses, signs and symptoms, allergies, and drugs.
- *Flow sheets and graphic sheets*—are used to record care measures, observations, and measurements made daily, every shift, or 3 to 4 times a day (Fig. 6-1). Information includes vital signs (blood pressure, temperature, pulse, respirations), weight, intake and output (Chapter 24), bowel movements, doctor visits, and every-day activities.
- *Progress notes and nurses' notes*—are used to describe observations, the care given, and the person's response and progress. They are used to record information about treatments, some drugs, and procedures. In long-term care, summaries of care describe the person's progress toward meeting goals and response to care.

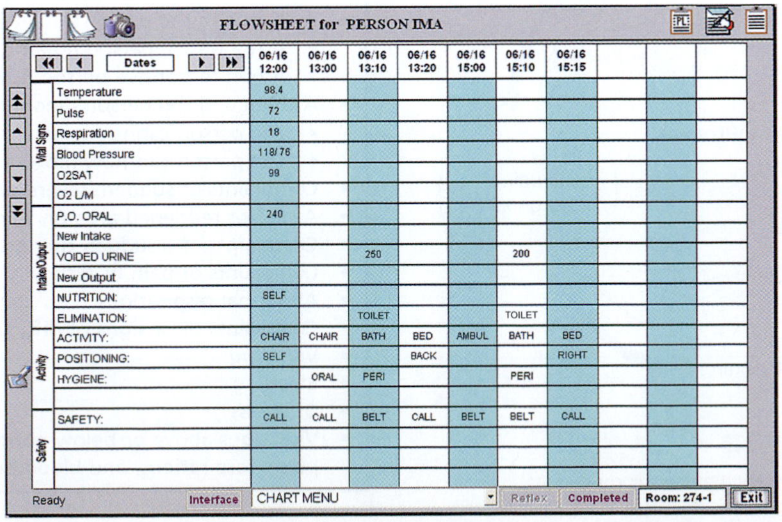

FIGURE 6-1 A sample flow sheet. (Courtesy Abraham Lincoln Memorial Hospital, Lincoln, Ill.)

THE NURSING PROCESS

The **nursing process** is the method nurses use to plan and deliver nursing care. It has 5 steps.

* *Assessment*
* *Nursing diagnosis*
* *Planning*
* *Implementation*
* *Evaluation*

The nursing process focuses on the person's nursing needs. All nursing team members do the same things for the person. They focus on the same goals for the person.

The nursing process is on-going. New information is gathered and the person's needs may change. However, the steps are the same. You will see how the nursing process is continuous as each step is explained (Fig. 6-2).

You have a key role in the nursing process. Your observations are used for nursing diagnoses and planning. You may help develop care plans. In the implementation step, you perform tasks in the care plan. Your assignment sheet (p. 57) tells you what to do. Your observations are used for the evaluation step.

Assessment

Assessment involves collecting information about the person. The nurse takes a health history about current and past health problems. The family's health history is important. Information from the doctor is reviewed. So are test results from past medical records.

An RN (registered nurse) assesses the person's body systems and mental status. You assist with assessment. You make observations as you give care and talk to the person.

Observation is using the senses of sight, hearing, touch, and smell to collect information.

* You *see* how the person lies, sits, or walks. You see flushed or pale skin. You see red and swollen body areas.
* You *listen* to the person breathe, talk, and cough. You use a stethoscope to measure blood pressure.
* Through *touch*, you feel if the skin is hot or cold, or moist or dry. You use touch to take a pulse.
* *Smell* is used to detect body, wound, and breath odors. You also smell odors from urine and bowel movements (BMs).

Objective data (signs) are seen, heard, felt, or smelled by an observer. You can feel a pulse. You can see urine color. *Subjective data (symptoms)* are things a person tells you about that you cannot observe through your senses. You cannot feel or see the person's pain, fear, or nausea.

Box 6-1 lists the observations to report at once. Box 6-2 lists the basic observations to make and report to the nurse. Make notes of your observations. Use them to report and record observations. Carry a note pad and pen in your pocket. Note your observations as you make them. Many agencies use electronic devices for recording (p. 61).

The Minimum Data Set.

The Centers for Medicare & Medicaid Services (CMS) requires the *Minimum Data Set (MDS)* for nursing center residents (Appendix C, p. 555). The MDS is an assessment tool. It provides information about the person. Examples include memory, communication, hearing and vision, physical function, and activities.

The nurse uses your observations for the MDS. The MDS is started when the person is admitted to the center. The MDS is updated before each care conference (p. 56). A new MDS is done once a year and for a significant change (decline or improvement) in the person's health status.

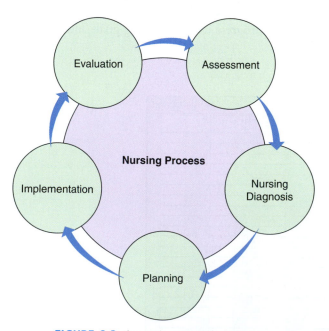

FIGURE 6-2 The nursing process is continuous.

BOX 6-1	Observations to Report at Once

* A change in the person's ability to respond
    * A responsive person no longer responds.
    * A non-responsive person now responds.
* A change in the person's mobility
    * The person cannot move a body part.
    * The person can now move a body part.
* Complaints of sudden, severe pain
* A sore or reddened area on the skin
* Complaints of a sudden change in vision
* Complaints of pain or difficulty breathing
* Abnormal respirations
* Complaints of or signs of difficulty swallowing
* Vomiting
* Bleeding
* Dizziness
* Vital signs above or below normal ranges—temperature, pulse, respirations, and blood pressure (Chapter 25)

BOX 6-2	Basic Observations

Ability to Respond
- Is the person easy or hard to wake up?
- Can the person give his or her name, the time, and location when asked?
- Does the person identify others correctly?
- Does the person answer questions correctly?
- Does the person speak clearly?
- Are instructions followed correctly?
- Is the person calm, restless, or excited?
- Is the person conversing, quiet, or talking a lot?

Movement
- Can the person squeeze your fingers with each hand?
- Can the person move arms and legs?
- Are movements shaky or jerky?
- Does the person complain of stiff or painful joints?

Pain or Discomfort
- Where is the pain located? (Have the person point to the pain.)
- Does the pain go anywhere else?
- How does the person rate the severity of the pain—mild, moderate, severe?
- How does the person rate the pain on a scale of 0 to 10 (Chapter 25)?
- When did the pain begin?
- What was the person doing when the pain began?
- How long does the pain last?
- How does the person describe the pain?
  - Sharp
  - Severe
  - Knife-like
  - Dull
  - Burning
  - Aching
  - Comes and goes
  - Depends on position
- Was a pain-relief drug given?
- Did the pain-relief drug relieve pain? Is pain still present?
- Can the person sleep and rest?
- What is the position of comfort?

Skin
- Is the skin pale or flushed?
- Is the skin cool, warm, or hot?
- Is the skin moist or dry?
- Does the skin appear mottled (blotchy, spotted with color)?
- What color are the lips and nail beds?
- Is the skin intact? Are there broken areas? If so, where?
- Are sores or reddened areas present? If yes, where?
- Are bruises present? If yes, where?
- Does the person complain of itching? If yes, where?

Eyes, Ears, Nose, and Mouth
- Is there drainage from the eyes? Drainage color?
- Are the eyelids closed? Do they stay open?
- Are the eyes reddened?
- Does the person complain of spots, flashes, or blurring?
- Is the person sensitive to bright lights?
- Is there drainage from the ears? Drainage color?
- Can the person hear? Is repeating necessary? Are questions answered correctly?

Eyes, Ears, Nose, and Mouth—cont'd
- Is there drainage from the nose? Drainage color?
- Can the person breathe through the nose?
- Is there breath odor?
- Does the person complain of a bad taste in the mouth?
- Does the person complain of painful gums or teeth?
- Do the person's gums bleed with oral hygiene (Chapter 18)?

Respirations
- Do both sides of the chest rise and fall with respirations?
- Is breathing noisy?
- Does the person complain of pain or difficulty breathing?
- What is the amount and color of sputum?
- How often does the person cough? Is the cough dry or productive?

Bowels and Bladder
- Is the abdomen firm or soft?
- Does the person complain of gas?
- Which does the person use: toilet, commode, bedpan, or urinal?
- What are the amount, color, and consistency of bowel movements (BMs)?
- What is the frequency of BMs?
- Can the person control BMs?
- Does the person have pain or difficulty urinating?
- What is the amount of urine?
- What is the color of urine?
- Is the urine clear? Are there particles in the urine?
- Does urine have a foul smell?
- Can the person control the passage of urine?
- What is the frequency of urination?

Appetite
- Does the person like the food served?
- How much of the meal is eaten?
- What foods does the person like?
- Can the person chew food?
- What is the amount of fluid taken?
- What fluids does the person like?
- How often does the person drink fluids?
- Can the person swallow food and fluids?
- Does the person complain of nausea?
- What is the amount and color of vomitus?
- Does the person have hiccups?
- Is the person belching?
- Does the person cough when swallowing?

Activities of Daily Living
- Can the person perform personal care without help?
  - Bathing?
  - Brushing teeth?
  - Combing and brushing hair?
  - Shaving?
- Does the person feed himself or herself?
- Can the person walk?
- What amount and kind of help is needed?

Bleeding
- Is the person bleeding? If yes, from where and how much?

BOX 6-3	Sample Nursing Diagnoses and Definitions
Nursing Diagnosis	**Definition**
Bathing self-care deficit	Inability to independently complete cleansing activities
Constipation	Decrease in normal frequency of defecation accompanied by difficult or incomplete passage of stool and/or passage of excessively hard, dry stool (*defecation means bowel movement*)
Diarrhea	Passage of loose, unformed stools
Dressing self-care deficit	Inability to independently put on or remove clothing
Impaired bed mobility	Limitation of independent movement from one bed position to another
Impaired memory	Persistent inability to remember or recall bits of information or skills
Impaired skin integrity	Altered epidermis and/or dermis
Impaired walking	Limitation of independent movement within the environment on foot
Insomnia	A disruption in amount and quality of sleep that impairs functioning
Urinary retention	Inability to empty bladder completely

T. Heather Herdman/Shigemi Kamitsuru (Eds.), NANDA International, Inc. Nursing Diagnoses: Definitions and Classification 2018-2020, Eleventh Edition © 2017 NANDA International, ISBN 978-1-62623-929-6. Used by arrangement with the Thieme Group, Stuttgart/New York.

Nursing Diagnosis

The RN uses assessment information to make a nursing diagnosis. A **nursing diagnosis** *describes a health problem that can be treated by nursing measures.* See Box 6-3 for examples.

Nursing diagnoses and medical diagnoses are not the same. A *medical diagnosis* is the identification of a disease or condition by a doctor. Cancer, stroke, heart attack, and diabetes are examples.

A person can have many nursing diagnoses. They may change as assessment information changes. Or new ones are added.

Planning

Planning *involves setting priorities and goals.* Priorities are what is most important for the person. Goals are aimed at the person's highest level of well-being and function—physical, emotional, social, and spiritual. Goals promote health and prevent health problems.

Nursing interventions are chosen after goals are set. A *nursing intervention* (*nursing action*, *nursing measure*) is an action or measure taken by the nursing team to help the person reach a goal. A nursing intervention does not need a doctor's order.

The **nursing care plan** (care plan) *is a written guide about the person's nursing care.* It has the person's nursing diagnoses and goals. It also has the nursing measures or actions for each goal. A communication tool, the care plan:

- Communicates what care to give
- Helps ensure that nursing team members give the same care

The care plan is found in the written or electronic medical record. The plan is carried out. It may change as nursing diagnoses change.

See *Focus on Surveys: Planning.*

FOCUS ON SURVEYS

Planning

During a survey, you may be asked about the person's care plan. Give honest and complete answers. You may be asked about:

- The person's goals
- Care measures
- How the care measures are carried out
- How you give input about the person's care needs and your observations

Care Conferences. Care conferences are held to share information and ideas about the person's care. The purpose is to develop or revise the nursing care plan. Effective care is the goal. Nursing assistants may take part in the conference.

See *Focus on Communication: Care Conferences.*

FOCUS ON COMMUNICATION

Care Conferences

You see what patients and residents like and do not like and what they can and cannot do. They talk to you. They tell you about their families and interests. You make observations when you are with them. Share this information in care conferences. Also share ideas about care. For example, you can say:

- "Mr. Antonio misses the fresh green beans and broccoli from his garden. Can he have those more often?"
- "Mrs. Clark can propel her wheelchair with her feet. Why do we push her wheelchair?"
- "Miss Walsh never talks when her family visits. She talks to her roommate often."

The Comprehensive Care Plan. The CMS requires a *comprehensive care plan*. It is a written guide about the person's care. The plan has the person's problems, nursing diagnoses, goals, and actions to take.

For example, the MDS shows that Mr. Woo cannot do activities of daily living (ADL). A care plan is developed to solve the problem. The goal is for Mr. Woo to do his own ADL. Actions to help Mr. Woo reach the goal are:

- Occupational therapy for ADL daily
- Physical therapy for exercises daily
- Nursing staff to walk Mr. Woo 20 yards twice daily

The care plan also has the person's strengths. For example, Mr. Woo can feed himself. The health team helps Mr. Woo continue to feed himself.

Implementation

To *implement* means *to perform or carry out*. In the *implementation* step, nursing interventions (nursing measures, nursing actions) in the care plan are performed or carried out. Care is given. The nurse delegates tasks within your legal limits and job description.

FOCUS ON COMMUNICATION

Assignment Sheets

Assignment sheets provide a summary of the information you need to give care. The sheets communicate information clearly and in an organized way.

Use your assignment sheets to receive a report from the nurse. Add new information. Ask the nurse if you have questions. For example:

> *I have a question about Mr. Parker. My assignment sheet does not mention assistive devices. Last week physical therapy was helping him use a walker instead of his cane. Which is he using now?*

Assignment Sheets. The nurse uses an assignment sheet to communicate delegated tasks to you (Fig. 6-3). The assignment sheet tells you about:

- Each person's care.
- What nursing measures and tasks to do.
- Which nursing unit tasks to do. Cleaning utility rooms and stocking shower rooms are examples.

Talk to the nurse about an unclear assignment. Also check the care plan for more information.

See *Focus on Communication: Assignment Sheets.*

Evaluation

Evaluate means *to measure*. The *evaluation* step involves measuring if the goals in the planning step were met. Progress is evaluated. Changes in nursing diagnoses, goals, and the care plan may result.

Assignment Sheet

Date: 9–10
Shift: Day
Nursing assistant: John Reed
Supervisor: Mary Garcia, RN

Breaks: 1000   1400
Lunch: 1230
Unit Tasks: *Pass drinking water at 0900*
Clean utility room at 1430

*****Check the care plan for other care measures and information**

Room # 501A Name: Mrs. Ann Lopez	Functional status/ care measures and procedures
ID Number: S1514491530 Date of birth: 11/04/1932	Total assist with ADL
VS: Daily at 0700	Stand-pivot transfers
T _____ P _____ R _____ BP _____	Uses w/c
Wt: Weekly (Monday at 0700)	Incontinent of bowel and bladder – uses briefs
Intake _____ Output _____ BM _____	Passive ROM exercises to extremities twice daily
Bath: Portable tub	Turn and re-position q2h when in bed
Shampoo Bed rails	Wears eyeglasses and dentures
	Diet: High fiber (Total Assist)
Room # 510B Name: Mr. Mark Lee	Functional status/ care measures and procedures
ID Number: D4468947762 Date of birth: 12/29/1938	Independent with ADL
VS: 2 times daily, at 0700 and 1500	Independent with ambulation
0700: T _____ P _____ R _____ BP _____	Attends exercise group every morning
1500: T _____ P _____ R _____ BP _____	Continent of bowel and bladder – q4h bathroom schedule
Wt: Daily at 0700	to maintain continence
Intake _____ Output _____ BM _____	Wears eyeglasses
Bath: Shower	Coughing and deep-breathing exercises q4h
	Diet: Sodium-controlled (Independent)

FIGURE 6-3 A sample assignment sheet. NOTE: This assignment sheet is a computer printout.

REPORTING AND RECORDING

The health team communicates by reporting and recording. **Reporting** *is the oral account of care and observations.* **Recording** *(charting) is the written account of care and observations.*

Reporting and Recording Time

The 24-hour clock (military time or international time) has 4 digits (Fig. 6-4). The first 2 digits are for the hours. The last 2 digits are for the minutes: 0110 = 1:10 AM. Colons and AM and PM are not used. Box 6-4 shows how *conventional time* is written in *24-hour time*.

See *Focus on Math: Reporting and Recording Time.*

See *Focus on Communication: Reporting and Recording Time.*

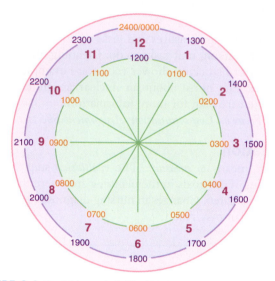

FIGURE 6-4 The 24-hour clock. The AM times are in orange. The PM times are in purple. NOTE: 12 noon is 1200; 12 midnight is 2400 or 0000.

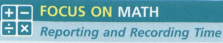

FOCUS ON MATH
Reporting and Recording Time

A *digit* is any number from 0 to 9. With *conventional time*, 3 or 4 digits are used. With *24-hour time*, 4 digits are used. To change conventional time to 24-hour time with 4 digits, do the following.

- When an AM time has 3 digits (1:00 AM to 9:59 AM), remove the colon and add a 0 as the first digit. For example:
  - Add a 0 to 1:00 AM for 0100.
  - Add a 0 to 7:30 AM for 0730.
  - Add a 0 to 9:59 AM for 0959.
- When an AM or 12:00 PM time has 4 digits (10:00 AM to 12:59 PM), simply remove the colon. For example:
  - 10:00 AM becomes 1000.
  - 11:15 AM becomes 1115.
  - 12:59 PM becomes 1259.
- For PM times, remove the colon and add 1200 to the time. For example:
  - 1:00 PM becomes 1300 by adding 100 and 1200.

    $$100 + 1200 = 1300$$

  - 4:30 PM becomes 1630 by adding 430 and 1200.

    $$430 + 1200 = 1630$$

  - 10:40 PM becomes 2240 by adding 1040 and 1200.

    $$1040 + 1200 = 2240$$

Some agencies use 0000 for midnight. Others use 2400. For example:
- 12:05 AM may be written as 0005 or 2405.
- 12:58 AM may be written as 0058 or 2458.
  Follow agency policy.

BOX 6-4	24-Hour Clock		
AM		**PM**	
Conventional Time	**24-Hour Time**	**Conventional Time**	**24-Hour Time**
12:00 MIDNIGHT	0000 or 2400	12:00 NOON	1200
1:00 AM	0100	1:00 PM	1300
2:00 AM	0200	2:00 PM	1400
3:00 AM	0300	3:00 PM	1500
4:00 AM	0400	4:00 PM	1600
5:00 AM	0500	5:00 PM	1700
6:00 AM	0600	6:00 PM	1800
7:00 AM	0700	7:00 PM	1900
8:00 AM	0800	8:00 PM	2000
9:00 AM	0900	9:00 PM	2100
10:00 AM	1000	10:00 PM	2200
11:00 AM	1100	11:00 PM	2300

Reporting

Report care and observations to the nurse.

- When there is a change from normal or a change in the person's condition. Report these changes at once.
- When the nurse asks you to do so.
- Before leaving the unit for meals, breaks, or other reasons.
- Before the end-of-shift report.
- After the end-of-shift report and before reporting off duty.

When reporting, follow the rules in Box 6-5.

End-of-Shift Report. *The nurse gives a report at the end of the shift to the on-coming shift. This is called the end-of-shift report or change-of-shift report.* The nurse reports about:

- The care given
- The care to give during other shifts
- The person's current condition
- Likely changes in the person's condition

Some agencies have the entire nursing team hear the end-of-shift report as they come on duty. In other agencies, only nurses hear the report. After the report, nursing assistants receive needed information.

See *Promoting Safety and Comfort: End-of-Shift Report.*

Recording

When recording (charting), you must communicate clearly and thoroughly. Follow the rules in Box 6-6. Figure 6-5 shows an electronic charting sample. Anyone reading your charting should know:

- What you observed
- What you did
- The person's response

  See *Focus on Communication: Recording.*

Electronic Recording.

Electronic health records (EHRs) and electronic medical records (EMRs) improve access to medical records. In many agencies, recording is done in patients' or residents' rooms, in hallways, at the nurses' station, or on portable devices (Fig. 6-6). Users log in to access the record. You will be trained to use your agency's system.

FOCUS ON COMMUNICATION

Recording

"Small," "moderate," "large," "long," and "short" mean different things to different people. Is small the size of a dime or the size of a quarter? In health care, different meanings can cause serious problems. Give accurate descriptions and measurements. If you have a question, ask the nurse to look at what you are trying to describe.

BOX 6-6	Rules for Recording

General Rules

- Follow agency policies and procedures for recording. Ask for needed training.
- Check the name and identifying information on the chart. You must record on the correct chart.
- Include the date and time for each recording. Use 24-hour time or conventional time (AM or PM) according to agency policy.
- Use only agency-approved abbreviations (p. 66).
- Use correct spelling, grammar, and punctuation.
- Do not use ditto (") marks.
- Record only what you observed and did yourself. Do not record for another person.
- Never chart a procedure, treatment, or care measure until after it is completed.
- Be accurate, concise, and factual. Do not record judgments or interpretations. For example, "The person felt sad" is a judgment. "The person was crying" is factual.
- Record in a logical manner and in sequence.
- Be descriptive. Avoid terms with more than 1 meaning.
- Use the person's exact words when possible. Use quotation marks ("...") for a direct quote.
- Chart changes from normal or changes in the person's condition. Also chart that you told the nurse (include the nurse's name), what you said, and the time you made the report.
- Do not omit information.
- Record safety measures. Examples include placing the call light within reach, assisting the person when up, or reminding a person not to get out of bed.
- Sign or save all entries as required by agency policy. For paper entries, include your name and title.

On Computer

- Log in using your username and password. Do not use another person's username.
- Check the time your entry is made. Make sure it is the right time.
- Check for accuracy. Review your entry before saving.
- Save your entries. Un-saved data will be lost.
- Follow the manufacturer's instructions to change or un-chart a mistaken entry. Most electronic systems keep a record of original entries and changes.
- Log off after charting. This prevents others from charting under your username.
- See "Electronic Devices."

On Paper

- Make sure each form has the person's name and other identifying information.
- Always use ink. Use the ink color required by the agency.
- Make sure writing is readable and neat.
- Never erase or use correction fluid (white out). Draw a line through the incorrect part. Date and initial the line. Write "mistaken entry" over it if this is agency policy. Then re-write the part. Follow agency policy for correcting errors.
- Do not skip lines. Draw a line through the blank space of a partially completed line or to the end of the page. This prevents others from recording in a space with your signature.

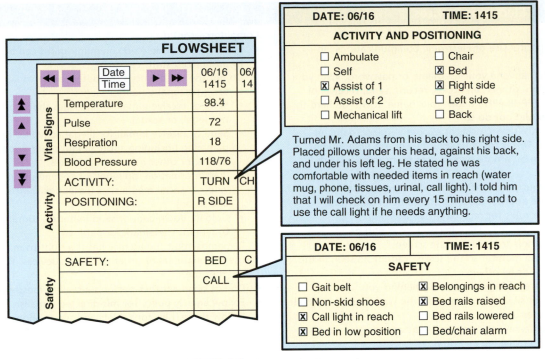

FLOWSHEET		06/16 1415	06/ 14
◀◀ ◀	Date Time ▶ ▶▶		
Vital Signs	Temperature	98.4	
	Pulse	72	
	Respiration	18	
	Blood Pressure	118/76	
Activity	ACTIVITY:	TURN	CH
	POSITIONING:	R SIDE	
Safety	SAFETY:	BED	C
		CALL	

DATE: 06/16   **TIME: 1415**

ACTIVITY AND POSITIONING

☐ Ambulate   ☐ Chair
☐ Self   ☒ Bed
☒ Assist of 1   ☒ Right side
☐ Assist of 2   ☐ Left side
☐ Mechanical lift   ☐ Back

Turned Mr. Adams from his back to his right side. Placed pillows under his head, against his back, and under his left leg. He stated he was comfortable with needed items in reach (water mug, phone, tissues, urinal, call light). I told him that I will check on him every 15 minutes and to use the call light if he needs anything.

DATE: 06/16   **TIME: 1415**

SAFETY

☐ Gait belt   ☒ Belongings in reach
☐ Non-skid shoes   ☒ Bed rails raised
☒ Call light in reach ☐ Bed rails lowered
☒ Bed in low position ☐ Bed/chair alarm

FIGURE 6-5 Electronic charting sample.

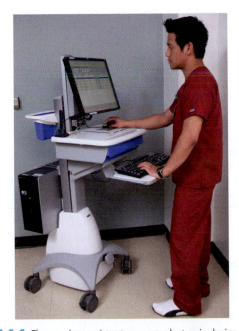

FIGURE 6-6 The nursing assistant uses an electronic device to record.

ELECTRONIC DEVICES

Computer systems collect, send, record, and store information (data). Data are retrieved when needed.

Computers and faxes are used to send messages and reports to the nursing unit. Information is sent with speed and accuracy.

Computers and other electronic devices save time. Quality care and safety are increased. Fewer errors are made in recording. Records are more complete. Staff are more efficient.

Each staff member using computers and other electronic devices has a username and password. They are used to access, send, receive, or store protected health information (PHI).

Follow agency policies when using computers and other electronic devices. You must keep PHI and electronic protected health information (ePHI; EPHI) confidential. Follow the rules in Box 6-7 (p. 62) and the ethical and legal rules about privacy, confidentiality, and defamation (Chapters 4 and 5) when using computers and other electronic devices.

BOX 6-7	Electronic Devices

Computers

- See "Wrongful Use of Electronic Communications" in Chapter 4.
- Do not tell anyone your username or password. With your information, others can access, record, send, receive, or store PHI (EPHI; ePHI) under your name. It will be hard to prove you did not do so.
- Do not write down, post, or expose your username or password. This is for your security. For example, do not write them on a note pad or post them at your work station.
- Change your password often. Follow agency policy.
- Do not use another person's username or password.
- Follow the rules for recording (see Box 6-6).
- Enter data carefully. Double-check your entries.
- Prevent others from seeing the screen.
  - Place the monitor so the screen cannot be seen in the hallway or by others.
  - Be aware of anyone standing behind you.
  - Stand or sit with your back to the wall if using a mobile computer unit.
  - Do not leave the computer unattended.
- Log off after making an entry.
- Do not leave printouts where others can read or pick them up.
- Shred or destroy computer printouts or worksheets. Place such documents in a wastebasket marked CONFIDENTIAL INFORMATION for shredding. Follow agency policy.
- Send e-mail and messages only to those needing the information.
- Do not e-mail information or messages that require immediate reporting. Give the report in person. The person may not read the e-mail in a timely manner.
- Do not use e-mail or messages to report confidential information. This includes addresses, phone numbers, and Social Security numbers. The computer system may not be secure.
- Remember that any communication can be read or heard by someone other than the intended person.

Computers—cont'd

- Remember that deleted communications can be retrieved by authorized staff.
- Do not use the agency's computer for personal use. Do not:
  - Send personal e-mail messages.
  - Send or receive e-mail or messages that are offensive, not legal, or sexual.
  - Send or receive e-mail for illegal activities, jokes, politics, gambling (including football and other pools), chain letters, or other non-work activities.
  - Post information, opinions, or comments on websites or video or social media sites (Facebook, Twitter, YouTube, and so on).
  - Upload, download, or send materials containing a copyright, trademark, or patent.
- Remember that the agency has the right to monitor your use of computers or other electronic devices. This includes Internet use.
- Do not open another person's e-mail or messages.
- Follow agency policy for mis-directed e-mails.
- Follow these rules for tablets and smart phones.

Faxes

- See "Wrongful Use of Electronic Communications" in Chapter 4.
- Use the agency's "cover sheet." The sheet has instructions about:
  - The confidentiality of PHI (EPHI; ePHI)
  - The receiver's responsibilities about PHI (EPHI; ePHI)
  - The receiver's responsibilities for a fax received in error (mis-directed fax)
- Complete the "cover sheet" according to agency policy. The following are common.
  - Name of the person to receive the fax
  - Receiver's fax number
  - Date
  - Number of pages being faxed
  - Department name
  - Name and phone number of the person sending the fax
- Follow agency policy for a mis-directed fax.
- Do not leave sent or received faxes unattended in the fax machine or lying around.

PHONE COMMUNICATIONS

You will answer phones at the nurses' station or in the person's room. You need good communication skills. The caller cannot see you. But you give much information by your tone of voice, how clearly you speak, and your attitude. Act as if speaking face-to-face. Be professional and courteous. Also practice good work ethics. Follow the agency's policy and the guidelines in Box 6-8.

MEDICAL TERMS AND ABBREVIATIONS

Medical terms and abbreviations are used in health care. Like all words, medical terms are made up of parts of words or *word elements*—prefixes, roots, and suffixes (Box 6-9). Most are from Greek or Latin. The word elements are combined to form medical terms.

Prefixes, Roots, and Suffixes

A *prefix* is a word element at the beginning of a word. It changes the meaning of the word. Prefixes are used with other word elements. Prefixes are never used alone.

The *root* is the word element that contains the basic meaning of the word. It is combined with another root, prefixes, or suffixes. A vowel (an *o* or an *i*) may be added when 2 roots are combined or when a suffix is added to a root. The vowel makes the word easier to pronounce.

A *suffix* is a word element at the end of a word. It changes the meaning of the word. Suffixes are not used alone.

BOX 6-8	Answering Phones

- Answer the call after the first ring if possible. Be sure to answer by the fourth ring.
- Do not answer in a rushed or hasty manner.
- Give a courteous greeting. Identify the agency or nursing unit and give your name and title. For example: "Good morning, 3 center. Mark Wills, nursing assistant." Follow agency policy for answering phones in patient or resident rooms.
- Write this information to take a message.
  - The caller's name and phone number (include the area code and extension number)
  - The date and time
  - Who the message is for
  - The message
- Repeat the message and phone number back to the caller.
- Ask the caller to "Please hold" if necessary. First find out who is calling and the caller's number. Then ask if the caller can hold. Do not put callers with an emergency on hold.

- Do not lay the phone down or cover the receiver with your hand when not speaking to the caller. The caller may over-hear confidential conversations.
- Return to a caller on hold within 30 seconds. Ask if the caller can wait longer or if the call can be returned.
- Do not give confidential information to any caller. Patient, resident, and employee information is confidential. Refer such calls to the nurse.
- Transfer the call if appropriate.
  - Tell the caller that you are going to transfer the call.
  - Give the name of the department or the name of the person who should answer the phone if appropriate.
  - Get the caller's name and number in case the call gets disconnected.
  - Give the caller the phone number to call in case the call gets disconnected or the line is busy.
- End the conversation politely. Thank the person for calling and say good-bye.
- Give the message to the appropriate person.

BOX 6-9	Medical Terminology

Prefix	Meaning
a-, an-	without, not, lack of
ab-	away from
ad-	to, toward, near
ante-	before, forward, in front of
anti-	against
auto-	self
bi-	double, two (2), twice
brady-	slow
circum-	around
contra-	against, opposite
cyan-	blue
de-	down, from
dia-	across, through, apart
dis-	apart, free from
dys-	bad, difficult, abnormal, painful
ecto-	outer, outside
en-	in, into, within
endo-	inner, inside
epi-	over, on, upon
erythro-	red
eu-	normal, good, well, healthy
ex-	out, out of, from, away from
hemi-	half
hyper-	excessive, too much, high
hypo-	under, decreased, less than normal
in-	in, into, within, not
inter-	between
intra-	within
intro-	into, within
leuko-	white
macro-	large
mal-	bad, illness, disease
meg-	large
micro-	small
mono-	one (1), single
neo-	new

Prefix	Meaning
non-	not
olig-	small, scant
para-	beside, beyond, after
per-	by, through
peri-	around
poly-	many, much
post-	after, behind
pre-	before, in front of, prior to
pro-	before, in front of
re-	again, backward
retro-	backward, behind
semi-	half
sub-	under, beneath
super-	above, over, excess
supra-	above, over
tachy-	fast, rapid
trans-	across
uni-	one (1)

Root (Combining Vowel)	Meaning
abdomin (o)	abdomen
aden (o)	gland
adren (o)	adrenal gland
angi (o)	vessel
arteri (o)	artery
arthr (o)	joint
bronch (o)	bronchus, bronchi
card, cardi (o)	heart
cephal (o)	head
chole, chol (o)	bile
chondr (o)	cartilage
colo	colon, large intestine
cost (o)	rib
crani (o)	skull
cyst (o)	bladder, cyst
cyt (o)	cell

Continued

BOX 6-9	Medical Terminology—cont'd

Root (Combining Vowel)	Meaning
dent (o)	tooth
derma	skin
duoden (o)	duodenum
electr (o)	electricity
encephal (o)	brain
enter (o)	intestines
fibr (o)	fiber, fibrous
gastr (o)	stomach
gloss (o)	tongue
gluc (o)	sweetness, glucose
glyc (o)	sugar
gyn, gyne, gyneco	woman
hem, hema, hemo, hemat (o)	blood
hepat (o)	liver
hydr (o)	water
hyster (o)	uterus
ile (o), ili (o)	ileum
laparo	abdomen, loin, flank
laryng (o)	larynx
lith (o)	stone
mamm (o)	breast, mammary gland
mast (o)	mammary gland, breast
meno	menstruation
my (o)	muscle
myel (o)	spinal cord, bone marrow
necro	death
nephr (o)	kidney
neur (o)	nerve
ocul (o)	eye
oophor (o)	ovary
ophthalm (o)	eye
orth (o)	straight, normal, correct
oste (o)	bone
ot (o)	ear
ped (o)	child, foot
pharyng (o)	pharynx
phleb (o)	vein
pneum (o)	lung, air, gas
proct (o)	rectum
psych (o)	mind
pulmo	lung
py (o)	pus
rect (o)	rectum
rhin (o)	nose
salping (o)	eustachian tube, fallopian tube
splen (o)	spleen
sten (o)	narrow, constriction
stern (o)	sternum
stomat (o)	mouth
therm (o)	heat
thoraco	chest
thromb (o)	clot, thrombus
thyr (o)	thyroid

Root (Combining Vowel)	Meaning
toxic (o)	poison, poisonous
toxo	poison
trache (o)	trachea
urethr (o)	urethra
urin (o)	urine
uro	urine, urinary tract, urination
uter (o)	uterus
vas (o)	blood vessel, vas deferens
ven (o)	vein
vertebr (o)	spine, vertebrae

Suffix	Meaning
-algia	pain
-asis	condition, usually abnormal
-cele	hernia, herniation, pouching
-centesis	puncture and aspiration of
-cyte	cell
-ectasis	dilation, stretching
-ectomy	excision, removal of
-emia	blood condition
-genesis	development, production, creation
-genic	producing, causing
-gram	record
-graph	a diagram, a recording instrument
-graphy	making a recording
-iasis	condition of
-ism	a condition
-itis	inflammation
-logy	the study of
-lysis	destruction of, decomposition
-megaly	enlargement
-meter	measuring instrument
-oma	tumor
-osis	condition
-pathy	disease
-penia	lack, deficiency
-phagia	to eat or consume, swallowing
-phasia	speaking
-phobia	an exaggerated fear
-plasty	surgical repair or re-shaping
-plegia	paralysis
-pnea	breathing, respiration
-ptosis	falling, sagging, dropping down
-rrhage, rrhagia	excessive flow
-rrhaphy	stitching, suturing
-rrhea	flow, discharge
-scope	examination instrument
-scopy	examination using a scope
-stasis	maintenance, maintaining a constant level
-stomy, -ostomy	creation of an opening
-tomy, -otomy	incision, cutting into
-uria	urine

TABLE 6-1	Defining Medical Terms	
Term	**Word Parts**	**Meaning**
Dyspnea	*dys-* (difficult, painful) + *-pnea* (breathing) [prefix] [suffix]	Difficult or painful breathing
Electrocardiogram	*electr (o)* (electricity) + *cardi (o)* (heart) + *-gram* (record) [root] [root] [suffix]	Record of the electricity in the heart
Endocarditis	*endo-* (inner) + *card* (heart) + *-itis* (inflammation) [prefix] [root] [suffix]	Inflammation of the inner part of the heart
Mastectomy	*mast* (breast) + *-ectomy* (excision or removal) [root] [suffix]	Removal of a breast
Nephritis	*nephr* (kidney) + *-itis* (inflammation) [root] [suffix]	Inflammation of the kidney
Oliguria	*olig-* (scant, small amount) + *-uria* (urine) [prefix] [suffix]	A small amount of urine

Defining Medical Terms. Medical terms are formed by combining word elements. Remember, prefixes are at the beginning. Suffixes are at the end. A root can be combined with prefixes, roots, and suffixes. Some words only have a prefix and suffix.

To define a term, separate the word into its elements (Table 6-1). To read the meaning:

1 Begin with the suffix. Read the meaning of the suffix.
2 Then go to the beginning of the word. Read the meaning of each word part up to the suffix.

For terms with only a prefix and suffix, read the meaning of the prefix. Then read the meaning of the suffix.

Directional Terms

Certain terms describe the position of 1 body part in relation to another. These terms give the direction of the body part when a person is standing and facing forward (Fig. 6-7).

- *Anterior (ventral)*—at or toward the front of the body or body part
- *Posterior (dorsal)*—at or toward the back of the body or body part
- *Proximal*—the part nearest to the center or to the point of attachment
- *Distal*—the part farthest from the center or from the point of attachment
- *Lateral*—away from the mid-line; at the side of the body or body part
- *Medial*—at or near the middle or mid-line of the body or body part

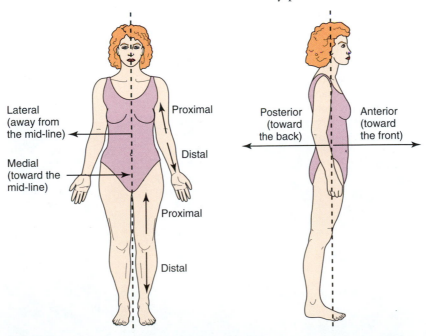

FIGURE 6-7 Directional terms describe the position of 1 body part in relation to another.

Abbreviations

Abbreviations are shortened forms of words or phrases. They save time and space when recording. Each agency has a list of allowed abbreviations. Obtain the list when you are hired. Use only those on the list. If not sure about an abbreviation, write the term out in full. This promotes clear communication.

Common abbreviations are on the inside of the back cover for easy use.

FOCUS ON P R I D E

The Person, Family, and Yourself

P **ersonal and Professional Responsibility**

You are responsible for what you report and record. It must be accurate. False or incomplete information can harm the person. If your agency allows you to chart:

- Chart what you did. If not charted, it is assumed that the task was not done. There is no proof that you completed a task.
- Never falsify charting. Never chart that something was done when it was not.
- Chart only after completing a task. If events change, your charting is wrong.
- Ask the nurse if you have questions about what or how to chart.

R **ights and Respect**

Employee satisfaction surveys allow you to share thoughts about your job with supervisors and managers. Comments are used to make changes and improve care and health team communication. When filling out a survey:

- Be honest. Positive and negative comments are important.
- Take the survey seriously. Do not rush. Answer questions completely.
- Complete and return the form in a timely manner.
  You have the right to voice your true thoughts on a survey. Take pride in your ideas. Your thoughts matter.

I **ndependence and Social Interaction**

Health team communications are not limited to reporting and recording. You interact in the nurses' station, patient and resident rooms, hallways, break room, cafeteria, parking lot, and so on. Treat co-workers with kindness and respect. Have a good attitude. Be someone others enjoy working with!

D **elegation and Teamwork**

You are responsible for your speech, actions, and charting. This is called being *accountable*. For example, you must complete a delegated task and report or record its completion. If the task was not done, you must tell the nurse why.

Do not be offended when asked if you completed a task or charted. This is part of being accountable. The nurse must know what was done and what was not done. To show you are accountable:

- Complete tasks in a timely manner
- Record accurately
- Report and record when you complete a task
- Tell the nurse if a task was not done and why

E **thics and Laws**

Assignment sheets have confidential information. Always keep your sheets with you. Do not leave them lying around for others to find. This violates the *Health Insurance Portability and Accountability Act of 1996* (Chapter 4). Before leaving work, place your assignment sheets in a wastebasket marked CONFIDENTIAL INFORMATION for shredding. Take pride in protecting the privacy and security of protected health information.

FOCUS ON PRIDE: *Application*

Explain why accurate and timely reporting and recording are important. What problems may occur from incorrect or delayed reporting or recording?

REVIEW QUESTIONS

Circle **T** *if the statement is TRUE or* **F** *if it is FALSE.*

1 **T F** You help with a person's care. Recording on the person's medical record violates the right to privacy.

2 **T F** Medical records can be used to prove the care given.

3 **T F** You can access all medical records in the agency.

4 **T F** You can take your assignment sheet home.

5 **T F** You can give information about the person over the phone.

Circle the BEST answer.

6 To communicate well, you should
   a Use terms with many meanings
   b Give long descriptions
   c Use unfamiliar terms
   d Give facts and be specific

7 A person is discharged from the agency. The medical record is
   a Destroyed
   b Sent home with the family
   c Permanent
   d No longer private

8 What happens during assessment?
   a Goals are set.
   b Information is collected.
   c Nursing measures are carried out.
   d Progress is evaluated.

9 Which is a symptom?
   a Redness
   b Vomiting
   c Pain
   d Pulse rate of 78

10 Which should you report at once?
   a The person complains of sudden, severe pain.
   b The person had a bowel movement.
   c The person does not like the food served.
   d The person complains of stiff, painful joints.

11 The care plan is
   a Written by the doctor
   b The measures to help the person
   c The same for all persons
   d Not changed after it is developed

12 To communicate delegated tasks to you, the nurse uses
   a The care plan
   b The Minimum Data Set
   c An assignment sheet
   d Care conferences

13 Which statement about recording is *correct?*
   a Avoid using the person's exact words.
   b Record only what you did and observed.
   c Use correction fluid for a mistaken entry.
   d Chart a procedure before completing it.

14 In the evening, the clock shows 9:26. In 24-hour clock time this is
   a 9:26 PM
   b 1926
   c 0926
   d 2126

15 In the morning, the clock shows 7:45. In 24-hour clock time this is
   a 0745
   b 1945
   c 745
   d 7:45 AM

16 You have access to the agency's computer. Which is *true?*
   a You should log off after making an entry.
   b E-mail is used for reports the nurse needs at once.
   c You can use another person's username.
   d You can use the computer for your personal needs.

17 A phone rings at the nurses' station. Which greeting is *best?*
   a "Good morning. This is Tammy."
   b "North hall."
   c "Good morning, North hall. Tammy Brown, nursing assistant, speaking."
   d "Hello."

18 A suffix is
   a Placed at the beginning of a word
   b Placed after a root
   c A shortened form of a word or phrase
   d The main meaning of the word

19 Which word means a blood condition involving too much sugar?
   a Hepatitis (hepat-itis)
   b Tachycardia (tachy-cardia)
   c Hyperglycemia (hyper-glyc-emia)
   d Aphasia (a-phasia)

20 Which word means an excessive flow of blood?
   a Hemiplegia (hemi-plegia)
   b Cyanosis (cyan-osis)
   c Laparoscopy (laparo-scopy)
   d Hemorrhage (hemo-rrhage)

21 Which term relates to the side of the body?
   a Anterior
   b Lateral
   c Posterior
   d Proximal

22 You must complete a task *stat*. "Stat" means
   a At once, immediately
   b As desired
   c Without moving the person
   d When necessary, as needed

Answers to Chapter 6 questions are on p. 551.

FOCUS ON PRACTICE

Problem Solving

A resident's daughter says: "No one does Mom's hair the way she likes it." How will you respond?

Explain your role in planning and implementing care. How are the person's needs and preferences communicated to staff?

CHAPTER 7

Understanding the Person

OBJECTIVES

- Define the key terms in this chapter.
- Identify the parts that make up the whole person.
- Explain how to properly address the person.
- Explain Abraham Maslow's theory of basic needs.
- Explain how culture and religion influence health and illness.
- Identify the elements needed for good communication.
- Describe how to use verbal and nonverbal communication.
- Explain the methods and barriers to good communication.
- Explain how to communicate with persons who have special needs.
- Explain why family and visitors are important to the person.
- Identify courtesies given to the person, family, and friends.
- Explain how to communicate with persons who have behavior problems.
- Explain how to promote PRIDE in the person, the family, and yourself.

KEY TERMS

body language Messages sent through facial expressions, gestures, posture, hand and body movements, gait, eye contact, and appearance

comatose Being unable to respond to stimuli

culture The characteristics of a group of people—language, values, beliefs, habits, likes, dislikes, and customs—passed from 1 generation to the next

disability Any lost, absent, or impaired physical or mental function

holism A concept that considers the whole person; the whole person has physical, social, psychological, and spiritual parts that are woven together and cannot be separated

need Something necessary or desired for maintaining life and mental well-being

nonverbal communication Communication that does not use words

religion Spiritual beliefs, needs, and practices

verbal communication Communication that uses written or spoken words

The patient or resident is the most important person in the agency. Each person has value. Each has needs, fears, and rights. Each has suffered losses—loss of home, family, friends, and body functions.

CARING FOR THE PERSON

Holism means *whole*. *Holism is a concept that considers the whole person. The whole person has physical, social, psychological, and spiritual parts. These parts are woven together and cannot be separated* (Fig. 7-1).

Each part relates to and depends on the others. As a social being, a person speaks and communicates with others. Physically, the brain, mouth, tongue, lips, and throat structures must function for speech. Communication is also psychological. It involves thinking and reasoning.

To consider only the physical part is to ignore the person's ability to think, make decisions, and interact with others. It also ignores the person's experiences, life-style, culture, religion, joys, sorrows, and needs.

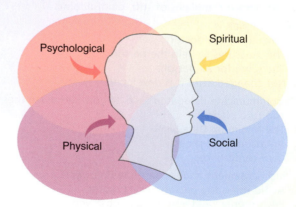

FIGURE 7-1 A person is a physical, psychological, social, and spiritual being. The parts over-lap and cannot be separated.

Addressing the Person

You must know and respect the whole person for effective, quality care. Too often a person is referred to as a room number. For example: "12A needs the bedpan" rather than "Mrs. Olson in 12A needs the bedpan." This strips the person of his or her identity.

To address patients and residents with dignity and respect:

- Greet the person by title—Mrs. Jones, Mr. Wills, Miss Parker, Ms. Norris, or Dr. Gonzalez. Then ask what name the person prefers.
- Do not call them by their first names or any other name unless they ask you to.
- Do not call them Grandma, Papa, Sweetheart, Honey, or other names.

BASIC NEEDS

A ***need** is something necessary or desired for maintaining life and mental well-being.* According to psychologist Abraham Maslow, basic needs must be met for a person to survive and function. The needs are arranged in order of importance (Fig. 7-2). Lower-level needs must be met before higher-level needs. Basic needs, from the lowest level to the highest level, are:

- *Physical needs.* Oxygen, food, water, elimination, rest, and shelter are needed to live and survive. A person dies within minutes without oxygen. Without food or water, weakness and illness occur within a few hours. The kidneys and intestines must function. If not, poisonous wastes build up in the blood and can cause death. Without enough rest and sleep, a person becomes very tired. Without shelter, the person is exposed to extremes of heat and cold.
- *Safety and security needs.* The person needs to feel safe from harm, danger, and fear. Many people are afraid of health care. Some care involves strange equipment, pain, or discomfort. People feel safe and more secure if they know what will happen. For every task, even a simple bath, the person should know:
  - Why it is needed
  - Who will do it
  - How it will be done
  - What sensations or feelings to expect

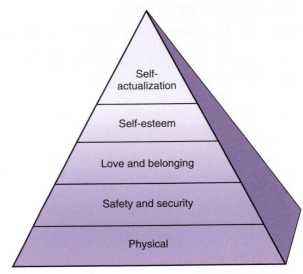

FIGURE 7-2 Basic needs for life as described by Maslow. (Redrawn from Maslow AH, Frager RD (Editor), Fadiman J (Editor): *Motivation and personality,* ed 3. © 1987. Reprinted with permission of Ann Kaplan.)

- *Love and belonging needs.* These needs relate to love, closeness, affection, and meaningful relationships with others. Some people become weaker or die from the lack of love and belonging. This is seen in children and in older persons who have out-lived family and friends.
- *Self-esteem needs.* Self-esteem means *to think well of oneself and to see oneself as useful and having value.* People often lack self-esteem when ill, injured, older, or disabled.
- *The need for self-actualization.* Self-actualization means *experiencing one's potential.* It involves learning, understanding, and creating to the limit of a person's ability. This is the highest need. Rarely, if ever, is it totally met. Most people constantly try to learn and understand more. This need can be postponed and life will continue.

CULTURE AND RELIGION

Culture is the characteristics of a group of people—language, values, beliefs, habits, likes, dislikes, and customs. They are passed from 1 generation to the next. The person's culture influences health beliefs and practices. Culture also affects thinking and behavior during illness.

People come from many cultures, races, and nationalities. Their family practices and food choices may differ from yours. So might their hygiene habits and clothing styles. Some speak a foreign language. Some cultures have beliefs about what causes and cures illness. They may perform rituals to rid the body of disease. Many cultures have health beliefs and rituals about dying and death (Chapter 37). Culture also is a factor in communication.

See *Caring About Culture: Health Care Beliefs and Sick Care Practices.*

Religion relates to spiritual beliefs, needs, and practices. Religions may have beliefs about daily living, behaviors, relationships with others, diet, healing, days of worship, birth and birth control, drugs, and death.

Many people find comfort and strength from religion during illness. They may want to pray and observe religious practices. Hospitals and nursing centers offer religious services and have areas for prayer. Assist the person to attend services as needed.

A person may not follow all the beliefs and practices of his or her culture or religion. Some people do not practice a religion. Each person is unique. Do not judge the person by your standards. And do not force your ideas on the person.

See *Focus on Communication: Culture and Religion.*

CARING ABOUT CULTURE

Health Care Beliefs and Sick Care Practices

Health Care Beliefs
Some *Mexican Americans* believe that illness is caused by prolonged exposure to hot or cold. If hot causes illness, cold is used for cure. Likewise, hot is used for illnesses caused by cold. Hot conditions include fever, infection, rashes, sore throat, diarrhea, and constipation. Cold conditions include cancer, joint pain, earache, and stomach cramps.

The hot-cold balance is also a belief of some *Vietnamese Americans*. Illnesses, food, drugs, and herbs are hot or cold. Hot is given to balance cold illnesses. Cold is given for hot illnesses.

Sick Care Practices
Folk practices are common among some *Vietnamese Americans*. They include *cao gio* ("rub wind")—rubbing the skin with a coin to treat the common cold. Skin pinching (*bat gio*—"catch wind") is for headaches and sore throats. Herbs, oils, and soups are used for many signs and symptoms.

Some *Russian Americans* practice folk medicine. Herbs are taken through drinks or enemas. For headaches, an ointment is placed behind the ears and temples and at the back of the neck. Treatment for back pain involves placing a dough of dark rye flour and honey on the spine.

Some *Mexican Americans* use folk healers. A *yerbero* uses herbs and spices to prevent or cure disease. A *curandero* (*curandera* if female) deals with serious physical and mental illnesses. Witches use magic. A *brujos* is a male witch. A *brujas* is a female witch.

(NOTE: Each person is unique. A person may not follow all of the beliefs and practices of his or her culture. Follow the care plan.)

Modified from Giger JN: *Transcultural nursing: assessment and intervention*, ed 6, St Louis, 2013, Mosby.

FOCUS ON COMMUNICATION

Culture and Religion

The person's care plan communicates practices to include in his or her care. Check the care plan for the person's preferences. You can also ask: "Do you have any cultural or religious practices that should be part of your care?"

FOCUS ON OLDER PERSONS

Communicating With the Person

Communicating with persons who have dementia is often hard. The Alzheimer's Disease Education and Referral Center (ADEAR) recommends the following. Also see Chapter 35.
- Gain the person's attention before speaking. Say the person's name. Make eye contact.
- Choose simple words and short sentences.
- Use a gentle, calm voice.
- Do not talk to the person as you would a baby.
- Do not talk about the person as if he or she is not there.
- Keep distractions and noise to a minimum.
- Help the person focus on what you are saying.
- Give the person time to respond. Do not interrupt.
- Try to provide the word the person is struggling to find.
- State questions and instructions in a positive way.

COMMUNICATING WITH THE PERSON

You communicate with the person. You give information to the person. The person gives information to you. For effective communication between you and the person, follow the rules in Box 7-1.

See *Focus on Older Persons: Communicating With the Person.*

BOX 7-1	Communicating With the Person

- Follow the rules of communication (Chapter 6).
  - Use words that have the same meaning for you and the person.
  - Avoid medical terms and words not familiar to the person.
  - Communicate in a logical and orderly manner. Do not wander in thought.
  - Give facts and be specific.
  - Be brief and concise.
- Understand and respect the patient or resident as a person.
- View the person as a physical, psychological, social, and spiritual human being.
- Appreciate the person's problems and frustrations.
- Respect the person's rights, religion, and culture.
- Give the person time to understand the information that you give.
- Repeat information as often as needed. Repeat what you said. Use the exact same words. Do not give the person a new message to process. If the person does not seem to understand after repeating, re-phrase the message. This is very important for persons with hearing problems.
- Ask questions to see if the person understood you.
- Be patient. People with memory problems may ask the same question many times. Do not say that you are repeating information.
- Include the person in conversations when others are present. This includes when a co-worker is assisting with care.

Verbal Communication

Verbal communication uses written or spoken words. You talk to the person. You share information and find out how the person feels. Most verbal communication involves the spoken word. Follow these rules.

- Face the person. Look directly at the person.
- Position yourself at the person's eye level. Sit or squat by the person as needed.
- Control the loudness and tone of your voice.
- Speak clearly, slowly, and distinctly.
- Do not use slang or vulgar words.
- Repeat information as needed.
- Ask 1 question at a time. Wait for an answer.
- Do not shout, whisper, or mumble.
- Be kind, courteous, and friendly.

You use the written word when the person cannot speak or hear but can read. The nurse and care plan tell you how to communicate with the person. The devices shown in Figure 7-3 (p. 72) are often used. The person may have poor vision. When writing messages:

- Keep them simple and brief.
- Use a black felt pen on white paper.
- Print in large letters.
- Use black and a large font (print size) if using a computer or other electronic device.

Some persons cannot speak or read. Ask questions that have "yes" or "no" answers. The person can nod, blink, or use other gestures for "yes" and "no." Follow the care plan. Persons who are deaf may use sign language. See Chapter 32.

Nonverbal Communication

Nonverbal communication does not use words. Gestures, facial expressions, posture, body movements, touch, and smell are used. Nonverbal messages more accurately reflect a person's feelings than words do. They are usually involuntary and hard to control. A person may say one thing but act another way. Watch the person's eyes, hand movements, gestures, posture, and other actions. They may tell you more than words.

Touch. Touch is an important form of nonverbal communication. It conveys comfort, caring, love, affection, interest, trust, concern, and reassurance. Touch means different things to different people. The meaning depends on age, gender (male or female), experiences, and culture. (See *Caring About Culture: Touch Practices,* p. 72.)

Some people do not like being touched. However, stroking or holding a hand can comfort a person. Touch should be gentle—not hurried, rough, or sexual. To use touch, follow the person's care plan. Remember to maintain professional boundaries.

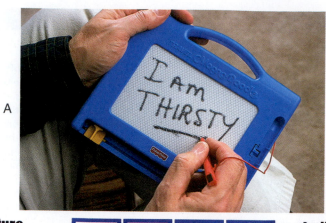

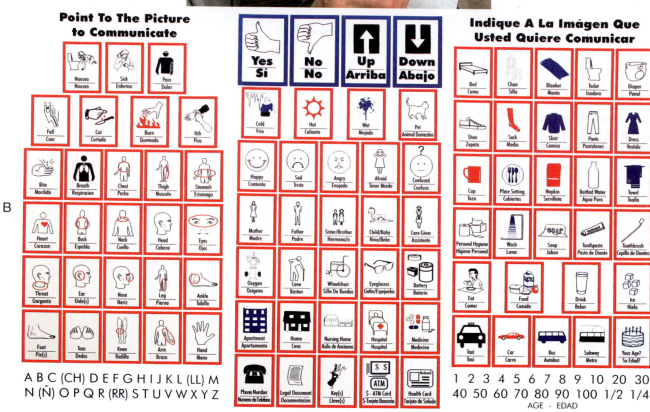

FIGURE 7-3 Communication aids. **A,** Magic Slate. **B,** Picture board in English and Spanish.

CARING ABOUT CULTURE

Touch Practices

Touch practices vary among cultural groups. Touch is a friendly gesture in the *Philippine* culture. Touch is often used in *Mexico.* Some people believe that using touch while complimenting a person is important. It is thought to neutralize the power of the evil eye *(mal de ojo).*

Persons from the *United Kingdom* tend to reserve touch for persons they know well. Within limits, touch is acceptable in *Poland.* Its use depends on age, gender, and relationship.

In *India,* men shake hands with other men but not with women. For women, they place their palms together and bow slightly. As a sign of respect or to seek a blessing, people touch the feet of older adults.

In *Vietnam,* a person's head is touched by others. It is considered the center of the soul. Men do not touch women they do not know. Men commonly shake hands with men.

People from *China* do not like being touched by strangers. A nod or slight bow is given during introductions. Health care workers of the same gender are preferred.

In *Ireland,* a firm handshake is preferred. Only family and close friends are embraced.

(NOTE: Each person is unique. A person may not follow all of the beliefs and practices of his or her culture. Follow the care plan.)

Modified from D'Avanzo CE: *Pocket guide to cultural health assessment,* ed 4, St Louis, 2008, Mosby.

Body Language. People send messages through their *body language.*

- *Facial expressions* (See *Caring About Culture: Facial Expressions.*)
- *Gestures*
- *Posture*
- *Hand and body movements*
- *Gait*
- *Eye contact*
- *Appearance* (dress, hygiene, jewelry, perfume, cosmetics, body art and piercings, and so on)

Many messages are sent through body language. Slumped posture may mean the person is not happy or not feeling well. A person may deny pain. Yet he or she protects the affected body part by standing, lying, or sitting in a certain way.

Your actions, movements, and facial expressions send messages. So do how you stand, sit, walk, and look at the person. Your body language should show interest, caring, respect, and enthusiasm.

Often you will need to control your body language. Control reactions to odors from body fluids, secretions, excretions, or the person's body. The person cannot control some odors. Embarrassment increases if you react to odors.

Communication Methods

Certain methods help you communicate with others. They result in better relationships. More information is gained for the nursing process.

Listening. Listening means to focus on verbal and nonverbal communication. You use sight, hearing, touch, and smell. You focus on what the person is saying. You observe nonverbal clues. They can support or not support what the person says. For example, a person says: "I want to stay here so my family won't have to care for me." You see tears and the person looks away from you. The person's verbal says *happy*; nonverbal shows *sadness.*

Listening requires that you care and have interest. Follow these guidelines.

- Face the person.
- Have good eye contact with the person. See *Caring About Culture: Eye Contact Practices.*
- Lean toward the person (Fig. 7-4, p. 74). Do not sit back with your arms crossed.
- Respond to the person. Nod your head. Say: "uh huh," "mmm," and "I see." Repeat what the person says. Ask questions.
- Avoid the communication barriers (p. 74).

CARING ABOUT CULTURE

Facial Expressions

Through facial expressions, *Americans* may communicate:

- *Coldness*—there is a constant stare. Face muscles do not move.
- *Fear*—eyes are wide open. Eyebrows are raised. The mouth is tense with the lips drawn back.
- *Anger*—eyes are fixed in a hard stare. Upper lids are lowered. Eyebrows are drawn down. Lips are slightly compressed.
- *Tiredness*—eyes are rolled upward.
- *Disapproval*—eyes are rolled upward.
- *Disgust*—narrowed eyes. The upper lip is curled. There are nose movements.
- *Embarrassment*—eyes are turned away or down. The face is flushed. The person pretends to smile. He or she rubs the eyes, nose, or face. He or she twitches the hair, beard, or mustache.
- *Surprise*—direct gaze with raised eyebrows.

Italian, Jewish, African-American, and *Hispanic* persons are known to smile readily. They may use many facial expressions and gestures for happiness, pain, or displeasure. *Irish, English,* and *Northern European* persons tend to have less facial expression.

In some cultures, facial expressions mean the opposite of what the person feels. For example, *Asians* may conceal negative emotions with a smile.

(NOTE: Each person is unique. A person may not follow all of the beliefs and practices of his or her culture. Follow the care plan.)

Modified from Giger JN: *Transcultural nursing: assessment and intervention,* ed 6, St Louis, 2013, Mosby.

CARING ABOUT CULTURE

Eye Contact Practices

In the *American* culture, eye contact usually signals a good self-concept. It also shows openness, interest in others, attention, honesty, and warmth. Lack of eye contact can mean:

- Shyness
- Lack of interest
- Humility
- Guilt
- Embarrassment
- Low self-esteem
- Rudeness
- Dishonesty

For some *Asian* and *American Indian* cultures, eye contact is impolite. It is an invasion of privacy. In certain *Indian* cultures, eye contact is avoided with persons of higher or lower socio-economic class.

Long, direct eye contact may be considered rude in *Mexico.* In some parts of *Vietnam,* it is not respectful to look at another person while talking. Blinking means that a message is received. In the *United Kingdom,* looking directly at a speaker usually means the listener is paying attention.

(NOTE: Each person is unique. A person may not follow all of the beliefs and practices of his or her culture. Follow the care plan.)

Modified from Giger JN: *Transcultural nursing: assessment and intervention,* ed 6, St Louis, 2013, Mosby. Modified from D'Avanzo CE: *Pocket guide to cultural health assessment,* ed 4, St Louis, 2008, Mosby.

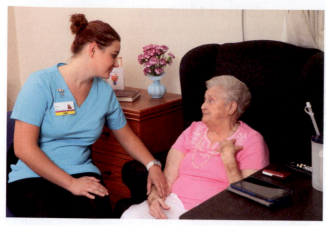

FIGURE 7-4 Listen by facing the person. Have good eye contact. Lean toward the person.

Paraphrasing. *Paraphrasing* is re-stating the person's message in your own words. You use fewer words than the person did. The person usually responds to your statement. For example:

Mrs. Hayes: My son was crying after talking to the doctor. I don't know what they said.
You: Your son was crying?
Mrs. Hayes: They must have talked about my tumor.

Direct Questions. Direct questions focus on certain information. You ask what you need to know. Some direct questions have "yes" or "no" answers. Others require more information. For example:

You: Mr. Walker do you want to shower this morning?
Mr. Walker: Yes.
You: Mr. Walker, when would you like to do that?
Mr. Walker: Could we start in 15 minutes? I want to call my son first.
You: Yes, we can start in 15 minutes. Did you have a bowel movement today?
Mr. Walker: No.
You: You said you didn't eat much breakfast. What did you eat?
Mr. Walker: I had toast and coffee. I didn't feel like eating.

Open-Ended Questions. Open-ended questions lead or invite the person to share thoughts, feelings, or ideas. The person controls the topic and the information given. Answers require more than a "yes" or "no." For example:
- "What do you like about living with your son?"
- "What was your husband like?"
- "What do you like about being retired?"

Clarifying. Clarifying lets you make sure that you understand the message. You can ask the person to repeat the message, say you do not understand, or re-state the message. For example:
- "Could you say that again?"
- "I'm sorry. I don't understand what you mean."
- "Are you saying that you want to go home?"

Focusing. Focusing is dealing with a certain topic. It is useful when a person rambles or wanders in thought. For example, a person talks at length about places to eat. You need to know why the person did not eat much breakfast. To focus on breakfast you say: "Let's talk about breakfast. You said you didn't feel like eating."

Silence. Silence is a powerful way to communicate. Sometimes you do not need to say anything. This is true during sad times. Just being there shows you care. At other times, silence gives time to think, organize thoughts, or choose words. It also helps when the person is upset and needs to gain control. Silence on your part shows caring and respect for the person's situation and feelings.

Pauses or long silences may seem uncomfortable. You do not need to talk when the person is silent. The person may need silence.

See *Caring About Culture: The Meaning of Silence.*

CARING ABOUT CULTURE

The Meaning of Silence

In some *English* and *Arabic* cultures, silence is used for privacy. Among *Russian, French,* and *Spanish* cultures, silence may mean agreement between parties. In some *Asian* cultures, silence is a sign of respect, particularly to an older person.

(NOTE: *Each person is unique. A person may not follow all of the beliefs and practices of his or her culture. Follow the care plan.*)

Modified from Giger JN: *Transcultural nursing: assessment and intervention,* ed 6, St Louis, 2013, Mosby.

Communication Barriers

Communication barriers prevent the sending and receiving of messages. Communication fails.
- *Unfamiliar language.* You and the person must use and understand the same language. If not, messages are not accurately interpreted. See *Evolve Student Learning Resources* for useful "Spanish Vocabulary and Phrases."
- *Cultural differences.* The person may attach different meanings to verbal and nonverbal communication. See *Caring About Culture: Communicating With Persons From Other Cultures.*
- *Changing the subject.* Someone changes the subject when the topic is uncomfortable.
- *Giving your opinion.* Opinions involve judging values, behaviors, or feelings. Let others express feelings and concerns without adding your opinion. Do not make judgments or jump to conclusions.

CARING ABOUT CULTURE

Communicating With Persons From Other Cultures

To communicate with persons from other cultures:
- Learn about the beliefs and values of the person's culture. You can ask the nurse, the person, and the family. The person's care plan includes cultural beliefs and customs.
- Do not judge the person by your attitudes, values, beliefs, and ideas.
- Do the following when communicating with foreign-speaking persons.
  - Convey comfort by your tone of voice and body language.
  - Do not speak loudly or shout. It will not help the person understand English.
  - Speak slowly and distinctly.
  - Keep messages short and simple.
  - Be alert for words the person seems to understand.
  - Use gestures and pictures.
  - Repeat the message in other ways.
  - Avoid using medical terms and abbreviations.
  - Be alert for signs the person is pretending to understand. Nodding and "yes" to all questions are signs that the person does not understand what you are saying.

(NOTE: Each person is unique. A person may not follow all of the beliefs and practices of his or her culture. Follow the care plan.)

Modified from Giger JN: *Transcultural nursing: assessment and intervention*, ed 6, St Louis, 2013, Mosby.

- *Talking a lot when others are silent.* Talking too much is usually from nervousness and discomfort with silence.
- *Failure to listen.* Do not pretend to listen. It shows lack of interest and caring. This causes poor responses. You miss important complaints or symptoms to report to the nurse.
- *Pat answers.* "Don't worry." "Everything will be okay." "Your doctor knows best." These make the person feel that you do not care about his or her concerns, feelings, and fears.
- *Illness and disability.* Speech, hearing, vision, cognitive function, and body movements are often affected. Verbal and nonverbal communication is affected.
- *Age.* Values and communication styles vary among age-groups.
  See *Focus on Communication: Communication Barriers.*

FOCUS ON COMMUNICATION

Communication Barriers

Persons from other cultures may not speak English. Normally family or friends may translate. However, the nurse may prefer to use a translator from the agency.

Trained translators know medical terms. Family or friends may state something other than what was meant. Receiving wrong information is a risk. Also, having family or friends translate violates the right to privacy. The *Health Insurance Portability and Accountability Act of 1996 (HIPAA)* protects the right to privacy and security of a person's health information (Chapter 4). Privacy is protected when using the agency's translator.

PERSONS WITH SPECIAL NEEDS

Each person is unique. Special knowledge and skills may be required to meet the person's needs.

Persons With Disabilities

A *disability is any lost, absent, or impaired physical or mental function.* It may be temporary or permanent. A person may acquire a disability any time from birth through old age. Disease and injury are common causes. Common courtesies and manners *(etiquette)* apply to any person with a disability. See Box 7-2 for disability etiquette.

The Person Who Is Comatose

Comatose means being unable to respond to stimuli. The person who is comatose is unconscious. The person cannot respond to others. Often the person can hear and can feel touch and pain. Pain may be shown by grimacing or groaning. Assume that the person hears and understands you. Use touch and give care gently. Practice these measures.
- Knock before entering the person's room.
- Tell the person your name, the time, and the place every time you enter the room.
- Give care on the same schedule every day.
- Explain what you are going to do. Explain care measures step-by-step as you do them.
- Tell the person when you are completing care.
- Use touch to communicate care, concern, and comfort.
- Tell the person what time you will be back to check on him or her.
- Tell the person when you are leaving the room.

BOX 7-2	Disability Etiquette

- Show the same courtesies to the person as you would to anyone else.
- Provide for privacy.
- Touch or handle the person's wheelchair only with his or her consent.
- Do not hang on or lean on a person's wheelchair.
- Treat adults as adults. Use the person's first name only if he or she asks you to do so. Do the same for others present.
- Do not pat a person who is in a wheelchair on the head.
- Speak directly to the person. Do not direct questions for the person to his or her companion.
- Do not be embarrassed for using words related to the disability. For example, you say: "Did you see that?" to a person with a vision problem.
- Sit or squat to talk to a person in a wheelchair or in a chair. You and the person are at eye level.
- Ask if help is needed before acting. If the person says "no," respect the person's wishes. If the person wants help, ask what to do and how to do it.
- Think before giving directions to a person in a wheelchair. Think about distances, weather conditions, stairs, curbs, steep hills, and other obstacles.
- Let the person set the pace in walking, talking, or other activities.
- See Chapter 32 for persons with hearing or vision problems.

Modified from Easter Seals, *Disability etiquette*, 2017.

Persons With Bariatric Needs

Bariatrics focuses on *the treatment and control of obesity.* Obesity means *having an excess amount of total body fat.* Bariatric persons are at risk for many serious health problems. Heart disease, high blood pressure, stroke, cancer, and diabetes are examples. Physical and emotional needs are common. Special equipment and furniture are needed to meet the person's needs.

FAMILY AND FRIENDS

Family and friends help meet basic needs. They offer support and comfort. The presence or absence of family or friends affects the person's quality of life.

The person has the right to visit with others in private and without unneeded interruptions. You may need to give care when visitors are there. Protect the right to privacy. Do not expose the person's body in front of them. Politely ask them to leave the room. Show them where to wait. Promptly tell them when they can return. A partner or family member may want to help you. If the patient or resident consents, you can let the person stay.

Treat family and friends with courtesy and respect. They have concerns about the person's condition and care. They need support and understanding. However, do not discuss the person's condition with them. Refer their questions to the nurse.

Visiting rules depend on agency policy and the person's condition. Know your agency's visiting policies and what is allowed for the person.

Visitors may have questions about the chapel, gift shop, lounge, dining room, or business office. Know the location, special rules, and hours of these areas.

A visitor may upset or tire a person. Report your observations to the nurse. The nurse will speak with the visitor about the person's needs.

See *Caring About Culture: Family Roles in Sick Care.*

🌸 CARING ABOUT CULTURE

Family Roles in Sick Care

In *Vietnam*, family members may be involved in the person's hospital care. They stay at the bedside and sleep in the person's bed or on straw mats. In *Vietnam* and *China*, family members may provide food, hygiene, and comfort.

(NOTE: *Each person is unique. A person may not follow all of the beliefs and practices of his or her culture. Follow the care plan.*)

Modified from D'Avanzo CE: *Pocket guide to cultural health assessment*, ed 4, St Louis, 2008, Mosby.

BEHAVIOR ISSUES

Many patients, residents, and families accept illness, injury, and disability. Others do not adjust well. They have some of the following behaviors.

- *Anger.* Causes include fear, pain, and dying and death. Loss of function and loss of control over health and life are causes. Anger is a symptom of some diseases that affect thinking and behavior. Some people are generally angry. Anger is communicated verbally and nonverbally. Verbal outbursts, shouting, raised voices, and rapid speech are common. Some people are silent. Others are not cooperative. Nonverbal signs include rapid movements, pacing, clenched fists, and a red face. Glaring and getting close to you when speaking are other signs. Violent behaviors can occur.

- *Demanding behavior.* Nothing seems to please the person. The person is critical of others. He or she wants care at a certain time and in a certain way. Loss of independence, loss of health, and loss of control of life are causes. So are unmet needs.

- *Self-centered behavior.* Only the person's needs are important. The needs of others are ignored. The person demands the time and attention of others. The person becomes impatient if needs are not met.

- *Aggressive behavior.* The person may swear, bite, hit, pinch, scratch, or kick. Fear, anger, pain, and dementia (Chapter 35) are causes. Protect the person, others, and yourself from harm (Chapter 10).

- *Withdrawal.* The person has little or no contact with others. He or she spends time alone and does not take part in social or group events. This may signal physical illness or depression. Some people are not social. They prefer to be alone.

- *Inappropriate sexual behavior.* Some people make inappropriate sexual remarks. Or they touch others in the wrong way. Some disrobe or masturbate in public. These behaviors may be on purpose. Or they are caused by disease, confusion, dementia, or drug side effects.

You cannot avoid the person or lose control. Good communication is needed. Behaviors are addressed in the care plan. The care plan may include some of the guidelines in Box 7-3.

See *Focus on Communication: Behavior Issues.*

BOX 7-3   Dealing With Behavior Issues

- Recognize frustrating and frightening situations. Put yourself in the person's situation. How would you feel? How would you want to be treated?
- Treat the person with dignity and respect.
- Answer questions clearly and thoroughly. Ask the nurse to answer questions you cannot answer.
- Keep the person informed. Tell the person what you are going to do and when.
- Do not keep the person waiting. Answer call lights promptly. If you tell the person that you will do something, do it promptly.
- Explain the reason for long waits. Ask if you can get or do something to increase the person's comfort.
- Stay calm and professional, especially if the person is angry or hostile. Often the person is not angry at you. He or she is angry at another person or situation.
- Do not argue with the person.
- Listen and use silence. The person may feel better if able to express his or her feelings.
- Protect yourself from violent behaviors (Chapter 10).
- Report the person's behavior to the nurse. Discuss how to deal with the person.

FOCUS ON COMMUNICATION

Behavior Issues

Anger is a common response to illness and disability. The person may be angry with the situation. You might have problems dealing with anger directed at you. Act professionally. Stay calm. Do not yell at or insult the person. Listen to his or her concerns. Give needed care. Try not to take angry statements personally. If a person says hurtful things, you can kindly say: "Please don't say those things. I'm trying to help you." Tell the nurse about the person's behavior.

Caring for demanding or angry persons can be hard. Ask the nurse or co-workers to help if needed.

FOCUS ON P R I D E

The Person, Family, and Yourself

Personal and Professional Responsibility

Improving communication is on-going. You may be uncomfortable with patient or resident interactions at first. You are responsible for developing your communication skills.

- Use methods such as listening and clarifying.
- Pay attention to the nonverbal messages you send.
- Avoid the communication barriers.
- Know where your agency keeps communication aids. These may include the devices in Figure 7-3 or translation lists with useful words or phrases (see *Evolve Student Learning Resources*).
- Learn from your mistakes.

Rights and Respect

You may care for young and old persons, ill and disabled persons, persons who are obese, and persons from other cultures. Each person is different. Each has his or her own needs and concerns.

Do not label the person or make assumptions. For example, a person is obese. That does not mean the person is lazy or lacks control. Or a person is elderly. That does not mean the person is confused.

Each person is unique and has value. Try to understand the person. Listen and use good communication. Treat the person with dignity and respect.

Independence and Social Interaction

Nursing center residents may feel lonely or abandoned. Patients may fear loss of function that affects independence. Feeling abandoned or worthless affects self-esteem and health. To provide a sense of identity, worth, and belonging:

- Greet each person by name.
- Talk to the person while giving care.
- Take an extra minute to talk or just listen.
- Encourage as much independence as possible.
- Focus on the person's abilities, not the disabilities.
- Allow private time with visitors.

Delegation and Teamwork

Caring for persons with behavior issues requires teamwork. Staff may become frustrated. The health team works together to manage such persons. Care assignments may rotate to allow breaks. Help co-workers when they are assigned to persons with behavior issues.

The person's quality of care must not be lowered. Treat the person as you treat others. Show respect. Be kind. Often when treated kindly, the person's behavior will improve. A supportive and encouraging team makes caring for persons with behavior issues easier.

Ethics and Laws

You will care for persons with different ideas, values, and life-styles. These shape the person's character and identity. It is not ethical to:

- Force your views and beliefs on another person.
- Make negative comments or insult the person's customs.
- Argue with a person about health care or religious beliefs.

Respect the person as a whole. This includes his or her cultural and religious practices.

FOCUS ON PRIDE: *Application*

Imagine yourself as a patient or resident. What would you want the staff to know about you? Ask 1 or 2 others what would be important to them. How does understanding the person allow you to give better care?

Circle the BEST answer.

1 You apply holism when you focus on
   a The person's care plan
   b The person's physical, safety and security, and self-esteem needs
   c The person as a physical, psychological, social, and spiritual being
   d The person's cultural and spiritual needs

2 Which basic need is the *most* essential?
   a The need to feel safe
   b The need to feel valued
   c The need for affection
   d The need for food

3 A person says: "I'm falling!" Which needs are *most* important at the time?
   a Self-actualization needs
   b Safety and security needs
   c Love and belonging needs
   d Self-esteem needs

4 Which statement about culture and religion is *true*?
   a Cultural and religious practices are not allowed in nursing centers.
   b A person must follow all beliefs and practices of his or her culture or religion.
   c Culture and religion influence health and illness practices.
   d Culture and religion do not influence food choices.

5 Which is *true*?
   a Nonverbal communication uses the written or spoken word.
   b Verbal communication is the truest reflection of a person's feelings.
   c Body language cannot be controlled.
   d Touch means different things to different people.

6 To communicate with the person you should
   a Use medical words and phrases
   b Change the subject often
   c Give your opinions
   d Be quiet when the person is silent

7 Which shows that you are listening?
   a You sit with your arms crossed.
   b You have eye contact with the person.
   c You avoid asking questions.
   d You use communication barriers.

8 Which is an open-ended question?
   a "What hobbies do you enjoy?"
   b "Do you want to wear your red sweater?"
   c "Would you like eggs and toast for breakfast?"
   d "Do you want to sit in your chair?"

9 You ask: "What is your name?" This is
   a A communication barrier
   b A direct question
   c Paraphrasing
   d An open-ended question

10 Which promotes communication?
   a "Don't worry."
   b "Everything will be fine."
   c "This is a good nursing center."
   d "Why are you crying?"

11 Which is a barrier to communication?
   a Focusing
   b Asking questions
   c Pretending to listen
   d Using familiar language

12 A person uses a wheelchair. For effective communication, you should
   a Lean on the wheelchair
   b Pat the person on the head
   c Direct questions to the companion
   d Sit or squat next to the person

13 A person is comatose. Which action is *correct*?
   a You assume that the person cannot hear.
   b You explain what you are going to do.
   c You use listening and silence to communicate.
   d You enter the room without knocking.

14 A visitor seems to tire a person. What should you do?
   a Ask the person to leave.
   b Tell the nurse.
   c Stay in the room to observe the person and visitor.
   d Find out the visitor's relationship to the person.

15 A person wants care given at a certain time and in a certain way. Nothing seems to please the person. The person is most likely demonstrating
   a Angry behavior
   b Withdrawn behavior
   c Demanding behavior
   d Aggressive behavior

16 A person is demonstrating problem behavior. You should
   a Put yourself in the person's situation
   b Ignore the behavior
   c Ask the person to be nicer
   d Avoid the person

Answers to Chapter 7 questions are on p. 551.

FOCUS ON PRACTICE

Problem Solving

A resident was admitted to the center last month. The resident is withdrawn, impatient, and angry toward the staff. Explain possible reasons for the behaviors. How will you manage the behaviors and provide quality care?

Body Structure and Function

OBJECTIVES

- Define the key terms and key abbreviations in this chapter.
- Identify the basic structures of the cell.
- Explain how cells divide.
- Describe 4 types of tissues.

- Identify the structures and functions of each body system.
- Explain how to promote PRIDE in the person, the family, and yourself.

KEY TERMS

artery A blood vessel that carries blood away from the heart

capillary A very tiny blood vessel; food, oxygen, and other substances pass from capillaries into the cells

cell The basic unit of body structure

digestion The process that breaks down food physically and chemically so it can be absorbed for use by the cells

hemoglobin The substance in red blood cells that carries oxygen and gives blood its red color

hormone A chemical substance secreted by the endocrine glands into the bloodstream

immunity Protection against a disease or condition; the person will not get or be affected by the disease

joint The point at which 2 or more bones meet to allow movement

menstruation The process in which the lining of the uterus (endometrium) breaks up and is discharged from the body through the vagina

metabolism The burning of food for heat and energy by the cells

organ Groups of tissue with the same function

peristalsis Involuntary muscle contractions in the digestive system that move food down the esophagus through the alimentary canal

respiration The process of supplying the cells with oxygen and removing carbon dioxide from them

system Formed by organs that work together to perform special functions

tissue A group of cells with similar functions

vein A blood vessel that returns blood to the heart

KEY ABBREVIATIONS

CNS	Central nervous system	**RBC**	Red blood cell
GI	Gastro-intestinal	**WBC**	White blood cell
mL	Milliliter		

Ideally, the human body is in *homeostasis*—a steady state. (*Homeo* means *sameness*. *Stasis* means *standing still*.) Various body functions and processes work to promote health and survival. Homeostasis is affected by illness, disease, and injury.

You help patients and residents meet their basic needs. Your care promotes comfort, healing, and recovery.

Therefore you need to know the body's normal structure (*anatomy*) and function (*physiology*). They will help you understand signs, symptoms, and the reasons for care and procedures. You will give safe and more effective care.

See Chapter 9 for the changes in body structure and function that occur with aging.

CELLS, TISSUES, AND ORGANS

*The basic unit of body structure is the **cell.*** Cells have the same basic structure. Function, size, and shape may differ. Cells are very small. You need a microscope to see them. Cells need food, water, and oxygen to live and function.

Figure 8-1 shows the cell and its structures. The *cell membrane* is the outer covering. It encloses the cell and helps hold the cell's shape. The *nucleus* is the control center of the cell. It directs the cell's activities. The nucleus is in the center of the cell. The *cytoplasm* surrounds the nucleus. Cytoplasm contains smaller structures that perform cell functions. *Protoplasm* means "living substance." It refers to all structures, substances, and water within the cell. Protoplasm is a semi-liquid substance much like an egg white.

Chromosomes are thread-like structures in the nucleus. Each cell has 46 chromosomes. Chromosomes contain *genes.* Genes control the traits children inherit from their parents. Height, eye color, and skin color are examples.

The nucleus controls cell reproduction. Cells reproduce by dividing in half. The process of cell division is called *mitosis.* It is needed for tissue growth and repair. During mitosis, the 46 chromosomes arrange themselves in 23 pairs. As the cell divides, the 23 pairs are pulled in half. The 2 new cells are identical. Each has 46 chromosomes (Fig. 8-2).

Cells are the body's building blocks. *Groups of cells with similar functions combine to form **tissues.***

- *Epithelial tissue* covers internal and external body surfaces. Tissue lining the nose, mouth, respiratory tract, stomach, and intestines is epithelial tissue. So are the skin, hair, nails, and glands.
- *Connective tissue* anchors, connects, and supports other tissues. It is in every part of the body. Bones, tendons, ligaments, and cartilage are connective tissue. Blood is a form of connective tissue.
- *Muscle tissue* stretches and contracts to let the body move.
- *Nerve tissue* receives and carries impulses to the brain and back to body parts.

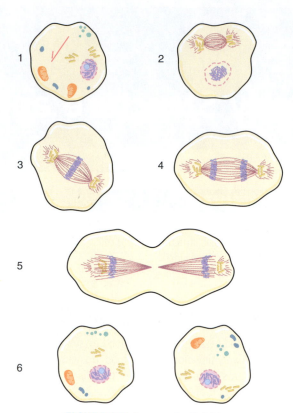

FIGURE 8-2 Process of cell division.

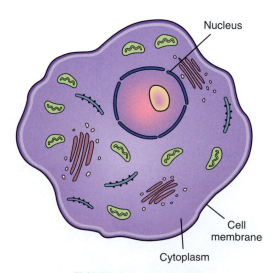

FIGURE 8-1 Parts of a cell.

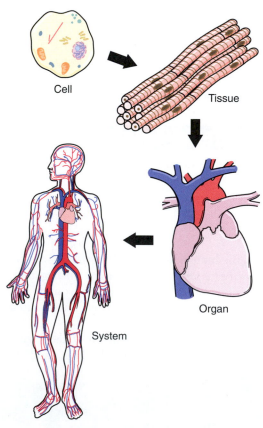

FIGURE 8-3 Organization of the body.

Groups of tissue with the same function form **organs.** An organ has 1 or more functions. Examples of organs are the heart, brain, liver, lungs, and kidneys. *Systems are formed by organs that work together to perform special functions* (Fig. 8-3).

THE INTEGUMENTARY SYSTEM

The *integumentary system*, or *skin*, is the largest system. *Integument* means *covering*. The skin covers the body. It has epithelial, connective, and nerve tissue. It also has oil glands and sweat glands. There are 2 skin layers (Fig. 8-4).

- The *epidermis* is the outer layer. It has living cells and dead cells. The dead cells were once deeper in the epidermis. They were pushed upward as the cells divided. Dead cells constantly flake off. They are replaced by living cells. Living cells die and flake off. Living cells of the epidermis contain *pigment*. Pigment gives skin its color. The epidermis has no blood vessels and few nerve endings.
- The *dermis* is the inner layer. It is made up of connective tissue. Blood vessels, nerves, sweat glands, and oil glands are found in the dermis. So are hair roots.

The epidermis and dermis are supported by *subcutaneous tissue*. The subcutaneous tissue is a thick layer of fat and connective tissue.

Oil glands and *sweat glands, hair,* and *nails* are skin appendages.

- Hair—covers the entire body, except the palms of the hands and the soles of the feet. Hair in the nose and ears and around the eyes protects these organs from dust, insects, and other foreign objects.
- Nails—protect the tips of the fingers and toes. Nails help fingers pick up and handle small objects.
- Sweat glands (*sudoriferous glands*)—help the body regulate temperature. Sweat consists of water, salt, and a small amount of wastes. Sweat is secreted through pores in the skin. The body is cooled as sweat evaporates.
- Oil glands (*sebaceous glands*)—lie near the hair shafts. They secrete an oily substance into the space near the hair shaft. Oil travels to the skin surface. This helps keep the hair and skin soft and shiny.

The skin has many functions.

- It is the body's protective covering.
- It prevents microorganisms and other substances from entering the body.
- It prevents excess amounts of water from leaving the body.
- It protects organs from injury.
- Nerve endings in the skin sense both pleasant and unpleasant stimulation. Nerve endings are over the entire body. They sense cold, pain, touch, and pressure to protect the body from injury.
- It helps regulate body temperature. Blood vessels *dilate* (widen) when temperature outside the body is high. More blood is brought to the body surface for cooling during evaporation. When blood vessels *constrict* (narrow), the body retains heat. This is because less blood reaches the skin.
- It stores fat and water.

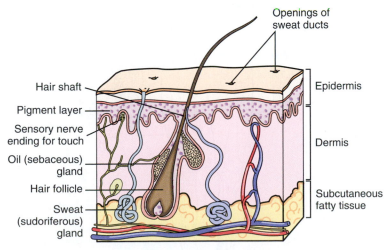

FIGURE 8-4 Layers of the skin.

THE MUSCULO-SKELETAL SYSTEM

The *musculo-skeletal system* provides the framework for the body. It lets the body move. This system also protects internal organs and gives the body shape.

Bones

The human body has 206 *bones* (Fig. 8-5). There are 4 types of bones.

- *Long bones* bear the body's weight. Leg bones are long bones.
- *Short bones* allow skill and ease in movement. Bones in the wrists, fingers, ankles, and toes are short bones.
- *Flat bones* protect the organs. They include the ribs, skull, pelvic bones, and shoulder blades.
- *Irregular bones* are the vertebrae in the spinal column. They allow various degrees of movement and flexibility.

Bones are hard, rigid structures. They are made up of living cells. Calcium and phosphorus are needed for bone formation and strength. Bones store these minerals for use by the body.

Bones are covered by a membrane called *periosteum*. Periosteum contains blood vessels that supply bone cells with oxygen and food. Inside the hollow centers of the bones is a substance called *bone marrow*. Blood cells are formed in the bone marrow.

Joints

A *joint* is the point at which 2 or more bones meet. Joints allow movement (Chapter 27). *Cartilage* is connective tissue at the end of the long bones. It cushions the joint so that the bone ends do not rub together. The *synovial membrane* lines the joints. It secretes *synovial fluid*. Synovial fluid acts as a lubricant so the joint can move smoothly. Bones are held together at the joint by strong bands of connective tissue called *ligaments*.

There are 3 major types of joints (Fig. 8-6).

- A *ball-and-socket joint* allows movement in all directions. It is made of the rounded end of 1 bone and the hollow end of another bone. The rounded end of 1 fits into the hollow end of the other. The joints of the hips and shoulders are ball-and-socket joints.
- A *hinge joint* allows movement in 1 direction. The elbow is a hinge joint.
- A *pivot joint* allows turning from side to side. A pivot joint connects the skull to the spine.

Some joints cannot move. They connect the bones of the skull.

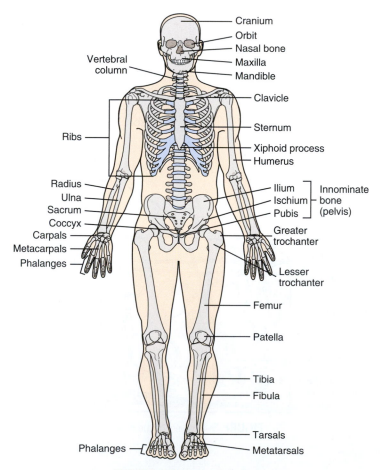

FIGURE 8-5 Bones of the body.

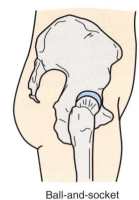

Ball-and-socket

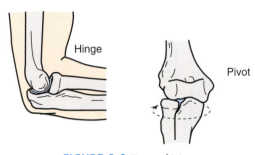

Hinge

Pivot

FIGURE 8-6 Types of joints.

Muscles

The body has over 500 *muscles* (Figs. 8-7 and 8-8). Some are voluntary. Others are involuntary.

- *Voluntary muscles* can be consciously controlled. Muscles attached to bones *(skeletal muscles)* are voluntary. Arm muscles do not work unless you move your arm; likewise for leg muscles. Skeletal muscles are *striated*. That is, they look striped or streaked.
- *Involuntary muscles* work automatically. You cannot control them. They control the action of the stomach, intestines, blood vessels, and other body organs. Involuntary muscles also are called *smooth muscles*. They look smooth, not streaked or striped.
- *Cardiac muscle* is in the heart. It is an involuntary muscle. However, it appears striated like skeletal muscle. Muscles have 3 functions.
- Movement of body parts
- Maintenance of posture or muscle tone
- Production of body heat

Strong, tough connective tissues called *tendons* connect muscles to bones. When muscles *contract* (shorten), tendons at each end of the muscle cause the bone to move. The body has many tendons. See the Achilles tendon in Figure 8-8. Some muscles constantly contract to maintain posture.

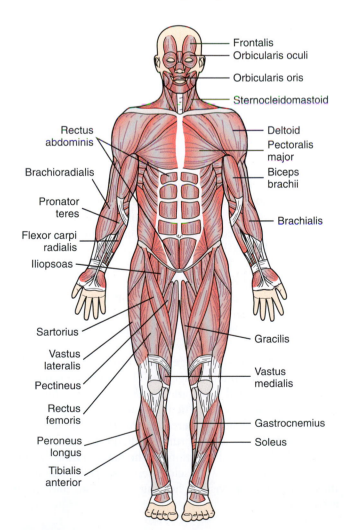

FIGURE 8-7 Anterior view of the muscles of the body. (From Herlihy B: *The human body in health and illness*, ed 5, St Louis, 2014, Elsevier.)

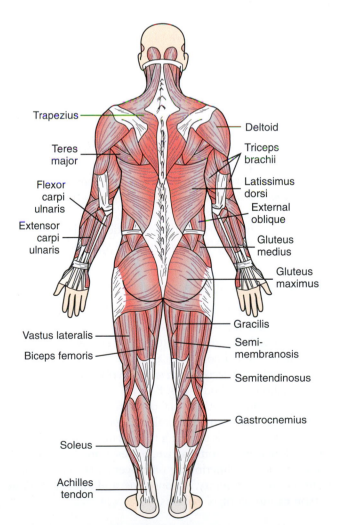

FIGURE 8-8 Posterior view of the muscles of the body. (From Herlihy B: *The human body in health and illness*, ed 5, St Louis, 2014, Elsevier.)

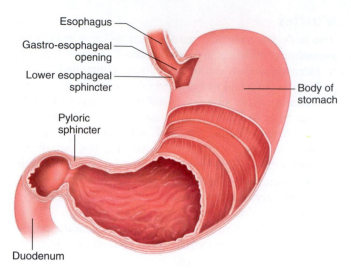

FIGURE 8-9 Pyloric sphincter. (Redrawn from Patton KT, Thibodeau GA: *The human body in health and disease*, ed 7, St Louis, 2018, Elsevier.)

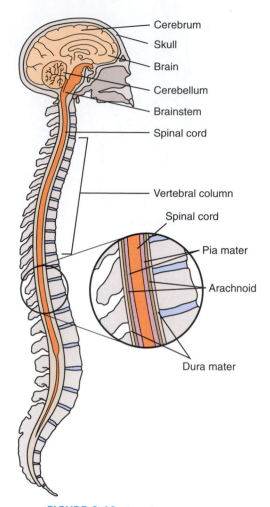

FIGURE 8-10 Central nervous system.

When muscles contract, they burn food for energy. Heat is produced. The more muscle activity, the greater the amount of heat produced. Shivering is how the body produces heat when exposed to cold. Shivering is from rapid, general muscle contractions.

Sphincters are circular bands of muscle fibers. They *constrict* (narrow) a passage. Or they close a natural body opening. For example:

- The *lower esophageal sphincter* (Fig. 8-9) is between the esophagus and the stomach. It prevents food from moving back up into the esophagus.
- The *pyloric sphincter* (see Fig. 8-9) is an opening from the stomach into the small intestine. Closed, it holds food in the stomach for partial digestion. It opens to allow partially digested food to enter the small intestine.
- The *anal sphincter* keeps the anus closed. It opens for a bowel movement.
- *Urethral sphincters* seal off the bladder. This allows urine to collect in the bladder. The sphincters open for urination.

THE NERVOUS SYSTEM

The *nervous system* controls, directs, and coordinates body functions. Its 2 main divisions are:

- The *central nervous system (CNS)*. It consists of the brain and spinal cord (Fig. 8-10).
- The *peripheral nervous system*. It involves the nerves throughout the body (Fig. 8-11).

Nerves connect to the spinal cord. Nerves carry messages or impulses to and from the brain. A *stimulus* causes a nerve impulse. A stimulus is anything that excites or causes a body part to function, become active, or respond. A *reflex* is the body's response (functioning or movement) to a stimulus. Reflexes are involuntary, unconscious, and immediate. The person cannot control reflexes.

Nerves are easily damaged and take a long time to heal. Some nerve fibers have a protective covering called a *myelin sheath*. The myelin sheath also insulates the nerve fiber. Nerve fibers covered with myelin conduct impulses faster than those fibers without it.

The Central Nervous System

The *brain* and *spinal cord* make up the central nervous system. The brain is covered by the skull. The 3 main parts of the brain are the *cerebrum*, the *cerebellum*, and the *brainstem* (Fig. 8-12).

The cerebrum is the largest part of the brain. It is the center of thought and intelligence. The cerebrum is divided into 2 halves called *right* and *left hemispheres*. The right hemisphere controls movement and activities on the body's left side. The left hemisphere controls the right side.

The outside of the cerebrum is called the *cerebral cortex*. It controls the highest functions of the brain. These include reasoning, memory, consciousness, speech, voluntary muscle movement, vision, hearing, sensation, and other activities.

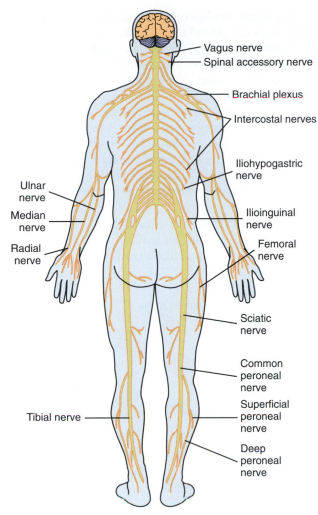

FIGURE 8-11 Peripheral nervous system.

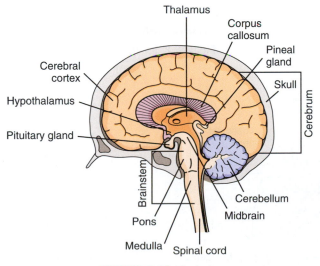

FIGURE 8-12 The brain.

The cerebellum regulates and coordinates body movements. It controls balance and the smooth movements of voluntary muscles. Injury to the cerebellum results in jerky movements, loss of coordination, and muscle weakness.

The brainstem connects the cerebrum to the spinal cord. The brainstem contains the *midbrain, pons,* and *medulla.* The midbrain and pons relay messages between the medulla and the cerebrum. The medulla is below the pons. The medulla controls heart rate, breathing, blood vessel size, swallowing, coughing, and vomiting. The brain connects to the spinal cord at the lower end of the medulla.

The spinal cord lies within the spinal column. The cord is 17 to 18 inches long. It contains pathways that conduct messages to and from the brain.

The brain and spinal cord are covered and protected by 3 layers of connective tissue called meninges.
- The outer layer lies next to the skull. It is a tough covering called the *dura mater.*
- The middle layer is the *arachnoid.*
- The inner layer is the *pia mater.*

The space between the middle layer (arachnoid) and inner layer (pia mater) is the *arachnoid space.* The space is filled with *cerebrospinal fluid.* It circulates around the brain and spinal cord. Cerebrospinal fluid protects the central nervous system. It cushions shocks that could easily injure brain and spinal cord structures.

The Peripheral Nervous System

The peripheral nervous system has 12 pairs of *cranial nerves* and 31 pairs of *spinal nerves.* Cranial nerves conduct impulses between the brain and the head, neck, chest, and abdomen. They conduct impulses for smell, vision, hearing, pain, touch, temperature, and pressure. They also conduct impulses for voluntary and involuntary muscles. Spinal nerves carry impulses from the skin, extremities, and internal structures not supplied by the cranial nerves.

Some peripheral nerves form the *autonomic nervous system.* This system controls involuntary muscles and certain body functions. The functions include the heartbeat, blood pressure, intestinal contractions, and glandular secretions. These functions occur automatically.

The autonomic nervous system is divided into the *sympathetic nervous system* and the *parasympathetic nervous system.* They balance each other. The sympathetic nervous system speeds up functions. The parasympathetic nervous system slows functions. When you are angry, scared, excited, or exercising, the sympathetic nervous system is stimulated. The parasympathetic system is activated when you relax or when the sympathetic system is stimulated for too long.

The Sense Organs

The 5 senses are *sight, hearing, taste, smell,* and *touch*. Receptors for taste are in the tongue. They are called *taste buds*. Receptors for smell are in the nose. Touch receptors are in the dermis, especially in the toes and fingertips.

The Eye. Receptors for vision are in the eyes (Fig. 8-13). The eye is easily injured. Bones of the skull, eyelids and eyelashes, and tears protect the eyes from injury. The eye has 3 layers.

- The *sclera,* the white of the eye, is the outer layer. It is made of tough connective tissue.
- The *choroid* is the second layer. Blood vessels, the *ciliary muscle,* and the *iris* make up the choroid. The iris gives the eye its color. The opening in the middle of the iris is the *pupil*. Pupil size varies with the amount of light entering the eye. The pupil constricts (narrows) in bright light. It dilates (widens) in dim or dark places.
- The *retina* is the inner layer. It has receptors for vision and the nerve fibers of the *optic nerve*.

Light enters the eye through the *cornea*. It is the transparent part of the outer layer that lies over the eye. Light rays pass to the *lens,* which lies behind the pupil. The light is then reflected to the retina. Light is carried to the brain by the optic nerve.

The *aqueous chamber* separates the cornea from the lens. The chamber is filled with a fluid called *aqueous humor*. The fluid helps the cornea keep its shape and position. The *vitreous humor* is behind the lens. It is a gelatin-like substance that supports the retina and maintains the eye's shape.

The Ear. The *ear* is a sense organ (Fig. 8-14). It functions in hearing and balance. The ear has 3 parts: the *external ear, middle ear,* and *inner ear*.

The external ear (outer part) is called the *pinna* or *auricle*. Sound waves are guided through the external ear into the *auditory canal*. Glands in the auditory canal secrete a waxy substance called *cerumen*. The auditory canal extends about 1 inch into the *eardrum*. The eardrum *(tympanic membrane)* separates the external and middle ear.

The middle ear is a small space. It contains the *eustachian tube* and 3 small bones called *ossicles*. The eustachian tube connects the middle ear and the throat. Air enters the eustachian tube so there is equal pressure on both sides of the eardrum. The ossicles amplify sound received from the eardrum and transmit the sound to the inner ear. The 3 ossicles are:

- The *malleus*. It looks like a hammer.
- The *incus*. It looks like an anvil.
- The *stapes*. It is shaped like a stirrup.

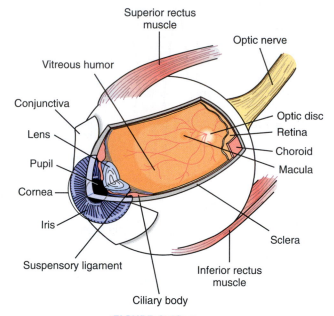

FIGURE 8-13 The eye.

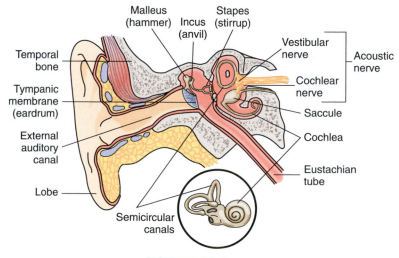

FIGURE 8-14 The ear.

The inner ear consists of *semicircular canals* and the *cochlea*. The cochlea looks like a snail shell. It contains fluid. The fluid carries sound waves from the middle ear to the *acoustic nerve*. The acoustic nerve then carries messages to the brain.

The 3 semicircular canals are involved with balance. They sense the head's position and changes in position. They send messages to the brain.

THE CIRCULATORY SYSTEM

The *circulatory system (cardiovascular system)* is made up of the *blood, heart,* and *blood vessels*. The heart pumps blood through the blood vessels. The circulatory system has many functions.

- Blood carries food, hormones, and other substances to the cells.
- Blood transports (carries) the gases of respiration (p. 89). It brings oxygen to the cells.
- Blood removes waste products from cells.
- Blood plays a role in maintaining the body's fluid balance.
- Blood and blood vessels help regulate body temperature. The blood carries heat from muscle activity to other body parts. Blood vessels in the skin dilate to cool the body. They constrict to retain heat.
- The system produces and carries cells that defend the body from microbes that cause disease.

The Blood

The *blood* consists of blood cells and *plasma*. Plasma is mostly water. It carries blood to other body cells. Plasma also carries substances that cells need to function. This includes food (proteins, fats, and carbohydrates), hormones (p. 94), and chemicals.

Red blood cells (RBCs) are called *erythrocytes*. **Hemoglobin is a substance in RBCs that carries oxygen and gives blood its red color.** As RBCs circulate through the lungs, hemoglobin picks up oxygen. Hemoglobin carries oxygen to the cells. When blood is bright red, hemoglobin in the RBCs is filled with oxygen. As blood circulates through the body, oxygen is given to the cells. Cells release carbon dioxide (a waste product). It is picked up by the hemoglobin. RBCs filled with carbon dioxide make the blood look dark red.

The body has about 25 trillion (25,000,000,000,000) RBCs. About $4\frac{1}{2}$ to 5 million cells are in a cubic millimeter of blood (the size of a tiny drop). RBCs live for 3 to 4 months. They are destroyed by the liver and spleen as they wear out. New RBCs are formed in the bone marrow. About 1 million RBCs are produced every second.

White blood cells (WBCs) are called *leukocytes*. They have no color. They protect the body against infection. There are about 5000 to 10,000 WBCs in a cubic millimeter of blood. At the first sign of infection, WBCs rush to the infection site. There they multiply rapidly. The number of WBCs increases when there is an infection. WBCs are formed by the bone marrow. They live about 9 days.

Platelets (thrombocytes) are needed for blood clotting. They are formed by the bone marrow. There are about 200,000 to 400,000 platelets in a cubic millimeter of blood. A platelet lives about 4 days.

The Heart

The *heart* is a muscle. It pumps blood through the blood vessels to the tissues and cells. The heart lies in the middle to lower part of the chest cavity toward the left side (Fig. 8-15). The heart is hollow and has 3 layers (Fig. 8-16).

- The *pericardium* is the outer layer. It is a thin sac covering the heart.
- The *myocardium* is the second layer. It is the thick, muscular part of the heart.
- The *endocardium* is the inner layer. A membrane, it lines the inner surface of the heart.

The heart has 4 chambers (see Fig. 8-16). Upper chambers receive blood and are called *atria*. The *right atrium* receives blood from body tissues. The *left atrium* receives blood from the lungs. Lower chambers are called *ventricles*. Ventricles pump blood. The *right ventricle* pumps blood to the lungs for oxygen. The *left ventricle* pumps blood to all parts of the body.

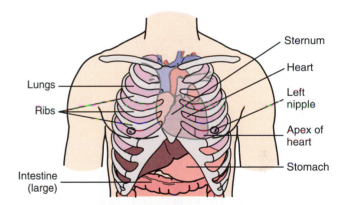

FIGURE 8-15 Location of the heart in the chest cavity.

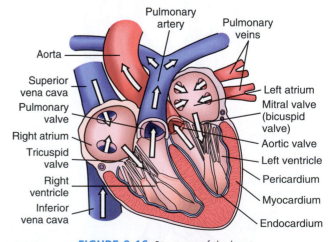

FIGURE 8-16 Structures of the heart.

Valves are between the atria and ventricles. The valves allow blood flow in 1 direction. They prevent blood from flowing back into the atria from the ventricles. The *tricuspid valve* is between the right atrium and the right ventricle. The *mitral valve (bicuspid valve)* is between the left atrium and left ventricle.

Heart action has 2 phases.

- *Diastole.* It is the resting phase. Heart chambers fill with blood.
- *Systole.* It is the working phase. The heart contracts. Blood is pumped through the blood vessels.

The Blood Vessels

Blood flows to body tissues and cells through the blood vessels. There are 3 groups of blood vessels: *arteries, capillaries,* and *veins.*

Arteries are blood vessels that carry blood away from the heart. Arterial blood is rich in oxygen. The *aorta* is the largest artery. It receives blood from the left ventricle. The aorta branches into other arteries that carry blood to all parts of the body (Fig. 8-17). These arteries branch into smaller parts within the tissues. The smallest branch of an artery is an *arteriole.*

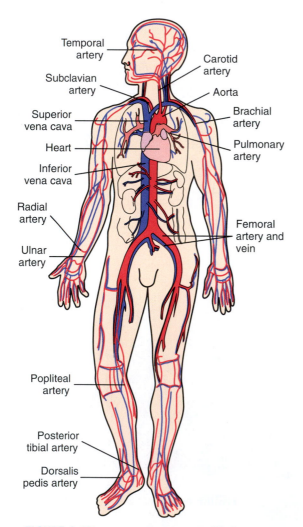

Arterioles connect to capillaries. *Capillaries are very tiny blood vessels. Food, oxygen, and other substances pass from capillaries into the cells.* The capillaries pick up waste products (including carbon dioxide) from the cells. Veins carry waste products back to the heart.

Veins are blood vessels that return blood to the heart. They connect to the capillaries by *venules.* Venules are small veins. Venules branch together to form veins. The many veins also branch together as they near the heart to form 2 main veins (see Fig. 8-17). The 2 main veins are the *inferior vena cava* and the *superior vena cava.* Both empty into the right atrium. The inferior vena cava carries blood from the legs and trunk. The superior vena cava carries blood from the head and arms. Venous blood is dark red. It has little oxygen and a lot of carbon dioxide.

Blood flow through the circulatory system is shown in Figure 8-16. The path of blood flow is as follows.

- Venous blood, poor in oxygen, empties into the right atrium.
- Blood flows through the tricuspid valve into the right ventricle.
- The right ventricle pumps blood into the lungs to pick up oxygen.
- Oxygen-rich blood from the lungs enters the left atrium.
- Blood from the left atrium passes through the mitral valve into the left ventricle.
- The left ventricle pumps the blood into the aorta. It branches off to form other arteries.
- Arterial blood is carried to the tissues by arterioles and to the cells by capillaries.
- Cells and capillaries exchange oxygen and nutrients for carbon dioxide and waste products.
- Capillaries connect with venules. Venules carry blood that has carbon dioxide and waste products.
- Venules form veins.
- Veins return blood to the heart.

THE LYMPHATIC SYSTEM

The lymphatic (lymph) system is a complex network that transports lymph throughout the body (Fig. 8-18). *Lymph* is a clear, thin, watery fluid. Lymph contains proteins and fats from the intestines. Lymph also contains white blood cells (WBCs). The lymphatic system:

- Collects extra lymph from the tissues and returns it to the blood. This helps maintain fluid balance. Water, proteins, and other substances normally leak out of the capillaries. The lymphatic system drains the extra fluid from the tissues. Otherwise, the tissues swell.
- Defends the body against infection by producing lymphocytes. *Lymphocytes* are a type of WBC that defends the body against microorganisms that cause infection (Chapter 13).
- Absorbs fats from the intestines and transports them to the blood.

FIGURE 8-17 Arterial (red) and venous (blue) systems.

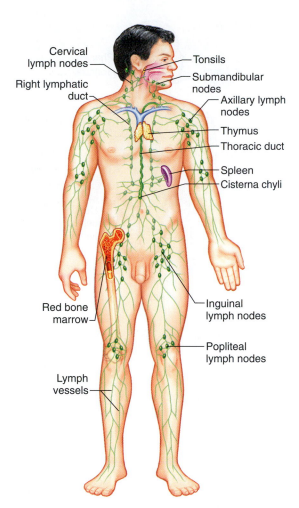

FIGURE 8-18 Lymphatic system. (From Patton KT, Thibodeau GA: *The human body in health and disease*, ed 7, St Louis, 2018, Elsevier.)

See Figure 8-18 for the location of the *thymus (thymus gland)*. Certain lymphocytes—T lymphocytes (T cells) develop in the thymus. Such lymphocytes are important for immune system function (p. 95). The thymus reaches full growth at puberty. Then thymus tissue is slowly replaced by fat and connective tissue. By age 80, it is usually gone.

The *tonsils* are in the back of the throat. *Adenoids* are behind the nose. These structures trap microorganisms in the mouth and nose to help prevent infection.

The *spleen* is the largest structure in the lymphatic system. It is about the size of a fist. The spleen has a rich blood supply—about 500 milliliters (mL) (1 pint) of blood. The spleen:

- Filters and removes bacteria and other substances.
- Destroys old RBCs.
- Saves the iron found in hemoglobin when RBCs are destroyed.
- Stores blood. When needed, the blood is returned to the circulatory system.

THE RESPIRATORY SYSTEM

Oxygen is needed to live. Every cell needs oxygen. Air contains about 21% oxygen. This meets the body's needs under normal conditions. The respiratory system (Fig. 8-19) brings oxygen into the lungs and removes carbon dioxide. *Respiration is the process of supplying the cells with oxygen and removing carbon dioxide from them.* Respiration involves *inhalation* (breathing in) and *exhalation* (breathing out). The terms *inspiration* (breathing in) and *expiration* (breathing out) also are used.

Lymph is formed in the tissues. Lymph is transported by *lymphatic vessels*—lymphatic capillaries to lymphatic venules to the right lymphatic duct and the thoracic duct. Lymph then enters the blood in veins near the neck.

- The *right lymphatic duct* collects lymph from the right arm and from the right side of the head, neck, and chest. It empties into a vein on the right side of the neck.
- The *thoracic duct (left lymphatic duct)* collects lymph from the pelvis, abdomen, lower chest, and rest of the body. It empties into a vein on the left side of the neck.

Lymph nodes are shaped like beans. They range from the size of a pinhead to as large as a lima bean. They are found in the neck, underarm, groin area, chest, abdomen, and pelvis. Usually, you cannot see or feel lymph nodes. They swell when producing more lymphocytes to fight infection.

Lymph enters lymph nodes through the lymphatic vessels. The lymph nodes filter bacteria, cancer cells, and damaged cells from the lymph. This prevents such substances from entering and circulating throughout the body.

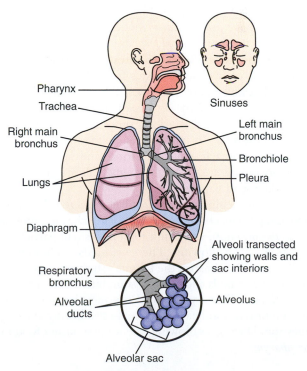

FIGURE 8-19 Respiratory system.

Air enters the body through the *nose*. The air then passes into the *pharynx* (throat). It is a tube-shaped passage-way for air and food. Air passes from the pharynx into the *larynx* (voice box). A piece of cartilage, the *epiglottis*, acts like a lid over the larynx. The epiglottis prevents food from entering the airway during swallowing. During inhalation the epiglottis lifts up to let air pass over the larynx. Air passes from the larynx into the *trachea* (windpipe).

The trachea divides at its lower end into the *right bronchus* and the *left bronchus*. Each bronchus enters a lung. Upon entering the lungs, the bronchi divide many times into smaller branches called *bronchioles*. Eventually the bronchioles subdivide. They end up in tiny 1-celled air sacs called *alveoli*.

Alveoli look like small clusters of grapes. They are supplied by capillaries. Oxygen and carbon dioxide are exchanged between the alveoli and capillaries. Blood in the capillaries picks up oxygen from the alveoli. Then the blood is returned to the left side of the heart and pumped to the rest of the body. Alveoli pick up carbon dioxide from the capillaries for exhalation.

The lungs are spongy tissues. They are filled with alveoli, blood vessels, and nerves. Each lung is divided into lobes. The right lung has 3 lobes; the left lung has 2. The lungs are separated from the abdominal cavity by a muscle called the *diaphragm*.

Each lung is covered by a 2-layered sac called the *pleura*. One layer is attached to the lung and the other to the chest wall. The pleura secretes a very thin fluid that fills the space between the layers. The fluid prevents the layers from rubbing together during inhalation and exhalation. A bony framework made up of the ribs, sternum, and vertebrae protects the lungs.

THE DIGESTIVE SYSTEM

Digestion is the process that breaks down food physically and chemically so it can be absorbed for use by the cells. The digestive system is also called the gastro-intestinal (GI) system. The system also removes solid wastes from the body.

The digestive system involves the *alimentary canal (GI tract)* and the accessory organs of digestion (Fig. 8-20). The alimentary canal is a long tube. It extends from the mouth to the anus. Its major parts are the mouth, pharynx, esophagus, stomach, small intestine, and large intestine. Accessory organs are the teeth, tongue, salivary glands, liver, gallbladder, and pancreas.

Digestion begins in the *mouth (oral cavity)*. It receives food and prepares it for digestion. Using chewing motions, the *teeth* cut, chop, and grind food into small particles for digestion and swallowing. The *tongue* aids in chewing and swallowing. *Taste buds* on the tongue's surface contain nerve endings. Taste buds allow sweet, sour, bitter, and salty tastes to be sensed. *Salivary glands* in the mouth secrete *saliva*. Saliva moistens food particles to ease swallowing and begin digestion. During swallowing, the tongue pushes food into the *pharynx*.

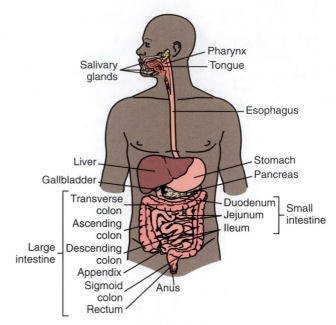

FIGURE 8-20 Digestive system.

The pharynx (throat) is a muscular tube. Swallowing continues as the pharynx contracts. Contraction of the pharynx pushes food into the *esophagus*. The esophagus is a muscular tube about 10 inches long. It extends from the pharynx to the *stomach*. *Involuntary muscle contractions in the digestive system move food down the esophagus through the alimentary canal* (**peristalsis**).

The stomach is a muscular, pouch-like sac. It is in the upper left part of the abdominal cavity. Strong stomach muscles stir and churn food to break it up into even smaller particles. A mucous membrane lines the stomach. It contains glands that secrete *gastric juices*. Food is mixed and churned with the gastric juices to form a semi-liquid substance called *chyme*. Through peristalsis, the chyme is pushed from the stomach into the small intestine.

The *small intestine* is about 20 feet long. It has 3 parts. The first part is the *duodenum*. There more digestive juices are added to the chyme. One is called *bile*. Bile is a greenish liquid made in the *liver*. Bile is stored in the *gallbladder*. Juices from the *pancreas* and small intestine are added to the chyme. Digestive juices chemically break down food so it can be absorbed.

Peristalsis moves the chyme through the 2 other parts of the small intestine: the *jejunum* and the *ileum*. Tiny projections called *villi* line the small intestine. Villi absorb the digested food into the capillaries. Most food absorption takes place in the jejunum and the ileum.

Some chyme is not digested. Undigested chyme passes from the small intestine into the *large intestine (large bowel or colon)*. The colon absorbs most of the water from the chyme. The remaining semi-solid material is called *feces*. Feces contain a small amount of water, solid wastes, and some mucus and germs. These are the waste products of digestion. Feces pass through the colon into the *rectum* by peristalsis. Feces pass out of the body through the *anus*.

THE URINARY SYSTEM

The digestive system rids the body of solid wastes. The lungs rid the body of carbon dioxide. Water and other substances leave the body through sweat. There are other waste products in the blood from cells burning food for energy. The urinary system (Fig. 8-21):

- Removes waste products from the blood.
- Maintains water balance within the body.
- Maintains electrolyte balance. *Electrolytes* are substances that dissolve in water—sodium, potassium, calcium, and magnesium.
  - Sodium is needed for fluid balance. The body retains water if sodium levels are high. Loss of sodium (through vomiting, diarrhea, some drugs, and so on) can result in dehydration.
  - Potassium is needed for the proper function of skeletal and cardiac muscles.
  - Calcium and magnesium are needed for normal nerve and muscle function and for bone and teeth formation.
- Maintains acid-base balance. A pH scale measures if a substance is acidic, neutral, or basic. A pH of 7 is neutral. Anything below 7 is acidic. Anything above 7 is basic. The blood must remain within a certain pH range (7.35–7.45) for the body to function normally.

The *kidneys* are 2 bean-shaped organs in the upper abdomen. They lie against the back muscles on each side of the spine. They are protected by the lower edge of the rib cage.

Each kidney has over a million tiny *nephrons* (Fig. 8-22). Each nephron is the basic working unit of the kidney. Each nephron has a *convoluted tubule*, which is a tiny coiled tubule. Each convoluted tubule has a *Bowman's capsule* at 1 end. The capsule partly surrounds a cluster of capillaries called a *glomerulus*. Blood passes through the glomerulus and is filtered by the capillaries. The fluid part of the blood is squeezed into the Bowman's capsule. The fluid then passes into the tubule. Most of the water and other needed substances are re-absorbed by the blood. The rest of the fluid and the waste products form *urine* in the tubule. Urine flows through the tubule to a *collecting tubule*. All collecting tubules drain into the *renal pelvis* in the kidney.

A tube called the *ureter* is attached to the renal pelvis of the kidney. Each ureter is about 10 to 12 inches long. The ureters carry urine from the kidneys to the *bladder*. The bladder is a hollow, muscular sac. It lies toward the front in the lower part of the abdominal cavity.

Urine is stored in the bladder until the need to urinate is felt. This usually occurs when there is about a half pint (250 mL) of urine in the bladder. Urine passes from the bladder through the *urethra*. The opening at the end of the urethra is called the *meatus*. Urine passes from the body through the meatus. Urine is a clear, yellowish fluid.

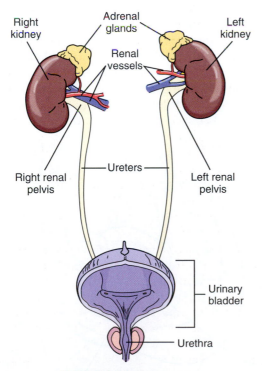

FIGURE 8-21 Urinary system.

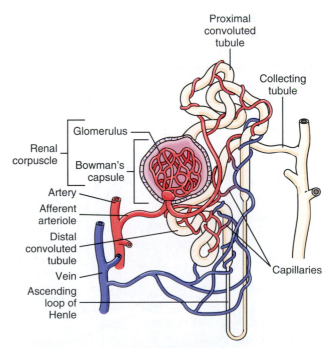

FIGURE 8-22 A nephron.

THE REPRODUCTIVE SYSTEM

Human reproduction results from the union of a male sex cell and a female sex cell. The male and female reproductive systems are different. This allows for the process of reproduction.

The Male Reproductive System

The male reproductive system is shown in Figure 8-23. The *testes (testicles)* are the male sex glands. Sex glands also are called *gonads*. The 2 testes are oval or almond-shaped glands. Male sex cells are produced in the testes. Male sex cells are called *sperm* cells.

Testosterone, the male hormone, is produced in the testes. This hormone is needed for reproductive organ function. It also is needed for the development of the male secondary sex characteristics. There is facial hair; pubic and axillary (underarm) hair; and hair on the arms, chest, and legs. Neck and shoulder sizes increase.

The testes are suspended between the thighs in a sac called the *scrotum*. The scrotum is made of skin and muscle.

Sperm travel from the testis to the *epididymis*. The epididymis is a coiled tube on top and to the side of the testis. From the epididymis, sperm travel through a tube called the *vas deferens*. Each vas deferens joins a *seminal vesicle*. The 2 seminal vesicles store sperm and produce *semen*. Semen is a fluid that carries sperm from the male reproductive tract. The ducts of the seminal vesicles unite to form the *ejaculatory duct*. It passes through the *prostate gland*.

The prostate gland lies just below the bladder. It is shaped like a donut. The gland secretes fluid into the semen. As the ejaculatory ducts leave the prostate, they join the *urethra*. The urethra runs through the prostate gland. The urethra is the outlet for urine and semen. The urethra is contained within the *penis*.

The penis is outside of the body. The *glans* is at the end of the penis. The urethra opens at the end of the glans. A fold of skin (*prepuce* or *foreskin*) is at the end of the penis (Chapter 18).

The penis has *erectile* tissue. When a man is sexually excited, blood fills the erectile tissue. The penis enlarges and becomes hard and erect. The erect penis can enter a female's vagina. *Cowper's glands* are 2 pea-sized glands under the prostate. They produce a clear, colorless fluid before ejaculation (release of semen). The fluid cleanses the urethra, protects sperm from damage, and provides some lubrication for intercourse. With ejaculation, semen—containing sperm—is released into the vagina.

The Female Reproductive System

Figure 8-24 shows the female reproductive system. The female gonads are 2 almond-shaped glands called *ovaries*. An ovary is on each side of the uterus in the abdominal cavity.

The ovaries contain *ova* or eggs. Ova are the female sex cells. One ovum (egg) is released monthly during the woman's reproductive years. Release of an ovum is called *ovulation*.

The ovaries secrete the female hormones *estrogen* and *progesterone*. These hormones are needed for reproductive system function. They also are needed for the development of secondary sex characteristics in the female. These include increased breast size, pubic and axillary (underarm) hair, slight deepening of the voice, and widening and rounding of the hips.

When an ovum is released from an ovary, it travels through a *fallopian tube*. There are 2 fallopian tubes, 1 on each side. The tubes are attached at 1 end to the *uterus*. The ovum travels through the fallopian tube to the uterus.

The uterus is a hollow, muscular organ shaped like a pear. It is in the center of the pelvic cavity behind the bladder and in front of the rectum. The main part of the uterus is the *fundus*. The neck or narrow section of the uterus is the *cervix*. Tissue lining the uterus is the *endometrium*. The endometrium has many blood vessels. If sex cells from the male and female unite into 1 cell, that cell implants into the endometrium. There the cell grows into a *fetus* (unborn baby) and receives nourishment.

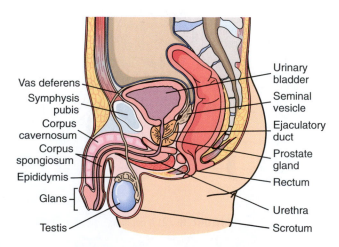

FIGURE 8-23 Male reproductive system.

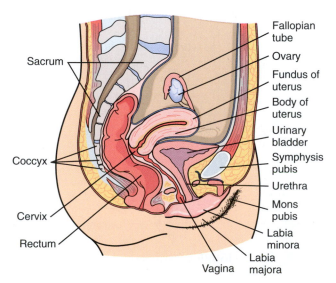

FIGURE 8-24 Female reproductive system.

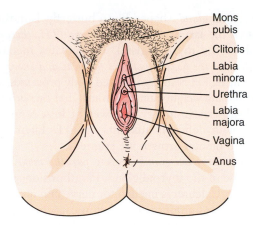

FIGURE 8-25 External female genitalia.

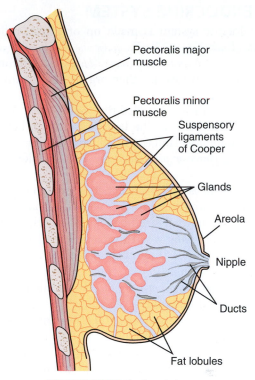

FIGURE 8-26 The female breast.

The cervix of the uterus projects into a muscular canal called the *vagina*. The vagina opens to the outside of the body. It is just behind the urethra. The vagina receives the penis during intercourse. It also is part of the birth canal. Glands in the vaginal wall keep it moistened with secretions. The Bartholin's glands are examples. The external vaginal opening is partially closed by a membrane called the *hymen*. The hymen can stretch or tear (rupture) from intercourse, injury, or surgery.

The external female genitalia are called the *vulva* (Fig. 8-25).
- The *mons pubis* is a rounded, fatty pad over a bone called the *symphysis pubis*. The mons pubis is covered with hair in the adult female.
- The *labia majora* and *labia minora* are 2 folds of tissue on each side of the vaginal opening.
- The *clitoris* is a small organ composed of erectile tissue. It becomes hard when sexually stimulated.

The *mammary glands (breasts)* secrete milk after childbirth. The glands are on the outside of the chest. They are made up of glandular tissue and fat (Fig. 8-26). The milk drains into ducts that open onto the *nipple*.

Menstruation. The endometrium is rich in blood to nourish the cell that grows into a fetus. If pregnancy does not occur, menstruation begins. *Menstruation is the process in which the lining of the uterus (endometrium) breaks up and is discharged from the body through the vagina.* It occurs about every 28 days. Therefore it is called the *menstrual cycle*.

The first day of the menstrual cycle begins with menstruation. Blood flows from the uterus through the vaginal opening. Menstrual flow usually lasts 3 to 7 days. Ovulation occurs during the next phase. An ovum matures in an ovary and is released. Ovulation usually occurs on or about day 14 of the cycle.

Meanwhile, estrogen and progesterone (the female hormones) are secreted by the ovaries. These hormones cause the endometrium to thicken for pregnancy. If pregnancy does not occur, the hormones decrease in amount. This causes the blood supply to the endometrium to decrease. The endometrium breaks up. It is discharged through the vagina. Another menstrual cycle begins.

Fertilization

To reproduce, a male sex cell (sperm) must unite with a female sex cell (ovum). The uniting of the sperm and ovum into 1 cell is called *fertilization*. A sperm has 23 chromosomes. An ovum has 23 chromosomes. When the 2 cells unite, the fertilized cell has 46 chromosomes.

During intercourse, millions of sperm are deposited into the vagina. Sperm travel up the cervix, through the uterus, and into the fallopian tubes. If a sperm and an ovum unite in a fallopian tube, fertilization results. Pregnancy occurs. The fertilized cell travels down the fallopian tube to the uterus. After a short time, the fertilized cell implants into the thick endometrium and grows during pregnancy.

THE ENDOCRINE SYSTEM

The endocrine system is made up of glands called the *endocrine glands* (Fig. 8-27). *The endocrine glands secrete chemical substances called* **hormones** *into the bloodstream.* Hormones regulate the activities of other organs and glands in the body.

The *pituitary gland* is called the *master gland.* About the size of a cherry, it is at the base of the brain behind the eyes. The pituitary gland is divided into the *anterior pituitary lobe* and the *posterior pituitary lobe.* The anterior pituitary lobe secretes:

- *Growth hormone (GH)*—needed for growth of muscles, bones, and other organs. It is needed throughout life to maintain normal-sized bones and muscles. Growth is stunted if a baby is born with deficient amounts of growth hormones. Too much of the hormone causes excessive growth.
- *Thyroid-stimulating hormone (TSH)*—needed for thyroid gland function.
- *Adrenocorticotropic hormone (ACTH)*—stimulates the adrenal glands.

The anterior lobe also secretes hormones that regulate growth, development, and function of the male and female reproductive systems.

The posterior pituitary lobe secretes *antidiuretic hormone (ADH)* and *oxytocin.* ADH prevents the kidneys from excreting excessive amounts of water. Oxytocin causes uterine muscles to contract during childbirth.

The *thyroid gland*, shaped like a butterfly, is in the neck in front of the larynx. *Thyroid hormone (TH, thyroxine)* is secreted by the thyroid gland. It regulates metabolism. **Metabolism** *is the burning of food for heat and energy by the cells.* Too little TH results in slowed body processes, slowed movements, and weight gain. Too much TH causes increased metabolism, excess energy, and weight loss. Some babies are born with deficient amounts of TH. Their physical growth and mental growth are stunted.

The 4 *parathyroid glands* secrete *parathormone.* Two lie on each side of the thyroid gland. Parathormone regulates calcium use. Calcium is needed for nerve and muscle function. Insufficient amounts of calcium cause *tetany.* Tetany is a state of severe muscle contraction and spasm. If untreated, tetany can cause death.

The *thymus* secretes the hormone *thymosin.* This hormone is important for the development and function of the immune system.

The *pancreas* secretes *insulin.* Insulin regulates the amount of sugar in the blood available for use by the cells. Insulin is needed for sugar to enter the cells. If there is too little insulin, sugar cannot enter the cells. If sugar cannot enter the cells, excess amounts build up in the blood. This condition is called *diabetes.*

There are 2 *adrenal glands.* An adrenal gland is on the top of each kidney. The adrenal gland has 2 parts: the *adrenal medulla* and the *adrenal cortex.* The adrenal medulla secretes *epinephrine* and *norepinephrine.* These hormones stimulate the body to quickly produce energy during emergencies. Heart rate, blood pressure, muscle power, and energy all increase.

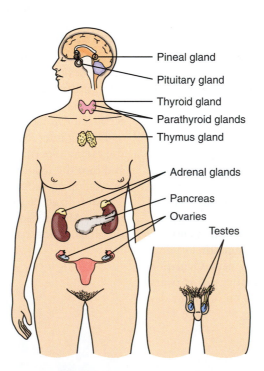

FIGURE 8-27 Endocrine system.

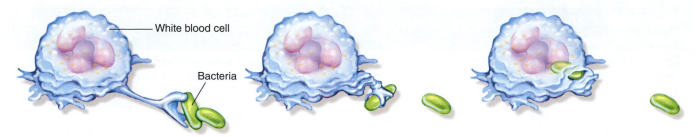

FIGURE 8-28 A phagocyte digests and destroys a microorganism. (Barbara Cousins; from Patton KT, Thibodeau GA: *Structure & function of the body*, ed 15, St Louis, 2016, Elsevier.)

The adrenal cortex secretes 3 groups of hormones needed for life.

- *Glucocorticoids*—regulate metabolism of carbohydrates. They also control the body's response to stress and inflammation.
- *Mineralocorticoids*—regulate the amount of salt and water that is absorbed and lost by the kidneys.
- Small amounts of male and female sex hormones are secreted.

The *gonads* are the glands of human reproduction. Male sex glands (testes) secrete *testosterone*. Female sex glands (ovaries) secrete *estrogen* and *progesterone*.

THE IMMUNE SYSTEM

The immune system protects the body from disease and infection. Abnormal body cells can grow into tumors. Sometimes the body produces substances that cause the body to attack itself. Microorganisms (bacteria, viruses, and other germs) can cause an infection. The immune system defends against threats inside and outside the body.

The immune system gives the body immunity. *Immunity means that a person has protection against a disease or condition. The person will not get or be affected by the disease.*

- *Specific immunity* is the body's reaction to a certain threat.
- *Non-specific immunity* is the body's reaction to anything it does not recognize as a normal body substance.

Special cells and substances function to produce immunity.

- *Antibodies*—normal body substances that recognize other substances. They are involved in destroying abnormal or unwanted substances.
- *Antigens*—substances that cause an immune response. Antibodies recognize and bind with unwanted antigens. This leads to the destruction of unwanted substances and the production of more antibodies.
- *Phagocytes*—white blood cells (WBCs) that digest and destroy microorganisms and other unwanted substances (Fig. 8-28).
- *Lymphocytes*—WBCs that produce antibodies. Lymphocyte production increases as the body responds to an infection.
  - *B lymphocytes (B cells)*—cause the production of antibodies that circulate in the plasma. The antibodies react to specific antigens.
  - *T lymphocytes (T cells)*—destroy invading cells. *Killer T cells* produce poisons near the invading cells. Some T cells attract other cells. The other cells destroy the invaders.

When the body senses an antigen from an unwanted substance, the immune system acts. Phagocyte and lymphocyte production increases. Phagocytes destroy the invaders through digestion. The lymphocytes produce antibodies that identify and destroy the unwanted substances.

Personal and Professional Responsibility

Taking care of yourself is a personal and professional responsibility. To care for others you need a strong and healthy body.

- Eat a healthy diet (Chapter 23), exercise, and get enough rest.
- See your doctor for a check-up at least once a year. Or do so sooner if you have a concern.
- Take prescription or over-the-counter drugs only as instructed.
- Keep your immunizations up to date. For example, get a tetanus booster every 10 years.
- Protect your bones and muscles from injury by using good body mechanics (Chapter 14).
- Protect yourself from infection. Follow Standard Precautions and practice good hand hygiene (Chapter 13).

Rights and Respect

Patients and residents have the right to make decisions about their bodies. You may not agree with those decisions. But you must respect the person's choices. If the decision will cause no harm, comply with the request. For example, a person does not want to wear a sweater today.

If the person's decision may cause harm, tell the nurse at once. For example, a person goes to dialysis 3 times a week. (*Dialysis* is the process of artificially removing wastes from the blood when the kidneys do not function.) The person does not want to go today. You know the importance of the urinary system. Without dialysis, the person will become very sick. You tell the nurse. The person cannot be forced to go to dialysis. But the nurse can talk with the person about the decision, the consequences, and possible solutions.

Independence and Social Interaction

The body does not always work right. People become ill or injured. Some illnesses cannot be cured. Sometimes the health team cannot prevent loss of function. To help maintain the person's optimal level of function:

- Do not treat the person as a sick, dependent person.
- Encourage the person to be as independent as possible.
- Always focus on the person's abilities, not disabilities.
- Tell the person when you notice progress.
- Promote social interaction. This improves mental performance.

Take pride in helping each person regain or maintain the highest level of functioning possible.

Delegation and Teamwork

The body works like a team. Each system has independent functions. But all systems interact and depend on each other. They work together to keep the body functioning. When a person has a problem with 1 body system, other systems are affected. Understanding each system and how the systems interact helps you provide better care.

Ethics and Laws

Sometimes a person is not able to make decisions about his or her own body. For example, the person has dementia. Or the person is unconscious or affected by drugs or alcohol. Or the person is a child. Ethical issues may arise over who makes decisions for such persons.

Spouses, parents, family members, or legal representatives may make decisions. Some persons have an advance directive (Chapter 37). Sometimes the court appoints a guardian for a short time. Finally, the agency's ethics committee may address complex issues. The person's safety and best interests must guide the care given.

FOCUS ON PRIDE: *Application*

Body systems interact for normal function. Explain how the body systems below interact with other systems. How might a problem in 1 system affect another?

- Nervous system
- Circulatory system
- Respiratory system
- Endocrine system

REVIEW QUESTIONS

Circle the BEST answer.

1 The basic unit of body structure is the
   a Cell
   b Neuron
   c Nephron
   d Ovum

2 The outer layer of the skin is called the
   a Dermis
   b Epidermis
   c Integument
   d Myelin

3 Which is a function of the skin?
   a Provides the protective covering for the body
   b Transports lymph
   c Forms blood cells
   d Provides the shape and framework for the body

4 Which allows movement?
   a Bone marrow
   b Synovial membrane
   c Joints
   d Ligaments

5 Skeletal muscles
  a Are under involuntary control
  b Appear smooth
  c Are under voluntary control
  d Appear striped and smooth

6 The highest functions in the brain take place in the
  a Cerebral cortex
  b Medulla
  c Brainstem
  d Spinal nerves

7 The ear is involved with
  a Regulating body movements
  b Balance
  c Smoothness of body movements
  d Controlling involuntary muscles

8 The liquid part of blood is the
  a Hemoglobin
  b Red blood cell
  c Plasma
  d White blood cell

9 Which part of the heart pumps blood to the body?
  a Right atrium
  b Left atrium
  c Right ventricle
  d Left ventricle

10 Which carry blood away from the heart?
  a Capillaries
  b Veins
  c Venules
  d Arteries

11 Which statement about the lymphatic system is *true*?
  a The tonsils are the largest structures in the lymphatic system.
  b Lymph transports oxygen and nutrients to cells.
  c The spleen filters bacteria and damaged cells.
  d Extra lymph from the blood is moved to the tissues.

12 Oxygen and carbon dioxide are exchanged
  a In the bronchi
  b Between the alveoli and capillaries
  c Between the lungs and pleura
  d In the trachea

13 Digestion begins in the
  a Mouth
  b Stomach
  c Small intestine
  d Colon

14 Most food absorption takes place in the
  a Stomach
  b Small intestine
  c Colon
  d Large intestine

15 Urine is formed by the
  a Jejunum
  b Kidneys
  c Bladder
  d Liver

16 Urine passes from the body through the
  a Ureters
  b Urethra
  c Anus
  d Nephrons

17 The male sex gland is called the
  a Penis
  b Semen
  c Testis
  d Scrotum

18 The male sex cell is the
  a Semen
  b Ovum
  c Gonad
  d Sperm

19 The female sex gland is the
  a Ovary
  b Cervix
  c Uterus
  d Vagina

20 The discharge of the lining of the uterus is called
  a The endometrium
  b Ovulation
  c Fertilization
  d Menstruation

21 The endocrine glands secrete
  a Hormones
  b Mucus
  c Semen
  d Antibodies

22 The immune system protects the body from
  a Low blood sugar
  b Disease and infection
  c Loss of fluid
  d Stunted growth

Answers to Chapter 8 questions are on p. 551.

FOCUS ON PRACTICE

Problem Solving

A patient has a disorder that affects the immune system. How does this affect body function? How will you provide care in a way that protects the person?

CHAPTER 9

The Older Person

OBJECTIVES

- Define the key terms and key abbreviation in this chapter.
- Identify the developmental tasks of each age-group.
- Identify the psychological and social changes common in older adulthood.
- Describe the physical changes from aging and the care required.
- Describe the gains and losses related to long-term care.
- Describe the sexual changes and needs of older persons.
- Explain how to deal with sexually aggressive persons.
- Explain how to promote PRIDE in the person, the family, and yourself.

KEY TERMS

development Changes in mental, emotional, and social function

developmental task A skill that must be completed during a stage of development

geriatrics The care of aging people

gerontology The study of the aging process

growth The physical changes that are measured and that occur in a steady, orderly manner

menopause When menstruation stops and menstrual cycles end; there has been at least 1 year without a menstrual period

sexuality The physical, emotional, social, cultural, and spiritual factors that affect a person's feelings and attitudes about his or her sex

KEY ABBREVIATION

OBRA Omnibus Budget Reconciliation Act of 1987

People live longer than ever before. They are healthier and more active. Late adulthood ranges from 65 years of age and older. The oldest-old are 85 years of age and older. Many older persons have at least 1 disability. Disabilities can interfere with daily activities.

Most older people live with a spouse, partner, children, brothers or sisters, other family, or friends. Still others live in assisted living residences or nursing centers.

Gerontology is the study of the aging process. Geriatrics is the care of aging people. Aging is normal. It is not a disease. Normal changes occur in body structure and function. The risk for illness, injury, and disability increases. Psychological and social changes also occur. Often changes are slow. Most people adjust well and lead happy, meaningful lives.

GROWTH AND DEVELOPMENT

Growth is the physical changes that are measured and that occur in a steady, orderly manner. Growth is measured in weight, height, and changes in appearance and body functions.

Development relates to changes in mental, emotional, and social function. A person behaves and thinks in certain ways in each stage of development. For example, babies depend on adults for basic needs. Adults can meet most of their basic needs without help.

Growth and development occur in a sequence, order, and pattern. Certain skills are completed during each stage. A *developmental task is a skill that must be completed during a stage of development.* A stage cannot be skipped. Each stage is the basis for the next stage. See Box 9-1.

BOX 9-1   Developmental Tasks

Infancy (Birth to 1 Year)
- Learning to walk
- Learning to eat solid foods
- Beginning to talk and communicate with others
- Learning to trust
- Beginning to have emotional relationships with parents, brothers, and sisters
- Developing stable sleep and feeding patterns

Toddlerhood (1 to 3 Years)
- Tolerating separation from the primary caregiver
- Gaining control of bowel and bladder function
- Using words to communicate
- Becoming less dependent on the primary caregiver

Preschool (3 to 6 Years)
- Increasing the ability to communicate and understand others
- Performing self-care
- Learning gender differences and developing sexual modesty
- Learning right from wrong and good from bad
- Learning to play with others
- Developing family relationships

School Age (6 to 9 or 10 Years)
- Developing the social and physical skills needed for playing games
- Learning to get along with persons of the same age-group and background (peers)
- Learning gender-appropriate behaviors and attitudes
- Learning basic reading, writing, and math skills
- Developing a conscience and morals
- Developing a good feeling and attitude about oneself

Late Childhood (9 or 10 to 12 Years)
- Becoming independent of adults and learning to depend on oneself
- Developing and keeping friendships with peers
- Understanding physical, psychological, and social changes
- Developing moral and ethical behavior
- Developing greater muscular strength, coordination, and balance
- Learning how to study

Adolescence (12 to 18 Years)
- Accepting changes in the body and appearance
- Developing appropriate relationships with others and beginning to attract partners
- Becoming independent from parents and adults
- Preparing for marriage and family life
- Preparing for a career
- Developing morals, attitudes, and values needed to function in society

Young Adulthood (18 to 40 Years)
- Choosing education and a career
- Selecting a partner
- Learning to live with a partner
- Becoming a parent and raising children
- Developing a satisfactory sex life

Middle Adulthood (40 to 65 Years)
- Adjusting to physical changes
- Having grown children
- Developing leisure-time activities
- Adjusting to aging parents

Late Adulthood (65 Years and Older)
- Adjusting to decreased strength and loss of health
- Adjusting to retirement and reduced income (Fig. 9-1)
- Coping with a partner's death
- Developing new friends and relationships
- Preparing for one's own death

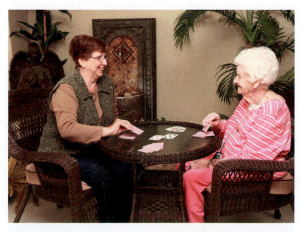

FIGURE 9-1 This retired woman is a nursing center volunteer.

PSYCHOLOGICAL AND SOCIAL CHANGES

Graying hair, wrinkles, and slow movements are physical reminders of aging. They threaten self-esteem, self-image, self-worth, and independence.

Social roles change. For example, a parent may rely on an adult child for care. Social changes include:

- *Retirement.* Retirement allows time to relax and enjoy life. Some people retire because of poor health or disability. Others have part-time jobs or do volunteer work. Work helps meet love, belonging, and self-esteem needs. The person feels useful and forms friendships.
- *Reduced income.* Retirement often means reduced income. Social Security may provide the only income. House or rent payments continue. Food, clothing, utility bills, and taxes are other expenses. Car expenses, home repairs, drugs, and health care are other costs. Severe money problems can result. Some people have income from savings, investments, retirement plans, and insurance.
- *Social relationships.* Social relationships change throughout life. Children grow up, leave home, and have families. Some live far away. Older family members and friends die, move away, or are disabled. Yet most older people have regular contact with children, grandchildren, family, and friends. Others are lonely. Separation from children is a common cause. So is lack of companionship with people their own age (Fig. 9-2). Hobbies, religious and community events, and new friends help prevent loneliness.
- *Children as caregivers.* Sometimes parents and children change roles. The child cares for the parent. Some older persons feel more secure. Others feel unwanted, in the way, and useless. Some lose dignity and self-respect. Tensions may occur among the child, parent, and other household members. Lack of privacy is a cause. So are disagreements and criticisms about housekeeping, raising children, cooking, and friends.
- *Death and grieving.* A person may try to prepare for a partner's death. When death occurs, the loss is crushing. No amount of preparation is ever enough for the emptiness and changes that result. The person loses a lover, friend, companion, and confidant. Grief may be very great. The person's life will likely change. Serious physical and mental health problems result. Some lose the will to live. Some attempt suicide.
  - *Death of a child.* Parents of any age experience great grief when a child dies. As people live longer, some out-live their adult children. Their emotional needs are great. Sadly, often few family and friends are left to provide support and comfort.

See *Focus on Communication: Psychological and Social Changes.*

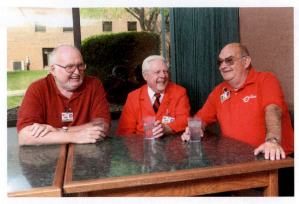

FIGURE 9-2 Older people enjoy being with others of their own age.

FOCUS ON COMMUNICATION

Psychological and Social Changes

The social changes of aging can cause loneliness. With nursing center care, the loneliness can seem greater. You can help the person feel less lonely.

- Suggest calling a family member or friend. Offer to help with phone numbers and dialing. Many residents have wireless phones.
- Keep the phone within reach. Calls can be placed or answered with greater ease.
- Suggest reading cards and letters. Offer to assist.
- Visit with the person a few times during your shift.
- Introduce new residents to other residents and staff.
- Encourage e-mailing or having video calls with family and friends. Some residents have computers with center-provided Internet access.

PHYSICAL CHANGES

Physical changes of aging happen to everyone (Table 9-1). Body processes slow. Energy level and body efficiency decline. The rate and degree of changes vary with each person. They depend on diet, health, exercise, stress, environment, heredity, and other factors. Changes are slow over many years. Often they are not seen for a long time.

TABLE 9-1	The Aging Process—Physical Changes and Care Measures
Physical Changes	**Care Measures**

Nervous System

Physical Changes:
- Brain and spinal cord lose nerve cells
- Nerve cells send messages at a slower rate
- Reflexes slow
- Reduced blood flow to the brain
- Abnormal structures can form in the brain
- Brain tissue may shrink (atrophy)
- Changes in brain cells affect personality and mental function
- Shorter memory
- Forgetfulness
- Trouble recalling recent events; long-ago events are easier to recall
- Slower ability to respond
- Confusion may occur
- Dizziness
- Sleep patterns change
  - Difficulty falling asleep
  - Waking during the night
  - Less sleep is needed
  - Going to sleep early and waking early are common
- Reduced sensitivity to pain, pressure, and touch
- Smell and taste decrease
- Eyelids thin and wrinkle
- Less tear secretion
- Pupils less responsive to light
- Decreased vision at night or in dark rooms
- Problems seeing green and blue colors
- Poor vision; problems focusing on close objects
- Changes in acoustic nerve
- Eardrums atrophy
- High-pitched sounds are hard to hear
- Earwax hardens and thickens; earwax impacted (wedged in the ear) can cause hearing loss
- Hearing loss

Care Measures:
- Practice safety measures to prevent injuries and falls.
- Remind the person to get up slowly from bed or chair.
- Follow the care plan to assist with memory, personality, or mental changes.
- Follow safety measures for heat and cold.
- Check for signs of skin breakdown and pressure injuries.
- Give good skin care.
- Prevent skin tears and pressure injuries.
- Follow the care plan to promote sleep. Day-time naps and rest may be needed.
- Have the person wear eyeglasses, contact lenses, and hearing aids as needed.
- Provide good room lighting and night-lights.
- See the following chapters for care measures.
  - Chapters 10 and 11—safety and preventing falls
  - Chapter 15—turning and moving
  - Chapter 16—getting in and out of bed or chair
  - Chapter 17—sleep
  - Chapter 28—heat and cold
  - Chapter 32—eyeglasses, contact lenses, and hearing aids
  - Chapters 34 and 35—confusion and mental changes

Integumentary System

Physical Changes:
- Skin becomes less elastic
- Skin loses strength
- Brown spots (age spots or liver spots) on the wrists and hands
- Fewer nerve endings affect temperature, pressure, and pain sensation
- Fewer blood vessels
- Fatty tissue layer is lost
- Skin thins and sags
- Skin is fragile and easily injured or burned
- Folds, lines, and wrinkles appear
- Blood vessels become more fragile
- Decreased secretion of oil and sweat glands
- Dry, itchy skin
- More sensitive to cold
- Nails become thick and tough
- Whitening or graying hair
- Facial hair in some women
- Loss or thinning of hair
- Drier hair

Care Measures:
- Protect from drafts and cold.
- Provide sweaters, lap blankets, socks, and extra blankets.
- Check thermostat settings. Higher settings are helpful.
- Provide for hygiene—shower or bath 2 times a week; partial baths on other days.
- Use mild soaps or soap substitutes to clean the underarms, genitals, and under the breasts. Soap is often avoided on the face, arms, legs, back, chest, and abdomen.
- Apply lotions and creams to prevent drying and itching.
- Provide nail and foot care.
- Prevent burns. Do not use hot water bottles or heating pads on the feet.
- Brush and shampoo hair as needed for hygiene and comfort. Shampoo frequency often decreases with age.
- Protect from prolonged sun exposure.
- See the following chapters for care measures.
  - Chapter 10—preventing burns
  - Chapters 18 and 19—hygiene, skin care, and grooming
  - Chapter 28—skin tears
  - Chapter 29—pressure injuries

Continued

TABLE 9-1	The Aging Process—Physical Changes and Care Measures—cont'd
Physical Changes	**Care Measures**
Musculo-Skeletal System • Muscles shrink (atrophy) • Muscle strength, tone, and contractility decrease • Bone mass decreases • Bones become weaker • Bones become brittle; can break easily • Vertebrae shorten • Joints become stiff and painful • Hip and knee joints become flexed (bent) • Gradual loss of height; trunk becomes shorter • Decreased mobility	• Promote exercise and activity as ordered to prevent atrophy and loss of strength. • Assist with range-of-motion exercises as ordered (Chapter 27). • Encourage a diet high in protein, calcium, and vitamins as ordered. • Practice safety measures to prevent injuries and falls (Chapters 10 and 11). • Turn and move the person gently and carefully. • Assist the person in getting out of bed or chair as needed. • Provide support when walking as needed (Chapter 27).
Circulatory System • Heart pumps with less force • Heart valves thicken and become stiff • Heart rate may slow • Abnormal heart rhythms may occur • Heart may enlarge slightly • Heart walls thicken • Arteries narrow and become stiffer • Less blood flows through narrowed arteries • Weakened heart works harder to pump blood through narrowed vessels • Number of red blood cells decreases • Fatigue	• Follow the person's activity limits. • Promote exercise as ordered. Encourage the person to be as active as possible. Moderate daily exercise helps maintain health and well-being. • Assist with range-of-motion exercises as ordered. • Avoid over-exertion. The person should not walk far, climb many stairs, or carry heavy things. Encourage rest periods. • Encourage bedrest if ordered. Bedrest means being confined to bed. • Keep personal care items, TV controls, phone, and other needed items within reach.
Respiratory System • Respiratory muscles weaken • Some lung tissue is lost • Lung tissue becomes less elastic • Chest is less able to stretch to breathe • Difficulty breathing (dyspnea) • Decreased strength for coughing and clearing the airway	• Promote normal breathing. • Position the person for easier breathing. Semi-Fowler's or Fowler's position (Chapter 14) may be preferred. • Assist with coughing and deep-breathing exercises as ordered (Chapter 30). • Avoid heavy bed linens over the chest. • Turn and position the person according to the care plan. Persons on bedrest are re-positioned often. • Encourage activity as ordered.
Digestive System • Decreased saliva production • Difficulty swallowing (dysphagia) • Decreased appetite • Decreased secretion of digestive juices • Difficulty digesting fried and fatty foods • Indigestion • Loss of teeth • Decreased peristalsis causing flatulence (gas) and constipation	• Provide oral hygiene and denture care to improve taste. • Encourage diet as ordered (Chapter 23). Dry, fried, fatty, and hard-to-chew foods are avoided. The person may need food ground, chopped, or pureed. • Promote fluid intake as ordered (Chapter 24). Thickened liquids may be needed for persons with swallowing problems. • Follow the care plan to prevent flatulence (gas) and constipation (Chapter 22). High-fiber foods help prevent constipation. Some are hard to chew and irritate the intestines. Apricots, celery, and fruits and vegetables with skins and seeds are avoided.
Urinary System • Kidney function decreases • Reduced blood supply to kidneys • Kidneys atrophy • Bladder tissues less able to stretch • Bladder muscles weaken • Bladder may not empty completely • Urinary tract infections may occur • Urinary frequency, urgency, incontinence (loss of bladder control), or night-time urination may occur • Prostate gland enlarges (men)	• Answer call lights promptly. • Promote normal urination (Chapter 20). • Provide the bedpan, urinal, or commode as needed. • Follow the care plan to manage incontinence. • Provide catheter care according to the care plan (Chapter 21). • Encourage fluids as ordered to prevent urinary tract infections. Most fluids should be taken before 5:00 PM (1700) to reduce the need to urinate at night. • Follow the person's bladder training program (Chapter 20).

TABLE 9-1	The Aging Process—Physical Changes and Care Measures—cont'd
Physical Changes	**Care Measures**
Reproductive System	

• Men
  • Testosterone decreases slightly
  • Erections take longer
  • Longer phase between erection and orgasm
  • Less forceful orgasms
  • Erections lost quickly
  • Longer time between erections
• Women
  • *Menopause—when menstruation stops and menstrual cycles end; there has been at least 1 year without a menstrual period*
  • Estrogen and progesterone decrease
  • Uterus, vagina, and genitalia atrophy
  • Thinning of vaginal walls
  • Vaginal dryness
  • Arousal takes longer
  • Less intense orgasms
  • Quicker return to pre-excitement state
	• Follow the care plan for the person with reproductive changes.

NURSING CENTER CARE

Some older persons cannot care for themselves. Nursing centers are options for them (Chapter 1). Some people stay in nursing centers until death. Others return home. The nursing center is the person's temporary or permanent home. The setting is as home-like as possible (Fig. 9-3).

The person needing nursing center care may suffer some or all of these losses.
- Loss of identity as a productive member of a family and community
- Loss of possessions—home, household items, car, and so on
- Loss of independence
- Loss of real-world experiences—shopping, traveling, cooking, driving, hobbies, and so on
- Loss of health and mobility

The person may feel useless, powerless, and hopeless. The health team helps the person cope with loss and improve quality of life. Treat the person with dignity and respect. Also practice good communication skills. Follow the care plan.

SEXUALITY

Sex is the physical activities involving the body and reproductive organs. *Sexuality is the physical, emotional, social, cultural, and spiritual factors that affect a person's feelings and attitudes about his or her sex.* Sexuality involves the personality and the body—how a person behaves, thinks, dresses, and responds to others.

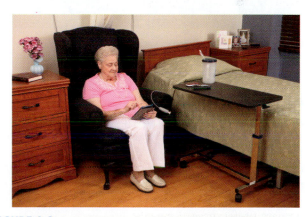

FIGURE 9-3 A nursing center is as home-like as possible. Some centers allow residents to bring their own bed and furniture from home.

Love, affection, and intimacy are needed throughout life (Fig. 9-4, p. 104). Older persons love, fall in love, hold hands, and embrace. Many have intercourse.

Frequency of sex may decrease. Besides life events, reasons relate to weakness, fatigue, and pain. Reduced mobility, aging, and chronic illness are other factors.

Some older people do not have intercourse. This does not mean loss of sexual needs or desires. Often needs are expressed in other ways. They hold hands, touch, caress, and embrace. These bring closeness and intimacy.

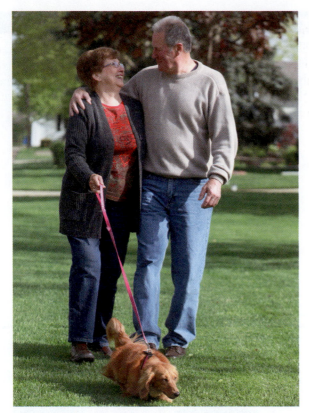

FIGURE 9-4 Love and affection are important to persons of all ages.

BOX 9-2	Promoting Sexuality

- Let the person practice grooming routines. Assist as needed. See Chapter 19.
- Let the person choose clothing. Patient gowns can embarrass the person. Street clothes are worn if the person's condition permits.
- Protect the right to privacy. Do not expose the person. Drape and screen the person.
- Treat the person with dignity and respect. The person may not share your sexual attitudes, values, or practices. The person may have a pre-marital or extra-marital relationship. Do not judge or gossip about the person.
- Allow privacy. If the person has a private room, close the door for privacy. Some agencies have DO NOT DISTURB signs for doors. Let the person and partner know how much time they have alone. For example, remind them about meal times and care measures. Tell other staff that the person wants time alone.
- Knock before you enter any room. This simple courtesy shows respect for privacy.
- Consider the person's roommate. Privacy curtains do not block sound. Arrange for privacy when the roommate is out of the room. A roommate may offer to leave for a while. Or the nurse finds a private area.
- Allow privacy for masturbation. It is a normal form of sexual expression. Close the privacy curtain and the door. Knock before you enter the room. This saves you and the person embarrassment. Sometimes confused persons masturbate in public areas. Lead the person to a private area. Or distract him or her with an activity.

Meeting Sexual Needs

The nursing team promotes the meeting of sexual needs. The measures in Box 9-2 may be part of the person's care plan.

Married couples in nursing centers can share the same room. This is a requirement of the *Omnibus Budget Reconciliation Act of 1987 (OBRA)*. Non-married persons may have roommate preferences.

Sometimes relationships develop between residents. They are allowed time together, not kept apart. To protect against sexual abuse, relationships must be consensual (Chapter 4). *Consensual* involves *giving consent*.

The Sexually Aggressive Person

Some persons flirt or make sexual advances or comments. Some expose themselves, masturbate, or touch staff. Often there are reasons for the person's behavior. Understanding this helps you deal with the matter.

Causes of sexually aggressive behaviors include:
- Nervous system disorders
- Confusion, disorientation, and dementia
- Drug side effects
- Fever
- Poor vision

The person may confuse someone with his or her partner. Or the person cannot control the behavior. The healthy person controls sexual urges. Changes in the brain and mental function make control difficult. Sexual behavior in these cases is usually innocent.

Sometimes touch is used to gain attention. For example, a person cannot speak or move the right side. Your buttocks are near the person. To get your attention, the person touches your buttocks. The behavior is not sexual.

Sometimes masturbation is a sexually aggressive behavior. However, touching the genitals may signal a health problem. Urinary or reproductive system disorders can cause genital soreness and itching. So can poor hygiene and being wet or soiled from urine or feces.

Touch can have a sexual purpose. For example, a person wants to prove he or she is attractive and can perform sexually. You must be professional about the matter.

- Ask the person not to touch you. State the places where you were touched.
- Tell the person that you will not do what he or she wants.
- Tell the person what behaviors make you uncomfortable. Politely ask the person not to act that way.
- Allow privacy if the person is becoming aroused. Provide for safety. Complete a safety check of the room (see the inside of the front cover). Tell the person when you will return.
- Discuss the matter with the nurse. The nurse can help you understand the behavior.
- Follow the care plan. It has measures to deal with sexually aggressive behaviors. They are based on the cause of the behavior.

See *Focus on Communication: The Sexually Aggressive Person.*

Protecting the Person

The person must be protected from unwanted sexual comments and advances. This is sexual abuse (Chapter 4). Tell the nurse right away. No one is allowed to sexually abuse another person. This includes staff members, patients, residents, family members or other visitors, and volunteers.

Circle the BEST answer.

1 Which is a developmental task of late adulthood?
   a Accepting changes in appearance
   b Adjusting to decreased strength
   c Developing a satisfactory sex life
   d Performing self-care

2 Retirement usually means
   a Lowered income
   b Changes from aging
   c Less free time
   d Financial security

3 Which causes loneliness in older persons?
   a Having hobbies
   b Children moving away
   c Attending community events
   d Contact with other older persons

4 Which statement about a partner's death is *true?*
   a The surviving partner's life will not likely change.
   b Preparing for the event lessens grief.
   c Grief cannot cause physical problems.
   d Feelings of loss and emptiness occur.

5 Skin changes occur with aging. Care should include
   a Keeping the room cool
   b A daily bath with soap
   c Applying lotion
   d Bathing in hot water

6 Musculo-skeletal changes occur with aging. Which is *true?*
   a Bones become firm.
   b Exercise promotes muscle atrophy.
   c Joints become stiff and painful.
   d Bedrest prevents loss of strength.

7 Changes occur in the nervous system. Which is *true?*
   a Less sleep is needed than when younger.
   b The person forgets events from long ago.
   c Sensitivity to pressure increases.
   d Confusion occurs in all older persons.

8 Changes occur in the eye with aging. Which is *true?*
   a Tear secretion increases.
   b There is no change in seeing colors.
   c There is more trouble focusing on far objects.
   d Vision is poor at night and in dark rooms.

9 Which is *true* of hearing loss in older persons?
   a Low-pitched sounds are hard to hear.
   b Acoustic nerve changes affect hearing.
   c Earwax cannot affect hearing.
   d Ear infections often cause hearing loss.

10 An older person has circulatory changes. Which care measure would you question?
   a Keep needed items nearby
   b Get a moderate amount of daily exercise
   c Avoid over-exertion
   d Take long walks

11 Respiratory changes occur with aging. Which is *true?*
   a Heavy bed linens are used.
   b The person is turned often if on bedrest.
   c The side-lying position is best for breathing.
   d Deep breathing is avoided.

12 Older persons should avoid dry foods because of
   a Decreases in saliva
   b Decreased appetite
   c Increased amounts of digestive juices
   d Increased peristalsis

13 An older person is at risk for a urinary tract infection. The doctor ordered increased fluid intake. You should
   a Give most of the fluid before 1700 (5:00 PM)
   b Question the order
   c Start a bladder training program
   d Insert a catheter

14 Reproductive organs change with aging.
   a True
   b False

15 A person is masturbating in the dining room. You should
   a Do nothing
   b Scold the person
   c Quietly take the person to his or her room
   d Restrain the person

16 A person touches you sexually. You should
   a Ignore the behavior
   b Push the person away from you
   c Tell your co-workers
   d Ask the person not to touch you

Answers to Chapter 9 questions are on p. 551.

FOCUS ON PRACTICE

Problem Solving

A person has urinary incontinence and swallowing problems due to changes from aging. A co-worker uses the term "diaper" to describe incontinence products and "bib" for clothing protectors. The co-worker threatens to with-hold privileges if the person does not finish meals.

   Why should you treat the person as an adult and not a child? Describe ways to provide age-appropriate care. How will you respond to your co-worker's statements and actions?

Safety Needs

CHAPTER 10

OBJECTIVES

- Define the key terms and key abbreviations in this chapter.
- Describe accident risk factors.
- Explain why you identify a person before giving care.
- Explain how to correctly identify a person.
- Describe the safety measures to prevent burns, poisoning, and suffocation.
- Identify the signs and causes of choking.
- Explain how to prevent equipment accidents.
- Explain how to handle hazardous chemicals.

- Identify natural and human-made disasters.
- Describe fire prevention measures and oxygen safety.
- Explain what to do during a fire.
- Explain how to protect yourself from workplace violence.
- Describe your role in risk management.
- Perform the procedures described in this chapter.
- Explain how to promote PRIDE in the person, the family, and yourself.

KEY TERMS

coma A state of being unaware of one's setting and being unable to react or respond to people, places, or things

dementia The loss of cognitive and social function caused by changes in the brain

disaster A sudden, catastrophic event in which people are injured and killed and property is destroyed

elopement When a patient or resident leaves the agency without staff knowledge

hazardous chemical Any chemical that is a physical hazard or a health hazard

paralysis Loss of muscle function, sensation, or both

poison Any substance harmful to the body when ingested, inhaled, injected, or absorbed through the skin

suffocation When breathing stops from the lack of oxygen

workplace violence Violent acts (including assault or threat of assault) directed toward persons at work or while on duty

KEY ABBREVIATIONS

AED	Automated external defibrillator
CPR	Cardiopulmonary resuscitation
EMS	Emergency Medical Services
FBAO	Foreign-body airway obstruction
ID	Identification

PASS	*Pull* the safety pin, *aim* low, *squeeze* the lever, *sweep* back and forth
RACE	Rescue, alarm, confine, extinguish
RRT	Rapid Response Team
SDS	Safety data sheet

Safety is a basic need. Patients and residents are at great risk for accidents and falls. (See Chapter 11 for falls.) Some accidents and injuries cause death.

You must protect patients, residents, visitors, co-workers, and yourself. The goal is to decrease the person's risk of accidents and injuries without limiting mobility and independence. The care plan lists other safety measures for the person.

See *Focus on Surveys: Safety Needs*, p. 108.
See *Promoting Safety and Comfort: Safety Needs*, p. 108.

ACCIDENT RISK FACTORS

Some people cannot protect themselves. They rely on others for safety. Certain factors increase the risk of accidents and injuries. Follow the person's care plan.

- *Age.* Children and older persons are at risk for injuries. Changes from aging increase the risk for falls and other injuries. Many older persons have decreased strength and move slowly. Some are unsteady. Older persons also are less sensitive to heat and cold. Vision and hearing problems are common. Confusion, poor judgment, memory problems, and disorientation may occur (Chapter 35). See *Focus on Older Persons: Accident Risk Factors (Age).*
- *Awareness of surroundings.* Confused and disoriented persons may not understand what is happening to and around them. A coma can occur from illness or injury. **Coma** *is a state of being unaware of one's setting and being unable to react or respond to people, places, or things.*
- *Agitated and aggressive behaviors.* Pain can cause these behaviors. So can confusion, decreased awareness of surroundings, and fear of what may happen.
- *Vision loss.* Persons with poor vision can fall or trip over toys, rugs, equipment, furniture, and cords. Some cannot read container labels. Poisoning can result.
- *Hearing loss.* Persons with hearing loss have problems hearing the spoken word. They may not hear warning signals or fire alarms. Some cannot hear approaching meal carts, drug carts, stretchers, or wheelchairs. They do not know to move to safety.
- *Impaired smell and touch.* Illness and aging affect smell and touch. The person may not detect smoke or gas odors. Burns are a risk from impaired touch. The person has problems sensing heat and cold. Some people have a decreased sense of pain. They may be unaware of injury.
- *Impaired mobility.* Some diseases and injuries affect mobility. Aware of a danger, the person may not be able to move to safety. Some persons cannot walk or propel wheelchairs. Some persons are paralyzed. **Paralysis** *means loss of muscle function, sensation, or both.*
- *Drugs.* Drug side effects may include loss of balance, drowsiness, and lack of coordination. Reduced awareness, confusion, and disorientation may occur.

IDENTIFYING THE PERSON

Each person has different treatments, therapies, and activity limits. Life and health are threatened from the wrong care.

The person may receive an identification (ID) bracelet when admitted to the agency (Fig. 10-1). The bracelet has the person's name, ID number, room and bed number, birth date, age, doctor, and other identifying information.

You use the bracelet to identify the person before giving care. Your assignment sheet states what care to give. To identify the person:

- Compare identifying information on the assignment sheet with that on the ID bracelet (Fig. 10-2). Carefully check the information. Some people have the same first and last names. For example, John Smith is a very common name.
- Use at least 2 identifiers. An identifier cannot be the person's room or bed number. Some agencies require the person to state and spell his or her name and give his or her birth date. Others require using the person's ID number. Always follow agency policy.
- Call the person by name when checking the ID bracelet. This is a courtesy as you touch the person and before giving care. Just calling the person by name is not enough for identification. Confused, disoriented, drowsy, hard-of-hearing, or distracted persons may answer to any name.

See *Focus on Communication: Identifying the Person.*
See *Promoting Safety and Comfort: Identifying the Person.*

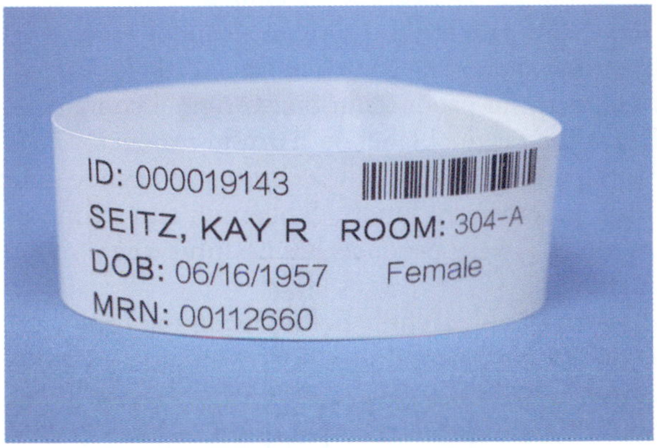

FIGURE 10-1 ID bracelet.

FOCUS ON COMMUNICATION
Identifying the Person

To identify the person, call the person by name. Ask to see the ID bracelet. For example: "Hello, Mr. Hall. May I see your ID bracelet?" Then ask for 2 identifiers. You can say: "Please tell me your full name and birth date." Compare the identifiers with the information on the ID bracelet and your assignment sheet.

For some persons, identifying themselves is annoying. The person may say: "Do I have to say it again? You know who I am." Be polite. Explain why you check the person's identity. You can say: "It is important to check so I give care to the right person. It is for your safety." Thank the person. Use his or her title and name. For example: "Thank you, Mr. Hall."

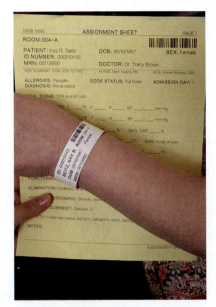

FIGURE 10-2 The ID bracelet is checked against the assignment sheet to accurately identify the person.

PROMOTING SAFETY AND COMFORT
Identifying the Person

Safety

Always identify the person before starting a task or procedure. Do not identify the person and then leave the room for supplies and equipment. You could go to the wrong room and give care to the wrong person. And the person for whom the care was intended would not receive it. This too could cause harm.

Sometimes ID bracelets are damaged from water, spilled food and fluids, and every-day wear and tear. If you cannot read the information on the ID bracelet, tell the nurse. The nurse can have a new bracelet made.

Comfort

Make sure ID bracelets are not too loose or too tight. You should be able to slide 1 or 2 fingers under a bracelet. If it is too loose or too tight, tell the nurse.

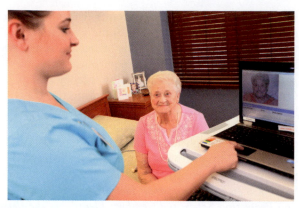

FIGURE 10-3 The nursing assistant uses the photo to identify the person.

Identifying Nursing Center Residents

Alert and oriented residents may choose not to wear ID bracelets. This is noted on the person's care plan. Follow center policy and the care plan to identify the person.

Some nursing centers use photo ID systems (Fig. 10-3). The person's photo is taken on admission for his or her medical record. If your center uses such a system, learn to use it safely.

PREVENTING BURNS

Smoking, spilled hot liquids, electrical items, and very hot water (sinks, tubs, showers) are common causes of burns. The safety measures in Box 10-1 can prevent burns.

See *Focus on Older Persons: Preventing Burns.*

PREVENTING POISONING

A *poison* is any substance harmful to the body when ingested, inhaled, injected, or absorbed through the skin. Drugs and household products are common poisons. Poisoning in adults may be from carelessness, confusion, or poor vision when reading labels. As a result, a person may take too much of a drug. To prevent poisoning:

- Make sure patients and residents cannot reach hazardous materials and chemicals (p. 115).
- Keep harmful products in their original containers.
- Leave the original label on harmful products.
- Store personal care items according to agency policy. Soap, mouthwash, lotion, deodorant, and shampoo are examples. These products are harmful when swallowed.
- Read all labels carefully before using the product.
- Do not leave harmful products unattended when in use.
- Store harmful products according to agency policy.

See *Promoting Safety and Comfort: Preventing Poisoning.*

PREVENTING SUFFOCATION

Suffocation is when breathing stops from the lack of oxygen. Death occurs if the person does not start breathing. Common causes include choking, drowning, inhaling gas or smoke, strangulation, and electrical shock (p. 114).

Measures to prevent suffocation are listed in Box 10-2. Clear the airway if the person is choking.

Choking

Foreign bodies can obstruct the airway. This is called *choking* or *foreign-body airway obstruction (FBAO)*. Air cannot pass through the airways into the lungs. The body does not get enough oxygen. Death can result.

Choking often occurs during eating. A large, poorly chewed piece of meat is the most common cause. Laughing and talking while eating also are common causes. So is excessive alcohol intake.

Unconscious persons can choke. Common causes are aspiration of vomitus and the tongue falling back into the airway.

Foreign bodies can cause mild or severe airway obstruction. With *mild airway obstruction*, some air moves in and out of the lungs. The person is conscious and usually can speak. Often forceful coughing can remove the object. Breathing may sound like wheezing between coughs. For mild airway obstruction:

- Stay with the person.
- Encourage the person to keep coughing to expel the object.
- Do not interrupt the person's efforts to clear the airway. If the person is breathing and coughing, abdominal thrusts are not needed.
- If the obstruction persists, call for help.

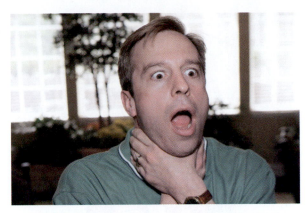

FIGURE 10-4 A choking person clutches at the throat.

A person with *severe airway obstruction* has difficulty breathing. Air does not move in and out of the lungs. The person may not be able to breathe, speak, or cough. If able to cough, the cough is of poor quality. When the person tries to inhale (breathe in), there is no noise or a high-pitched noise. The person may appear pale and *cyanotic* (bluish color).

The conscious person usually clutches at the throat (Fig. 10-4). Clutching at the throat is often called the *universal sign of choking*. The conscious person is very frightened. If the obstruction is not removed, the person will die. Severe airway obstruction is an emergency.

See *Focus on Older Persons: Choking.*

FOCUS ON OLDER PERSONS

Choking

Older persons are at risk for choking. Weakness, dentures that fit poorly, *dysphagia* (difficulty swallowing), and chronic illness are common causes.

Relieving Choking. *Abdominal thrusts* are used to relieve severe airway obstruction. Abdominal thrusts are quick, upward thrusts to the abdomen. This is also known as the *Heimlich maneuver*. The thrusts force air out of the lungs and create an artificial cough. They are done to try to expel the foreign body from the airway.

You may observe a person choking. And you may perform emergency measures to relieve choking. Relief of choking occurs when the foreign body is removed. Or it occurs when you feel air move and see the chest rise and fall when giving rescue breaths. The person may still be unresponsive.

If you assist a choking person, report and record what happened. Include what you did and the person's response.

Chest thrusts are used for obese or pregnant persons (Fig. 10-5, p. 112). If you are alone and choking, perform self-administered abdominal thrusts. See Box 10-3, p. 112.

See procedure: *Relieving Choking—Adult or Child (Over 1 Year of Age)*, p. 112.

BOX 10-2 Preventing Suffocation

- Cut foods into small, bite-sized pieces for persons who cannot do so themselves.
- Make sure dentures fit properly and are in place.
- Make sure the person can chew and swallow the food served.
- Report loose teeth or dentures.
- Check the care plan for swallowing problems before serving food (including snacks) or fluids. The person may ask for something that he or she cannot swallow.
- Tell the nurse at once if the person has swallowing problems.
- Do not give oral foods or fluids to persons with feeding tubes (Chapter 23).
- Follow aspiration precautions (Chapter 23).
- Do not leave a person unattended in a bathtub or shower.
- Move all persons from the area if you smell smoke.
- Position the person in bed properly (Chapter 17).
- Use bed rails correctly (Chapter 11).
- Use restraints correctly (Chapter 12).
- Prevent entrapment in the bed system (Chapter 17).
- Do not use power strips for care equipment.
- See "Preventing Equipment Accidents" (p. 114).

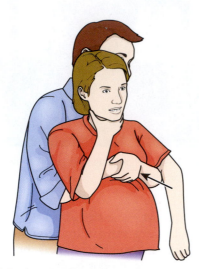

FIGURE 10-5 Chest thrusts to relieve choking in a pregnant woman.

BOX 10-3	Relieving Choking

Chest Thrusts for Obese or Pregnant Persons
1 Stand behind the person.
2 Place your arms under the person's underarms. Wrap your arms around the person's chest.
3 Make a fist. Place the thumb side of the fist on the middle of the sternum (breastbone).
4 Grasp the fist with your other hand.
5 Give chest thrusts until the object is expelled or the person becomes unresponsive.
6 If the person becomes unresponsive, have someone activate the Emergency Medical Services (EMS) system or the agency's Rapid Response Team (RRT) if not already done. This team quickly responds to give care in life-threatening situations. Start cardiopulmonary resuscitation (CPR). See Chapter 36.

Self-Administered Abdominal Thrusts
1 Make a fist with 1 hand.
2 Place the thumb side of the fist above your navel and below the lower end of the sternum.
3 Grasp your fist with your other hand.
4 Press inward and upward quickly.
5 Press the upper abdomen against a hard surface if the thrust did not relieve the obstruction. Use the back of a chair, a table, or a railing.
6 Use as many thrusts as needed.

Basic Life Support guidelines are updated as new information becomes available. You are responsible for following current guidelines. Updates can be found on-line at the American Heart Association's website.

Relieving Choking—Adult or Child (Over 1 Year of Age)

PROCEDURE

1 Ask the person if he or she is choking.
   a *If the person can cough or talk,* see p. 111 for mild airway obstruction.
   b *If the person is unresponsive,* you may not know the cause. Call for help and begin CPR. See Chapter 36.
   c *If the person nods "yes" and cannot talk,* continue to step 2.
2 Have someone call for help.
   a *In a public area,* have someone activate the EMS system by calling 911. Send someone to get an automated external defibrillator (AED) (Chapter 36).
   b *In an agency,* have someone call the agency's RRT and get a defibrillator (AED).
3 Give abdominal thrusts.
   a Stand or kneel behind the person.
   b Wrap your arms around the person's waist.
   c Make a fist with 1 hand.
   d Place the thumb side of the fist against the abdomen. The fist is slightly above the navel in the middle of the abdomen and well below the end of the sternum (breastbone). See Figure 10-6, *A*.
   e Grasp your fist with your other hand (Fig. 10-6, *B*).
   f Press your fist into the abdomen with a quick, upward thrust (Fig. 10-7).
   g Repeat thrusts until the object is expelled or the person becomes unresponsive.
4 *If the object is dislodged,* encourage hospital care. Injuries can occur from abdominal thrusts.

5 *If the person becomes unresponsive:*
   a Lower the person to the floor or ground. Position the person supine (lying flat on the back).
   b Make sure the EMS or RRT was called.
      1 *If alone with a phone,* use it while giving care.
      2 *If alone without a phone,* give about 2 minutes of CPR first. Then call the EMS or RRT and get an AED.
   c Start CPR. See Chapter 36. Do not check for a pulse.
      1 Begin with compressions. Give 30 compressions.
      2 Use the head tilt–chin lift method to open the airway (Fig. 10-8). Open wide the person's mouth. Look for an object. Remove the object if you can see it and can remove it easily.
      3 Give 2 breaths.
      4 Continue cycles of 30 compressions and 2 breaths. Look for an object every time you open the airway.
   d *If choking is relieved,* check for a response, breathing, and a pulse. (NOTE: Choking is relieved when you feel air move and see the chest rise and fall when giving breaths.)
      1 *If no response, no normal breathing, and no pulse*—continue CPR. Use the AED as soon as possible (Chapter 36).
      2 *If no response and no normal breathing but there is a pulse*—give rescue breaths. For an adult, give 1 breath every 5 to 6 seconds. For a child, give 1 breath every 3 to 5 seconds. Check for a pulse about every 2 minutes. If no pulse, begin CPR.
      3 *If the person has normal breathing and a pulse*—place the person in the recovery position if there is no response (Chapter 36). Continue to check the person until help arrives. Encourage hospital care.

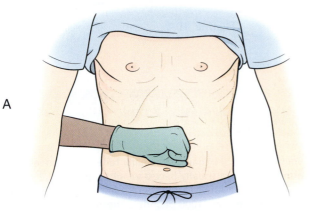

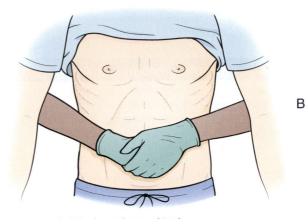

FIGURE 10-6 Hand positioning for abdominal thrusts. **A,** The fist is slightly above the navel in the mid-line of the abdomen. **B,** The other hand clasps the fist.

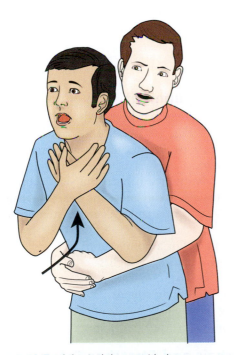

FIGURE 10-7 Abdominal thrusts with the person standing.

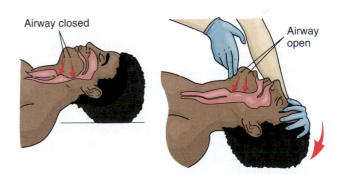

Airway closed

Airway open

FIGURE 10-8 The head tilt–chin lift method opens the airway. One hand is on the person's forehead. Pressure is applied to tilt the head back. The chin is lifted with the fingers of the other hand.

PREVENTING EQUIPMENT ACCIDENTS

All equipment is unsafe if broken, not used correctly, or not working properly. This includes hospital beds. Inspect all equipment before use. Check all items for cracks, chips, and sharp or rough edges. They can cause cuts, stabs, or scratches. Follow the Bloodborne Pathogen Standard (Chapter 13). Also practice the safety measures in Box 10-4.

See *Promoting Safety and Comfort: Preventing Equipment Accidents.*

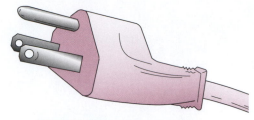

FIGURE 10-9 A three-pronged plug.

BOX 10-4	Preventing Equipment Accidents

General Safety
- Follow agency policies and procedures.
- Follow the manufacturer's instructions. Use equipment correctly.
- Read all caution and warning labels.
- Do not use an unfamiliar item. Ask for training. Also ask a nurse to supervise you the first time you use the item.
- Use an item only for its intended purpose.
- Make sure the item works before you begin.
- Have all needed equipment before you begin. For example, you need an outlet to plug in an item.
- Show a broken or damaged item to the nurse. Follow the nurse's instructions and agency policies for discarding items or sending them for repair.
- Do not try to repair broken or damaged items.
- Do not use broken or damaged items.

Electrical Safety
- Check cords and equipment for damage. Make sure they are in good repair.
- Use 3-pronged plugs on all electrical devices (Fig. 10-9). Make sure all prongs are intact.
- Avoid using extension cords. If you need one, use it for only 1 device. This prevents over-loading a circuit.
- Do not use power strips for care equipment.
- Do not cover or run any cord under rugs, carpets, linens, or other materials.
- Connect a bed power cord directly to a wall outlet. Do not connect a bed power cord to an extension cord or power strip.
- Do not use electrical items owned by the person until they are safety checked. The maintenance staff does this.
- Keep electrical items away from water.
- Keep work areas clean and dry. Wipe up spills right away.
- Do not touch electrical items if you are wet, if your hands are wet, if you are in water, or if you are standing in water. This includes using a phone when it is plugged into a charger.
- Do not put a finger or any item into an outlet.
- Turn off equipment before unplugging it. Sparks occur when electrical items are unplugged while turned on.
- Hold on to the plug (not the cord) when removing it from an outlet.
- Do not give showers or tub baths during storms. Lightning can travel through pipes.
- Do not use electrical items or phones during storms.
- Do not use water to put out an electrical fire. If possible, turn off or unplug the item.
- Do not touch a person having an electrical shock. If possible, turn off or unplug the item. Call for help at once.
- Keep electrical cords away from heating vents and other heat sources.
- Turn off the device when done using the item.
- Unplug all devices when not in use.

PROMOTING SAFETY AND COMFORT
Preventing Equipment Accidents

Safety

Beds, chairs, wheelchairs, stretchers, toilets, commodes, and other equipment usually have a weight capacity of 250 to 350 pounds. Bariatric patients and residents can weigh from 250 pounds to over 1000 pounds. Bariatric equipment is labeled:
- BARIATRIC
- "EC" for "expanded capacity"
- With the weight limit suggested by the manufacturer

Do not use the item if the person's weight is greater than the weight capacity. Follow the nurse's directions and the care plan.

Electrical Equipment

Electrical items must work properly and be in good repair. Frayed cords (Fig. 10-10, *A*) and over-loaded electrical outlets (Fig. 10-10, *B*) can cause fires, burns, and electrical shocks. *Electrical shock* is when electrical current passes through the body. It can burn the skin, muscles, nerves, and other tissues. It can affect the heart and cause death.

Warning signs of a faulty electrical item include:
- Shocks
- Loss of power or a power surge
- Dimming or flickering lights
- Sparks
- Sizzling or buzzing sounds
- Burning odor
- Loose plugs

Wheelchair and Stretcher Safety

Wheelchairs are useful for people who cannot walk or who have severe problems walking. Stretchers are used to transport persons who cannot use wheelchairs. They cannot sit up or must lie down.

The person can fall from the wheelchair or stretcher. Or the person can fall during transfers to and from the wheelchair or stretcher. See Chapter 16 for wheelchair and stretcher safety.

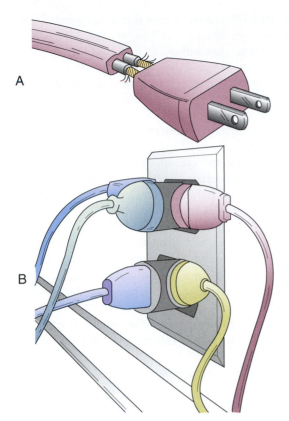

FIGURE 10-10 A, A frayed electrical cord. **B,** An over-loaded electrical outlet.

Health Hazard	Flame
• Carcinogen • Mutagenicity • Reproductive Toxicity • Respiratory Sensitizer • Target Organ Toxicity • Aspiration Toxicity	• Flammables • Pyrophorics • Self-Heating • Emits Flammable Gas • Self-Reactives • Organic Peroxides
Exclamation Mark	**Gas Cylinder**
• Irritant (skin and eye) • Skin Sensitizer • Acute Toxicity • Narcotic Effects • Respiratory Tract Irritant • Hazardous to Ozone Layer (Non-Mandatory)	• Gases Under Pressure
Flame Over Circle	**Skull and Crossbones**
• Oxidizers	• Acute Toxicity (fatal or toxic)

FIGURE 10-11 Some pictograms from the Occupational Safety and Health Administration. Depending on the chemical, the warning label contains the necessary pictograms and associated health hazards. (Redrawn from OSHA Quick Card™, OSHA® Occupational Safety and Health Administration, U.S. Department of Labor, Washington, DC.)

HAZARDOUS CHEMICALS

A *hazardous chemical is any chemical that is a physical hazard or a health hazard. Physical hazards* can cause fires or explosions. *Health hazards* can cause health problems. Health hazards can:

* Cause cancer.
* Affect blood cell formation and function.
* Damage the kidneys, nervous system, lungs, skin, eyes, or mucous membranes.
* Cause birth defects, miscarriages, and fertility problems.

Exposure to hazardous chemicals can occur from equipment failures, container ruptures, or the release of a hazard into the workplace. Workplace hazards include:

* Latex gloves (Chapter 13)
* Thermometers and blood pressure equipment containing mercury (Chapter 25)
* Cleaners and disinfectants (Chapter 13)

Your agency provides hazardous chemical training. It also provides eyewash and total body wash stations where hazardous chemicals are used.

Labeling

Hazardous chemical containers have warning labels. The warning labels contain *pictograms*—symbols used to communicate specific information about a chemical hazard. See Figure 10-11 for examples.

If a warning label is removed or damaged, do not use the substance. Show the container to the nurse and explain the problem. Do not leave the container unattended.

Safety Data Sheets

Every hazardous chemical has a *safety data sheet (SDS)*. Some agencies use the term *material safety data sheet (MSDS)*. Information provided includes:

* Name and common names
* Hazards about the chemical
* First aid measures
* Fire-fighting measures
* Safe handling and storage measures
* Personal protection measures

Check the SDS before using a hazardous chemical, cleaning up a leak or spill, or disposing of the substance. Call for the nurse about a leak or spill right away. Do not leave a leak or spill unattended.

DISASTERS

A *disaster is a sudden, catastrophic event. People are injured and killed. Property is destroyed.* Natural disasters include tornadoes, hurricanes, blizzards, earthquakes, volcano eruptions, floods, and some fires. Human-made disasters include auto, bus, train, and airplane accidents. They also include fires, bombings, nuclear power plant accidents, gas or chemical leaks, explosions, and wars.

Communities, fire and police departments, and health care agencies have disaster plans. They include caring for people needing treatment. The disaster plan includes agency evacuation procedures.

See *Focus on Surveys: Disasters*, p. 116.

Bomb Threats

Follow agency procedures for a bomb threat or if you find an item that looks or sounds strange. Bomb threats can be sent by phone, mail, e-mail, text message, messenger, or other means. Or the person can leave a bomb in the agency. If you see a stranger or strange item or package in the agency, tell the nurse at once. You cannot be too safe.

Fire Safety

Faulty electrical equipment and wiring, over-loaded electrical circuits, and smoking are major causes of fires. The health team must prevent fires and act quickly during a fire. See Box 10-5.

BOX 10-5   Fire Prevention Measures

- Follow the safety measures:
  - For oxygen use (See "Fire and Oxygen.")
  - To prevent equipment accidents (p. 114)
  - To prevent burns (p. 110)
- Practice smoking and ashtray safety.
  - Supervise persons who smoke. This is very important for persons who are confused, disoriented, or sedated.
  - Provide ashtrays.
  - Empty ashtrays only when sure that all ashes, cigars, cigarettes, and other smoking materials are out.
  - Empty ashtrays into a metal container partially filled with sand or water. Do not empty ashtrays into plastic containers or wastebaskets lined with paper or plastic bags.
  - Smoke only where allowed to do so.
- Keep matches, lighters, flammable liquids and materials away from children and confused or disoriented persons.
- Light matches carefully.
  - Be alert for sparks when lighting a match. The sparks can ignite materials that can burn.
  - Keep your hair, clothing, and anything that will burn away from the match and flame.
- Do not leave cooking unattended on stoves, in ovens, or in microwave ovens.
- Do not smoke or light matches or lighters around flammable liquids or materials.

Fire and Oxygen. Three things are needed for a fire.

- A spark or flame
- A material that will burn
- Oxygen

Air has some oxygen. However, some people need extra oxygen (Chapter 30). Safety measures are needed where oxygen is used and stored.

- NO SMOKING signs are placed on the door and near the bed.
- The person and visitors cannot smoke in the room.
- Smoking materials (cigarettes, cigars, and pipes), matches, and lighters are removed from the room.
- Safety measures to prevent equipment accidents are followed (see Box 10-4).
- Wool blankets and synthetic fabrics that cause static electricity are removed from the person's room.
- The person wears a cotton gown or pajamas.
- Lit candles, incense, and other open flames are not allowed.
- Materials that ignite easily are removed from the room. They include oil, grease, nail polish remover, and so on.

See Focus on Communication: Fire and Oxygen.

What to Do During a Fire. Know your agency's fire emergency and evacuation procedures. Know where to find fire alarms, fire extinguishers, and emergency exits. Fire drills are held to practice emergency fire procedures. Remember the word RACE (Fig. 10-12).

- R—for rescue. Rescue persons in immediate danger. Move them to a safe place.
- A—for alarm. Sound the nearest fire alarm. Call 911 or the operator.
- C—for confine. Close doors and windows to confine the fire. Turn off oxygen or electrical items used in the general area of the fire.
- E—for extinguish. Use a fire extinguisher on a small fire that has not spread to a larger area.

Clear equipment from all normal and emergency exits. Do not use elevators if there is a fire.

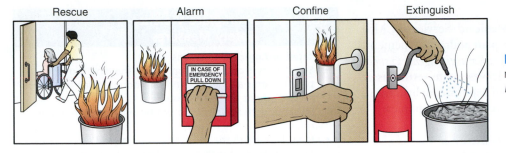

FIGURE 10-12 During a fire, remember *RACE*: *Rescue, Alarm, Confine, Extinguish.*

Rescue   Alarm   Confine   Extinguish

IN CASE OF EMERGENCY PULL DOWN

Using a Fire Extinguisher. Different extinguishers are used for different kinds of fires.
- Oil and grease fires
- Electrical fires
- Paper and wood fires

A general procedure for using a fire extinguisher follows. See procedure: *Using a Fire Extinguisher.*

Using a Fire Extinguisher

PROCEDURE

1 Pull the fire alarm.
2 Get the nearest fire extinguisher.
3 Carry it upright.
4 Take it to the fire.
5 Follow the word *PASS*.
  a P—for *pull the safety pin* (Fig. 10-13, A). This unlocks the handle.
  b A—for *aim low* (Fig. 10-13, B). Direct the hose or nozzle at the base of the fire. Do not try to spray the tops of the flames.

  c S—for *squeeze the lever* (Fig. 10-13, C). Squeeze or push down on the lever, handle, or button to start the stream. Release the lever, handle, or button to stop the stream.
  d S—for *sweep back and forth* (Fig. 10-13, D). Sweep the stream back and forth (side to side) at the base of the fire.

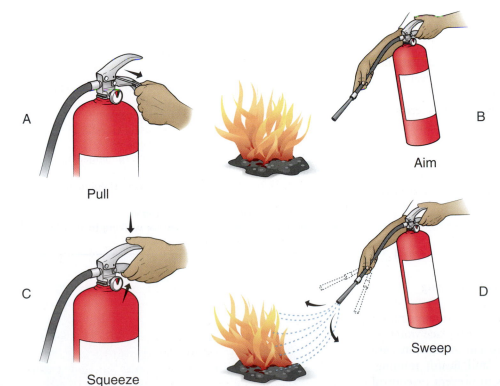

A   Pull

B   Aim

C   Squeeze

D   Sweep

FIGURE 10-13 Using a fire extinguisher. **A,** *Pull* the safety pin. **B,** *Aim* the hose at the base of the fire. **C,** *Squeeze* the top handle down. **D,** *Sweep* back and forth.

Elopement

The Centers for Medicare & Medicaid Services (CMS) requires that an agency's disaster plan address elopement. *Elopement is when a patient or resident leaves the agency without staff knowledge.* The person who leaves a safe setting is at risk for many dangers. Heat or cold exposure, dehydration, drowning, and being struck by a vehicle are examples.

The agency must:

- Identify persons at risk for elopement.
- Monitor and supervise persons at risk.
- Address elopement in the person's care plan.
- Have a plan to find a missing patient or resident.

WORKPLACE VIOLENCE

Workplace violence is violent acts (including assault or threat of assault) directed toward persons at work or while on duty. It includes:

- Murders
- Beatings, stabbings, and shootings
- Rapes and sexual assaults
- Use of weapons—firearms, bombs, knives, and so on
- Kidnapping
- Robbery
- Threats—obscene phone calls; threatening oral, written, or body language; and harassment of any nature (being followed, sworn at, or shouted at)
- Terrorism

Violence occurs in health care settings. Nurses and nursing assistants are at risk. They have the most contact with patients, residents, and visitors. Risk factors include:

- People with weapons.
- Police holds—persons arrested or convicted of crimes.
- Acutely disturbed and violent persons seeking health care.
- Alcohol and drug abuse.
- Persons with mental health disorders who do not take needed drugs, do not have follow-up care, and are not in hospitals unless they are an immediate threat to themselves or others.
- Agencies have drugs and are a target for robberies.
- Gang members and substance abusers are patients, residents, or visitors.
- Upset, agitated, and disturbed family and visitors.
- Long waits for emergency care or other services.
- Being alone with the person during care or transport to other areas.
- Low staff levels during meals, emergencies, and at night.
- Poor lighting in hallways, rooms, parking lots, and other areas.
- Lack of training in recognizing and managing potentially violent situations.

The Occupational Safety and Health Administration (OSHA) has guidelines for preventing workplace violence. Work-site hazards are identified. Prevention measures are followed. Also, staff receive safety and health training. Box 10-6 has some safety measures to prevent or control workplace violence.

BOX 10-6	Workplace Violence— Safety Measures

Agitated or Aggressive Persons

- Stand away from the person. Judge the length of the person's arms and legs. Stand far enough away that the person cannot hit or kick you.
- Stand close to the door. Do not become trapped in the room.
- Identify items in the room that can be used as weapons. Move away from such objects. Vases, phones, radios, letter openers, paper weights, and belts are examples.
- Know where to find panic buttons, call lights, alarms, closed-circuit monitors, and other security devices.
- Keep your hands free.
- Stay calm. Talk to the person in a calm manner. Do not raise your voice or argue, scold, or interrupt the person.
- Be aware of your body language. Do not point a finger or glare at the person. Do not put your hands on your hips.
- Do not touch the person.
- Tell the person that you will get the nurse to speak to him or her.
- Leave the room as soon as you can. Make sure the person is safe.
- Tell the nurse and security officer about the matter at once. Report items in the room that can be used as weapons.

Weapons

- Jewelry and scarves are not worn. They can be used as weapons. For example, a person can grab earrings and bracelets. Or a person can strangle someone with a necklace or scarf.
- Long hair is worn up and off the collar (Chapter 5). A person can pull long hair and cause head injuries.
- Keys, scissors, pens, or other items that can serve as weapons are not visible.
- Pictures, vases, and other items that can serve as weapons are few in number.
- Tools or items left by maintenance staff or visitors are removed if they can serve as weapons.

Staff Safety Measures

- Staff are not alone when caring for persons with agitated or aggressive behaviors.
- Staff wear ID badges that prove employment.
- Staff use a "buddy system" when using elevators, stairways, restrooms, and low traffic areas.
- Uniforms fit well. Tight uniforms limit running. An attacker can grab loose uniforms.
- Shoes have good soles. Shoes that cause slipping limit running.
- Vehicles are locked and in good repair.
- Security escort services are used for walking to vehicles, bus stops, or train stations.

RISK MANAGEMENT

Risk management involves identifying and controlling risks and safety hazards affecting the agency. The intent is to:

- Protect all in the agency—patients, residents, visitors, and staff.
- Protect agency property from harm or danger.
- Protect the person's valuables.
- Prevent accidents and injuries.
  Risk management deals with these and other safety issues.
- Accident and fire prevention
- Negligence and malpractice
- Abuse
- Workplace violence
- Federal and state requirements

Risk managers look for patterns and trends in incidents, complaints (patients, residents, staff), and accident and injury investigations. Unsafe situations are corrected. Procedure changes and training recommendations are made as needed.

Color-Coded Wristbands

Color-coded wristbands promote the person's safety and prevent harm. They quickly communicate an alert or warning (Fig. 10-14). The type of alert is printed on the band. The printing is useful in dim lighting and for persons who are color blind. These colors are common.

- Red—for an "allergy alert." Red is a warning to "stop." A red wristband warns of allergies to food, drugs, treatment supplies such as tape or latex gloves, dust, plants, grass, and so on. Allergies are not listed on the wristband.
- Yellow—for a "fall risk." Yellow implies "caution." Yellow wristbands are used for persons with a history of falls. Or they are used for persons at risk for falls because of dizziness, balance problems, confusion, and so on.
- Purple—for a "Do Not Resuscitate" (DNR) order. See Chapter 37.

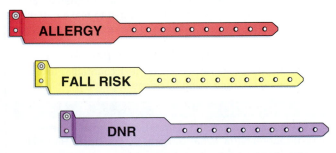

FIGURE 10-14 Color-coded wristbands. The alert is printed on the band.

Some agencies have colors for other alerts. For example, pink is for a "limb alert." This means that an arm or leg is not used for blood pressure measurements, blood draws, or intravenous infusions. To safely use color-coded wristbands:

- Know the wristband colors used in your agency. Colors may vary among agencies.
- Check the care plan and your assignment sheet when you see a color-coded wristband. You need to know the reason for the wristband and the care measures needed. Ask the nurse if you have questions.
- Do not confuse "social cause" bands with your agency's color-coded wristbands. "Live Strong" is an example.
- Check for wristbands on persons transferred from another agency. That agency may use different colors. Or the meanings may differ from those in your agency. The nurse needs to remove wristbands from another agency.
- Tell the nurse if you think a person needs a color-coded wristband.

Personal Belongings

The person's belongings must be kept safe. A personal belongings list is completed. Each item is listed and described. The staff member and the person sign the completed list.

A valuables envelope is used for jewelry and money. Each jewelry item is listed and described on the envelope. Describe what you see. For example, describe a ring as having a white stone with 4 prongs in a yellow setting. Do not assume the stone is a diamond in a gold setting. For valuables:

- Count money with the person.
- Put money and each jewelry item in the envelope. Have the person watch. Seal and sign the envelope like a personal belongings list.
- Give the envelope to the nurse. Have a witness. The nurse takes it to the safe or sends it home with the family.

Dentures, eyeglasses, hearing aids, watches, some jewelry, radios and music players, computers, and other electronic devices are kept at the bedside. Items kept at the bedside are listed in the person's record. Some people keep money for newspapers and personal items. The amount kept is noted in the person's record.

In nursing centers, clothing and shoes are labeled with the person's name. So are other items brought from home. Follow center procedures to label items.

Reporting Incidents

An *incident* is any event that has harmed or could harm a patient, resident, visitor, or staff member. This includes:

- Accidents involving patients, residents, visitors, or staff.
- Errors in care—giving the wrong care, giving care to the wrong person, not giving care.
- Broken or lost items owned by the person. Dentures, hearing aids, and eyeglasses are examples.
- Lost money or clothing.
- Hazardous chemical incidents.
- Workplace violence incidents.

Report accidents and errors at once. Complete an *incident report* as soon as possible. Incident reports are reviewed by a risk management committee. They look for patterns and trends in accidents or errors. For example, are falls occurring on the same shift and on the same unit? Are lost or missing items being reported on the same shift or same unit? Are residents being injured on the same shift or same unit? There may be new policies and procedures to prevent future incidents.

FOCUS ON P R I D E

The Person, Family, and Yourself

Personal and Professional Responsibility

Some persons are at risk for choking. Persons with developmental disabilities, young children, and older persons are examples. Safety measures must be taken to avoid harm.

You can help prevent choking. Know who is at risk. Ask the nurse or check the care plan. Monitor those persons closely. Check that they have the right diet. See Chapter 23 for more precautions.

Rights and Respect

Respect for others' well-being affects your actions. If you value the person's safety, you will perform safety measures. For example, you will:

- Identify the person before giving care.
- Check water temperature before bathing.
- Use and store harmful products safely.
- Cut food into small pieces.
- Observe for swallowing problems and signs of choking.
- Use equipment correctly.
- Know what to do during a fire or disaster.
- Report concerns and incidents.

Show respect for the person in how you give care. Take pride in providing safe care.

Independence and Social Interaction

Older persons often cannot do things they used to do. They still may try. To promote safety:

- Know who you need to protect.
- Know common safety hazards and the causes of accidents.
- Practice safety measures to prevent accidents and injuries.
- Respect their desire to maintain independence. Listen to them. Discuss letting them try a task with help. Let them do as much as they safely can. Kindly communicate safety limits.

Delegation and Teamwork

Personal safety practices protect you and co-workers. Work as a team for the safety of all staff arriving and leaving the agency.

- Wait for a person finishing work a few minutes late. Ask if you can help the person.
- Walk with others to and from the parking area.
- Walk in well-lit areas at night.
- Do not leave the parking area until your co-workers are safely in their vehicles. Have them do the same for you.
- Offer to call security escort services for a co-worker going to a different location. For example, a person is walking to a bus stop.

Take pride in caring about the safety of all team members.

Ethics and Laws

Accidents happen. Errors occur. No matter how much you try, mistakes are made. Do not lie or try to hide the incident. You must:

- Be honest.
- Tell the nurse.
- Fill out an incident report.

Incident reports are used to improve systems and promote safety, not for punishment. Information gained signals areas for improvement. Processes may be changed to make mistakes more difficult. Or they are changed to make it easier to do the right thing.

Always do your best to give safe care. When errors or accidents happen, take responsibility. Be accountable. Take pride in doing the right thing by honest reporting.

FOCUS ON PRIDE: *Application*

As a student or new nursing assistant, it is normal to have fears of causing harm. What concerns do you have? How will you overcome your fears?

Circle the BEST answer.

1 Which is *safe*?
   a Not wearing needed eyeglasses
   b Hearing problems
   c Memory problems
   d Oriented to person, time, and place

2 A person in a coma
   a Has suffered an electrical shock
   b Has dementia
   c Is unaware of surroundings
   d Has stopped breathing

3 To identify a person, you
   a Call the person by name
   b Ask the person his or her name
   c Compare information on the ID bracelet against your assignment sheet
   d Ask both roommates their names

4 To prevent burns
   a Keep smoking materials at the person's bedside
   b Pour hot liquids near a person
   c Turn on hot water first
   d Check water temperature before the person enters the shower

5 Which prevents poisoning?
   a Keeping harmful products in low storage areas
   b Keeping harmful products in the original containers
   c Removing product labels
   d Storing harmful products near food

6 Which can cause suffocation?
   a Reporting loose teeth or dentures
   b Using electrical items that are in good repair
   c Cutting food into small, bite-sized pieces
   d Restraints

7 The most common cause of choking in adults is
   a A loose denture
   b Meat
   c Marbles
   d Candy

8 If severe airway obstruction occurs, the person usually
   a Clutches at the throat
   b Can speak, cough, and breathe
   c Is calm
   d Has a seizure

9 These statements are about FBAO. Which is *true?*
   a A person is coughing forcefully. Give abdominal thrusts.
   b A person is pregnant. Give abdominal thrusts.
   c Injuries can occur from abdominal or chest thrusts.
   d Unconscious persons cannot choke.

10 Before using a new resident's electric shaver,
   a Fill the sink with water
   b The maintenance staff must check the device
   c Check the SDS
   d Get an extension cord

11 You are using electrical equipment. Which measure is *unsafe?*
   a Following the manufacturer's instructions
   b Keeping electrical items away from water and spills
   c Pulling on the cord to remove a plug from an outlet
   d Turning off electrical items after using them

12 A person's weight exceeds a chair's weight capacity. The chair is safe to use.
   a True
   b False

13 You spilled a hazardous substance. You should
   a Follow the instructions on the safety data sheet
   b Cover the spill and go tell the nurse
   c Wipe up the spill with paper towels
   d Leave the spill for housekeeping

14 The fire alarm sounds. Which action is *correct?*
   a Leave oxygen on.
   b Use elevators.
   c Open doors and windows.
   d Move residents to a safe place.

15 You work in a nursing center. In a severe weather alert, you should
   a Take cover
   b Follow the center's disaster plan
   c Make sure your family is safe
   d Pull the fire alarm

16 A person is agitated and aggressive. Which is *unsafe?*
   a Standing away from the person
   b Standing close to the door
   c Using touch to show you care
   d Talking to the person without raising your voice

17 Risk managers
   a Look for patterns or trends in accidents and errors
   b Prevent legal problems when injuries occur
   c Are only responsible for staff safety
   d Are the same as surveyors

18 You see a color-coded wristband. You should
   a Read the wristband for special instructions or care measures
   b Ask the person what it means
   c Check your assignment sheet and the person's care plan
   d Remove the wristband when the risk is no longer present

19 A resident brought a computer from home. To prevent property loss
   a Send the item home with the family
   b Label the item with the person's name
   c Put the item in a safe
   d Use a wheelchair pouch for the item

20 You gave a person the wrong treatment. Which is *true?*
   a Report the error at the end of the shift.
   b Take action only if the person was injured.
   c You are guilty of negligence.
   d You must complete an incident report.

Answers to Chapter 10 questions are on p. 551.

FOCUS ON PRACTICE

Problem Solving

A person begins to cough loudly during a meal. The person can speak a few words. You hear wheezing between breaths. What do you do? The person is suddenly unable to cough, speak, or breathe. What do you do?

OBJECTIVES

- Define the key terms and key abbreviations in this chapter.
- Identify the causes and risk factors for falls.
- Describe the safety measures that prevent falls.
- Explain how to use bed and chair alarms safely.
- Explain how to use bed rails safely.
- Explain the purpose of hand rails and grab bars.

- Explain how to use wheel locks safely.
- Describe how to use transfer/gait belts.
- Explain how to help the person who is falling.
- Perform the procedures described in this chapter.
- Explain how to promote PRIDE in the person, the family, and yourself.

KEY TERMS

bed rail A device that serves as a guard or barrier along the side of the bed; side rail
gait belt See "transfer belt"

transfer belt A device applied around the waist and used to support a person who is unsteady or disabled; gait belt

KEY ABBREVIATIONS

CDC Centers for Disease Control and Prevention

CMS Centers for Medicare & Medicaid Services

The risk of falling increases with age. Persons older than 65 years are at risk. A history of falls increases the risk of falling again. Falls are the most common accidents in nursing centers.

According to the Centers for Disease Control and Prevention (CDC):

- Falls are the main cause of injuries and injury-related deaths in older adults.
- Falls can cause serious injury. Fractures of the spine, hip, forearm, leg, ankle, pelvis, upper arm, and hand are the most common. Hip fractures and head trauma increase the risk of death.
- Falls result in disability, decline in function, and reduced quality of life.

See *Focus on Surveys: Preventing Falls.*

FOCUS ON SURVEYS

Preventing Falls

The Centers for Medicare & Medicaid Services (CMS) defines a *fall* as:

- Unintentionally coming to rest on the ground, floor, or other lower level. Force, such as being pushed, was not involved.
- When a person loses his or her balance and would have fallen if staff did not act to prevent the fall.
- When a person is found on the floor unless matters suggest otherwise.
  The survey team will observe and interview staff about:
- Fall risk factors described in this chapter.
- The hazards described in this chapter and in Chapter 10.
- Safety measures to prevent falls.
- The safe use of bed rails, hand rails and grab bars, and wheel locks.
- The safe use of assistive (adaptive) devices. Canes, walkers, and transfer/gait belts (p. 127) are examples.
- Safe transfer (Chapter 16) and ambulation (Chapter 27) procedures.
- Answering call lights promptly.
- Following the person's care plan and meeting care needs.

CAUSES AND RISK FACTORS FOR FALLS

Most falls are caused by many risk factors. The more risk factors present, the greater the risk of falling. Most falls occur in patient and resident rooms.

The accident risk factors described in Chapter 10 can lead to falls. The problems listed in Box 11-1 increase a person's risk of falling.

See *Focus on Older Persons: Causes and Risk Factors for Falls.*

BOX 11-1 Fall Risk Factors

Care Setting
- Bed height: too low or too high
- Care equipment: IV (intravenous) poles, drainage tubes and bags, and others
- Floors: cluttered, wet, slippery, or uneven
- Furniture out-of-place
- No hand rails or grab bars
- Lighting: poor or glares
- Restraint use
- Setting: new, strange, and unfamiliar
- Throw rugs or other tripping hazards
- Wet and slippery bathtubs and showers
- Wheelchairs, walkers, canes, and crutches: improper use or fit

The Person
- Age: over 65 years
- Alcohol: over-use
- Balance problems
- Blood pressure: low or high
- Confusion; disorientation
- Depression
- Dizziness or light-headedness; dizziness on standing
- Drug side effects
  - Confusion and disorientation
  - Coordination: poor
  - Diarrhea
  - Dizziness
  - Drowsiness
  - Fainting
  - Low blood pressure when standing or sitting
  - Unsteadiness
  - Urination: frequent
- Elimination: urinary incontinence, frequency, urgency, urinating at night (*nocturia*); fecal incontinence
- Falls: history of; fear of falling
- Foot problems
- Gait: unsteady
- Joint pain and stiffness
- Judgment: poor
- Memory problems
- Mobility: impaired
- Muscle weakness
- Reaction time: slow
- Shoes that fit poorly
- Sleep problems
- Vision problems
- Weakness

FOCUS ON OLDER PERSONS

Causes and Risk Factors for Falls

Nursing center residents are at increased risk for falls. According to the CDC:
- Residents are often older and more frail than older adults in the community.
- Residents tend to have problems with their health, thinking and memory, and ability to perform activities of daily living (ADL).
- Many residents have trouble walking and need help with mobility (ability to move about).

FALL PREVENTION PROGRAMS

Agencies have fall prevention programs. The measures listed in Box 11-2 (pp. 124-125) are part of the program and the person's care plan. The care plan also lists measures for the person's risk factors.

See *Focus on Communication: Fall Prevention Programs.*
See *Promoting Safety and Comfort: Fall Prevention Programs.*

FOCUS ON COMMUNICATION

Fall Prevention Programs

A person can fall when reaching for needed items. The person reaches too far and falls. Or the person tries to get up without help. To prevent falls, ask the person these questions.
- "What things would you like near you?"
- "Can I move this closer to you?"
- "Can you reach the call light?"
- "Can you reach your cane?" (Walker and wheelchair are other examples.)
- "Do you need to use the bathroom?"
- "Do you need anything else before I leave the room?"

PROMOTING SAFETY AND COMFORT

Fall Prevention Programs

Safety
Some people have vision problems. Besides the measures in Box 11-2, other safety measures are needed to prevent falls. See Chapter 32.

BOX 11-2	Preventing Falls

Basic Needs
- Fluid needs are met.
- Eyeglasses and hearing aids are worn as needed. Reading glasses are not worn when up and about.
- Tasks are explained before and while performing them.
- Help is given with elimination needs. Assist the person to the bathroom. Or provide the bedpan, urinal, or commode.
- The bedpan, urinal, or commode is kept within reach if the person can use the device without help.
- A warm drink, soft lights, or a back massage is used to calm the person who is agitated.
- Barriers are used to prevent wandering (Fig. 11-1).
- The person is properly positioned when in bed, a chair, or a wheelchair. Use pillows, wedge pads, seats, or other positioning devices as directed (Chapter 14).
- Correct procedures and equipment are used for transfers (Chapter 16). Follow the care plan.
- The person is involved in meaningful activities.
- Exercise programs are followed. They help improve balance, strength, walking, and physical function.

Bathrooms and Shower/Tub Rooms
- Tubs and showers have non-slip surfaces or non-slip bath mats.
- The person uses grab bars (safety bars) in bathrooms and showers (p. 126).
- Shower chairs are used (Chapter 18).
- Safety measures for tub baths and showers are followed (Chapter 18).

Floors, Stairs, and Hallways
- Carpeting (if used) is wall-to-wall or tacked down.
- Scatter, area, and throw rugs are not used.
- Floor covers are 1 color. Bold designs can cause dizziness in older persons.
- Floors have non-glare, non-slip surfaces.
- Non-skid wax is used on hardwood, tiled, or linoleum floors.
- Non-slip strips are on the floor next to the bed and in the bathroom. They are intact.
- Loose floor boards and tiles are reported. So are frayed rugs and carpets.
- Floors and stairs are free of clutter, cords, and other items that can cause tripping.
- Floors are free of spills. Wipe up spills at once. Put a WET FLOOR sign by the wet area.
- Floors are free of excess furniture and equipment.
- Electrical and extension cords are out of the way. This includes power strips.
- Equipment and supplies are kept on 1 side of the hallway.
- Hand rails (p. 126) are on both sides of stairs and hallways.
- The person uses hand rails when walking or using stairs.

Furniture
- Furniture is placed for easy movement.
- Furniture is kept in place. It is not re-arranged.
- Chairs have armrests. Armrests give support when standing or sitting.
- A phone, lamp, and personal belongings are within reach.

Beds and Other Equipment
- The bed is at the correct height for the person. Follow the care plan. The bed is raised for bedside care. Then it is lowered to a safe and comfortable level for the person. The distance from the bed to the floor is reduced if the person falls or gets out of bed.

Beds and Other Equipment—cont'd
- Bed rails (p. 126) are used according to the care plan.
- A mattress, special mat, or floor cushion is on the floor by the bed (Fig. 11-2). This reduces the chance of injury if the person falls or gets out of bed.
- Wheelchairs, walkers, canes, and crutches fit properly. They are in good repair. Another person's equipment is not used.
- Crutches, canes, and walkers have non-skid tips.
- Wheelchair and stretcher safety is followed (Chapter 16).
- Wheel locks on beds (p. 127), wheelchairs, and stretchers are in working order.
- Bed and wheelchair or stretcher wheels are locked for transfers.
- Linens are checked for sharp objects and for the person's property (dentures, eyeglasses, hearing aids, and so on).

Lighting
- Rooms, hallways, and stairways have good lighting. So do bathrooms and shower/tub rooms.
- Light switches are within reach and easy to find.
- Night-lights are in bedrooms, hallways, and bathrooms.

Shoes and Clothing
- Non-skid footwear is worn. Socks, bedroom slippers, and long shoelaces are avoided.
- Shoes fit well. They do not slip up and down on the feet. All shoelaces and straps are fastened.
- Clothing fits properly. Clothing is not loose or dragging on the floor.
- Belts are tied or secured in place.

Call Lights and Alarms
- The person is taught how to use the call light (Chapter 17).
- The call light is always within the person's reach. This includes when sitting in the chair or on the commode and when in the bathroom and shower/tub room.
- The person is asked to use the call light when help is needed.
  - To get out of bed or a chair or return to bed
  - To walk
  - To get to or from the bathroom
  - To get on or off the bedpan, toilet, or commode
  - To stand to use the urinal
- Call lights are answered promptly. The person may need help right away. He or she may not wait for help.
- Bed, chair, door, floor mat, and belt alarms are used. They sense when the person tries to get up, get out of bed, or open a door.
- Alarms are responded to at once.

Observation
- The person is checked often. This may be every 15 minutes or as required by the care plan. Careful and frequent observation is important.
- Frequent checks are made on persons with poor judgment or memory. This may be every 15 minutes or as required by the care plan.
- Persons at risk for falls are close to the nurses' station.
- Family and friends are asked to visit during busy times. Meal times and shift changes are examples. They are also asked to visit during the evening and night shifts.
- Companions are provided. Sitters, companions, or volunteers are with the person.

BOX 11-2	Preventing Falls—cont'd

Other

- Color-coded alerts warn of a fall risk. Yellow is common for a fall alert. Besides wristbands (Chapter 10), some agencies also use color-coded blankets, non-skid footwear, socks, and magnets or stickers on room doors.
- Caution is used when turning corners, entering corridor intersections, and going through doors. You could injure a person coming from the other direction.

Other—cont'd

- Pull (do not push) wheelchairs, stretchers, carts, and other wheeled equipment through doorways. You lead the way and can see where you are going.
- A safety check is made of the room after visitors leave. (See the inside of the front cover.) They may have lowered a bed rail, moved a call light, or moved a walker out of reach. Or they may have brought an item that could harm the person.

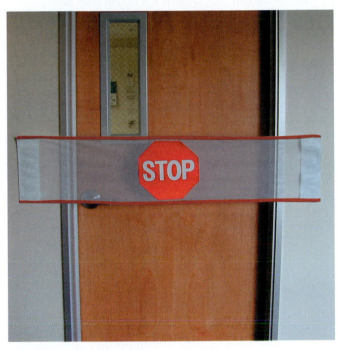

FIGURE 11-1 Barriers are used to prevent wandering. (Image courtesy Posey Co., Arcadia, Calif.)

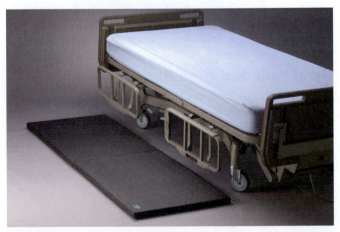

FIGURE 11-2 Floor cushion. NOTE: Two half-length bed rails are shown. (Image courtesy Posey Co., Arcadia, Calif.)

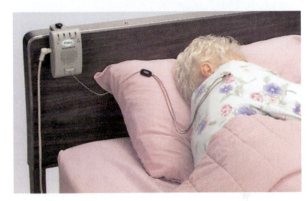

FIGURE 11-3 Bed alarm. The alarm attaches to clothing at the back near the shoulder. (Image courtesy Posey Co., Arcadia, Calif.)

Bed and Chair Alarms

Bed and chair alarms alert that a person is moving from the bed or chair. See Figure 11-3. The device attaches to clothing. Or the person sits or lies on a flat sensor. To alert staff, the device makes a sound—alarm, beep, chime, music, and so on. Some play a recorded message. For example: "Please do not get up. Sit down and use your call light for help."

To use bed and chair alarms safely:

- Follow the manufacturer's instructions.
- Test the alarm before leaving the person. If the device does not work, stay with the person. Call for the nurse.
- Respond to alarms at once.
  For alarms that attach to clothing:
- Mount the alarm securely out of the person's reach.
- Place the alarm at least 2 feet away from the person's ear. Alarms close to the ear may cause hearing loss or injury.
- Attach the clip securely out of the person's reach. The clip is at the back near the shoulder. Check that clothing is not frayed or torn.
- Check the cord. The cord should allow enough movement for comfort but be short enough to sound the alarm if the person moves from the safe area. The cord must not be tangled in bed rails, linens, chair parts, and so on.

Alarms do not replace close observation. Persons at risk for falls are checked often. Careful and frequent observation is important.

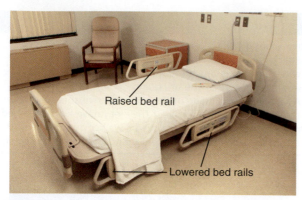

FIGURE 11-4 Bed rails. A far bed rail is raised. The near bed rails are lowered.

Bed Rails

A *bed rail* (side rail) is a device that serves as a guard or barrier along the side of the bed. Bed rails are raised and lowered (Fig. 11-4). They lock in place with levers, latches, or buttons. Bed rails are half ($\frac{1}{2}$), three quarters ($\frac{3}{4}$), or the full length of the bed. When half-length rails are used, each side has 1 or 2 rails (see Fig. 11-4).

The nurse and the care plan tell you when to raise bed rails. They are needed by persons who are unconscious or sedated with drugs. Some confused or disoriented people need them. When bed rails are needed, keep them up at all times except when giving bedside care.

Bed rails present hazards. When raised, the person cannot get out of bed. He or she can fall if trying to climb over them. *Entrapment* is a risk (Chapter 17). That is, the person can get caught, trapped, entangled, or strangled.

Bed rails are considered to be restraints (Chapter 12) if:
- The person cannot get out of bed.
- They cannot or will not be lowered to allow the person to leave the bed.

Bed rails cannot be used unless needed to treat a medical symptom. They must be in the person's best interest. Some people feel safer with bed rails up. Others use them for position changes in bed. The person or legal representative must give written consent for raised bed rails. The need for bed rails is carefully noted in the person's medical record and care plan.

The procedures in this book include bed rails. This helps you learn to use them correctly. The nurse, the care plan, and your assignment sheet tell you who uses bed rails. If a person does not use them, omit the "raise bed rails" and "lower bed rails" steps.

Check the person often. Tell the nurse that you checked the person. If allowed to chart, record when you checked the person and your observations.

See *Promoting Safety and Comfort: Bed Rails.*

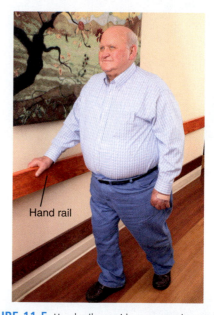

FIGURE 11-5 Hand rails provide support when walking.

Hand Rails and Grab Bars

Hand rails are in hallways and stairways (Fig. 11-5). They give support to persons who are weak or unsteady when walking.

Grab bars (safety bars) are in bathrooms and in shower/tub rooms (Fig. 11-6). They provide support to sit down or get up from a toilet. They also are used to get in and out of the shower or tub.

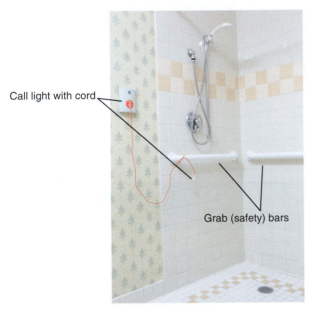

FIGURE 11-6 Grab bars (safety bars) in a shower.

Call light with cord

Grab (safety) bars

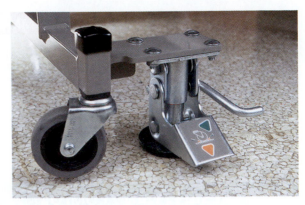

FIGURE 11-7 Bed wheel lock.

Wheel Locks

Bed wheels let the bed move easily. Wheels have locks to prevent the bed from moving (Fig. 11-7). Wheels are locked at all times except when moving the bed. Make sure bed wheels are locked:

- When giving bedside care
- When you transfer a person to and from bed
  Wheelchair and stretcher wheels also are locked during transfers (Chapter 16). You or the person can be injured if the bed, wheelchair, or stretcher moves.

TRANSFER/GAIT BELTS

A *transfer belt (gait belt) is a device applied around the waist and used to support a person who is unsteady or disabled* (Fig. 11-8). It helps prevent falls and injuries.

- When used to transfer a person (Chapter 16), it is called a *transfer belt.*
- When used to help a person walk, it is called a *gait belt.*

The belt goes around the waist. Grasp the belt from underneath for support during the transfer or when assisting the person to walk. If the belt has handles, grasp the belt by the handles (Fig. 11-9).

See *Focus on Communication: Transfer/Gait Belts,* p. 128.

See *Promoting Safety and Comfort: Transfer/Gait Belts,* p. 128.

See procedure: *Using a Transfer/Gait Belt,* p. 129.

Text continued on p. 130.

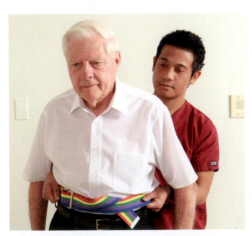

FIGURE 11-8 Transfer/gait belt. The buckle is off-center. Excess strap is tucked into the belt. The nursing assistant grasps the belt from underneath.

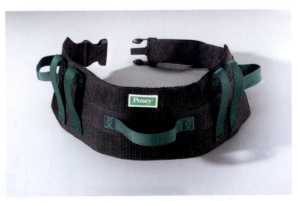

FIGURE 11-9 A transfer/gait belt with handles. (Image courtesy Posey Co., Arcadia, Calif.)

PROMOTING SAFETY AND COMFORT

Transfer/Gait Belts

Safety

Transfer/gait belts are routinely used in nursing centers. If the person needs help, a belt is required. For safe use, always follow the manufacturer's instructions.

Some transfer/gait belts have a quick-release buckle (Fig. 11-10). Position the quick-release buckle at the back where the person cannot reach or release it. Injury could result if the buckle is released.

Do not leave excess strap dangling. Tuck the excess strap into the belt (see Fig. 11-8).

Remove the belt after the procedure. Do not leave the person alone while wearing a transfer/gait belt.

The standard-sized transfer/gait belt fits waist sizes up to 51 inches. Bariatric-sized belts fit waist sizes up to 71 inches. The nurse and care plan tell you what size to use. If the person's waist size is greater than 71 inches, follow the nurse's directions and the care plan.

Safety—cont'd

Using a transfer/gait belt is unsafe for some persons. The belt could cause pressure or rub against care equipment. Check with the nurse and the care plan before using a transfer/gait belt if the person has:

- An ostomy—colostomy or ileostomy (Chapter 22)
- A gastrostomy tube (Chapter 23)
- Chronic obstructive pulmonary disease (Chapter 33)
- An abdominal or chest wound, incision, or drainage tube
- Monitoring equipment
- A hernia (Part of an organ protrudes or projects through an opening in a muscle wall. Hernias often involve a loop of bowel or the stomach.)
- Other conditions or equipment involving the chest or abdomen

Comfort

A transfer/gait belt is always applied over clothing—never over bare skin. Also, it is applied around the waist and under the breasts. Breasts must not be caught under the belt. The belt buckle is never positioned over the person's spine.

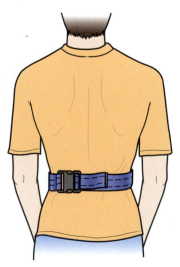

FIGURE 11-10 A transfer/gait belt with a quick-release buckle. The buckle is positioned off-center at the back.

Using a Transfer/Gait Belt

QUALITY OF LIFE

- Knock before entering the person's room.
- Address the person by name.
- Introduce yourself by name and title.

- Explain the procedure before starting and during the procedure.
- Protect the person's rights during the procedure.
- Handle the person gently during the procedure.

PRE-PROCEDURE

1 See *Promoting Safety and Comfort: Transfer/Gait Belts.*
2 Practice hand hygiene.
3 Obtain a transfer/gait belt of the correct type and size.

4 Identify the person. Check the identification (ID) bracelet against the assignment sheet. Use 2 identifiers (Chapter 10). Also call the person by name.
5 Provide for privacy.

PROCEDURE

6 Assist the person to a sitting position.
7 Apply the belt. Hold the belt by the buckle. Wrap the belt around the person's waist over clothing. Do not apply it over bare skin.
   a For a belt with a metal buckle:
      1 Insert the belt's metal tip into the buckle. Pass the belt through the side with the teeth first (Fig. 11-11, *A*).
      2 Bring the belt tip across the front of the buckle. Insert the tip through the buckle's smooth side (Fig. 11-11, *B*).
   b For a belt with a quick-release buckle, push the belt ends together to secure the buckle.
8 Tighten the belt so it is snug. It should not cause discomfort or impair breathing. You should be able to slide your open, flat hand under the belt. Ask about the person's comfort.

9 Make sure that the person's breasts are not caught under the belt.
10 Place the buckle off-center in the front (Fig. 11-11, *C*) or off-center in the back (see Fig. 11-10) for the person's comfort. A quick-release buckle is turned around to the back out of the person's reach. The buckle is not over the spine.
11 Tuck any excess strap into the belt (see Fig. 11-11, *C*).
12 Complete the transfer (Chapter 16) or ambulation procedure (Chapter 27). Grasp the belt from underneath with 2 hands (see Fig. 11-8). Or grasp the belt by the handles.

POST-PROCEDURE

13 Remove the belt after the procedure in step 12. The person is not left alone wearing the belt.
   a For a belt with a metal buckle:
      1 Bring the belt strap back through the buckle's smooth side.
      2 Pull the belt through the side with the teeth.
   b For a belt with a quick-release buckle, push inward on the quick-release buttons.
   c Remove the belt from the person's waist. Avoid dragging the belt across the waist.

14 Provide for comfort. (See the inside of the front cover.)
15 Place the call light and other needed items within reach.
16 Unscreen the person.
17 Complete a safety check of the room. (See the inside of the front cover.)
18 Return the transfer/gait belt to its proper place.
19 Practice hand hygiene.
20 Report and record your observations.

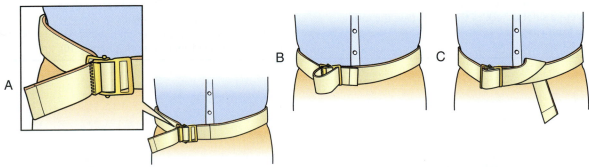

FIGURE 11-11 Applying a transfer/gait belt at the waist. **A,** The belt is inserted into the buckle. The belt goes through the side with the teeth first. **B,** The belt is inserted into the buckle's smooth side. **C,** The buckle is off-center in the front. Excess strap is tucked into the belt.

THE FALLING PERSON

A person may start to fall when standing or walking. See p. 123 for the causes and risk factors for falls.

Do not try to prevent the fall. You could injure yourself and the person while twisting and straining to prevent the fall. You could lose your balance trying to prevent the fall. You both could fall. Head, wrist, arm, hip, knee, and back injuries could occur.

If a person starts to fall, ease him or her to the floor. This lets you control the direction of the fall. You can also protect the person's head. Do not let the person move or get up before the nurse checks for injuries.

If you find a person on the floor, do not move the person. Stay with the person and call for the nurse.

See *Focus on Older Persons: The Falling Person.*
See *Promoting Safety and Comfort: The Falling Person.*
See procedure: *Helping the Falling Person.*

FOCUS ON OLDER PERSONS

The Falling Person

Some older persons are confused. A confused person may not understand why you do not want him or her to move or get up after a fall. Forcing a person not to move may injure the person and you. You may need to let the person move for his or her safety and your own. Never use force to hold a person down. Stay calm and protect the person from injury. Talk to the person in a quiet, soothing voice. Call for help.

PROMOTING SAFETY AND COMFORT

The Falling Person

Safety

If a bariatric person starts to fall, there is little that you can do. For the person's safety and yours:
- Do *not* use the procedure: *Helping the Falling Person.*
- Move items that could cause injury out of the way. Do so as fast as possible.
- Try to protect the person's head from striking the floor, equipment, or other objects.
- Call for the nurse at once. Stay with the person.
- Assist the health team to return the person to bed.

Helping the Falling Person

PROCEDURE

1 Stand behind the person with your feet apart. Keep your back straight.
2 Bring the person close to your body as fast as possible (Fig. 11-12, *A*). Use the transfer/gait belt. Or wrap your arms around the person's waist. If necessary, hold the person under the arms.
3 Move your leg so the person's buttocks rest on it (Fig. 11-12, *B*). Move your leg that is near the person.
4 Lower the person to the floor. The person slides down your leg to the floor (Fig. 11-12, *C*). Bend at your hips and knees as you lower the person.
5 Call a nurse to check the person. Stay with the person.
6 Help the nurse return the person to bed. Ask other staff to help if needed.

POST-PROCEDURE

7 Provide for comfort. (See the inside of the front cover.)
8 Place the call light and other needed items within reach.
9 Raise or lower bed rails. Follow the care plan.
10 Complete a safety check of the room. (See the inside of the front cover.)
11 Practice hand hygiene.
12 Report and record the following.
   - How the fall occurred
   - How far the person walked
   - How activity was tolerated before the fall
   - Complaints before the fall
   - How much help the person needed while walking
13 Complete an incident report (Chapter 10).

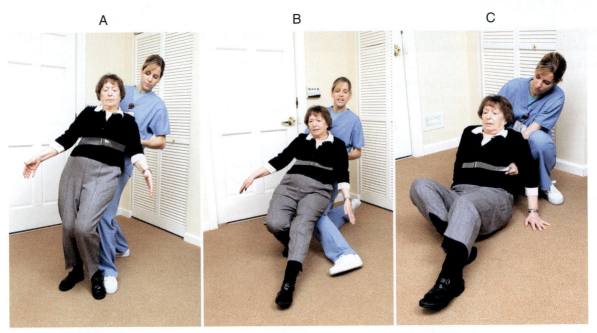

FIGURE 11-12 Helping the falling person. **A,** The falling person is supported with the gait belt. **B,** The person's buttocks rest on the nursing assistant's leg. **C,** The person is eased to the floor on the nursing assistant's leg.

FOCUS ON PRIDE
The Person, Family, and Yourself

Personal and Professional Responsibility

Safety measures can take time. Resist the urge to take short cuts. Take the time to:
- Find and use assistive (adaptive) devices.
- Put proper footwear on the person.
- Raise or lower the bed and bed rails as appropriate.
- Lock wheels on beds, stretchers, and wheelchairs.
- Ask for help if needed.

Take time for safety (see Box 11-2). Take pride in doing the right thing.

Rights and Respect

Safety and security are not only rights, but basic needs (Chapter 7). Fear of falling does not make a person feel safe. Before moving a person, explain what you are going to do and what he or she needs to do. Also give step-by-step instructions as you progress. Tell the person before you move him or her. Good communication supports the person's right to safety and security. See Chapters 15 and 16 for how to safely move and transfer the person.

Independence and Social Interaction

Some people feel that safety devices limit independence. For example, a person says: "I feel trapped. Do these bed rails have to be up?" The person fell out of bed during the night. The care plan includes raised bed rails while in bed.

Listen to the person's concerns. Kindly explain the reason for the safety device. If the person still refuses, tell the nurse. Do not be talked out of a safety measure or using a safety device. Safety is always a priority.

Delegation and Teamwork

Helping co-workers is part of teamwork. However, you may not know a person and his or her care plan. Communication is essential for safety. When assisting with the transfer of a co-worker's patient or resident, you must have certain information.
- Is the person at risk for falls?
- Is the person weak? Can he or she bear weight?
- Are there activity limits?
- How many staff are needed for the transfer?
- Are assistive (adaptive) devices needed? A cane, transfer belt, wheelchair, and walker are examples.
- Is other equipment needed? Oxygen and a chair alarm are examples.

Ethics and Laws

Falls are a serious matter. Failing to prevent falls can result in legal action. You must prevent falls. Follow the safety measures in this chapter. Take pride in protecting the person, yourself, and the agency.

FOCUS ON PRIDE: *Application*

A person is embarrassed about needing a transfer/gait belt and walker. How will you promote the person's safety and dignity? What if the person refuses to use the devices?

Circle the BEST answer.

1 These statements are about falls. Which is *true?*
 a Most are caused by many risk factors.
 b Serious injuries are unlikely.
 c Most occur outdoors.
 d Nursing center residents are at decreased risk.

2 Which person has the lowest risk of falls?
 a A 75-year-old with confusion
 b A 68-year-old with a history of falls
 c A 60-year-old with a hearing aid
 d An 80-year-old with urinary incontinence

3 A person's care plan includes fall prevention measures. Which should you question?
 a Assist with elimination needs.
 b Keep phone, lamp, and TV controls within reach.
 c Check the person every 2 hours.
 d Complete a safety check after visitors leave the room.

4 You observe the following in the person's room. Which is *unsafe?*
 a The lamp cord is by the chair.
 b The chair has armrests.
 c The night-light is on.
 d The bed is in a low position.

5 You note the following after a person is dressed. Which is *safe?*
 a Pant cuffs are dragging on the floor.
 b The person is wearing non-skid shoes.
 c The belt is not fastened.
 d The shirt is too big.

6 A resident's chair alarm goes off. What should you do?
 a Find the resident's nursing assistant.
 b Tell the nurse.
 c Assist the resident.
 d Wait for someone to respond to the alarm.

7 To help prevent falls, you need to report
 a Equipment and supplies being on 1 side of the hallway
 b A floor cushion beside the bed
 c A co-worker pulling a wheelchair through a doorway
 d Clutter on stairways

8 Bed rails are used
 a When you think they are needed
 b According to the care plan
 c When the bed is raised
 d To support persons who are weak or unsteady

9 Before transferring a person to the bed, you must
 a Raise the bed rails
 b Get a grab bar
 c Lock the bed wheels
 d Remove the person's shoes

10 A transfer/gait belt is applied
 a To the skin
 b Over clothing at the waist
 c Over the breasts
 d Under the robe

11 To safely use a transfer/gait belt, you must
 a Follow the manufacturer's instructions
 b Be able to slide a closed fist under the belt
 c Leave the belt on if the person is left alone
 d Position the buckle over the person's spine

12 You apply a transfer/gait belt. What should you do with the excess strap?
 a Cut it off.
 b Wrap it around the person's waist.
 c Tuck it into the belt.
 d Let it dangle.

13 A person starts to fall. Your *first* action is to
 a Try to prevent the fall
 b Call for help
 c Bring the person close to your body as fast as possible
 d Lower the person to the floor

14 When a bariatric person falls, you should
 a Try to stop the fall
 b Try to protect the person's head
 c Quickly pull the person close to you
 d Do nothing

15 You found a person lying on the floor. What should you do?
 a Lock the bed wheels.
 b Help the person back to bed.
 c Apply a transfer belt.
 d Call for the nurse.

Answers to Chapter 11 questions are on p. 551.

FOCUS ON PRACTICE

Problem Solving

You are assisting a resident in the bathroom. The resident is not to be left alone while in the bathroom. You hear a chair alarm sound in the hallway outside the door. What will you do?

Restraint Alternatives and Restraints

- Define the key terms and key abbreviations in this chapter.
- Describe the purpose of restraints.
- Identify restraint alternatives.
- Identify the risk factors related to restraint use.
- Explain the legal aspects of restraint use.

- Explain how to use restraints safely.
- Perform the procedure described in this chapter.
- Explain how to promote PRIDE in the person, the family, and yourself.

KEY TERMS

chemical restraint Any drug used for discipline or convenience and not required to treat medical symptoms
enabler A device that limits freedom of movement but is used to promote independence, comfort, or safety
freedom of movement Any change in place or position of the body or any part of the body that the person is able to control
medical symptom An indication or characteristic of a physical or psychological condition

physical restraint Any manual method or physical or mechanical device, material, or equipment attached to or near the person's body that he or she cannot remove easily and that restricts freedom of movement or normal access to one's body
remove easily The manual method, device, material, or equipment used to restrain the person that can be removed intentionally by the person in the same manner it was applied by the staff

KEY ABBREVIATIONS

CMS	Centers for Medicare & Medicaid Services	**ROM**	Range-of-motion
FDA	Food and Drug Administration	**TJC**	The Joint Commission
OBRA	Omnibus Budget Reconciliation Act of 1987		

Chapters 10 and 11 have many safety measures. Some persons need extra protection. They may present dangers to themselves or others (including staff).

The Centers for Medicare & Medicaid Services (CMS) has rules for using restraints. Like the *Omnibus Budget Reconciliation Act of 1987 (OBRA)*, CMS rules protect the person's rights and safety. This includes the right to be free from restraint. Restraints may be used only to treat a medical symptom or for the immediate physical safety of the person or others. Restraints may be used only when less restrictive measures fail to protect the person or others. They must be discontinued as soon as possible.

The CMS uses these terms.

- *Physical restraint*—any manual method or physical or mechanical device, material, or equipment attached to or near the person's body that he or she cannot remove easily and that restricts freedom of movement or normal access to one's body.

- *Chemical restraint*—any drug used for discipline or convenience and not required to treat medical symptoms. The drug or dosage is not a standard treatment for the person's condition.
  - *Discipline*—any action taken by the agency to punish or penalize a patient or resident.
  - *Convenience*—any action taken to control or manage a person's behavior that requires less effort by the staff; the action is not in the person's best interests.
- *Freedom of movement*—any change in place or position of the body or any part of the body that the person is able to control.
- *Remove easily*—the manual method, device, material, or equipment used to restrain the person that can be removed intentionally by the person in the same manner it was applied by the staff. For example, the person can put bed rails down, untie a knot, or open a buckle.

HISTORY OF RESTRAINT USE

Restraints were once used to *prevent* falls. Research shows that restraints *cause* falls. Falls occur while trying to get free of the restraints. Injuries are more serious from falls in restrained persons than in those not restrained.

Restraints also were used to prevent wandering or interfering with treatment. They were often used for confusion, poor judgment, or behavior problems. Older persons were restrained more often than younger persons were. Restraints were viewed as necessary to protect a person. However, they can cause serious harm, even death. See "Risks From Restraint Use" on p. 136.

Besides the CMS, the Food and Drug Administration (FDA), state agencies, and The Joint Commission (TJC—an accrediting agency) have restraint guidelines. They do not forbid restraint use. *They require considering or trying all other appropriate alternatives first.*

Every agency has policies and procedures for restraints. They include identifying persons at risk for harm, harmful behaviors, restraint alternatives, and proper restraint use. Staff training is required.

RESTRAINT ALTERNATIVES

Often there are causes and reasons for harmful behaviors. Knowing and treating the cause can prevent restraint use. The nurse tries to learn what the behavior means.

- Is the person in pain, ill, or injured?
- Is the person short of breath?
- Is the person afraid in a new setting?
- Does the person need to use the bathroom?
- Is clothing or a wound dressing (Chapter 28) tight or causing discomfort?
- Is the person's position uncomfortable?
- Are body fluids, secretions, or excretions causing skin irritation?
- Is the person too hot or too cold? Hungry or thirsty?
- What are the person's life-long habits?
- Does the person have problems communicating?
- Is the person seeing, hearing, or feeling things that are not real (Chapters 34 and 35)?
- Is the person confused or disoriented (Chapter 35)?
- Are drugs causing the behaviors?

Restraint alternatives are identified in the care plan (Box 12-1). The care plan is changed as needed. Restraint alternatives may not protect the person. The doctor may need to order restraints.

BOX 12-1	Restraint Alternatives

Physical Needs
- Life-long habits and routines are in the care plan. For example, showers before breakfast; reads in the bathroom; walks outside before lunch; watches TV after lunch.
- Pillows, wedge cushions, and posture and positioning devices are used.
- Food, fluid, hygiene, and elimination needs are met.
- The bedpan, urinal, or commode is within reach.
- Back massages are given.
- A calm, quiet setting is provided.
- Exercise programs are provided.
- Outdoor time is planned for nice weather.
- Furniture meets the person's needs—lower bed, reclining chair, rocking chair, chair or wheelchair with lap-top tray (Fig. 12-1).
- Observations and visits are made at least every 15 minutes or more often. Follow the care plan.
- The person's room is close to the nurses' station.
- Lighting meets the person's needs and preferences.
- Staff assignments are consistent.
- Sleep is not interrupted.
- Noise levels are reduced.

Safety and Security Needs
- The call light is within reach.
- Call lights are answered promptly.
- The person wanders in safe areas.
- All staff are aware of persons who tend to wander. This includes staff in other departments.
- Knob guards are used on doors.

Safety and Security Needs—cont'd
- Falls and injuries are prevented (Chapter 11).
  - Padded hip protectors are worn under clothing (Fig. 12-2).
  - Floor cushions are placed next to beds (Chapter 11).
  - Roll guards are attached to the bed frame (Fig. 12-3).
- Bed, chair, and door alarms are used.
- Walls and furniture corners are padded.
- Procedures and care measures are explained.
- Frequent explanations are given about equipment or devices.
- Confused persons are oriented to person, time, and place. (To *orient* means to *remind the person of his or her name and the date, time, and setting*.) Calendars and clocks are provided. See Chapter 35.

Love, Belonging, and Self-Esteem Needs
- Diversion is provided—TV, videos, music, games, relaxation, and so on.
- The person watches videos of family and friends and of their visits.
- Time is spent in supervised areas (dining room, lounge, by the nurses' station).
- Family, friends, and volunteers visit.
- The person has companions or sitters.
- Time is spent with the person.
- Extra time is spent with a person who is restless.
- Reminiscing is done with the person.
- The person does jobs or tasks he or she consents to.

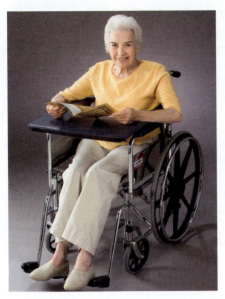

FIGURE 12-1 This lap-top tray is a restraint alternative. It is a restraint when used to prevent freedom of movement. (Image courtesy Posey Company, Arcadia, Calif.)

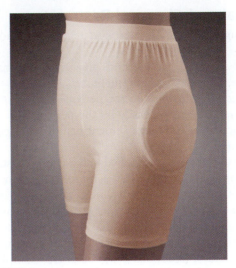

FIGURE 12-2 Hip protector. (Image courtesy Posey Company, Arcadia, Calif.)

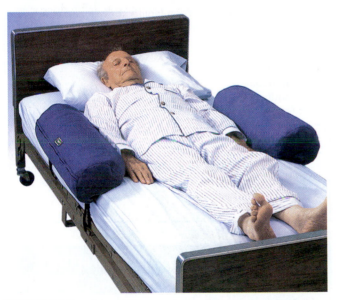

FIGURE 12-3 Roll guard. (Image courtesy Posey Company, Arcadia, Calif.)

SAFE RESTRAINT USE

Restraints can cause serious injury and death. CMS, OBRA, FDA, and TJC rules and guidelines are followed. So are state laws. They are part of the agency's policies and procedures for restraint use.

Restraints are not used to discipline a person or for staff convenience. Restraints are used only when necessary to treat medical symptoms. A *medical symptom is an indication or characteristic of a physical or psychological condition.* Symptoms may relate to physical, emotional, or behavioral problems. Sometimes restraints are needed to protect the person or others. That is, a person may have violent or aggressive behaviors that are harmful to self or others or that are threatening to others.

See *Focus on Surveys: Safe Restraint Use.*

FOCUS ON SURVEYS

Safe Restraint Use

Agencies must have a policy about restraint use. Surveyors will try to learn if restraints were used:
- For discipline or staff convenience
- Only for a certain time for the person's well-being
Surveyors may interview staff about:
- How staff members define "restraint."
- The medical symptoms leading to restraint use. Could they be reversed or reduced?
- Were medical symptoms caused by failure to:
  - Meet the person's needs
  - Provide rehabilitation
  - Provide meaningful activities
  - Change the person's setting for safety
- What restraint alternatives were used.
- If the least restrictive restraints were used.
- How long the restraints were used.

Physical and Chemical Restraints

According to the CMS, a *physical restraint* includes these points.

- May be any manual method, physical or mechanical device, material, or equipment.
- Is attached to or next to the person's body.
- Cannot be removed easily by the person.
- Restricts freedom of movement or normal access to one's body.

Physical restraints are applied to the chest, waist, elbows, wrists, hands, or ankles. They confine the person to a bed or chair. Or they prevent movement of a body part. Some furniture or barriers also prevent freedom of movement.

- A device used with a chair that the person cannot remove easily. The device prevents the person from rising. Trays, tables, bars, and belts are examples (see Fig. 12-1).
- Any chair that prevents the person from rising.
- Any bed or chair so close to the wall that the person cannot get out of the bed or chair.
- Bed rails (Chapter 11) that prevent the person from getting out of bed. They cannot or will not be lowered to allow the person to leave the bed.
- Tucking in or using Velcro (or other device) to hold a sheet, fabric, or clothing so tightly that freedom of movement is restricted.

Drugs or drug dosages are *chemical restraints* if they:

- Control behavior or restrict movement.
- Are not standard treatment for the person's condition.

Drugs cannot be used for discipline or staff convenience. They cannot be used if they affect physical or mental function.

Some drugs can help persons who are confused, disoriented, anxious, agitated, or aggressive. The doctor may order drugs to control such behaviors. The drugs should not make the person sleepy and unable to function at his or her highest level.

Enablers.

An *enabler is a device that limits freedom of movement but is used to promote independence, comfort, or safety.* Some devices can be restraints or enablers. When the person can easily remove the device and it helps the person function, it is an enabler. For example:

- A chair or wheelchair with a lap-top tray for meals, writing, and so on (see Fig. 12-1). The tray is an enabler. If used to limit freedom of movement, the tray is a restraint.
- A person wants raised bed rails. They are used to move in bed and to prevent falling out of bed. The bed rails are enablers, not restraints.

Risks From Restraint Use

Box 12-2 lists the risks from restraints. Injuries can occur as the person tries to get free of the restraint. Injuries also occur from using the wrong restraint, applying it wrong, or keeping it on too long. Cuts, bruises, and fractures are common. *The most serious risk is death from strangulation.*

Restraints are medical devices. The *Safe Medical Devices Act* applies if a restraint causes illness, injury, or death. Also, CMS requires the reporting of any death that occurs:

- While a person is in a restraint.
- Within 24 hours after a restraint was removed.
- Within 1 week after a restraint was removed. This is done if the restraint may have contributed directly or indirectly to the person's death.

See *Promoting Safety and Comfort: Risks From Restraint Use.*

BOX 12-2 Risks From Restraint Use

- Constipation
- Contractures
- Cuts and bruises
- Decline in physical function (ability to walk and muscle problems are examples)
- Dehydration
- Falls
- Fractures
- Head trauma
- Incontinence
- Infections: pneumonia and urinary tract
- Nerve injuries
- Pressure injuries
- Social and mental health problems: agitation, anger, delirium, depression, loss of dignity, embarrassment and humiliation, mistrust, loss of self-respect, reduced social contact, withdrawal
- Strangulation

PROMOTING SAFETY AND COMFORT

Risks From Restraint Use

Safety

If you find a person strangling from a restraint:

- Release the restraint. Or cut the strap if you have scissors in your pocket or within reach.
- Shout for help and a nurse as you are releasing the restraint.
- Stay with the person. If the person is not responding, provide Basic Life Support if allowed by agency policy (Chapter 36). Do so until help takes over. Assist the nurse as directed.

Laws, Rules, and Guidelines

Laws (federal and state) and rules (CMS, FDA) for restraint use are followed. So are accrediting agency (TJC) guidelines. Remember:

- *Restraints must protect the person.* They are not used for staff convenience or to discipline a person. Using restraints is not easier than properly supervising and observing the person. A restrained person requires more staff time for care, supervision, and observation.
- *A doctor's order is required.* The doctor gives the reason for the restraint, what body part to restrain, what to use, and how long to use it. This information is on the care plan and your assignment sheet. In an emergency, the nurse can decide to apply restraints before getting a doctor's order.
- *The least restrictive method is used.* It allows the greatest amount of movement or body access possible. Some restraints attach to the person's body and to a non-movable object. They restrict freedom of movement or body access. Vest, jacket, ankle, wrist, hand, and some belt restraints are examples. Other restraints are near but not attached to the person's body (bed rails or wedge cushions). They do not totally restrict freedom of movement. They allow access to certain body parts.
- *Restraints are used only after other measures fail to protect the person* (see Box 12-1). Some people can harm themselves or others. The care plan must include measures to protect the person and prevent harm to others. Many fall prevention measures are restraint alternatives (Chapter 11).
- *Unnecessary restraint is false imprisonment* (Chapter 4). You must understand the reason for the restraint and its risks. If not, politely ask about its use. If you apply an unneeded restraint, you could face false imprisonment charges.
- *Informed consent is required.* The person must understand the reason for the restraint. The person is told how the restraint will help medical treatment. The person is told about the risks of restraint use. If the person cannot give consent, his or her legal representative is given the information. Consent is needed before a restraint can be used. The doctor or nurse provides needed information and obtains consent.
  See *Focus on Communication: Laws, Rules, and Guidelines.*

Safety Guidelines

The restrained person must be kept safe. Follow the safety measures in Box 12-3, pp. 138-139. Also remember these key points.

- *Observe for increased confusion and agitation.* Restraints can increase confusion and agitation. Whether confused or alert, people are aware of restricted movements. They may try to get out of the restraint or struggle to pull at it. Some restrained persons beg others to free or to help release them. These behaviors often are viewed as signs of confusion. Some people become more confused because they do not understand what is happening to them. Restrained persons need repeated explanations and reassurance. Spending time with them has a calming effect.
- *Protect the person's quality of life.* Restraints are used for as short a time as possible. The care plan must show how to reduce restraint use. You must meet the person's physical, emotional, and social needs. Visit with the person and explain the reason for the restraint.
- *Follow the manufacturer's instructions to safely apply and secure the restraint.* Tight restraints affect circulation and breathing. The person must be comfortable and able to move the restrained part to a limited and safe extent. You could be negligent if you do not apply or secure a restraint properly.
- *Apply restraints with enough help to protect the person and staff from injury.* Persons in danger of harming themselves or others are restrained quickly. Combative and agitated people can hurt themselves and the staff when restraints are applied. Enough staff members are needed to complete the task safely and quickly.
- *Observe the person at least every 15 minutes or as often as directed by the nurse and the care plan.* Restraints are dangerous. Injuries and deaths can result from improper restraint use and poor observation. Prevent complications. Breathing and circulation problems are examples.
- *Remove or release the restraint, re-position the person, and meet basic needs at least every 2 hours. Or do so as often as noted in the care plan.*
  - Remove or release the restraint for at least 10 minutes.
  - Provide for food, fluid, comfort, safety, hygiene, and elimination needs. Also give skin care.
  - Perform range-of-motion (ROM) exercises or help the person walk (Chapter 27). Follow the care plan.
  See *Focus on Communication: Safety Guidelines,* p. 138.

Text continued on p. 142.

FOCUS ON COMMUNICATION

Safety Guidelines

Restraints can increase confusion. Remind the person of the reason for the restraint and to call for help when it is needed. Do so as often as needed. For example:

- "Your doctor ordered this restraint so you don't hurt yourself. If you need to get up, please call for help. I'll check on you every 15 minutes. Other staff will check on you too."
- "How does the restraint feel? Is it too tight? Is it too loose?"

- "Please put your call light on. I want to make sure that you can reach and use it with the restraint on."
- "Please call for help right away if the restraint is too tight."
- "Please call for help right away if you feel pain in your fingers or hands. Also call for me if you feel numbness or tingling."
- "Please call for help right away if you are having problems breathing."

BOX 12-3   Safety Measures for Using Restraints

Before Applying Restraints

- Do not use sheets, towels, tape, rope, straps, bandages, Velcro, or other items to restrain a person.
- Apply a restraint only after being instructed about its proper use.
- Demonstrate correct application of the restraint before applying it.
- Use the restraint noted in the care plan. Use the correct size. Small restraints are tight. They cause discomfort and agitation. They also restrict breathing and circulation. Strangulation is a risk from big or loose restraints.
- Use only restraints that have the manufacturer's instructions and warning labels.
  - Read the warning labels. Note the front and back of the restraint.
  - Follow the instructions. Some restraints are safe for bed, chair, and wheelchair use. Others are used only with certain equipment.
- Use intact restraints.
  - Look for broken stitches, tears, cuts, or frayed fabric or straps.
  - Look for missing or loose buckles, locks, hooks, loops, or straps or other damage. The restraint must hold securely.
- Test zippers, buckles, locks, hooks, loops, and other fasteners. The device must fasten securely.
- Do not use a restraint near a fire, a flame, or smoking materials.

Applying Restraints

- Follow agency policies and procedures.
- Do not use a restraint to position a person:
  - On a toilet
  - On furniture that does not allow for correct application
- Position the person in good alignment before applying the restraint (Chapter 14).
  - Semi-Fowler's position is usually preferred for a vest, jacket, or belt restraint.
  - When in a chair, position the person so the hips are well to the back of the chair.
- Pad bony areas and the skin as directed by the nurse. This prevents pressure and injury from the restraint.

Applying Restraints—cont'd

- Follow the manufacturer's instructions. A restraint applied wrong or backward may cause serious injury or death. Death may occur from suffocation or strangulation.
  - *Vest restraint*—The "V" neck is in front (Fig. 12-4).
  - *Jacket restraint*—The opening is in the back.
  - *Belt restraint when in a chair*—Apply the restraint at a 45-degree angle over the thighs (Fig. 12-5).
- Do not criss-cross straps in the back unless required by the manufacturer's instructions (Fig. 12-6, p. 140). Straps may loosen when the person moves and cause serious injury.
- Secure restraints according to agency policy. The policy should follow the manufacturer's instructions and allow for quick release in an emergency. Quick-release buckles or airline-type buckles are used (Fig. 12-7, p. 140). So are quick-release ties (Fig. 12-8, p. 140).
- Secure straps out of the person's reach.
- Leave 1 to 2 inches of slack in the straps if directed to do so by the nurse. This allows some movement of the part.
- Secure the restraint to the movable part of the bed frame (Fig. 12-9, p. 140). The restraint will not tighten or loosen when the head or foot of the bed is raised or lowered. For chairs, secure straps under the seat of the wheelchair or chair (Fig. 12-10, p. 140).
- Check for snugness after applying the restraint. The restraint should be snug but allow some movement of the restrained part. Follow the manufacturer's instructions. For example:
  - *If applied to the chest or waist*—Make sure the person can breathe easily. A flat hand should slide between the restraint and the person's body (Fig. 12-11, p. 141). Check with the nurse if you have very small or very large hands. Small or large hands could cause a tight or loose restraint.
  - *For wrist and mitt restraints*—You should be able to slide 1 finger under the restraint. Check with the nurse if you have very small or very large fingers. Small or large fingers could cause a tight or loose restraint.
- Make sure that the straps:
  - Cannot tighten, loosen, slip, or cause too much slack.
  - Will not slide in any direction. If straps slide, they change the restraint's position. The person can get suspended off the mattress or chair (Figs. 12-12 and 12-13, p. 141). Strangulation can result.

BOX 12-3 Safety Measures for Using Restraints—cont'd

Applying Restraints—cont'd

- Never secure restraints to the bed rails. The person can reach bed rails to release knots or buckles. Also, injury is likely when raising or lowering bed rails.
- Use bed rail covers or gap protectors as instructed by the nurse (Fig. 12-14, p. 141). They prevent entrapment between the rails or the bed rail bars (see Fig. 12-12). Entrapment can occur between:
  - The bars of a bed rail
  - The space between half-length (split) bed rails
  - The bed rail and mattress
  - The head-board or foot-board and mattress

After Applying Restraints

- Keep full bed rails up when using a vest, jacket, or belt restraint. Also use bed rail covers or gap protectors. Otherwise the person could fall off the bed and strangle on the restraint. Or the person can get caught between half-length bed rails.
- Do not use back cushions when a person is restrained in a chair. If the cushion moves out of place, slack occurs in the straps. Strangulation is a risk if the person slides forward or down from the extra slack.
- Do not cover the person with a sheet, blanket, bedspread, or other covering. The restraint must be within plain view at all times.
- Check the person at least every 15 minutes for safety, comfort, and signs of injury. Or check the person more often as directed by the nurse and the care plan.
- Monitor persons in the supine (back-lying) position constantly. Aspiration is a great risk if vomiting occurs (Chapter 23). Call for the nurse at once.

After Applying Restraints—cont'd

- Check the person's circulation at least every 15 minutes or more often as directed by the nurse and the care plan.
  - *For mitt, wrist, or ankle restraints*—You should feel a pulse at a pulse site below the restraint. Fingers or toes should be warm and pink. Tell the nurse at once if:
    - You cannot feel a pulse.
    - Fingers or toes are cold, pale, or blue in color.
    - The person complains of pain, numbness, or tingling in the restrained part.
    - The skin is red or damaged.
  - *For a belt, jacket, or vest restraint*—The person should be able to breathe easily. Also check the position of the restraint, especially in the front and back.
- Keep scissors in your pocket. In an emergency such as strangulation, cutting the tie may be faster than untying a knot or releasing a buckle. Never leave scissors where the person can reach them. Make sure the person cannot reach the scissors in your pocket.
- Remove or release the restraint and re-position the person every 2 hours or more often as noted in the care plan. The restraint is removed or released for at least 10 minutes. Meet the person's basic needs.
  - Measure vital signs.
  - Meet elimination needs.
  - Offer food and fluids.
  - Meet hygiene needs.
  - Give skin care.
  - Perform range-of-motion (ROM) exercises or help the person walk. Follow the care plan.
  - Provide for physical and emotional comfort. (See the inside of the front cover.)
- Keep the call light and other needed items within the person's reach. Record that this was done.
- Complete a safety check before leaving the room. (See the inside of the front cover.)
- Report to the nurse every time you checked the person and removed or released the restraint. Report your observations and the care given. Follow agency policy for recording.

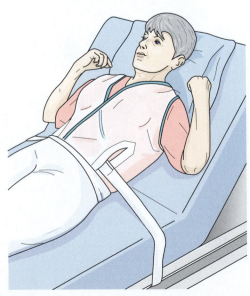

FIGURE 12-4 The vest restraint criss-crosses in front. The "V" neck is in front. (NOTE: The bed rails are raised after the restraint is applied.)

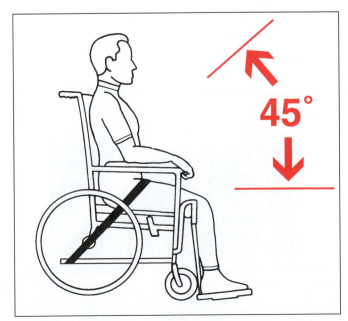

FIGURE 12-5 The belt restraint is at a 45-degree angle over the thighs. (Image courtesy Posey Company, Arcadia, Calif.)

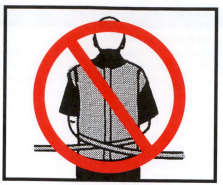

FIGURE 12-6 Never criss-cross vest or jacket straps in the back. (Image courtesy Posey Company, Arcadia, Calif.)

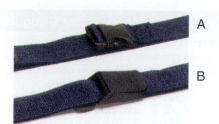

FIGURE 12-7 A, Quick-release buckle. **B,** Airline-type buckle. (Image courtesy Posey Company, Arcadia, Calif.)

How to Tie the Posey Quick-Release Tie

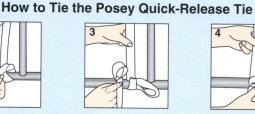
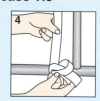

1. Wrap the strap once around a movable part of the bed frame leaving at least an 8" (20 cm) tail. Fold the loose end in half to create a loop and cross it over the other end.
2. Insert the folded strap where the straps cross over each other, as if tying a shoelace. Pull on the loop to tighten.
3. Fold the loose end in half to create a second loop.
4. Insert the second loop into the first loop.
5. Pull on the loop to tighten. Test to make sure strap is secure and will not slide in any direction.
6. Repeat on other side. Practice quick-release ties to ensure the knot releases with one pull on the loose end of the strap.

FIGURE 12-8 The Posey quick-release tie. (Image courtesy Posey Company, Arcadia, Calif.)

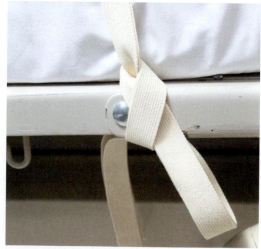

FIGURE 12-9 The restraint is secured to the movable part of the bed frame.

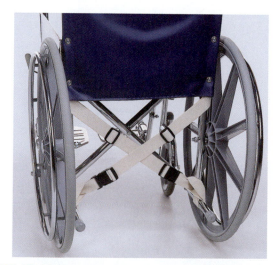

FIGURE 12-10 The restraint straps are secured to the wheelchair frame. (Image courtesy Posey Company, Arcadia, Calif.)

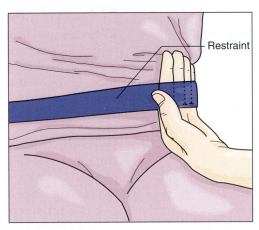

FIGURE 12-11 A flat hand slides between the restraint and the person.

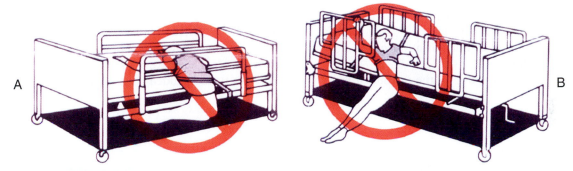

FIGURE 12-12 A, A person can get suspended and caught between bed rail bars. **B,** The person can get suspended and caught between half-length bed rails. (Images courtesy Posey Company, Arcadia, Calif.)

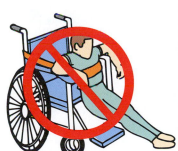

Straps to prevent sliding should always be over the thighs—NOT around the waist or chest. Straps should be at a 45° angle and secured to the chair under the seat, not behind the back. They should be snug but comfortable and not restrict breathing. If a belt or vest is too loose or applied around the waist, the person may slide partially off the seat—resulting in possible suffocation and death.

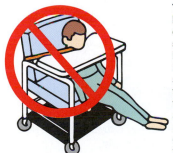

Tray tables (with or without a belt or vest) pose potential danger if the person should slide partly under the table and become caught. This could result in suffocation and death. Make sure the person's hips are positioned at the back of the chair—this may necessitate the use of an anti-slide material (Posey Grip), a pommel cushion, or a restrictive device if the person shows any tendency to slide forward.

FIGURE 12-13 Strangulation can result if the person slides forward or down because of extra slack in the restraint. (Images courtesy Posey Company, Arcadia, Calif.)

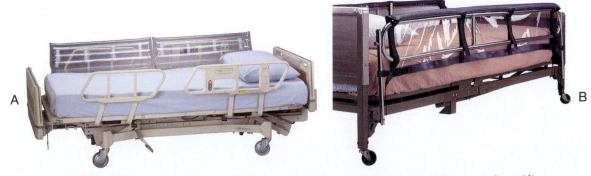

FIGURE 12-14 A, Bed rail protector. **B,** Guard rail pads. (Images courtesy Posey Company, Arcadia, Calif.)

Reporting and Recording

Restraint information is recorded in the person's medical record. If you apply restraints or care for a restrained person, report and record:

- The type of restraint applied
- The body part or parts restrained
- The reason for the application
- Safety measures taken (for example, bed rails padded and up, call light within reach)
- The time you applied the restraint
- The time you removed or released the restraint and for how long
- The person's vital signs
- The care given when the restraint was removed and for how long
- Skin color and condition
- Condition of the limbs
- The pulse felt in the restrained part
- Changes in the person's behavior
  Report the following complaints at once.
- Difficulty breathing
- Pain, numbness, or tingling in the restrained part
- Discomfort
- A tight restraint

Applying Restraints

Restraints are made of cloth or leather. Cloth restraints (soft restraints) are mitts, belts, straps, jackets, and vests. They are applied to the wrists, ankles, hands, waist, and chest. Leather restraints are applied to the wrists and ankles. Leather restraints are used for extreme agitation and combativeness.

Wrist Restraints. Wrist restraints (limb holders) limit arm movement (Fig. 12-15). They may be used when the person:

- Is at risk for pulling out tubes used for life-saving treatment (intravenous [IV] infusion, feeding tube).
- Is at risk for pulling at devices used to monitor vital signs.
- Scratches at, pulls at, or peels the skin, a wound, or a dressing. This can damage the skin or the wound.

Mitt Restraints. Hands are placed in mitt restraints. They prevent finger use. They allow hand, wrist, and arm movements. They have the same purpose as wrist restraints. Most mitts are padded (Fig. 12-16).

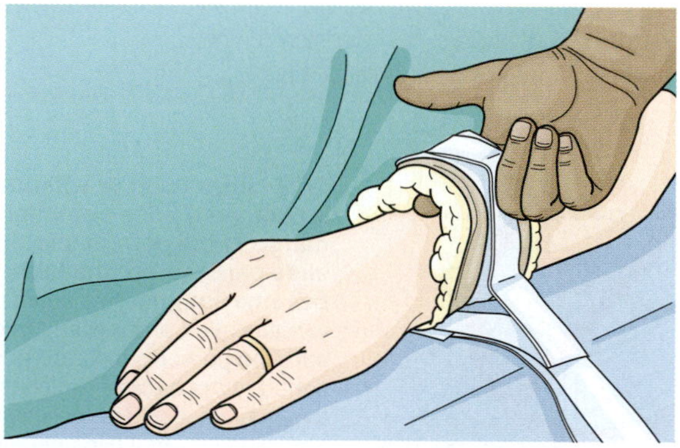

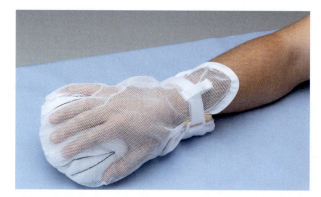

FIGURE 12-15 Wrist restraint. The soft part is toward the skin. Note that 1 finger fits between the restraint and the wrist.

FIGURE 12-16 Mitt restraint. (Image courtesy Posey Company, Arcadia, Calif.)

Belt Restraints. A belt restraint (Fig. 12-17) may be used when injuries from falls are risks or for positioning during a medical treatment. The person cannot get out of bed or out of a chair. However, a roll belt allows the person to turn from side to side or to sit up in bed.

The belt is applied around the waist and secured to the bed or chair (lap belt). It is applied over a garment. The person can release the quick-release type. It is less restrictive than those that only staff can release.

Vest Restraints and Jacket Restraints. Vest and jacket restraints are applied to the chest. They have the same purpose as belt restraints. The person cannot turn in bed or get out of a chair.

A jacket restraint is applied with the opening in the back. For a vest restraint, the "V" neck is in front and the vest crosses in the front (see Fig. 12-4). Vest and jacket restraints are never worn backward. Strangulation or other injuries are risks if the person slides down in the bed or chair. The restraint is always applied over a garment. (*NOTE: The straps of vest and jacket restraints cross in the front. A vest or jacket restraint may have a positioning slot in the back* [Fig. 12-18]. *Criss-cross straps following the manufacturer's instructions.*)

Vest and jacket restraints have life-threatening risks. Death can occur from strangulation. If caught in the restraint, it can become so tight that the person's chest cannot expand to inhale air. The person quickly suffocates and dies. Correct application is critical. You are advised to only assist the nurse in applying them. The nurse should have full responsibility for applying a vest or jacket restraint.

See *Focus on Communication: Applying Restraints,* p. 144.

See *Focus on Older Persons: Applying Restraints,* p. 144.

See *Delegation Guidelines: Applying Restraints,* p. 144.

See *Promoting Safety and Comfort: Applying Restraints,* p. 144.

See procedure: *Applying Restraints,* p. 145.

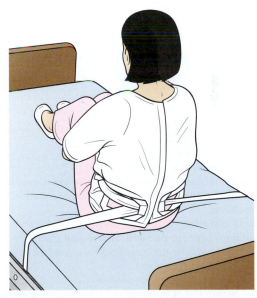

FIGURE 12-18 Jacket restraint. (NOTE: The bed rails are raised after the restraint is applied.)

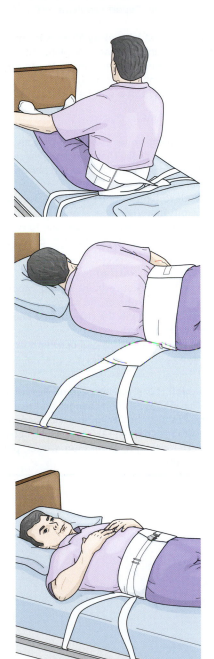

FIGURE 12-17 Belt restraint. (NOTE: The bed rails are raised after the restraint is applied.)

FOCUS ON COMMUNICATION
Applying Restraints

If you do not know how to apply a certain restraint, do not do so. Ask the nurse to show you the correct way. You can say: "I've never applied a restraint like this before. Would you please show me how and then watch me apply it?" Thank the nurse for helping you.

When applying a restraint, explain to the person what you are going to do. Then tell the person what you are doing step-by-step. Always check for safety and comfort. You can ask: "How does the restraint feel? Is it too tight? Is it too loose?"

Make sure the person can communicate with you after leaving the room. Place the call light within reach. Make sure the person can use it with the restraint on. Remind the person to call if uncomfortable or if anything is needed.

FOCUS ON OLDER PERSONS
Applying Restraints

Restraints may increase confusion and agitation in persons with dementia. They do not understand what you are doing. They may resist your efforts to apply a restraint. They may try to get free from the restraint. Serious injury and death are risks.

Never use force to apply a restraint. If a person is confused or agitated, ask a co-worker to help apply the restraint. Report problems to the nurse at once.

DELEGATION GUIDELINES
Applying Restraints

Before applying a restraint, you need this information from the nurse and the care plan.
- Why the doctor ordered the restraint.
- What type and size to use.
- Where to apply the restraint.
- How to safely apply the restraint. Have the nurse show you how to apply it. Then show correct application back to the nurse.
- How to correctly position the person.
- What bony areas to pad and how to pad them.
- If bed rail covers or gap protectors are needed.
- If bed rails are up or down.
- What special equipment is needed.
- If the person needs to be checked more often than every 15 minutes. If yes, how often?
- When to apply and release the restraint.
- What observations to report and record. See "Reporting and Recording," p. 142.
- When to report observations.
- What patient or resident concerns to report at once.

PROMOTING SAFETY AND COMFORT
Applying Restraints

Safety
Restraints can cause serious harm, even death. Always follow the manufacturer's instructions. The instructions for 1 restraint may not apply to another. Also, the manufacturer may have instructions for applying restraints on persons who are agitated.

Never use force. Ask a co-worker to help if a person is confused and agitated. Report problems to the nurse at once.

Check the person at least every 15 minutes or more often as directed by the nurse and the care plan. Make sure the call light is within reach. Ask the person to use the call light at the first sign of problems or discomfort.

Never use a restraint as a seat belt in a car or other vehicle.

Mitt Restraints
Mitt restraints prevent finger use. Often they are not secured to the bed or chair. Therefore the person can raise the mitt to his or her mouth. Observe the person closely to make sure that he or she does not:
- Use the teeth to remove or damage the device.
- Ingest any mitt material.

Persons with mitt restraints may be able to walk about. Falls are a risk. Practice safety measures to prevent falls (Chapter 11).

Belt, Vest, and Jacket Restraints
When a belt, vest, or jacket restraint is used, monitor the person to make sure that he or she cannot:
- Slide forward or down in the chair or bed and become suspended or entrapped.
- Fall off the chair or mattress and become suspended or entrapped.

Comfort
The person's comfort is always important. Restraints limit movement. This affects position changes and reaching needed items. Position the person in good alignment before applying a restraint (Chapter 14). Make sure needed items are within reach—call light, water mug, tissues, phone, bed controls, and so on.

Applying Restraints

QUALITY OF LIFE

- Knock before entering the person's room.
- Address the person by name.
- Introduce yourself by name and title.

- Explain the procedure before starting and during the procedure.
- Protect the person's rights during the procedure.
- Handle the person gently during the procedure.

PRE-PROCEDURE

1 Follow *Delegation Guidelines: Applying Restraints.* See *Promoting Safety and Comfort: Applying Restraints.*
2 Collect the following as instructed by the nurse.
   - Correct type and size of restraint
   - Padding for skin and bony areas
   - Bed rail pads or gap protectors (if needed)

3 Practice hand hygiene.
4 Identify the person. Check the ID (identification) bracelet against the assignment sheet. Use 2 identifiers (Chapter 10). Also call the person by name.
5 Provide for privacy.

PROCEDURE

6 Position the person for comfort and good alignment.
7 Put the bed rail pads or gap protectors (if needed) on the bed for the person in bed. Follow the manufacturer's instructions.
8 Pad bony areas. Follow the nurse's instructions and the care plan.
9 Read the manufacturer's instructions. Note the front and back of the restraint.
10 *For wrist restraints:*
   a Follow the manufacturer's instructions. Place the soft or foam part toward the skin.
   b Secure the restraint so it is snug but not tight. Make sure you can slide 1 finger under the restraint (see Fig. 12-15). Follow the manufacturer's instructions. Adjust the straps if the restraint is too loose or too tight. Check for snugness again.
   c Secure the straps to the movable part of the bed frame out of the person's reach. Use the buckle or a quick-release tie.
   d Repeat steps 10, a–c for the other wrist.
11 *For mitt restraints:*
   a Clean and dry the person's hands.
   b Insert the person's hand into the restraint with the palm down. Follow the manufacturer's instructions.
   c Wrap the wrist strap around the smallest part of the wrist. Secure the strap with the hook-and-loop or other closure.
   d Secure the restraint to the bed if directed to do so. Secure the straps to the movable part of the bed frame out of the person's reach. Use the buckle or a quick-release tie.
   e Check for snugness. Slide 1 finger between the restraint and the wrist. Follow the manufacturer's instructions. Adjust the straps if the restraint is too loose or too tight. Check for snugness again.
   f Repeat steps 11, b–e for the other hand.

12 *For a belt restraint:*
   a Assist the person to a sitting position.
   b Apply the restraint. Follow the manufacturer's instructions.
   c Remove wrinkles or creases from the front and back.
   d Bring the ties through the slots in the belt.
   e Position the straps at a 45-degree angle between the wheelchair seat and sides (see Fig. 12-5). If in bed, help the person lie down.
   f Make sure the person is comfortable and in good alignment.
   g Secure the straps to the movable part of the bed frame. Use the buckle or a quick-release tie. The buckle or tie is out of the person's reach. For a wheelchair, criss-cross and secure the straps as in Figure 12-10.
   h Check for snugness. Slide an open hand between the restraint and the person. Adjust the restraint if it is too loose or too tight. Check for snugness again.
13 *For a vest restraint:*
   a Assist the person to a sitting position. If in a wheelchair:
      1 Position him or her as far back in the wheelchair as possible.
      2 Make sure the buttocks are against the chair back.
   b Apply the restraint. Follow the manufacturer's instructions. The "V" neck is in the front.
   c Bring the straps through the slots.
   d Make sure side seams are under the arms. Remove wrinkles in the front and back. Close the zipper if the device opens in the back. Or fasten with other closures.
   e Position the straps at a 45-degree angle between the wheelchair seat and sides. If in bed, help the person lie down.
   f Make sure the person is comfortable and in good alignment.
   g Secure the straps to the movable part of the bed frame at waist level. Use the buckle or a quick-release tie. The buckle or tie is out of the person's reach. For a wheelchair, criss-cross and secure the straps as in Figure 12-10.
   h Check for snugness. Slide an open hand between the restraint and the person. Adjust the restraint if it is too loose or too tight. Check for snugness again.

Continued

Applying Restraints—cont'd

PROCEDURE—cont'd

14 *For a jacket restraint:*
a Assist the person to a sitting position. If in a wheelchair:
  1 Position him or her as far back in the wheelchair as possible.
  2 Make sure the buttocks are against the chair back.
b Apply the restraint. Follow the manufacturer's instructions. The jacket opening goes in the back.
c Make sure the side seams are under the arms. Remove wrinkles in the front and back.
d Close the back with the zipper or other closures.

e Position the straps at a 45-degree angle between the wheelchair seat and sides. If in bed, help the person lie down.
f Make sure the person is comfortable and in good alignment.
g Secure the straps to the movable part of the bed frame at waist level. Use the buckle or quick-release tie. The buckle or tie is out of the person's reach. For a wheelchair, criss-cross and secure the straps as in Figure 12-10.
h Check for snugness. Slide an open hand between the restraint and the person. Adjust the restraint if it is too loose or too tight. Check for snugness again.

POST-PROCEDURE

15 Position the person as the nurse directs.
16 Provide for comfort. (See the inside of the front cover.)
17 Place the call light and other needed items within the person's reach.
18 Raise or lower bed rails. Follow the care plan and the manufacturer's instructions for the restraint.
19 Unscreen the person.
20 Complete a safety check of the room. (See the inside of the front cover.)
21 Practice hand hygiene.
22 Check the person and the restraint at least every 15 minutes or more often as directed by the nurse and the care plan. Report and record your observations.
  a *For wrist or mitt restraints*: check the pulse, color, and temperature of the restrained parts.
  b *For a vest, jacket, or belt restraint*: check the person's breathing. Make sure the restraint is properly positioned in the front and back. Release the restraint and call for the nurse at once if the person is not breathing or is having problems breathing.

23 Do the following at least every 2 hours for at least 10 minutes.
  a Remove or release the restraint.
  b Measure vital signs.
  c Re-position the person.
  d Meet food, fluid, hygiene, and elimination needs.
  e Give skin care.
  f Perform ROM exercises or help the person walk. Follow the care plan.
  g Provide for physical and emotional comfort. (See the inside of the front cover.)
  h Re-apply the restraint.
24 Complete a safety check of the room. (See the inside of the front cover.)
25 Practice hand hygiene.
26 Report and record your observations and the care given (Fig. 12-19).

FIGURE 12-19 Charting sample.

Restraint Type				
☐ Wrist restraints	☒ Mitt restraints	☐ Belt restraint	☐ Vest restraint	☐ Jacket restraint

Care Measures		
☒ Restraints released/removed	☒ Food/fluid needs met	☒ Comfort measures
Duration: 15 minutes	☒ ROM/exercise/activity	☒ Skin care
☒ Restraints re-applied	☒ Urinary/bowel elimination	☒ Hygiene
☐ Measures refused	☒ Positioning	☐ Other:
Notified nurse: E. Scott, RN	☒ Call light and needed items in reach	

Vital Signs							
Temp 98.4 °F	Pulse 70	R 14	BP 116 / 72 mmHg	Pain 0 /10

Circulation Observations (Normal in blue)

Color: ☒ Pink ☐ Pale ☐ Cyanotic (bluish)	**Tell the nurse at once if any observations are abnormal.**
Temperature: ☐ Hot ☒ Warm ☐ Cool ☐ Cold	
Sensation: ☒ Good sensation ☐ Numbness/tingling ☐ No sensation	
Movement: ☒ Able to move extremities ☐ Unable to move extremities	Notified Nurse:
Pulses: ☒ Pulses present in all extremities ☐ Pulse faint/absent in any extremity	

Personal and Professional Responsibility

Restraints have many risks. See Box 12-2. Therefore restraint use brings many responsibilities. You must:

- Promote safety and comfort.
- Apply the restraint properly.
- Observe the person closely.
- Meet basic needs.
- Report any concerns to the nurse.

If you do not know how to apply a restraint, do not do so. Ask the nurse to show you. To use restraints safely and responsibly, follow the guidelines in Box 12-3.

Rights and Respect

Every person has the right to freedom from restraint. Restraints are used as a last resort to protect the person or others from harm. Other methods must be tried first. You may be asked to assist with restraint alternatives (see Box 12-1). Make a true effort. Be honest. Do not tell the nurse you tried if you did not. Do your best to allow the person the right to freedom from restraint.

Independence and Social Interaction

All restraints limit movement. Independence is restricted. To promote independence:

- Keep the call light within reach at all times. Make sure the person can use it. Tell the person to signal for you if anything is needed. Answer the call light and meet the person's needs promptly.
- Keep needed items within reach. This is most important with restraints that allow hand and arm use. Belt, vest, and jacket restraints are examples.
- Check the person at least every 15 minutes or more often as directed by the nurse and the care plan.
- Remove or release the restraint at least every 2 hours.
- Meet food, fluid, hygiene, and elimination needs.
- Assist the person with walks or ROM exercises.
- Allow choice. For example, let the person choose where to walk or what to eat and drink.
- Let the person do as much for himself or herself as safely possible.

Delegation and Teamwork

Care conferences are held to meet the person's safety needs. Every attempt is made to protect the person without restraints.

Your input has value. Share your observations and ideas. For example, a person does not try to get out of a chair when looking at photos or reading a book. You share this with the health team for the person's care plan.

Ethics and Laws

Imagine the following.

- Your nose itches. But your wrists are restrained. You cannot scratch your nose.
- You need to use the bathroom. You cannot get up or reach your call light. You soil yourself with urine or a bowel movement.
- You cannot answer your phone.
- You are uncomfortable. You have a vest restraint. You cannot move or turn in bed.
- You are thirsty. Your wrists are restrained. You cannot reach the water mug.
- You hear the fire alarm. You have on a restraint. You cannot get up to move to a safe place. You must wait to be rescued.

What would you do? Would you calmly lie or sit there? Would you try to get free from the restraint? Would you yell for help? Would the staff think that you are uncomfortable? Or would they think that you are agitated and uncooperative? Would you feel angry, embarrassed, or humiliated?

Ethics deals with how others are treated. Restraints lessen the person's dignity and freedom. A person should not be treated in this way. Put yourself in the person's situation. Then you can better understand how the person feels. Treat the person like you would want to be treated—with kindness, caring, respect, and dignity.

FOCUS ON PRIDE: *Application*

Describe 3 scenarios involving behavior that is dangerous or that interferes with treatment. List ideas for managing the behavior without using restraints.

Circle T if the statement is TRUE or F if it is FALSE.

1   T F   Restraint alternatives fail to protect a person. You can apply a restraint.

2   T F   A restraint restricts a person's freedom of movement.

3   T F   Some drugs are restraints.

4   T F   Restraints can be used for staff convenience.

5   T F   A device is a restraint only if it is attached to the person's body.

6   T F   Bed rails are restraints if they cannot be lowered. The person cannot leave the bed.

7   T F   Restraints are used only for a person's specific medical symptom.

8   T F   Unnecessary restraint is false imprisonment.

9   T F   You can apply restraints when you think they are needed.

10 T F   You can use a vest restraint to position a person on the toilet.

11 T F   Restraints are removed or released at least every 2 hours.

12 T F   Restraints are tied to bed rails.

13 T F   Wrist restraints are used to prevent falls.

14 T F   A vest restraint crosses in front.

15 T F   Bed rails are left down when a vest restraint is used.

Circle the BEST answer.

16 Which is a restraint alternative?
    a Positioning the person's chair close to the wall
    b Raising all bed rails
    c Giving a drug that restricts movement
    d Padding walls and corners of furniture

17 Physical restraints
    a Can be removed easily by the person
    b Are not allowed by OBRA
    c Require a doctor's order
    d Are safer than chemical restraints

18 The following can occur because of restraints. Which is the *most* serious?
    a Fractures
    b Strangulation
    c Pressure injuries
    d Urinary tract infections

19 A belt restraint is applied to a person in bed. Where should you secure the straps?
    a To the bed rails
    b To the head-board
    c To the movable part of the bed frame
    d To the foot-board

20 A person has a restraint. You should check the person and the position of the restraint at least every
    a 15 minutes
    b 30 minutes
    c Hour
    d 3 hours

21 A person has mitt restraints. Which will you report to the nurse at once?
    a The hands are clean, warm, and dry.
    b The person has numbness in the hands.
    c You removed the restraints for 10 minutes.
    d You felt a pulse in both arms.

22 When applying restraints, you should
    a Know when to apply and release them
    b Use force if the person is agitated
    c Allow plenty of slack in the straps
    d Apply a restraint you have not used before

23 A person has a vest restraint. To check for snugness, slide
    a A fist between the vest and the person
    b 1 finger between the vest and the person
    c An open hand between the vest and the person
    d 2 fingers between the vest and the person

24 The correct way to apply any restraint is to follow the
    a Nurse's directions
    b Doctor's orders
    c Care plan
    d Manufacturer's instructions

Answers to Chapter 12 questions are on p. 551.

FOCUS ON PRACTICE

Problem Solving

A person uses a wheelchair and often tries to get up without help. What are some alternatives to restraints that may be tried? If a restraint is needed, how will you provide for the person's basic needs?

Preventing Infection

OBJECTIVES

- Define the key terms and key abbreviations in this chapter.
- Identify what microbes need to live and grow.
- List the signs and symptoms of infection.
- Explain the chain of infection.
- Describe healthcare-associated infections and the persons at risk.
- Describe the principles of medical asepsis.
- Explain the rules of hand hygiene.

- Explain how to care for equipment and supplies.
- Describe disinfection and sterilization methods.
- Describe Standard Precautions and Transmission-Based Precautions.
- Explain the Bloodborne Pathogen Standard.
- Perform the procedures described in this chapter.
- Explain how to promote PRIDE in the person, the family, and yourself.

KEY TERMS

antibiotic A drug that kills certain microbes that cause infection

antisepsis The processes, procedures, and chemical treatments that kill microbes or prevent them from causing an infection; *anti* means *against* and *sepsis* means *infection*

asepsis The absence *(a)* of disease-producing microbes; *sepsis* means *infection*

biohazardous waste Items contaminated with blood, body fluids, secretions, or excretions; *bio* means *life* and *hazardous* means *dangerous* or *harmful*

carrier A human or animal that is a reservoir for microbes but does not develop the infection

clean technique See "medical asepsis"

communicable disease A disease caused by pathogens that spread easily; contagious disease

contagious disease See "communicable disease"

contamination The process of becoming unclean

cross-contamination Passing microbes from 1 person to another by contaminated hands, equipment, or supplies

disinfection The process of killing pathogens

healthcare-associated infection (HAI) An infection that develops in a person cared for in any setting where health care is given; the infection is related to receiving health care

infection A disease state resulting from the invasion and growth of microbes in the body

infection control Practices and procedures that prevent the spread of infection

medical asepsis Practices used to reduce the number of microbes and prevent their spread from 1 person or place to another person or place; clean technique

microbe See "microorganism"

microorganism A small *(micro)* living thing *(organism)* seen only with a microscope; microbe

non-pathogen A microbe that does not usually cause an infection

pathogen A microbe that is harmful and can cause an infection

sterile The absence of *all* microbes

sterilization The process of destroying *all* microbes

KEY ABBREVIATIONS

CDC	Centers for Disease Control and Prevention
E. coli	*Escherichia coli*
GI	Gastro-intestinal
HAI	Healthcare-associated infection
HBV	Hepatitis B virus
HIV	Human immunodeficiency virus
MDRO	Multidrug-resistant organism

MRSA	Methicillin-resistant *Staphylococcus aureus*
OPIM	Other potentially infectious materials
OSHA	Occupational Safety and Health Administration
PPE	Personal protective equipment
TB	Tuberculosis
VRE	Vancomycin-resistant *Enterococci*

An *infection is a disease state resulting from the invasion and growth of microbes in the body.* Infection is a major safety and health hazard. Minor infections are short-term. Some infections are serious and can cause death. Older and disabled persons are at risk. The health team follows certain *practices and procedures that prevent the spread of infection (infection control).* The goal is to protect patients, residents, visitors, and staff from infection.

This chapter includes measures of antisepsis. *Antisepsis is the processes, procedures, and chemical treatments that kill microbes or prevent them from causing an infection.* (Anti *means* against. Sepsis *means* infection.)

MICROORGANISMS

A *microorganism (microbe) is a small* (micro) *living thing* (organism). *It is seen only with a microscope.* Commonly called *germs,* microbes are everywhere—mouth, nose, respiratory tract, stomach, and intestines. They are on the skin and in the air, soil, water, and food. They are on animals, clothing, and furniture.

Microbes that are harmful and can cause infections are called **pathogens.** **Non-pathogens** *are microbes that do not usually cause an infection.*

Requirements of Microbes

Microbes need a *reservoir* (host). The reservoir is the place where the microbe lives and grows. People, plants, animals, the soil, food, and water are common reservoirs. Microbes need *water* and *nourishment* from the reservoir. Most need *oxygen* to live. A *warm* and *dark* environment is needed. Most grow best at body temperature. They are destroyed by heat and light.

Multidrug-Resistant Organisms

Multidrug-resistant organisms (MDROs) are microbes that can resist the effects of antibiotics. *Antibiotics are drugs that kill certain microbes that cause infections.* Some microbes can change their structures, making them harder to kill. They can live in the presence of antibiotics. Therefore the infections they cause are hard to treat.

MDROs are caused by prescribing antibiotics when not needed (over-prescribing). Not taking antibiotics for the length of time prescribed is another cause. Common MDROs are:

- *Methicillin-resistant Staphylococcus aureus (MRSA). Staphylococcus aureus* ("staph") is found in the nose and on the skin. MRSA is resistant to antibiotics often used for "staph" infections. MRSA can cause serious wound and bloodstream infections and pneumonia.
- *Vancomycin-resistant Enterococci (VRE). Enterococcus* is found in the intestines and in feces. It can be transmitted to others by contaminated hands, toilet seats, care equipment, and other items that the hands touch. When not in the intestines, enterococci can cause urinary tract, wound, pelvic, and other infections. Enterococci resistant to vancomycin (an antibiotic) are called *vancomycin-resistant Enterococci (VRE).*

INFECTION

A *local infection* is in a body part. A *systemic infection* involves the whole body. (*Systemic* means *entire.*) The person has some or all of the signs and symptoms listed in Box 13-1.

See *Focus on Older Persons: Infection.*
See *Focus on Surveys: Infection.*

BOX 13-1	Infection—Signs and Symptoms

- *Fever* (elevated body temperature)
- Pulse and respirations: increased
- Chills
- Pain, tenderness, or limited use of a body part
- Fatigue and loss of energy
- Appetite: loss of *(anorexia)*
- Nausea and vomiting
- Diarrhea
- Rash
- Sores on mucous membranes
- Redness and swelling of a body part
- Discharge or drainage from the infected area
- Heat or warmth in a body part
- Headache
- Muscle aches
- Joint pain
- Confusion

FOCUS ON OLDER PERSONS
Infection

The immune system protects the body from disease and infection (Chapter 8). Changes occur in this system with aging. Therefore older persons are at risk for infection.

An older person may not show the signs and symptoms listed in Box 13-1. The person may have only a slight fever or no fever at all. Redness and swelling may be very slight. The person may not complain of pain. Confusion and delirium may occur (Chapter 35).

An infection can become life-threatening before the older person has obvious signs and symptoms. Report minor changes in the person's behavior or condition at once.

Healing takes longer in older persons. Therefore an infection can prolong the rehabilitation process. Independence and quality of life are affected.

FOCUS ON SURVEYS
Infection

Infection control practices are a focus of surveys. You may be asked about signs and symptoms of infection.
- What you do when you observe them
- Who do you tell

The Chain of Infection

The chain of infection (Fig. 13-1) involves a:

- Source—A pathogen.
- Reservoir—The pathogen needs a place where it can grow and multiply. A *carrier is a human or animal that is a reservoir for microbes but does not develop the infection.* Carriers can pass pathogens to others.
- Portal of exit—The pathogen needs a way to leave the reservoir. Exits are the respiratory, gastro-intestinal (GI), urinary, and reproductive tracts; breaks in the skin; and blood.
- Method of transmission—The pathogen is *transmitted* to another host (Fig. 13-2).
- Portal of entry—The pathogen enters the body. Portals of entry and exit are the same—the respiratory, GI, urinary, and reproductive tracts; breaks in the skin; and blood.
- Susceptible host—The transmitted microbe needs a host where it can grow and multiply.

Susceptible Hosts. Susceptible hosts are at risk for infection. They include persons who:

- Are very young or who are older.
- Are ill.
- Were exposed to the pathogen.
- Do not follow practices to prevent infection.
- Are burn patients. When burns destroy the skin, the wound is a portal of entry for microbes.
- Are transplant patients. A *transplant* involves transferring an organ or tissue from 1 person to another person or from 1 body part to another body part. The body's normal immune response is to attack (reject) the new organ or tissue. Drugs are given to prevent rejection. They suppress (prevent) the immune system from producing antibodies. Antibodies are needed to fight infection.
- Are chemotherapy patients (Chapter 33). Some chemotherapy drugs affect the ability to produce white blood cells (WBCs). WBCs are needed to fight infection.

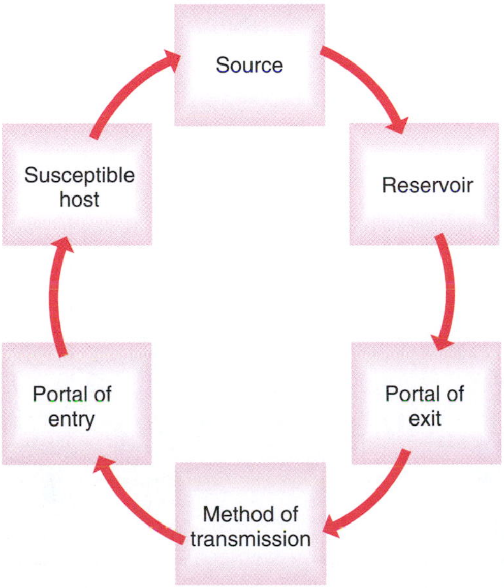

FIGURE 13-1 The chain of infection. (Redrawn and modified from Potter PA, Perry AG, Stockert PA, Hall AM: *Fundamentals of nursing,* ed 9, St Louis, 2017, Elsevier.)

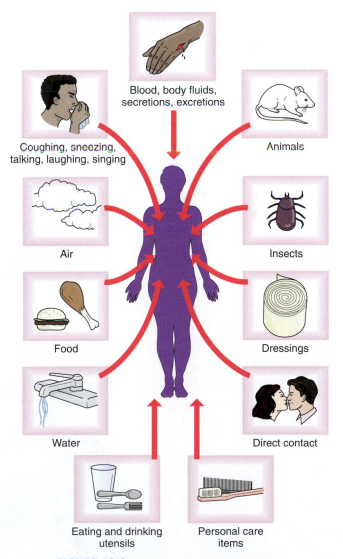

FIGURE 13-2 Methods of transmitting microbes.

Healthcare-Associated Infections

A *healthcare-associated infection (HAI)* *is an infection that develops in a person cared for in any setting where health care is given. The infection is related to receiving health care.* HAIs also are called nosocomial infections. (*Nosocomial* comes from the Greek word for *hospital.*)

HAIs are caused by microbes normally found in or on the body. Or they are caused by microbes transmitted to the person from other sources. For example, *Escherichia coli* (*E. coli*) is normally in the colon and feces. Poor wiping after bowel movements can cause *E. coli* to enter the urinary system. With poor hand-washing, *E. coli* spreads to any body part, thing, or person the hands touch.

Microbes can enter the body from care equipment and supplies. Such items must be free of microbes. Staff can transfer microbes from 1 person to another and from themselves to others. Common sites for HAIs are:

- The urinary system
- The respiratory system
- Wounds
- The bloodstream
  The health team must prevent infection by:
- Medical asepsis. This includes hand hygiene.
- Surgical asepsis, p. 171.
- Standard Precautions, p. 159.
- Transmission-Based Precautions, p. 161.
- The Bloodborne Pathogen Standard, p. 170.

MEDICAL ASEPSIS

Asepsis *is the absence* (a) *of disease-producing microbes. Sepsis means* infection. Microbes are everywhere. Measures are needed to achieve asepsis. *Medical asepsis (clean technique) is the practices used to:*

- *Reduce the number of microbes.*
- *Prevent microbes from spreading from 1 person or place to another person or place.*

Contamination *is the process of becoming unclean.* In medical asepsis, an item or area is *clean* when it is free of pathogens. The item or area is *contaminated* when pathogens are present. *Sterile* *means the absence of* all *microbes*—pathogens and non-pathogens. A *sterile* item or area is *contaminated* when pathogens or non-pathogens are present. *Cross-contamination* *is passing microbes from 1 person to another by contaminated hands, equipment, or supplies* (Fig. 13-3). Medical asepsis and *surgical asepsis* (the practices to remove all microbes) prevent cross-contamination.

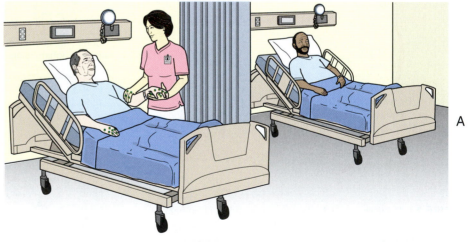

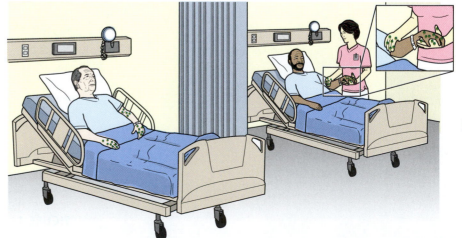

FIGURE 13-3 Cross-contamination. **A,** Microbes on the person's skin are transmitted to the nursing assistant's hands. **B,** The nursing assistant's contaminated hands transmit microbes from 1 person to another.

Common Aseptic Practices

Aseptic practices break the chain of infection. To prevent the spread of microbes, wash your hands:

- After elimination.
- After changing tampons or sanitary pads.
- After contact with your own or another person's blood, body fluids, secretions, or excretions. This includes saliva, vomitus, urine, feces, vaginal discharge, mucus, semen, wound drainage, pus, and respiratory secretions.
- After coughing, sneezing, or blowing your nose.
- Before and after handling, preparing, or eating food.
- After smoking.
  Also do the following.
- Provide all persons with their own linens and personal care items.
- Cover your nose and mouth when coughing, sneezing, or blowing your nose. If without tissues, cough or sneeze into your upper arm (Fig. 13-4). Do not cough or sneeze into your hands.
- Bathe, wash hair, and brush your teeth regularly.
- Wash fruit and raw vegetables before eating or serving them.
- Wash cooking and eating utensils with soap and water after use.
  See *Focus on Older Persons: Common Aseptic Practices.*

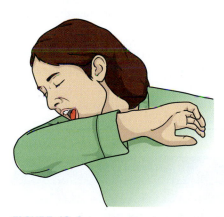

FIGURE 13-4 Sneezing into the upper arm.

Hand Hygiene

Hand hygiene is the easiest and most important way to prevent the spread of microbes and infection. You use your hands for almost everything. They are easily contaminated. They can spread microbes to other persons or items (see Fig. 13-3). *Practice hand hygiene before and after giving care.* See Box 13-2 (p. 154) for the rules of hand hygiene.

See *Focus on Surveys: Hand Hygiene.*
See *Promoting Safety and Comfort: Hand Hygiene.*
See procedure: *Hand-Washing*, p. 154.
See procedure: *Using an Alcohol-Based Hand Sanitizer,* p. 156.

Text continued on p. 157.

FOCUS ON SURVEYS

Hand Hygiene

Hand hygiene is a focus of surveys. A surveyor may:

- Observe you washing your hands or using an alcohol-based hand sanitizer according to agency policy.
- Observe if you practice hand hygiene:
  - After each direct patient or resident contact
  - Before and after all procedures
  - After removing gloves
  - When entering or leaving the room of a person on Transmission-Based Precautions (p. 161)
- Ask you questions about:
  - When you should wash your hands
  - When you can use an alcohol-based hand sanitizer

PROMOTING SAFETY AND COMFORT

Hand Hygiene

Safety
You use your hands for almost every task. They can pick up microbes from a person, place, or thing. Your hands transfer them to other people, places, or things. That is why hand hygiene is so very important. Always practice hand hygiene before and after giving care.

Comfort
You will practice hand hygiene frequently during your shift. Hand lotions and hand creams help prevent chapping and dry skin. Use an agency-approved lotion or cream.

FOCUS ON OLDER PERSONS

Common Aseptic Practices

Persons with dementia do not understand aseptic practices. The staff must protect them from infection. Assist them with hand-washing:

- After elimination
- After coughing, sneezing, or blowing the nose
- Before and after they eat or handle food
- Any time their hands are soiled
  Check and clean their hands and fingernails often. They may not or cannot tell you when soiling occurs.

BOX 13-2	Rules of Hand Hygiene

- Wash your hands (with soap and water):
  - When they are visibly dirty or soiled with blood, body fluids, secretions, or excretions
  - Before eating and after using a restroom
  - After known or suspected exposure to *Clostridium difficile* (Chapter 22) or to persons with infectious diarrhea
  - If exposure to the anthrax spore is suspected or proven
  - If an alcohol-based hand sanitizer is not available
- Use an alcohol-based hand sanitizer for hand hygiene if your hands are not visibly soiled.
  - Before direct contact with a person.
  - After contact with the person's intact skin. After taking a pulse or blood pressure or after moving a person are examples.
  - After contact with body fluids or excretions, mucous membranes, non-intact skin, and wound dressings if hands are not visibly soiled.
  - When moving from a contaminated body site to a clean body site.
  - After contact with items in the person's care setting.
  - After removing gloves.
- Follow these rules for washing your hands with soap and water. See procedure: *Hand-Washing.*
  - Wash your hands under warm running water. Do not use hot water.
  - Stand away from the sink. Do not let your hands, body, or uniform touch the sink. The sink is contaminated. See Figure 13-5.
  - Do not touch the inside of the sink at any time.
  - Keep your hands and forearms lower than your elbows. Hands are dirtier than elbows and forearms. If you hold your hands and forearms up, dirty water runs from your hands to your elbows. Those areas become contaminated.
- Rub your palms together (Fig. 13-6) and interlace your fingers (Fig. 13-7) to work up a good lather. The rubbing action helps remove microbes and dirt.
- Pay attention to areas often missed during hand-washing—thumbs, knuckles, sides of the hands, little fingers, and under the nails.
- Clean fingernails by rubbing the fingertips against your palms (Fig. 13-8).
- Use a nail file or orangewood stick to clean under fingernails (Fig. 13-9). Microbes grow easily under the fingernails.
- Wash your hands for at least 15 to 20 seconds. Wash your hands longer if they are dirty or soiled with blood, body fluids, secretions, or excretions. Use your judgment and follow agency policy.
- Use clean, dry paper towels to dry your hands.
- Dry your hands starting at the fingertips. Work up to your forearms (Fig. 13-10). You will dry the cleanest area first.
- Use a clean, dry paper towel for each faucet to turn the water off (Fig. 13-11, p. 156). Faucets are contaminated. The paper towels prevent you from contaminating your clean hands.
- Follow these rules when decontaminating your hands with an alcohol-based hand sanitizer. See procedure: *Using an Alcohol-Based Hand Sanitizer,* p. 156.
  - Apply the product to the palm of 1 hand. Follow the manufacturer's instructions for the amount to use.
  - Rub your hands together.
  - Cover all surfaces of your hands and fingers.
  - Continue rubbing your hands together until your hands are dry.
- Apply hand lotion or cream after hand hygiene. This prevents the skin from chapping and drying. Skin breaks can occur in chapped and dry skin. Skin breaks are portals of entry for microbes.

Modified from Centers for Disease Control and Prevention: Guidelines for hand hygiene in health-care settings, *Morbidity and Mortality Weekly,* Report 51 (RR-16), October 2002.

Hand-Washing

PROCEDURE

1 See *Promoting Safety and Comfort: Hand Hygiene,* p. 153.
2 Make sure you have soap, paper towels, an orangewood stick or nail file, and a wastebasket. Collect missing items.
3 Push your watch up your arm 4 to 5 inches. Push long uniform sleeves up too.
4 Stand away from the sink so your clothes do not touch the sink (see Fig. 13-5). Stand so the soap and faucet are easy to reach. Do not touch the inside of the sink at any time.
5 Turn on and adjust the water until it feels warm.
6 Wet your wrists and hands. Keep your hands lower than your elbows. Be sure to wet the area 3 to 4 inches above your wrists.
7 Apply about 1 teaspoon of soap to your hands.
8 Rub your palms together and interlace your fingers to work up a good lather (see Fig. 13-6). Lather your wrists, hands, and fingers. Keep your hands lower than your elbows. This step should last at least 15 to 20 seconds.

9 Wash each hand and wrist thoroughly. Clean the back of your fingers and between your fingers (see Fig. 13-7).
10 Clean under the fingernails. Rub your fingertips against your palms (see Fig. 13-8).
11 Clean under the fingernails with a nail file or orangewood stick (see Fig. 13-9). Do this for the first hand-washing of the day and when your hands are highly soiled.
12 Rinse your wrists, hands, and fingers well. Water flows from above the wrists to your fingertips.
13 Repeat steps 7 through 12, if needed.
14 Dry your wrists and hands with clean, dry paper towels. Pat dry starting at your fingertips (see Fig. 13-10).
15 Discard the paper towels into the wastebasket.
16 Turn off faucets with clean, dry paper towels. This prevents you from contaminating your hands (see Fig. 13-11). Use a clean paper towel for each faucet. Or use knee or foot controls to turn off the faucet.
17 Discard the paper towels into the wastebasket.

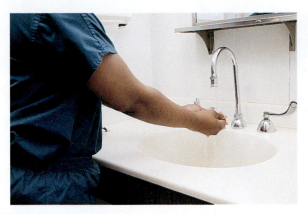

FIGURE 13-5 The uniform does not touch the sink. Hands are lower than the elbows. Hands do not touch the inside of the sink.

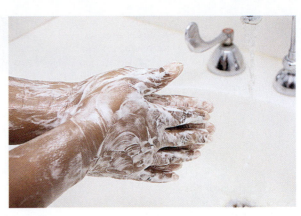

FIGURE 13-6 The palms are rubbed together to work up a good lather.

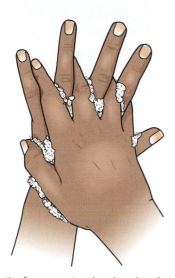

FIGURE 13-7 The fingers are interlaced to clean between the fingers.

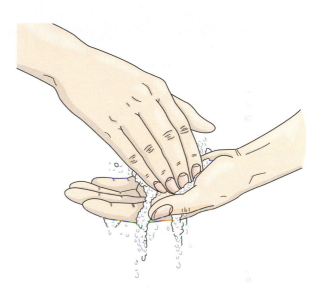

FIGURE 13-8 The fingertips are rubbed against the palms to clean under the fingernails.

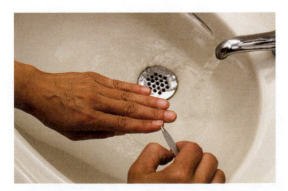

FIGURE 13-9 A nail file is used to clean under the fingernails.

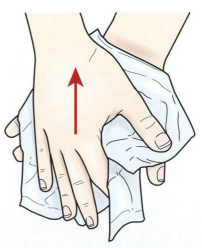

FIGURE 13-10 Hands are dried starting at the fingertips and working up to the forearms.

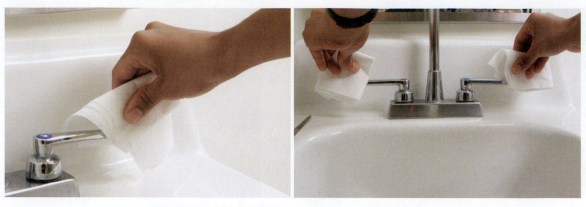

FIGURE 13-11 A paper towel is used to turn off each faucet.

Using an Alcohol-Based Hand Sanitizer

  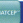

PROCEDURE

1 See *Promoting Safety and Comfort: Hand Hygiene,* p. 153.
2 Apply a palmful of an alcohol-based hand sanitizer into a cupped hand (Fig. 13-12, *A*).
3 Rub your palms together (Fig. 13-12, *B*).
4 Rub the palm of 1 hand over the back of the other (Fig. 13-12, *C*). Do the same for the other hand.
5 Rub your palms together with your fingers interlaced (Fig. 13-12, *D*).

6 Interlock your fingers as in Figure 13-12, *E*. Rub your fingers back and forth.
7 Rub the thumb of 1 hand in the palm of the other (Fig. 13-12, *F*). Do the same for the other thumb.
8 Rub the fingers of 1 hand into the palm of the other hand (Fig. 13-12, *G*). Use a circular motion. Do the same for the fingers of the other hand.
9 Continue rubbing your hands until they are dry.

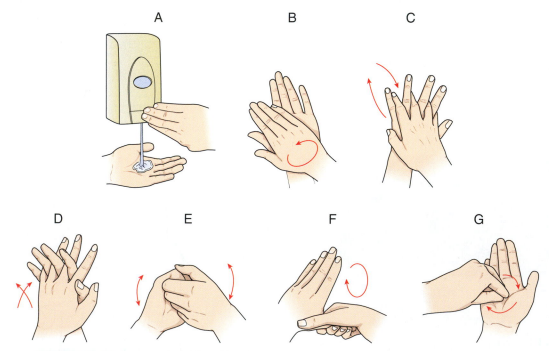

FIGURE 13-12 Using an alcohol-based hand sanitizer. **A,** A palmful of an alcohol-based hand sanitizer is applied into a cupped hand. **B,** The palms are rubbed together. **C,** The palm of 1 hand is rubbed over the back of the other. **D,** The palms are rubbed together with the fingers interlaced. **E,** The fingers are interlocked and rubbed back and forth. **F,** The thumb of 1 hand is rubbed in the palm of the other. **G,** The fingers of 1 hand are rubbed into the palm of the other hand with circular motions.

Supplies and Equipment

Disposable supplies and equipment help prevent the spread of infection. Discard single-use items after use. A person uses multi-use items many times. They include bedpans, urinals, wash basins, and water mugs. Label multi-use items with the person's name and room and bed number. Do not "borrow" them for another person.

Non-disposable items are cleaned and then disinfected. Then they are sterilized.

Cleaning. Cleaning reduces the number of microbes present. It also removes organic matter such as blood, body fluids, secretions, and excretions. *Organic matter* comes from living plants and animals and is able to decay.

To clean equipment:

- Wear personal protective equipment (PPE) to clean items contaminated with blood, body fluids, secretions, or excretions. PPE includes gloves, a mask, a gown, and goggles or a face shield.
- Work from *clean* to *dirty* areas. If you work from a *dirty* to *clean* area, the *clean* area becomes contaminated *(dirty)*.
- Rinse the item in cold water to remove organic matter. Heat makes organic matter thick, sticky, and hard to remove.
- Wash the item with soap and hot water.
- Scrub thoroughly. Use a brush if necessary.
- Rinse the item in warm water. Dry the item.
- Disinfect the item. Or have it sterilized.
- Disinfect equipment and the sink used for cleaning.
- Discard PPE.
- Practice hand hygiene.

Disinfection. *Disinfection is the process of killing pathogens.* Disinfectants are used to clean objects and surfaces. A *disinfectant* is a liquid chemical that can kill many or all pathogens. Disinfectants are used to clean counters, tubs, showers, and re-usable items. Such items include:

- Blood pressure cuffs
- Commodes and metal bedpans
- Wheelchairs and stretchers
- Furniture

See *Promoting Safety and Comfort: Disinfection.*

Sterilization. *Sterilization is the process of destroying all microbes* (pathogens and non-pathogens). Very high temperatures are used. Heat destroys microbes.

Boiling water, radiation, liquid or gas chemicals, dry heat, and *steam under pressure* are sterilization methods. An autoclave (Fig. 13-13) is a pressure steam sterilizer. Glass, surgical items, and metal objects are autoclaved. High temperatures destroy plastic and rubber items. They are not autoclaved.

Other Aseptic Measures

Hand hygiene, cleaning, disinfection, and sterilization are important aseptic measures. So are the measures listed in Box 13-3, p. 158. They are useful in home and health care settings and in every-day life.

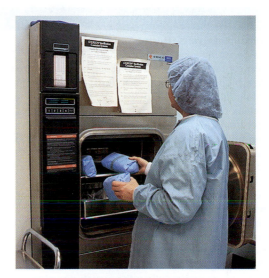

FIGURE 13-13 An autoclave.

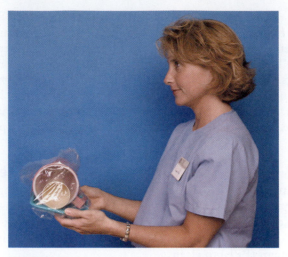

FIGURE 13-14 Hold equipment away from your uniform.

BOX 13-3 Aseptic Measures

Controlling Reservoirs (Hosts—You or the Person)
- Provide for hygiene needs (Chapter 18).
- Wash contaminated areas with soap and water. Feces, urine, blood, body fluids, secretions, and excretions can contain microbes.
- Use leak-proof plastic bags for soiled tissues, linens, and other items.
- Keep tables, counters, wheelchair trays, and other surfaces clean and dry.
- Label bottles with the person's name and the date the bottle was opened.
- Keep bottles and fluid containers tightly capped or covered.
- Keep drainage containers below the drainage site (Chapter 21).
- Empty drainage containers and dispose of drainage following agency policy. Usually drainage containers are emptied every shift. Follow the nurse's directions about emptying them more often.

Controlling Portals of Exit
- Cover your nose and mouth to cough or sneeze.
- Provide the person with tissues to use when coughing or sneezing.
- Wear PPE as needed (p. 162).

Controlling Transmission
- Provide all persons with their own personal care equipment. This includes wash basins, bedpans, urinals, commodes, and eating and drinking utensils.
- Do not take equipment from 1 person's room to use for another person. Even if un-used, do not take the item from 1 room to another.
- Hold equipment and linens away from your uniform (Fig. 13-14).
- Practice hand hygiene. See Box 13-2.
- Assist the person with hand-washing.
  - Before and after eating
  - After elimination
  - After changing tampons, sanitary napkins, or other personal hygiene products
  - After contact with blood, body fluids, secretions, or excretions

Controlling Transmission—cont'd
- Prevent dust movement. Do not shake linens or equipment. Use a damp cloth for dusting.
- Clean from *clean* to *dirty* areas. This prevents soiling a clean area.
- Clean away from your body. Do not dust, brush, or wipe toward yourself. Otherwise you transmit microbes to your skin, hair, and clothing.
- Flush urine and feces down the toilet. Avoid splatters and splashes.
- Pour contaminated liquids directly into sinks or toilets. Avoid splashing onto other areas.
- Do not sit on the person's bed or chair. You will pick up microbes and transfer them to surfaces that you sit on.
- Do not use items on the floor. The floor is contaminated.
- Follow agency disinfection procedures to clean:
  - Tubs, showers, and shower chairs after each use
  - Bedpans, urinals, and commodes after each use
- Report pests—ants, spiders, mice, and so on.

Controlling Portals of Entry
- Provide good skin care and oral hygiene (Chapter 18). This promotes intact skin and mucous membranes.
- Protect the skin from injury.
  - Do not let the person lie on tubes or other items.
  - Make sure linens are dry and wrinkle-free (Chapter 17).
  - Turn and re-position the person as directed by the nurse and care plan (Chapters 15 and 16).
- Assist with or clean the genital area after elimination. (See "Perineal Care" in Chapter 18.) Wipe and clean from the urethra (cleanest area) to the rectum (dirtiest area). This helps prevent urinary tract infections.
- Make sure drainage tubes are properly connected. This prevents microbes from entering the drainage system.

Protecting the Susceptible Host
- Follow the care plan to meet nutrition and fluid needs (Chapters 23 and 24). This helps prevent infection.
- Assist with deep-breathing and coughing exercises as directed (Chapter 30). This helps prevent respiratory infections.

ISOLATION PRECAUTIONS

Blood, body fluids, secretions, and excretions can transmit pathogens. Sometimes barriers are needed to keep pathogens in a certain area—usually the person's room. This requires isolation precautions.

The *Guideline for Isolation Precautions: Preventing Transmission of Infectious Agents in Healthcare Settings 2007* is followed. This is a guideline of the Centers for Disease Control and Prevention (CDC). Isolation precautions prevent the spread of *communicable diseases (contagious diseases). They are diseases caused by pathogens that spread easily.*

Isolation precautions are based on *clean* and *dirty. Clean* areas or objects have no pathogens. They are not contaminated or *dirty. Dirty* areas or objects are contaminated with pathogens. If a *clean* area or object has contact with something dirty, the clean area or object is now *dirty. Clean* and *dirty* also depend on how the pathogen is spread.

The CDC guideline has 2 tiers of precautions.
- Standard Precautions
- Transmission-Based Precautions (p. 161)

Standard Precautions

Standard Precautions (Box 13-4):
- Reduce the risk of spreading pathogens.
- Reduce the risk of spreading known and unknown infections. *Standard Precautions are used for all persons whenever care is given.* They prevent the spread of infection from:
  - Blood.
  - All body fluids, secretions, and excretions (except sweat) even if blood is not visible. Sweat is not known to spread infection.
  - Non-intact skin (skin with open breaks).
  - Mucous membranes.

BOX 13-4	Standard Precautions

Hand Hygiene
- Follow the rules for hand hygiene. See Box 13-2.
- Touch surfaces close to the person only when necessary. This prevents contaminating clean hands from room or care setting surfaces. It also prevents transmitting pathogens from contaminated hands to other surfaces.
- Do not wear fake nails or nail extenders for contact with persons at risk for infection or other adverse outcomes. (NOTE: Some agencies do not allow fake nails or nail extenders.)

Personal Protective Equipment (PPE) (p. 162)
- Wear PPE when contact with blood or body fluids is likely.
- Do not contaminate your clothing or skin when removing PPE.
- Remove and discard PPE before leaving the person's room or care setting.

Gloves (p. 163)
- Wear gloves when contact with the following is likely.
  - Blood
  - Potentially infectious materials (body fluids, secretions, and excretions are examples)
  - Mucous membranes
  - Non-intact skin
  - Skin that may be contaminated (for example, a person is incontinent of feces or urine)
- Wear gloves that fit and are needed for the task.
  - Wear disposable gloves for direct care.
  - Wear disposable gloves or utility gloves to clean equipment or care settings.
- Remove gloves after contact with:
  - The person
  - The person's care setting
  - Equipment used in the person's care or other care equipment
- Remove gloves after contact with a person and before going to another person.
- Do not wash gloves for re-use with different persons.
- Change gloves during care if your hands will move from a contaminated body site to a clean body site.

Gowns (p. 162)
- Wear a gown to protect your skin and clothing when contact with blood, body fluids, secretions, or excretions is likely.
- Wear a gown for direct contact with a person who has uncontained secretions or excretions.
- Remove the gown and perform hand hygiene before leaving the person's room or care setting.
- Do not re-use gowns, even for repeat contact with the same person.

Mouth, Nose, and Eye Protection (p. 162)
- Wear PPE—masks, goggles, face shields—for procedures and tasks that are likely to cause splashes and sprays of blood, body fluids, secretions, and excretions.
- Wear the correct PPE for the procedure or task.
- Wear gloves, a gown, and 1 of the following for procedures or tasks likely to cause sprays of respiratory secretions.
  - A face shield that fully covers the front and sides of the face
  - A mask with attached shield
  - A mask and goggles

Respiratory Hygiene/Cough Etiquette
- Instruct persons with respiratory symptoms to:
  - Cover the nose and mouth to cough or sneeze.
  - Use tissues to contain respiratory secretions.
  - Dispose of tissues in the nearest waste container.
  - Perform hand hygiene after contact with respiratory secretions.
- Provide visitors with masks according to agency policy.

Care Equipment
- Wear the correct PPE to handle:
  - Care equipment that is visibly soiled with blood, body fluids, secretions, or excretions
  - Care equipment that may have been in contact with blood, body fluids, secretions, or excretions
- Remove organic material before disinfection and sterilization procedures. Follow agency policy for using cleaning agents.

Continued

BOX 13-4 Standard Precautions—cont'd

Care of the Environment
- Follow agency procedures to clean and maintain surfaces. Care setting surfaces and care equipment are examples. Surfaces near the person may need frequent cleaning and maintenance—door knobs, bed rails, over-bed tables, walker and cane handles, toilet surfaces and areas, and so on.
- Follow agency procedures to clean and disinfect multi-use electronic equipment. This includes:
  - Items used by patients and residents
  - Items used to give care
  - Mobile devices that are moved in and out of patient or resident rooms
- Follow these rules for children's toys. This includes toys in waiting areas.
  - Select toys that are easy to clean and disinfect.
  - Do not allow stuffed, furry toys if they will be shared.
  - Clean and disinfect large stationary toys (for example, climbing equipment) at least weekly and when visibly soiled.
  - Rinse toys with water after disinfection if they are likely to be mouthed by children. Or wash them in a dishwasher.
  - Clean and disinfect a toy at once when it needs cleaning. Or store the toy in a labeled container away from toys that are clean and ready for use.

Textiles and Laundry
- Handle used textiles and fabrics (linens) with minimum agitation. This prevents contamination of air, surfaces, and other persons.

Worker Safety
- Protect yourself and others from exposure to bloodborne pathogens. This includes handling needles and other sharps. See "Bloodborne Pathogen Standard," p. 170.
- Use a mouthpiece, resuscitation bag, or other ventilation device for resuscitation to prevent contact with the person's mouth and oral secretions. See Chapter 36.

Patient or Resident Placement
- A private room is preferred if the person is at risk for transmitting the infection to others.
- Follow the nurse's directions if a private room is not available.

Modified from Siegel JD, Rhinehart E, Jackson M, Chiarello L, and the Healthcare Infection Control Practices Advisory Committee: Guideline for isolation precautions: preventing transmission of infectious agents in healthcare settings 2007, Atlanta, 2007, Centers for Disease Control and Prevention.

BOX 13-5 Transmission-Based Precautions

Contact Precautions
- Used for persons with known or suspected infections or conditions that increase the risk of contact transmission.
- Patient or resident placement:
  - A single room is preferred.
  - Do the following if a room is shared with another person not infected with the same agent.
    - Keep the privacy curtain between the beds closed.
    - Change PPE and practice hand hygiene between contact with persons in the same room. Do so regardless of whether 1 or both persons are on contact precautions.
- Gloves:
  - Don (put on) gloves upon entering the person's room or care setting.
  - Wear gloves to touch the person's intact skin.
  - Wear gloves to touch surfaces or items near the person.
- Gown:
  - Wear a gown when clothing may have direct contact with the person.
  - Wear a gown when contact is likely with surfaces or equipment near the person.
  - Don the gown upon entering the person's room.
  - Remove the gown and practice hand hygiene before leaving the person's room.
  - Make sure your clothing and skin do not touch potentially contaminated surfaces after removing the gown.

Contact Precautions—cont'd
- Patient or resident transport:
  - Limit transport and movement of the person outside of the room to medically-necessary purposes.
  - Cover the infected area of the person's body.
  - Remove and discard contaminated PPE and practice hand hygiene before transporting the person.
  - Don clean PPE to handle the person at the transport destination.
- Care equipment:
  - Follow Standard Precautions.
  - Use disposable equipment when possible. If possible, leave non-disposable equipment in the person's room.
  - Clean and disinfect non-disposable and multiple-use equipment before use on another person.

Droplet Precautions
- Used for persons known or suspected to be infected with pathogens transmitted by respiratory droplets. Such droplets come from coughing, sneezing, or talking.
- Patient or resident placement:
  - A single room is preferred.
  - Do the following if a room is shared with another person who is not infected with the same agent.
    - Keep the privacy curtain between the beds closed.
    - Change PPE and practice hand hygiene between contact with persons in the same room. Do so regardless of whether 1 or both persons are on droplet precautions.

BOX 13-5 Transmission-Based Precautions—cont'd

Droplet Precautions—cont'd
- PPE:
  - Don a mask upon entering the person's room.
- Patient or resident transport:
  - Limit transport and movement of the person outside of the room to medically-necessary purposes.
  - Have the person wear a mask.
  - Instruct the person to follow Respiratory Hygiene/Cough Etiquette (see Box 13-4).
  - No mask is required for staff transporting the person.

Airborne Precautions
- Used for persons known or suspected to be infected with pathogens transmitted person-to-person by the airborne route. Tuberculosis (TB), measles, chicken pox, smallpox, and severe acute respiratory syndrome (SARS) are examples.
- The person is placed in an airborne infection isolation room (AIIR). If not available, the person is transferred to an agency with an AIIR. AIIR practices include:
  - All persons entering the room wear a TB respirator.
  - The room door is kept closed except when someone enters or leaves the room.
  - Treatments and procedures are done in the room.
  - The person wears a mask during transport.

Airborne Precautions—cont'd
- Staff susceptible to the infection do not enter the room. This is if immune staff members are available.
- PPE:
  - A mask or respirator is applied before entering the person's room.
  - An approved respirator is worn on entering the room or home of a person with TB.
  - Respiratory protection is recommended for all staff when caring for persons with smallpox.
- Patient or resident transport:
  - Limit transport and movement of the person outside of the room to medically-necessary purposes.
  - Have the person wear a surgical mask.
  - Instruct the person to follow Respiratory Hygiene/Cough Etiquette (see Box 13-4).
  - Cover skin lesions infected with the microbe.
  - No mask or respirator is required for staff transporting the person.

Modified from Siegel JD, Rhinehart E, Jackson M, Chiarello L, and the Healthcare Infection Control Practices Advisory Committee: Guideline for isolation precautions: preventing transmission of infectious agents in healthcare settings 2007, Atlanta, 2007, Centers for Disease Control and Prevention.

Transmission-Based Precautions

Some infections require Transmission-Based Precautions (Box 13-5). They are commonly called "isolation precautions." Transmission-Based Precautions require wearing PPE—gloves, gown, mask, and goggles or face shield. You must understand how certain infections are spread (see Fig. 13-2). This helps you understand the 3 types of Transmission-Based Precautions.

Removing linens, trash, and equipment from the room may require double-bagging (p. 169). Follow agency procedures to collect specimens and transport persons.

Agency policies may differ from those in this text. The rules in Box 13-6 are a guide for giving safe care when using Transmission-Based Precautions.

See *Focus on Communication: Transmission-Based Precautions, p. 162.*

See *Focus on Surveys: Transmission-Based Precautions, p. 162.*

See *Delegation Guidelines: Transmission-Based Precautions, p. 162.*

See *Promoting Safety and Comfort: Transmission-Based Precautions, p. 162.*

BOX 13-6 Rules for Isolation Precautions

- Collect all needed items before entering the room.
- Do not contaminate equipment and supplies. Floors are contaminated. So is any object on the floor or that falls to the floor.
- Clean floors with mops wetted with a disinfectant solution. Floor dust is contaminated.
- Prevent drafts. Drafts can carry some microbes in the air.
- Use paper towels to handle contaminated items.
- Remove items from the room in leak-proof plastic bags.
- Double-bag items if the outside of the bag is or can be contaminated (p. 169).
- Follow agency policy to remove and transport disposable and re-usable items.
- Return re-usable dishes, drinking vessels, eating utensils, and trays to the food service (dietary) department. Discard disposable dishes, drinking vessels, eating utensils, and trays in the waste container in the person's room.
- Do not touch your hair, nose, mouth, eyes, or other body parts.
- Do not touch any clean area or object if your hands are contaminated.
- Wash your hands if they are visibly dirty or contaminated with blood, body fluids, secretions, or excretions.
- Place clean items on paper towels.
- Do not shake linens.
- Use paper towels to turn faucets on and off.
- Use a paper towel to open the door to the person's room. Discard it after use.
- Tell the nurse if you have any cuts, open skin areas, a sore throat, vomiting, or diarrhea.

Personal Protective Equipment

The PPE needed depends on tasks, procedures, care measures, and the type of Transmission-Based Precautions used. Sometimes only gloves are needed. The nurse tells you when a gown, goggles or a face shield, and a mask are needed.

Gowns. Gowns prevent the spread of microbes. They protect your clothes and body from contact with blood, body fluids, secretions, and excretions. They also protect against splashes and sprays.

A gown must completely cover you from your neck to your knees. The long sleeves have tight cuffs. The gown opens at the back. It is tied at the neck and waist. The gown front and sleeves are considered *contaminated*.

Gowns are used once. A wet gown is contaminated. Remove it and put on a dry one. Discard disposable gowns after use.

Masks and Respiratory Protection. You wear disposable masks:
- For protection from contact with infectious materials from the person. Respiratory secretions and sprays of blood or body fluids are examples.
- When assisting with sterile procedures. This protects the person from infectious agents carried in your mouth or nose.

A wet or moist mask is *contaminated*. Breathing can cause masks to become wet or moist. Apply a new mask when contamination occurs.

A mask fits snugly over your nose and mouth. Practice hand hygiene before putting on a mask. To remove a mask, touch only the ties or the elastic bands. The front of the mask is contaminated.

Goggles and Face Shields. Goggles and face shields protect your eyes, mouth, and nose from splashing or spraying of blood, body fluids, secretions, and excretions. Splashes and sprays can occur when you give care, clean items, or dispose of fluids.

The front (outside) of goggles or a face shield is *contaminated*. The headband, ties, or ear-pieces used to secure the device are *clean*. Use them to remove the device after hand hygiene. They are safe to touch with bare hands. Lift the ties or ear-pieces from the back when removing the device.

Discard disposable goggles or face shields after use. Re-usable eyewear is cleaned before re-use. It is washed with soap and water. Then a disinfectant is used.

See *Promoting Safety and Comfort: Goggles and Face Shields.*

PROMOTING SAFETY AND COMFORT
Goggles and Face Shields

PROMOTING SAFETY AND COMFORT
Goggles and Face Shields

Safety
Eyeglasses and contact lenses do not provide eye protection. The face shield must fit over glasses with minimal gaps.

Goggles do not provide splash or spray protection to other parts of your face.

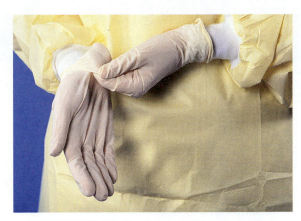

FIGURE 13-15 The gloves cover the gown cuffs.

Gloves. A natural barrier, the skin prevents microbes from entering the body. Small skin breaks on the hands and fingers are common. Disposable gloves act as a barrier. They protect:

- You from pathogens in the person's blood, body fluids, secretions, and excretions
- The person from microbes on your hands

Wear gloves when contact with blood, body fluids, secretions, excretions, mucous membranes, or non-intact skin is likely. Contact may be direct with blood, body fluids, secretions, or excretions. Or contact may be with contaminated items or surfaces.

Wearing gloves is the most common measure for Standard Precautions and Transmission-Based Precautions. When using gloves:

- Consider the outside of gloves to be *contaminated*.
- Apply to dry hands. Gloves are easier to put on dry hands.
- Do not tear gloves when putting them on. Carelessness, long fingernails, and rings can tear gloves. Blood, body fluids, secretions, and excretions can enter the glove through the tear. This contaminates your hand.
- Remove and discard torn, cut, or punctured gloves at once. Practice hand hygiene. Then put on a new pair.
- Apply a new pair for every person.
- Wear gloves once. Discard them after use.
- Put on new gloves just before touching mucous membranes or non-intact skin.
- Put on new gloves when gloves become contaminated with blood, body fluids, secretions, or excretions. A task may require more than 1 pair of gloves.
- Change gloves when moving from a contaminated body site to a clean body site.
- Change gloves when touching portable computer keyboards or other equipment that is moved from room to room.
- Put on gloves last when they are worn with other PPE.
- Make sure gloves cover your wrists. If you wear a gown, gloves cover the cuffs (Fig. 13-15).
- Remove gloves so the inside part is on the outside. The inside is *clean*.
- Practice hand hygiene after removing gloves.
See *Promoting Safety and Comfort: Gloves.*

PROMOTING SAFETY AND COMFORT
Gloves

Safety
No special method is needed to put on non-sterile gloves. To remove gloves, see procedure: *Donning and Removing Personal Protective Equipment*, p. 167.

Some gloves are made of latex (a rubber product). Latex allergies can cause skin rashes. Difficulty breathing and shock are more serious problems. Report skin rashes and breathing problems to the nurse at once.

You may have a latex allergy. Some patients and residents are allergic to latex. This is noted on the care plan and your assignment sheet. Latex-free gloves are worn for latex allergies.

Comfort
Gloves are needed when contact with blood, body fluids, secretions, excretions, mucous membranes, or non-intact skin is likely. Gloves are not needed when such contact is not likely. Back massages and brushing and combing hair are examples if the skin is intact. To reduce exposure to latex, wear gloves only when needed.

Donning and Removing PPE. The type of PPE worn depends on the type of precautions needed. According to the CDC's isolation guidelines, gloves are always worn when gowns are worn. Sometimes other PPE is needed when gowns are worn.

See *Promoting Safety and Comfort: Donning and Removing PPE*, p. 164.
See procedure: *Donning and Removing Personal Protective Equipment*, p. 167.

Text continued on p. 168.

PROMOTING SAFETY AND COMFORT
Donning and Removing PPE

Safety

According to the CDC, PPE is donned and removed in the following order.

- Donning PPE (Fig. 13-16, *A*):
  1. Gown
  2. Mask or respirator
  3. Eyewear (goggles or face shield)
  4. Gloves
- Removing PPE (removed at the doorway before leaving the person's room):
  - Method 1 (Fig. 13-16, *B*)
    1. Gloves
    2. Eyewear (goggles or face shield)
    3. Gown
    4. Mask or respirator (a respirator is removed after leaving the person's room and closing the door)
  - Method 2 (Fig. 13-16, *C*, p. 166)
    1. Gown and gloves
    2. Eyewear (goggles or face shield)
    3. Mask or respirator (a respirator is removed after leaving the person's room and closing the door)

Practice hand hygiene after removing PPE. Practice hand hygiene between steps if your hands become contaminated. Then practice hand hygiene again after removing all PPE.

(NOTE: Some state competency tests require hand hygiene after removing each PPE item. And some states use a different order for donning and removing PPE. Follow the procedures used in your state and agency.)

Some severe and deadly infections require additional PPE—full face shield, helmet, or headpiece; coveralls with socks or special gowns; double gloving; boot or shoe covers; and aprons. Special training is needed to care for such patients and for donning and removing the PPE.

SEQUENCE FOR PUTTING ON PERSONAL PROTECTIVE EQUIPMENT (PPE)

The type of PPE used will vary based on the level of precautions required, such as standard and contact, droplet or airborne infection isolation precautions. The procedure for putting on and removing PPE should be tailored to the specific type of PPE.

1. GOWN
- Fully cover torso from neck to knees, arms to end of wrists, and wrap around the back
- Fasten in back of neck and waist

2. MASK OR RESPIRATOR
- Secure ties or elastic bands at middle of head and neck
- Fit flexible band to nose bridge
- Fit snug to face and below chin
- Fit-check respirator

3. GOGGLES OR FACE SHIELD
- Place over face and eyes and adjust to fit

4. GLOVES
- Extend to cover wrist of isolation gown

A

USE SAFE WORK PRACTICES TO PROTECT YOURSELF AND LIMIT THE SPREAD OF CONTAMINATION

- Keep hands away from face
- Limit surfaces touched
- Change gloves when torn or heavily contaminated
- Perform hand hygiene

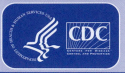

CS250672-E

FIGURE 13-16 A, Donning PPE.

HOW TO SAFELY REMOVE PERSONAL PROTECTIVE EQUIPMENT (PPE) EXAMPLE 1

There are a variety of ways to safely remove PPE without contaminating your clothing, skin, or mucous membranes with potentially infectious materials. Here is one example. **Remove all PPE before exiting the patient room** except a respirator, if worn. Remove the respirator **after** leaving the patient room and closing the door. Remove PPE in the following sequence:

1. GLOVES

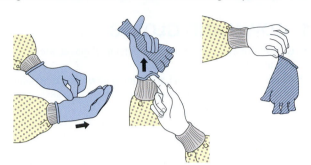

- Outside of gloves are contaminated!
- If your hands get contaminated during glove removal, immediately wash your hands or use an alcohol-based hand sanitizer
- Using a gloved hand, grasp the palm area of the other gloved hand and peel off first glove
- Hold removed glove in gloved hand
- Slide fingers of ungloved hand under remaining glove at wrist and peel off second glove over first glove
- Discard gloves in a waste container

2. GOGGLES OR FACE SHIELD

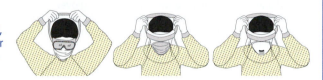

- Outside of goggles or face shield are contaminated!
- If your hands get contaminated during goggle or face shield removal, immediately wash your hands or use an alcohol-based hand sanitizer
- Remove goggles or face shield from the back by lifting head band or ear pieces
- If the item is reusable, place in designated receptacle for reprocessing. Otherwise, discard in a waste container

3. GOWN

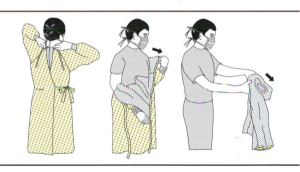

- Gown front and sleeves are contaminated!
- If your hands get contaminated during gown removal, immediately wash your hands or use an alcohol-based hand sanitizer
- Unfasten gown ties, taking care that sleeves don't contact your body when reaching for ties
- Pull gown away from neck and shoulders, touching inside of gown only
- Turn gown inside out
- Fold or roll into a bundle and discard in a waste container

B

4. MASK OR RESPIRATOR

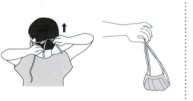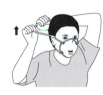

- Front of mask/respirator is contaminated — DO NOT TOUCH!
- If your hands get contaminated during mask/respirator removal, immediately wash your hands or use an alcohol-based hand sanitizer
- Grasp bottom ties or elastics of the mask/respirator, then the ones at the top, and remove without touching the front
- Discard in a waste container

5. WASH HANDS OR USE AN ALCOHOL-BASED HAND SANITIZER IMMEDIATELY AFTER REMOVING ALL PPE

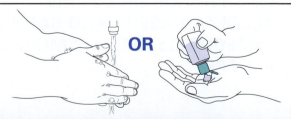

OR

PERFORM HAND HYGIENE BETWEEN STEPS IF HANDS BECOME CONTAMINATED AND IMMEDIATELY AFTER REMOVING ALL PPE

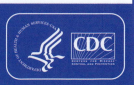

CS250672-E

FIGURE 13-16, cont'd B, Method 1: Removing PPE.

Continued

HOW TO SAFELY REMOVE PERSONAL PROTECTIVE EQUIPMENT (PPE) EXAMPLE 2

Here is another way to safely remove PPE without contaminating your clothing, skin, or mucous membranes with potentially infectious materials. **Remove all PPE before exiting the patient room** except a respirator, if worn. Remove the respirator **after** leaving the patient room and closing the door. Remove PPE in the following sequence:

1. GOWN AND GLOVES

- Gown front and sleeves and the outside of gloves are contaminated!
- If your hands get contaminated during gown or glove removal, immediately wash your hands or use an alcohol-based hand sanitizer
- Grasp the gown in the front and pull away from your body so that the ties break, touching outside of gown only with gloved hands
- While removing the gown, fold or roll the gown inside-out into a bundle
- As you are removing the gown, peel off your gloves at the same time, only touching the inside of the gloves and gown with your bare hands. Place the gown and gloves into a waste container

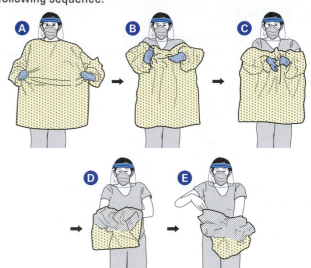

2. GOGGLES OR FACE SHIELD

- Outside of goggles or face shield are contaminated!
- If your hands get contaminated during goggle or face shield removal, immediately wash your hands or use an alcohol-based hand sanitizer
- Remove goggles or face shield from the back by lifting head band and without touching the front of the goggles or face shield
- If the item is reusable, place in designated receptacle for reprocessing. Otherwise, discard in a waste container

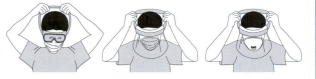

3. MASK OR RESPIRATOR

- Front of mask/respirator is contaminated — DO NOT TOUCH!
- If your hands get contaminated during mask/respirator removal, immediately wash your hands or use an alcohol-based hand sanitizer
- Grasp bottom ties or elastics of the mask/respirator, then the ones at the top, and remove without touching the front
- Discard in a waste container

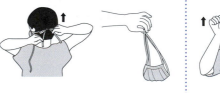
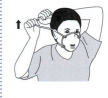

4. WASH HANDS OR USE AN ALCOHOL-BASED HAND SANITIZER IMMEDIATELY AFTER REMOVING ALL PPE

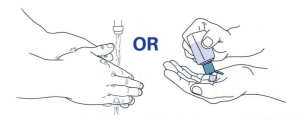

OR

PERFORM HAND HYGIENE BETWEEN STEPS IF HANDS BECOME CONTAMINATED AND IMMEDIATELY AFTER REMOVING ALL PPE

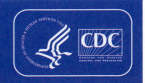

CS250672-E

FIGURE 13-16, cont'd C, Method 2: Removing PPE. (From Centers for Disease Control and Prevention, Department of Health and Human Services.)

Donning and Removing Personal Protective Equipment

PROCEDURE

1 Follow *Delegation Guidelines: Transmission-Based Precautions,* p. 162. See *Promoting Safety and Comfort:*
   a *Transmission-Based Precautions,* p. 162
   b *Goggles and Face Shields,* p. 163
   c *Gloves,* p. 163
   d *Donning and Removing PPE,* p. 164
2 Remove your watch and all jewelry.
3 Roll up uniform sleeves.
4 Practice hand hygiene.
5 Put on a gown (see Fig. 13-16, *A*).
   a Hold a clean gown out in front of you.
   b Unfold the gown. Face the back of the gown. Do not shake it.
   c Put your hands and arms through the sleeves.
   d Make sure the gown covers you from your neck to your knees. It must cover your arms to the end of your wrists.
   e Tie the strings at the back of the neck.
   f Over-lap the back of the gown. Make sure it covers your uniform. The gown should be snug, not loose.
   g Tie the waist strings. Tie them at the back or the side. Do not tie them in front.
6 Put on a mask or respirator (see Fig. 13-16, *A*).
   a Pick up a mask by its upper ties. Do not touch the part that will cover your face.
   b Place the mask over your nose and mouth (Fig. 13-17, *A*, p. 168).
   c Place the upper strings above your ears. Tie them at the back in the middle of your head (Fig. 13-17, *B*, p. 168).
   d Tie the lower strings at the back of your neck (Fig. 13-17, *C*, p. 168). The lower part of the mask is under your chin.
   e Pinch the metal band around your nose. The top of the mask must be snug over your nose. If you wear eyeglasses, the mask must be snug under the bottom of the eyeglasses.
   f Make sure the mask is snug over your face and under your chin.
7 Put on goggles or a face shield (if needed and if not part of the mask) (see Fig. 13-16, *A*).
   a Place the device over your face and eyes.
   b Adjust the device to fit.
8 Put on gloves. Make sure the gloves cover the wrists of the gown.
9 Provide care.
10 Remove and discard the PPE. Practice hand hygiene between each step if your hands become contaminated.
   a *Method 1: gloves, goggles or face shield, gown, mask or respirator* (see Fig. 13-16, *B*)
      1 Remove and discard the gloves.
         a Make sure that glove touches only glove.
         b Grasp a glove at the palm (Fig. 13-18, *A*, p. 168). Grasp it on the outside.
         c Pull the glove down over your hand so it is inside-out (Fig. 13-18, *B*, p. 168).
         d Hold the removed glove with your other gloved hand.
         e Reach inside the other glove. Use the first 2 fingers of the ungloved hand (Fig. 13-18, *C*, p. 168).
         f Pull the glove down (inside-out) over your hand and the other glove (Fig. 13-18, *D*, p. 168).
         g Discard the gloves.

2 Remove and discard the goggles or face shield if worn.
   a Lift the headband or ear-pieces from the back. Do not touch the front of the device.
   b Discard the device. If re-usable, follow agency policy.
3 Remove and discard the gown. Do not touch the outside of the gown.
   a Untie the neck and then the waist strings.
   b Pull the gown down and away from your neck and shoulders. Only touch the inside of the gown.
   c Turn the gown inside-out as it is removed. Hold it at the inside shoulder seams and bring your hands together.
   d Fold or roll up the gown away from you. Keep it inside-out. Do not let the gown touch the floor.
   e Discard the gown.
4 Remove and discard the mask if worn. (NOTE: Remove a respirator after leaving the room and closing the door.)
   a Untie the lower strings of the mask.
   b Untie the top strings.
   c Hold the top strings. Remove the mask without touching the front of the mask.
   d Discard the mask.
   b *Method 2: gown and gloves, goggles or face shield, mask or respirator* (see Fig. 13-16, *C*).
1 Remove and discard the gown and gloves.
   a Grasp the gown in front with your gloved hands. Pull away from your body so the ties break. Only touch the outside of the gown.
   b Fold or roll the gown inside-out into a bundle while removing the gown. Keep it inside-out. Do not let the gown touch the floor.
   c Peel off your gloves as you remove the gown. Only touch the inside of the gloves and gown with your bare hands.
   d Discard the gown and gloves.
2 Remove and discard the goggles or face shield.
   a Lift the headband or ear-pieces from the back. Do not touch the front of the device.
   b Discard the device. If re-usable, follow agency policy.
3 Remove and discard the mask if worn. (NOTE: Remove a respirator after leaving the room and closing the door.)
   a Untie the lower strings of the mask.
   b Untie the top strings.
   c Hold the top strings. Remove the mask without touching the front of the mask.
   d Discard the mask.
11 Practice hand hygiene after removing all PPE.

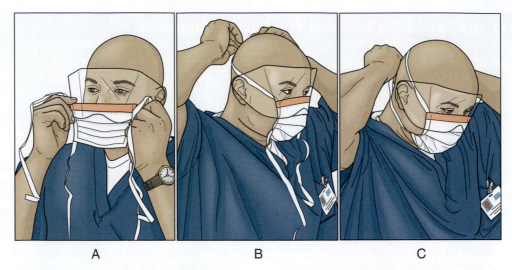

FIGURE 13-17 Donning a mask. (NOTE: The mask has a face shield.) **A,** The mask covers the nose and mouth. **B,** Upper strings are tied at the back of the head. **C,** Lower strings are tied at the back of the neck.

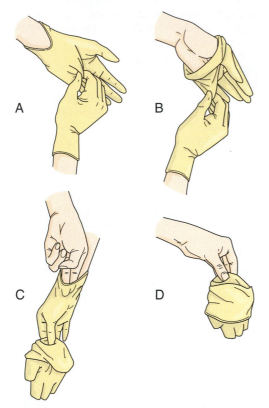

FIGURE 13-18 Removing gloves. **A,** Grasp the glove at the palm. **B,** Pull the glove down over the hand. The glove is inside-out. **C,** Insert the fingers of the ungloved hand inside the other glove. **D,** Pull the glove down and over the other hand and glove. The glove is inside-out.

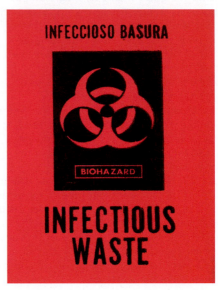

FIGURE 13-19 *BIOHAZARD* symbol.

Bagging Items

Contaminated items are bagged for removal from the person's room. Leak-proof plastic bags are used. They have the *BIOHAZARD* symbol (Fig. 13-19). *Biohazardous waste is items contaminated with blood, body fluids, secretions, or excretions.* (Bio *means* life. Hazardous *means* dangerous or harmful.)

Bag and transport linens following agency policy. Laundry bags with contaminated linens need a *BIOHAZARD* symbol. Melt-away bags dissolve in hot water. Once soiled linens are bagged, no one needs to handle them. Do not over-fill the bag. Tie the bag securely. Then place it in a laundry hamper lined with a biohazard plastic bag.

Trash is placed in a container labeled with the *BIOHAZARD* symbol. Follow agency policy for bagging and transporting trash, equipment, and supplies.

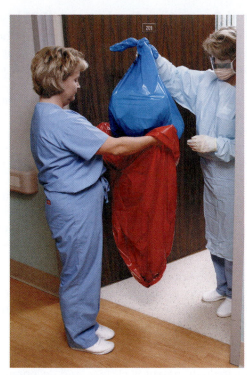

FIGURE 13-20 Double-bagging. One nursing assistant is in the room by the doorway. The other is outside the doorway. The *dirty* bag is placed inside the *clean* bag.

Double-Bagging. Usually 1 bag is needed. Double-bagging involves 2 bags. Double-bagging is needed if the outside of the bag is wet, soiled, or may be contaminated. To double-bag:

1 Ask a co-worker to stand outside the doorway. You are in the room.
2 Seal the *dirty* bag in the room.
3 Have your co-worker make a wide cuff on a *clean* bag and hold it wide open.
4 Place the *dirty* bag into the *clean* bag (Fig. 13-20). Do not touch the outside of the *clean* bag.
5 Ask your co-worker to seal and label the *clean* bag. It is labeled with the *BIOHAZARD* symbol.
6 Ask your co-worker to take the bag to the appropriate area for disposal, disinfection, or sterilization.

Collecting Specimens

Blood, body fluids, secretions, and excretions often require laboratory testing (Chapter 26). Specimens are transported to the laboratory in biohazard specimen bags. Follow agency procedures to collect and transport specimens when a person is on Transmission-Based Precautions.

Transporting Persons

Persons on Transmission-Based Precautions usually do not leave their rooms. Sometimes they go to other areas for treatments or tests.

Transport procedures vary among agencies. Some require transport by bed. This prevents contaminating wheelchairs and stretchers. Others use wheelchairs and stretchers. Follow agency procedures for a safe transport when a person is on Transmission-Based Precautions.

Meeting Basic Needs

The person has love, belonging, and self-esteem needs. Often they are unmet during Transmission-Based Precautions. Visitors and staff avoid the person. Putting on PPE takes extra effort before entering the room. Some are not sure what they can touch. They may fear getting the disease.

The person may feel lonely, unwanted, and rejected. The person knows the disease can be spread to others. He or she may feel dirty and undesirable. Without intending to, visitors and staff can make the person feel ashamed and guilty for having a contagious disease.

You can help meet love, belonging, and self-esteem needs.
- Remember that the pathogen is undesirable, not the person.
- Treat the person with respect, kindness, and dignity.
- Provide newspapers, magazines, books, a current TV guide, and other reading matter.
- Provide hobby materials if possible.
- Place a clock in the room.
- Suggest that the person call family and friends.
- Plan your work so you can stay to visit with the person.
- Say "hello" from the doorway often.

Items brought into the person's room become contaminated. Disinfect or discard the items according to agency policy.

See *Focus on Communication: Meeting Basic Needs.*
See *Focus on Older Persons: Meeting Basic Needs.*

FOCUS ON COMMUNICATION

Meeting Basic Needs

Some questions or statements can make the person feel dirty or ashamed. Be careful what you say. For example, do not say:
- "How did you get that?"
- "What were you doing?"
- "I'm afraid to touch you."
- "Don't breathe on me."

Always treat the person with respect, kindness, and dignity.

FOCUS ON OLDER PERSONS

Meeting Basic Needs

Persons with poor vision need to know who you are. Let them see your face before you put on a mask, goggles, or a face shield. State your name at the doorway and explain what you need to do. Then put on PPE.

Some older persons have dementia. Masks, gowns, goggles, and face shields may increase confusion and cause fear and agitation. These measures can help.
- Let the person see your face before putting on PPE.
- Tell the person who you are and what you need to do.
- Use a calm, soothing voice.
- Do not rush the person.
- Use touch to reassure the person.
- Follow the care plan and the nurse's instructions for other measures to help the person.
- Report signs of increased confusion or behavior changes.

BLOODBORNE PATHOGEN STANDARD

The human immunodeficiency virus (HIV) and the hepatitis B virus (HBV) are major health concerns (Chapter 33). The Bloodborne Pathogen Standard protects the health team from exposure to these viruses. It is a regulation of the Occupational Safety and Health Administration (OSHA).

Found in the blood, HIV and HBV are bloodborne pathogens. They exit the body through blood. They are spread to others by blood and other potentially infectious materials (OPIM). OPIM are contaminated with blood or with a body fluid that may contain blood. This includes semen, vaginal secretions, and saliva. Urine and feces may contain blood. OPIM also includes needles, suction equipment, soiled linens, dressings, and other care items.

Staff at risk for exposure to blood or OPIM receive free training. It occurs upon employment and yearly. Training is also done for new or changed tasks involving exposure to bloodborne pathogens.

Hepatitis B Vaccination

Hepatitis B is a liver disease caused by HBV. HBV is spread by the blood and sexual contact.

The hepatitis B vaccine produces immunity against hepatitis B. *Immunity* means that a person has protection against a certain disease. He or she will not get the disease.

A *vaccination* involves giving a vaccine to produce immunity against an infectious disease. A *vaccine* is a preparation containing dead or weakened microbes. The hepatitis B vaccination involves 3 injections (shots). Injection 2 is given 1 month after the first. Injection 3 is given at least 4 months after the first one. The vaccination can be given before or after HBV exposure.

The agency must offer the hepatitis B vaccination after you are trained about the vaccine and within 10 days of your first working day. The agency pays for it. You can refuse the vaccination. If so, you must sign a statement refusing the vaccine. You can have the vaccination at a later date if you want.

Engineering and Work Practice Controls

Engineering controls reduce employee exposure in the workplace. *Work practice controls* also reduce exposure risks. All tasks involving blood or OPIM are done in ways to limit splatters, splashes, and sprays. Producing droplets also is avoided.

- Do not eat, drink, smoke, apply cosmetics or lip balm, or handle contact lenses in areas of exposure.
- Do not store food or drinks where blood or OPIM are kept.
- Practice hand hygiene after removing gloves.
- Wash hands as soon as possible after skin contact with blood or OPIM.
- Never re-cap, bend, or remove needles by hand. Use a mechanical means (forceps) or a 1-handed method.
- Never shear or break needles.
- Discard needles and sharp instruments (such as razors) in containers that are closable, puncture-resistant, and leak-proof. *Containers are color-coded in red and have the BIOHAZARD symbol.* Containers must be upright and not allowed to over-fill.

Personal Protective Equipment (PPE)

This includes gloves, goggles, face shields, masks, laboratory coats, gowns, shoe covers, and surgical caps. Blood or OPIM must not pass through them. They protect your clothes, under-garments, skin, eyes, mouth, and hair.

PPE is free to staff. OSHA requires these measures.

- Remove PPE before leaving the work area.
- Remove PPE when it becomes contaminated.
- Place used PPE in marked areas or containers when being stored, washed, decontaminated, or discarded.
- Wear gloves for contact with blood or OPIM.
- Wear gloves to handle or touch contaminated items or surfaces.
- Replace worn, punctured, or contaminated gloves.
- Never wash or decontaminate disposable gloves for re-use.
- Discard utility gloves that show signs of cracking, peeling, tearing, or puncturing. Utility gloves are decontaminated for re-use if the process will not ruin them.

Equipment

Contaminated equipment is cleaned and decontaminated. Decontaminate equipment and work surfaces with a proper disinfectant.

- Upon completing tasks
- At once for obvious contamination
- At the end of your work shift when surfaces became contaminated since the last cleaning

Use a brush and dustpan or tongs to clean up broken glass. Never pick up broken glass with your hands, not even with gloves. Discard broken glass into a puncture-resistant container.

Laundry

OSHA requires these measures for contaminated laundry.

- Handle it as little as possible.
- Wear gloves or other needed PPE.
- Bag contaminated laundry where it is used.
- Mark laundry bags or containers with the *BIOHAZARD* symbol for laundry sent off-site.
- Place wet, contaminated laundry in leak-proof containers before transport. The containers are color-coded in red or have the *BIOHAZARD* symbol. See *Focus on Surveys: Laundry.*

FOCUS ON SURVEYS

Laundry

Surveyors will observe how staff handle, store, process, and transport linens. For example, do staff:

- Handle linens in a way that prevents exposure of urine or feces?
- Handle linens in a way that prevents the spread of infection?
- Handle linens according to agency policies and procedures?
- Store and transport linens properly?

Exposure Incidents

An *exposure incident* is any eye, mouth, other mucous membrane, non-intact skin, or parenteral contact with blood or OPIM. *Parenteral* means *piercing the mucous membranes or the skin.* Piercing occurs by needle-sticks, human bites, cuts, and abrasions.

Report exposure incidents at once. Medical evaluation, follow-up, and testing are free. Your blood is tested for HIV and HBV. If you refuse testing, the blood sample is kept for at least 90 days. Testing is done later if you desire.

You are told about any medical conditions that may need treatment. You receive a written opinion within 15 days after the evaluation is complete.

The *source individual* is the person whose blood or body fluids are the source of an exposure incident. His or her blood is tested for HIV or HBV. The agency informs you about laws affecting the source's identity and test results.

SURGICAL ASEPSIS

Surgical asepsis (sterile technique) is the practices used to remove *all* microbes. *Sterile* means *the absence of* all *microbes.* Surgical asepsis is required any time the skin or sterile tissues are entered.

Your state and agency may allow you to assist with or perform some sterile procedures. If so, make sure you receive the needed training.

FOCUS ON PRIDE
The Person, Family, and Yourself

Personal and Professional Responsibility
You are responsible for following the guidelines in this chapter. Practice good hand hygiene before and after giving care. Follow Standard Precautions and Transmission-Based Precautions.

Rights and Respect
Caring for persons who need Transmission-Based Precautions can be a challenge. Extra time and effort are needed to apply and remove PPE and clean equipment used in the room. You must plan carefully when gathering supplies before entering the room. If an item is forgotten, you must wait for help or remove and re-apply PPE. You may feel frustrated.

The person must not feel as if he or she is a burden. The person deserves the same kindness and respect you give others. You must:
- Watch your verbal and nonverbal communication (Chapter 7).
- Avoid complaining.
- Practice good teamwork and time management.
- Tell the nurse if you are feeling overwhelmed.

Independence and Social Interaction
Patients and residents often cannot perform their usual hygiene measures. Hand hygiene is an example. Ask patients and residents if they would like to wash their hands. Ask them often. Assist them to wash their hands before and after eating, after elimination, after coughing or sneezing, and any time the hands are dirty. Hand hygiene is important for you and for patients and residents. When independence is limited, protect the person and others by promoting hand hygiene.

Delegation and Teamwork
Before making delegation decisions, the nurse must assess and plan (Chapter 6). The nurse considers the person's needs and risks. If delegated care of persons at increased risk for infection, you must:
- Practice medical asepsis at all times.
- Practice hand hygiene.
- Follow Standard Precautions and the Bloodborne Pathogen Standard at all times.
- Follow any Transmission-Based Precautions ordered for the person.
- Wear PPE as directed by the nurse.
- Follow the person's care plan.
- Report any signs or symptoms of infection at once.
- Provide good oral hygiene and skin care (Chapter 18).
- Tell the nurse if you have any sign or symptom of an infection.

Ethics and Laws
The health team must prevent the spread of microbes and infection. Even one careless act can spread microbes. This affects the person's health and safety. Be very careful about your work.

When assisting with or performing a procedure, remove items that become contaminated. If necessary, stop and get new supplies. Do not use a contaminated item. You may be alone. Be honest with yourself. Be responsible. Do the right thing, even if other staff are not present. Take pride in providing care that prevents the spread of infection.

FOCUS ON PRIDE: Application
Consider your every-day actions. How do they affect infection control? Give some examples. Identify areas to improve. How might your attitude affect how you prevent infection at work?

REVIEW QUESTIONS

*Circle **T** if the statement is TRUE or **F** if it is FALSE.*

1 **T F** Microbes are pathogens in their natural sites.

2 **T F** A pathogen can cause an infection.

3 **T F** An infection results when microbes invade and grow in the body.

4 **T F** An item is sterile if non-pathogens are present.

5 **T F** You hold your hands and forearms up during hand-washing.

6 **T F** A towel falls to the floor. The towel is contaminated.

7 **T F** Un-used items in the person's room are used for another person.

8 **T F** A person received the hepatitis B vaccine. The person will develop the disease.

Circle the BEST answer.

9 Which area is *best* for a pathogen to live and grow?
   a A cold and wet area
   b A warm and dark area
   c A hot and bright area
   d A dry area without oxygen

10 Which is a sign of infection?
   a A bruise
   b Redness in a body part
   c Warm, dry, and intact skin
   d A bleeding wound

11 To control a portal of exit
   a Cover the mouth and nose when coughing
   b Position drainage containers above the drainage site
   c Clean the genital area from the rectum to the urethra
   d Leave an open wound uncovered

12 You have blood on your hand. What should you do?
   a Wash your hands with soap and water.
   b Use an alcohol-based hand sanitizer.
   c Rinse your hands.
   d Wash your hands with a disinfectant.

13 You move from a contaminated body site to a clean body site. Your hands are not visibly soiled. What should you do?
   a Disinfect your gloves.
   b Practice hand hygiene.
   c Rinse your hands.
   d Continue care without hand hygiene.

14 To use an alcohol-based hand sanitizer correctly
   a Wash your hands before applying the hand sanitizer
   b Rinse your hands after applying the hand sanitizer
   c Rub the product only on the palms of your hands
   d Rub your hands together until they are dry

15 When cleaning equipment
   a Rinse the item in hot water before cleaning
   b Wash the item with soap and cold water
   c Use a brush if necessary
   d Work from dirty to clean areas

16 Isolation precautions
   a Treat communicable diseases
   b Destroy pathogens
   c Keep pathogens within a certain area
   d Destroy all microbes

17 Which statement about Standard Precautions is *true*?
   a They are used for all persons.
   b The 3 types are contact, droplet, and airborne.
   c They are used only in hospitals.
   d They require a doctor's order.

18 You wear utility gloves for contact with
   a Blood
   b Body fluids
   c Secretions and excretions
   d Cleaning solutions

19 A mask
   a Can be re-used
   b Is clean on the inside
   c Is contaminated when moist
   d Should fit loosely for breathing

20 To use PPE correctly
   a Never change gloves in the person's room
   b Tie a gown's waist strings in front
   c Don gloves first when applying PPE
   d Apply new PPE for each person

21 Which task requires gloves?
   a Applying wrist restraints
   b Giving a back massage
   c Providing denture care
   d Moving the person up in bed

22 Goggles or a face shield is worn
   a When using Standard Precautions
   b When splashing body fluids is likely
   c If you have an eye infection
   d When assisting with sterile procedures

23 The Bloodborne Pathogen Standard involves microbes spread through
   a Blood and OPIM
   b Only blood
   c Droplets
   d Close contact

24 According to the Bloodborne Pathogen Standard, you should
   a Practice hand hygiene after removing gloves
   b Discard a used razor in a wastebasket
   c Tell the nurse about exposure to blood before washing your hands
   d Refuse the hepatitis B vaccine

25 You were exposed to a bloodborne pathogen. Which is *true?*
   a You do not have to report the exposure.
   b You pay for required tests.
   c You can refuse HIV and HBV testing.
   d The source individual can refuse testing.

Answers to Chapter 13 questions are on p. 551.

FOCUS ON PRACTICE

Problem Solving

A nurse enters the room of a person who requires contact precautions. The nurse is not wearing PPE. What do you do? What PPE is needed? What precautions are needed upon entering and leaving the room and while in the room?

OBJECTIVES

- Define the key terms and key abbreviations in this chapter.
- Explain the purpose and rules of body mechanics.
- Identify the risk factors for work-related injuries.
- Identify the signs, symptoms, and activities associated with back injuries.

- Explain how to prevent work-related injuries.
- Position persons in the basic bed positions and in a chair.
- Explain how to promote PRIDE in the person, the family, and yourself.

KEY TERMS

base of support The area on which an object rests
body alignment The way the head, trunk, arms, and legs are aligned with one another; posture
body mechanics Using the body in an efficient and careful way
dorsal recumbent position The back-lying or supine position
ergonomics The science of designing a job to fit the worker; *ergo* means *work*, *nomos* means *law*
Fowler's position A semi-sitting position; the head of the bed is raised between 45 and 60 degrees
lateral position The person lies on 1 side or the other; side-lying position

musculo-skeletal disorders (MSDs) Injuries and disorders of the muscles, tendons, ligaments, joints, and cartilage
posture See "body alignment"
prone position The person lies on the abdomen with the head turned to 1 side
semi-prone side position See "Sims' position"
side-lying position See "lateral position"
Sims' position A left side-lying position in which the upper leg (right leg) is sharply flexed so it is not on the lower leg (left leg) and the lower arm (left arm) is behind the person; semi-prone side position
supine position The back-lying or dorsal recumbent position

KEY ABBREVIATIONS

MSD   Musculo-skeletal disorder

OSHA   Occupational Safety and Health Administration

Body mechanics *means using the body in an efficient and careful way.* It involves good posture, balance, and using your strongest and largest muscles for work. Fatigue, muscle strain, and injury can result from the incorrect use and positioning of the body during activity or rest.

PRINCIPLES OF BODY MECHANICS

Body alignment (posture) is the way the head, trunk, arms, and legs are aligned with one another. Good alignment lets the body move and function with strength and efficiency. Standing, sitting, and lying down require good alignment.

Base of support is the area on which an object rests. A good base of support is needed for balance (Fig. 14-1). When standing, your feet are your base of support. Stand with your feet apart for a wider base of support and more balance.

Your strongest and largest muscles are in your shoulders, upper arms, hips, and thighs. Use these muscles to handle and move persons and heavy objects. Otherwise, you place strain and exertion on the smaller and weaker muscles. This causes fatigue and injury. *Back injuries are a major risk.* For good body mechanics:

- Bend your knees and squat to lift a heavy object (Fig. 14-2). Do not bend from your waist. Bending from the waist places strain on small back muscles.
- Hold items close to your body and base of support (see Fig. 14-2). This involves upper arm and shoulder muscles. Holding objects away from the body places strain on small muscles in the lower arms.

All activities require good body mechanics. Follow the rules in Box 14-1.

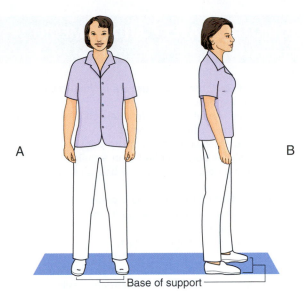

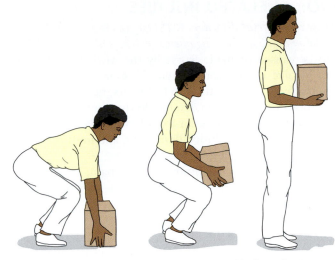

FIGURE 14-2 Picking up a box using good body mechanics.

FIGURE 14-1 A, Anterior (front) view of an adult in good body alignment. The feet are apart for a wide base of support. **B,** Lateral (side) view of an adult with good posture and alignment.

BOX 14-1	Rules for Body Mechanics

- Keep your body in good alignment with a wide base of support. Your feet are at least 12 inches apart or shoulder-width apart.
- Use an upright working posture. Bend your legs. Do not bend your back.
- Use the stronger and larger muscles in your shoulders, upper arms, thighs, and hips.
- Keep objects close to your body to lift, move, or carry them (see Fig. 14-2).
- Avoid unnecessary bending and reaching. Raise the bed and over-bed table to waist level or to a comfortable working height.
- Face your work area. This prevents unnecessary twisting.
- Push, slide, or pull heavy objects when you can rather than lifting them. Pushing is easier than pulling.
- Widen your base of support to push or pull. Move your front leg forward when pushing. Move your rear leg back when pulling (Fig. 14-3).
- Use both hands and arms to lift, move, or carry objects.
- Turn your whole body to change the direction of the turn. Do not twist your body.
- Work with smooth and even movements. Avoid sudden or jerky motions.
- Do not lean over a person to give care.
- *Get help from a co-worker to move persons or heavy objects. Do not lift or move them by yourself.*
- Bend your hips and knees to lift heavy objects from the floor (see Fig. 14-2). Straighten your back as the object reaches thigh level. Your leg and thigh muscles work to raise the item off the floor and to waist level.
- Do not lift objects higher than chest level. Do not lift above your shoulders. Use a step stool or ladder to reach an object higher than chest level.

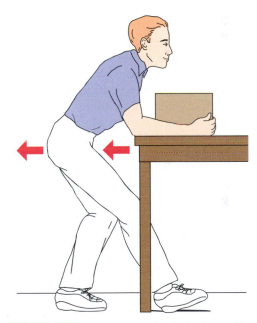

FIGURE 14-3 Move your rear leg back when pulling.

WORK-RELATED INJURIES

Musculo-skeletal disorders (MSDs) are injuries and disorders of the muscles, tendons, ligaments, joints, and cartilage. They can be caused or made worse by the work setting. They can involve the nervous system. The arms and back are often affected. So are the hands, fingers, neck, wrists, legs, and shoulders. MSDs can develop slowly over weeks, months, and years. Or they can occur from 1 event. Pain, numbness, tingling, stiff joints, difficulty moving, and muscle loss can occur. Sometimes there is paralysis.

Early signs and symptoms include pain, limited joint movement, or soft tissue swelling. Time off work is often needed.

MSD Risk Factors

The Occupational Safety and Health Administration (OSHA) has identified MSD risk factors. An MSD is more likely if risk factors are combined. For example, a task involves both force and repeating actions.

- *Force*—the amount of physical effort needed for a task. Lifting or transferring heavy persons, preventing falls, and sudden motions are examples.
- *Repeating action*—doing the same motion or series of motions often or continually. Re-positioning persons and transfers to and from beds, chairs, and commodes without adequate rest breaks are examples.
- *Awkward postures*—assuming positions that place stress on the body. Examples are reaching above shoulder height, kneeling, squatting, leaning over a bed, bending, or twisting the torso while lifting.
- *Heavy lifting*—manually lifting people who cannot move themselves.
  According to the U.S. Department of Labor, nursing assistants are at great risk.

Back Injuries. Back injuries are major threats. Back injuries can occur from repeated activities or from 1 event. Signs and symptoms include:

- Pain when trying to assume a normal posture
- Decreased mobility
- Pain when standing or rising from a seated position

Follow the rules and safety measures in this chapter to prevent back injuries. Be very careful during tasks associated with back injuries.

See *Promoting Safety and Comfort: Back Injuries.*

PROMOTING SAFETY AND COMFORT
Back Injuries

Safety

According to OSHA, these activities are related to back injuries in nursing centers.

- Moving a person who depends totally on others for care.
- Moving a person who is combative.
- Transferring a person on the floor to the bed or chair.
- Re-positioning a person in bed or in a chair.
- Transferring a person to or from a bed, chair, wheelchair, or toilet.
- Bending to bathe, dress, or feed a person.
- Bending to make a bed or change linens.
- Weighing a person.
- Changing an incontinence product.
- Trying to stop a person from falling.
  Use good body mechanics to protect yourself from injury.

Do not work alone. Avoid lifting whenever possible.

Preventing MSDs

Ergonomics is the science of designing a job to fit the worker. (Ergo *means* work. Nomos *means* law.) It involves changing the task, work station, equipment, and tools to help reduce stress on the worker's body. The goal is to eliminate a serious work-related MSD.

The work setting must be free of hazards that cause or may cause death or serious physical harm to staff. The employer must make reasonable attempts to prevent or reduce the hazard.

Always report a work-related injury as soon as possible. Early attention can prevent the problem from becoming worse. Also, injuries are often less serious and less costly to treat with early attention.

To prevent work-related MSDs, follow the rules in Box 14-1 and Box 14-2.

See *Promoting Safety and Comfort: Preventing MSDs.*

PROMOTING SAFETY AND COMFORT
Preventing MSDs

Safety

According to OSHA, injuries commonly occur from manually lifting, transferring, and re-positioning persons. Proper body mechanics alone do not reduce MSDs. Policies and procedures that minimize manual lifting must be followed to prevent injuries. Use assist devices and mechanical lifts (Chapters 15 and 16) when possible.

BOX 14-2   Preventing Work-Related Injuries

General Guidelines

- Wear shoes with good traction. Avoid shoes with worn-down soles or sides. Good traction helps prevent slips or falls.
- Use assist equipment and devices (Chapters 15 and 16) when possible instead of lifting and moving the person manually. Follow the care plan.
- Get help from other staff. The nurse and care plan tell you the number of staff needed for a task.
- Plan and prepare for the task. For example, know what equipment is needed, where to place chairs or wheelchairs, and what side of the bed to work on.
- Schedule harder tasks early in your shift.
- Balance lighter and harder tasks. Plan to complete a lighter task after a harder one.
- Lock (brake) bed wheels and wheelchair or stretcher wheels.
- Tell the person how he or she can help. Give clear, simple instructions. Give the person time to respond.
- Do not hold or grab the person under the underarms.
- Do not let the person hold or grasp you around your neck.

Manual Lifting

- Minimize or eliminate manual lifting when possible.
- Stand with good posture. Keep your back straight.
- Bend your legs, not your back.
- Use the large muscles in your legs to do the work.
- Face the person.
- Do not twist or turn. Pick up your feet and pivot your whole body in the direction of the move.
- Keep what you are moving close to you.
- Move the person toward you, not away from you.
- Use a wide, balanced base of support. Stand with 1 foot slightly ahead of the other.
- Use smooth, even movements. Avoid jerking movements.
- Lift on the "count of 3" when lifting with others. Everyone lifts at the same time.

Lifting or Moving the Person in Bed

- Adjust the bed height to a safe and comfortable level.
- Lower the bed rail.
- Work on the side where the person will be closest to you.
- Place equipment or other items close to you at waist level or at a comfortable working height.
- Use friction-reducing devices—drawsheets, turning pads, large re-usable waterproof under-pads, slide sheets (Chapters 15 and 16).

Transfer/Gait Belts

- Keep the person as close to you as possible.
- Avoid bending, reaching, or twisting to:
  - Apply or remove a transfer/gait belt.
  - Lower the person to the chair, bed, toilet, or floor.
  - Help the person walk.
- Use a gentle rocking motion to help the person stand. The rocking motion gives strength and force as you help the person stand.
- See Chapter 11.

Stand and Pivot Transfers (Chapter 16)

- Use assist devices as directed. Follow the care plan.
- Use a transfer belt as directed. The nurse may have you use a transfer belt with handles. See Chapter 11.
- Plan the transfer so the person's strong side moves first.

Stand and Pivot Transfers—cont'd

- Lower the bed so the person can place his or her feet on the floor.
- Get the person close to the edge of the bed or the chair. Ask the person to lean forward as he or she stands.
- Block the person's weak leg with your legs or knees. If the position is awkward:
  - Use a transfer belt with handles.
  - Straddle your legs around the person's weak leg.
- Keep your feet at least shoulder-width apart.
- Bend your legs. Do not bend your back.
- Use a gentle rocking motion to help the person stand. The rocking motion gives strength and force as you help the person stand.
- Pivot with your feet to turn.

Lateral Transfers (Chapter 16)

- Position surfaces close to each other.
- Adjust surfaces to about waist height or to a comfortable working height. Do 1 of the following as directed by the nurse and care plan.
  - Adjust the surfaces to the same level.
  - Adjust the receiving surface so it is slightly lower (about ½ inch) than the surface the person is on. This allows the use of gravity. For example, for a bed to stretcher transfer, the stretcher surface is lower than the bed.
- Lower bed rails and stretcher side rails.
- Use friction-reducing devices.
- Get a good hand-hold. Roll up drawsheets, turning pads, large re-usable waterproof under-pads, and slide sheets. Or use assist devices with handles.
- Kneel on the bed or stretcher. This prevents extended reaches and bending your back.
- Have staff on both sides of the bed or the other surface. Move the person on the "count of 3." Use a smooth, push-pull motion. Do not reach across the person.

Transporting the Person and Equipment

- Push, do not pull.
- Keep the load close to your body.
- Use an upright posture.
- Push with your whole body, not just your arms.
- Move down the center of the hallway. This helps avoid collisions.
- Watch out for door handles and high thresholds on floors. These can cause abrupt stops.

Transferring the Person From the Floor

- Assist as the nurse directs. Stand by to monitor persons able to stand alone. For no injuries or minor injuries, the nurse uses 1 of these methods.
  - *Method 1:* Use a full-sling mechanical lift (Chapter 16). Two or more staff are needed. The lift must reach the floor.
  - *Method 2:* See "Manual Lifting" if a manual lift is required.
    - Roll the person onto the side.
    - Position an assist device. A blanket or drawsheet (Chapter 17) are examples. Avoid reaching across the person.
    - Have at least 2 staff members on each side. The larger the person, the more staff needed.
    - Kneel on 1 knee. Grasp the assist device.
    - Lift smoothly with your legs as you stand. Staff stand together on the "count of 3."

Modified from Cal/OSHA: *A back injury prevention guide for health care providers,* Sacramento, Calif, 1997, Author; and Occupational Safety and Health Administration: *Guidelines for nursing homes: ergonomics for the prevention of musculoskeletal disorders,* Washington, DC, revised March 2009, Author.

POSITIONING THE PERSON
The person must be positioned correctly at all times. Regular position changes and good alignment promote comfort and well-being. Breathing is easier. Circulation is promoted. Pressure injuries and contractures are prevented. A *contracture* is the lack of joint mobility caused by the abnormal shortening of a muscle (Chapter 27).

Whether in bed or chair, the person is re-positioned at least every 2 hours or more often. Follow the nurse's instructions and the care plan. To safely position a person:
- Use good body mechanics.
- Ask a co-worker to help you if needed.
- Explain the procedure to the person.
- Provide for privacy.
- Be gentle when moving the person.
- Use pillows as directed by the nurse for support and alignment.
- Provide for comfort after positioning. (See the inside of the front cover.)
- Place the call light and other needed items within reach after positioning.
- Complete a safety check before leaving the room. (See the inside of the front cover.)
  See *Focus on Communication: Positioning the Person.*
  See *Delegation Guidelines: Positioning the Person.*
  See *Promoting Safety and Comfort: Positioning the Person.*

Fowler's Positions
Fowler's position is a semi-sitting position. The head of the bed is raised between 45 and 60 degrees (Fig. 14-4). The knees may be slightly elevated. Other forms of Fowler's position include:
- *Semi-Fowler's position*—the head of the bed is raised 30 degrees (Chapter 17). Some agencies define semi-Fowler's position as the head of the bed raised 30 degrees and the knee portion raised 15 degrees.
- *High-Fowler's position*—the head of the bed is raised 60 to 90 degrees (Chapter 17).
  For good alignment:
- The spine is straight.
- The head is supported with a small pillow.
- The arms are supported with pillows.

The nurse may have you place small pillows under the lower back, thighs, and ankles. Persons with heart and respiratory disorders usually breathe easier in Fowler's position.

See *Focus on Math: Fowler's Positions.*

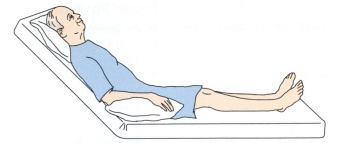

FIGURE 14-4 Fowler's position.

FOCUS ON MATH

Fowler's Positions

When 2 lines meet, an angle is formed. Angles measure how much 1 line has to turn to be in the same position as the other line. Angles are measured in degrees (°). Degrees range from 0 to 360. With bed positions, you need a basic understanding of angle measurements between 0° and 90°.

To estimate the angle:

1 Use the bed frame and the head of the bed as the 2 lines.
2 Estimate the angle from the bed frame to the head of the bed. See Figure 14-5.

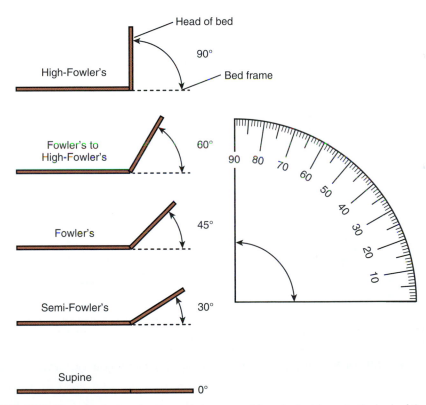

FIGURE 14-5 Measuring bed angles. The angle is measured from the bed frame to the back of the head of the bed. As the head of the bed rises, the angle increases.

Supine Position

The *supine position (dorsal recumbent position) is the back-lying position* (Fig. 14-6).

- The bed is flat.
- The head and shoulders are supported on a pillow.
- Arms and hands are at the sides. You can support the arms with regular pillows. Or you can support the hands on small pillows with the palms down.

The nurse may have you place a folded or rolled towel under the lower back and a small pillow under the thighs. A pillow under the lower legs lifts the heels off of the bed. This prevents the heels from rubbing on the sheets.

Prone Position

In the *prone position, the person lies on the abdomen with the head turned to 1 side.*

- The bed is flat.
- Small pillows are under the head, abdomen, and lower legs (Fig. 14-7).
- Arms are flexed at the elbows with the hands near the head.

You also can position a person with the feet hanging over the end of the mattress (Fig. 14-8). A pillow is not needed under the feet.

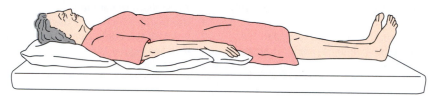

FIGURE 14-6 Supine position.

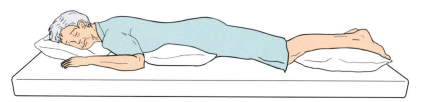

FIGURE 14-7 Prone position.

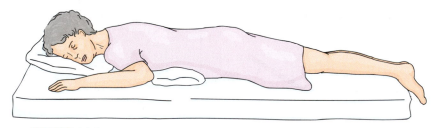

FIGURE 14-8 Prone position with the feet hanging over the edge of the mattress.

Lateral Position

In the *lateral position (side-lying position),* the person lies on 1 side or the other (Fig. 14-9).

- The bed is flat.
- A pillow is under the head and neck.
- The upper leg is in front of the lower leg. (The nurse may ask you to position the upper leg behind the lower leg, not on top of it.)
- The ankle, upper leg, and thigh are supported with pillows.
- A small pillow is against the person's back. The person rolls back against the pillow so that his or her back is at a 45-degree angle with the mattress.
- A small pillow is under the upper hand and arm.

Sims' Position

The *Sims' position (semi-prone side position)* is a left side-lying position. The upper leg (right leg) is sharply flexed so it is not on the lower leg (left leg). The lower arm (left arm) is behind the person (Fig. 14-10).

- The bed is flat.
- A pillow is under the person's head and shoulder.
- The upper leg (right leg) is supported with a pillow.
- A pillow is under the upper arm (right arm) and hand (right hand).

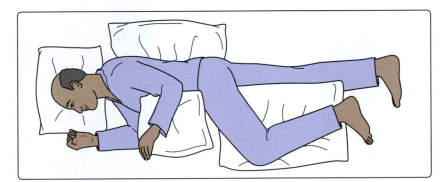

FIGURE 14-9 Lateral position.

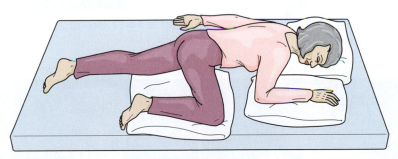

FIGURE 14-10 Sims' position.

Chair Position

Persons who sit in chairs must hold their upper bodies and heads erect. If not, poor alignment results. For good alignment:

- The person's back and buttocks are against the back of the chair.
- Feet are flat on the floor or wheelchair footplates. Never leave feet unsupported.
- Backs of the knees and calves are slightly away from the edge of the seat (Fig. 14-11).

The nurse may have you put a small pillow between the person's lower back and the chair. This supports the lower back. *Remember, a pillow is not used behind the back if restraints are used* (Chapter 12).

Paralyzed arms are supported on pillows. Some persons have positioners (Fig. 14-12). Ask the nurse about their correct use. The nurse may have you position the wrists at a slight upward angle.

Some people need postural supports if they cannot keep their upper bodies erect (Fig. 14-13). Postural supports promote good alignment. The health team selects the best product for the person's needs. Safety, dignity, and function are considered.

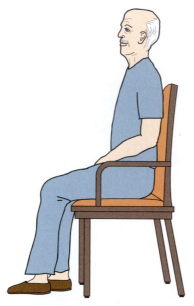

FIGURE 14-11 Chair position.

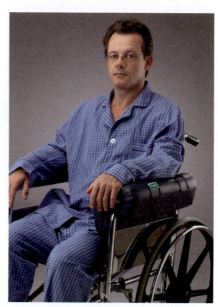

FIGURE 14-12 Elevated armrest. (Image courtesy Posey Co., Arcadia, Calif.)

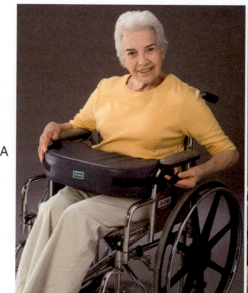 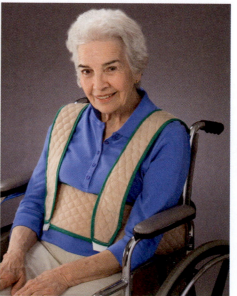

A | B

FIGURE 14-13 Postural supports. **A,** Posey Hugger. **B,** Torso support. (Images courtesy Posey Co., Arcadia, Calif.)

Personal and Professional Responsibility

You make decisions daily about protecting yourself.

- Do you bend at the waist or the hips and knees to pick up objects?
- Do you reach or use a step stool to get high objects?
- Do you exercise for strength and endurance?
- Do you raise the bed for good body mechanics when giving bedside care?
- Do you move a person alone or get help?

Your decisions affect the safety of yourself and others. Use good judgment at home and in the workplace. Protect yourself from harm.

Rights and Respect

OSHA requires a safe work setting. You have the right to ask employers about safety plans to reduce your risk of injury. Ask about training or orientation programs related to body mechanics, safe handling of persons, and workplace hazards. Know and follow agency procedures to report problems.

Independence and Social Interaction

Independence to the extent possible promotes dignity, self-esteem, and pride. Let the person choose bed or chair positions as allowed by the nurse and the care plan. Let the person help as much as safely possible. Talk with the person while moving him or her. Ask what he or she prefers. Doing so promotes comfort, independence, and social interaction.

Delegation and Teamwork

Many tasks strain your body. Injuries can occur. Some tasks increase your risk for injury. See "MSD Risk Factors," p. 176. Know which tasks often cause harm. Use caution when doing them. Get help when needed.

Thinking that injuries happen only to others is dangerous. Anyone can be injured. Your safety is important. Take pride in working carefully.

Ethics and Laws

Proper body mechanics help prevent injuries that could affect health and function. Failure to move and position the person correctly places the person at risk. For example:

- A person is slumped in a chair for 3 hours. The person develops a pressure injury.
- A person is not re-positioned according to the care plan. The person's contracture worsens.
- A person is moved without enough help. The move is rough. The person is injured.

You must provide care in a manner that maintains or improves each person's quality of life, health, and safety. It is the right thing to do.

FOCUS ON PRIDE: *Application*

What changes will you make in your daily life to protect yourself from injury? How do you plan to protect yourself in the workplace?

REVIEW QUESTIONS

Circle the BEST answer.

1 Good body mechanics involve
   a Having an upright posture
   b Having a narrow base of support
   c Using the muscles in the back and lower arms
   d Lifting a heavy object alone

2 Good alignment means
   a The area on which an object rests
   b Having the head, trunk, arms, and legs aligned with one another
   c Using muscles, tendons, ligaments, and joints correctly
   d The back-lying or supine position

3 Which action shows poor body mechanics?
   a Holding an object close to your body
   b Facing the direction you are working to prevent twisting
   c Leaning over a raised bed rail to give care
   d Using both hands and arms to lift an object

4 You need to move a large chair in a resident's room. You should
   a Push or slide the chair
   b Lift and carry the chair
   c Ask the nurse to move the chair for you
   d Pull the chair using quick, jerking motions

5 The purpose of ergonomics is to
   a Reduce stress on the worker's body
   b Safely position the person
   c Promote quality of life
   d Use good body mechanics

6 Risk of MSDs decreases with
   a Repeating actions
   b Awkward postures
   c Avoiding manual lifting when possible
   d Greater force

7 Which statement about back injuries is *true?*
   a Back injuries cannot be prevented.
   b Pain when assuming normal posture is a symptom.
   c Nursing center staff are at low risk.
   d Bending to change bed linens is not a cause of back injuries.

8 Which statement about positioning is *true?*
   a Re-positioning prevents pressure injuries and contractures.
   b Circulation is not affected by positioning.
   c Position changes are avoided if moving causes pain.
   d Persons in chairs are re-positioned less often than those in bed.

Continued

9 You position a resident in the lateral position. Where do you place the call light?
   a At the foot of the bed
   b At the head of the bed
   c Behind the person
   d Within the person's reach

10 Patients and residents are re-positioned at least every
   a 15 minutes
   b 30 minutes
   c 2 hours
   d 3 hours

11 The back-lying position is called
   a Fowler's position
   b The supine position
   c The lateral position
   d Sims' position

12 For Fowler's position
   a The bed is flat
   b The head of the bed is raised 45 to 60 degrees
   c The person's head is turned to 1 side
   d The feet hang over the edge of the mattress

13 A pillow is placed against the person's back in
   a A chair while restraints are used
   b The prone position
   c The lateral position
   d Sims' position

14 When in a chair, the person's feet
   a Must be flat on the floor
   b Are positioned on footplates
   c Dangle
   d Are positioned on pillows

Answers to Chapter 14 questions are on p. 551.

FOCUS ON PRACTICE

Problem Solving

You are a new nursing assistant. To complete tasks quickly, you do not adjust the bed height to a comfortable working level. You move persons alone instead of getting help. You do not use bed rails correctly. Why do these actions put you at increased risk for injury?

You now have back pain and numbness in a leg. Your walking is affected. How does this affect your work and daily life? How could you have avoided this problem?

Moving the Person

KEY TERMS

bed mobility How a person moves to and from a lying position, turns from side to side, and re-positions in a bed or other furniture

friction The rubbing of 1 surface against another

logrolling Turning the person as a unit, in alignment, with 1 motion

shearing When the skin sticks to a surface while muscles slide in the direction the body is moving

KEY ABBREVIATION

ID Identification

You assist with bed mobility. *Bed mobility is how a person moves to and from a lying position, turns from side to side, and re-positions in a bed or other furniture.* You must work carefully to protect yourself and the person from injury.

See *Focus on Communication: Moving the Person.*
See *Promoting Safety and Comfort: Moving the Person.*

FOCUS ON COMMUNICATION

Moving the Person

Moving can be painful from injury, surgery, or painful joints. Provide for comfort and avoid causing pain. You can say:

- "Please tell me when you feel pain or discomfort."
- "Are you comfortable? Do you need a pillow adjusted?"
- "How can I make you more comfortable?"

Before a procedure, tell the person what you and your co-workers will do. Also explain what the person needs to do. Before the move, remind the person what will happen.

The procedures in this chapter move the person on the "count of 3." Staff smoothly move the person at the same time. One co-worker leads by counting. Decide who will count before the move. Be sure the person and staff know who is leading and what to do. You can say:

We will help you move up in bed. I will count "1, 2, 3." When I say "3," push against the bed with your feet and pull up with the trapeze. We will help move your body to the head of the bed when I say "3."

PROMOTING SAFETY AND COMFORT

Moving the Person

Safety

Many older persons have fragile bones and joints. To prevent injuries:

- Follow the rules of body mechanics (Chapter 14).
- Always have help to move the person.
- Move the person carefully.
- Keep the person in good alignment during and after the procedure.
- Make sure the face, nose, and mouth are not obstructed by a pillow or other device.

Comfort

To promote mental comfort when moving the person:

- Explain what you will do and how the person can help.
- Screen and cover the person to provide for privacy.

To promote physical comfort:

- Keep the person in good alignment.
- Do not let the person's head hit the head-board when being moved up in bed. If the person can be without a pillow, place it upright against the head-board.
- Use pillows and other positioning devices to position the person as directed by the nurse and the care plan. If a pillow is allowed under the person's head, position it under the head and shoulders.

PREVENTING WORK-RELATED INJURIES

Moving procedures involve lifting, awkward postures, and repeated motions. These increase your risk for injury. You must prevent work-related injuries during moving procedures. See Chapter 14.

Good body mechanics alone will not prevent injury. The Occupational Safety and Health Administration (OSHA) recommends:

- Minimizing manual lifting in all cases
- Eliminating manual lifting when possible

Each person is different. Careful planning is needed to move the person safely. You must know about the person's physical abilities and the number of staff needed. The number of staff depends on the person's height, weight, cognitive function, and physical abilities. The nurse and care plan tell you what procedure to use and the equipment needed. Always follow the manufacturer's instructions. Ask for training to use equipment and devices safely.

See *Focus on Older Persons: Preventing Work-Related Injuries.*

See *Delegation Guidelines: Preventing Work-Related Injuries.*

See *Promoting Safety and Comfort: Preventing Work-Related Injuries.*

DELEGATION GUIDELINES
Preventing Work-Related Injuries

Many tasks involve moving persons. Before doing so, you need this information from the nurse and the care plan.

- The person's height and weight.
- The person's physical abilities. Does the person have strength in the arms and legs?
- If the person has a weak side. If yes, which side?
- If the person has problems that increase the risk of injury. Dizziness, confusion, hearing or vision problems, recent surgery, and fragile skin are examples.
- Any doctor's orders for moving the person.
- The person's ability to follow directions.
- If behavior problems are likely. Combative, agitated, uncooperative, and unpredictable behaviors are examples.
- The amount of assistance needed.
- The number of staff needed to complete the task safely.
- What procedure to use.
- What equipment to use.

FOCUS ON OLDER PERSONS
Preventing Work-Related Injuries

Persons with dementia may not understand what you are doing. They may resist your efforts. The person may shout, grab you, or try to hit you. Always have a co-worker help you. Do not force the person. The person's care plan has measures for safe care. For example:

- Proceed slowly.
- Use a calm, pleasant voice.
- Distract the person. For example, let the person hold a washcloth or other soft object. This helps distract the person and keeps the hands busy.

Tell the nurse at once if you have problems moving the person.

PROMOTING SAFETY AND COMFORT
Preventing Work-Related Injuries

Safety

Decide how to move the person before starting the procedure. Ask needed staff to help before you begin. Also plan how to protect drainage tubes or containers connected to the person.

Beds are raised to move persons in bed. This reduces bending and reaching. You must:

- Use the bed correctly.
- Protect the person from falling when the bed is raised.
- Follow the rules of body mechanics (Chapter 14).

PROTECTING THE SKIN

Protect the person's skin during moving procedures. Friction and shearing injure the skin. Both cause infection and pressure injuries (Chapter 29).

- *Friction is the rubbing of 1 surface against another.* When moved in bed, the person's skin rubs against the sheet.
- *Shearing is when the skin sticks to a surface while muscles slide in the direction the body is moving* (Fig. 15-1). It occurs when the person slides down in bed or is moved in bed.

To reduce friction and shearing when moving the person in bed:

- Roll the person.
- Use friction-reducing devices. Such devices include a lift sheet (turning sheet). Drawsheets (Chapter 17) serve as lift sheets (turning sheets). Turning pads (Fig. 15-2), large re-usable waterproof under-pads (Chapter 17), and slide sheets (p. 190) are other friction-reducing devices.

See *Focus on Older Persons: Protecting the Skin.*
See *Focus on Surveys: Protecting the Skin.*

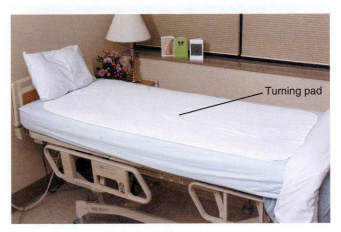

FIGURE 15-2 Turning pad.

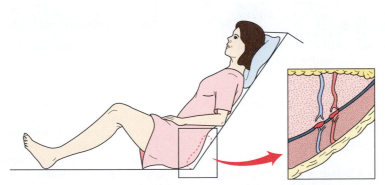

FIGURE 15-1 Shearing. When the head of the bed is raised to a sitting position, skin on the buttocks stays in place. However, internal structures move forward as the person slides down in bed. This pinches the skin between the mattress and the hip bones.

MOVING PERSONS IN BED

Some persons can move and turn in bed. Others need help from at least 1 person. Those who are weak, unconscious, paralyzed, or in casts need help. Sometimes 2 or 3 people or a mechanical lift (Chapter 16) is needed. Follow the guidelines in Box 15-1 to lift or move persons in bed.

See *Delegation Guidelines: Moving Persons in Bed.*

BOX 15-1	Guidelines for Moving Persons in Bed

- Follow the rules to prevent work-related injuries (Chapter 14).
- Know how much help and what equipment or friction-reducing devices you need. Follow the nurse's directions and the care plan. The nurse uses the person's weight as a guide to plan a safe move.
  - *Persons fully able to assist*—staff assistance is not needed. Staff stand by for safety and provide cues as needed. (To *cue* means *to remind the person what to do.*)
  - *Persons partially able to assist:*
    - *The person weighs less than 200 pounds*—2 to 3 staff members and a friction-reducing device are used.
    - *The person weighs more than 200 pounds*—at least 3 staff members and a friction-reducing device are used.
  - *Persons unable to assist*—a mechanical lift and at least 2 staff members are needed. See "Using a Mechanical Lift" in Chapter 16.

Modified from Occupational Safety and Health Administration: *Guidelines for nursing homes: ergonomics for the prevention of musculoskeletal disorders*, Washington, DC, revised March 2009, Author.

Moving the Person Up in Bed

When the head of the bed is raised, it is easy to slide down toward the middle and foot of the bed (Fig. 15-3). You move the person up in bed for good alignment and comfort.

You can sometimes move light-weight adults up in bed alone if they assist using a trapeze. However, it is best done with help and an assist device (p. 190). For heavy, weak, and older persons, 2 or more staff members are needed. Always protect the person and yourself from injury.

See *Promoting Safety and Comfort: Moving the Person Up in Bed.*

See procedure: *Moving the Person Up in Bed.*

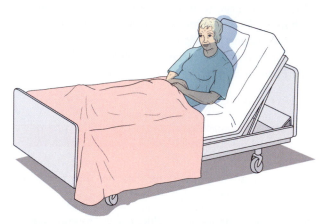

FIGURE 15-3 A person in poor alignment after sliding down in bed.

DELEGATION GUIDELINES

Moving Persons in Bed

Before moving a person in bed, you need this information from the nurse and the care plan.
- What procedure to use
- The number of staff needed to safely move the person
- Position limits and restrictions
- How far you can lower the head of the bed
- Any limits in the person's ability to move or be re-positioned
- What pillows you can remove before moving the person
- What equipment is needed—trapeze, lift sheet, slide sheet, mechanical lift

- How to position the person
- If the person uses bed rails
- What observations to report and record:
  - Who helped you with the procedure
  - How much help the person needed
  - How the person tolerated the procedure
  - How you positioned the person
  - Complaints of pain or discomfort
- When to report observations
- What patient or resident concerns to report at once

PROMOTING SAFETY AND COMFORT

Moving the Person Up in Bed

Safety

This procedure is best done with at least 2 staff members. Work from the side of the bed. *Do not pull the person from the head of the bed.* Use assist devices as directed by the nurse and the care plan. Ask any questions before you begin the procedure.

Perform the procedure alone only if all of the following conditions are met.

- The person is small in size.
- The person can follow directions.
- The person can assist with much of the moving.
- The person uses a trapeze.
- The person can push against the mattress with the feet.
- The nurse says it is safe to do so.
- You are comfortable doing so.

 ## Moving the Person Up in Bed

QUALITY OF LIFE

- Knock before entering the person's room.
- Address the person by name.
- Introduce yourself by name and title.

- Explain the procedure before starting and during the procedure.
- Protect the person's rights during the procedure.
- Handle the person gently during the procedure.

PRE-PROCEDURE

1 Follow *Delegation Guidelines:*
   a *Preventing Work-Related Injuries*, p. 186
   b *Moving Persons in Bed*
   See *Promoting Safety and Comfort:*
   a *Moving the Person*, p. 185
   b *Preventing Work-Related Injuries*, p. 186
   c *Moving the Person Up in Bed*
2 Ask a co-worker to help you.

3 Practice hand hygiene.
4 Identify the person. Check the ID (identification) bracelet against the assignment sheet. Use 2 identifiers (Chapter 10). Also call the person by name.
5 Provide for privacy.
6 Lock (brake) the bed wheels.
7 Raise the bed for body mechanics. Bed rails are up if used.

PROCEDURE

8 Lower the head of the bed to a level appropriate for the person. It is as flat as possible.
9 Stand on 1 side of the bed. Your co-worker stands on the other side.
10 Lower the bed rails if up.
11 Remove pillows as directed by the nurse. Place a pillow upright against the head-board if the person can be without it.
12 Stand with a wide base of support. Point the foot near the head of the bed toward the head of the bed. Face the head of the bed.
13 Bend your hips and knees. Keep your back straight.
14 Place 1 arm under the person's shoulder and 1 arm under the thighs. Your co-worker does the same. Grasp each other's forearms (Fig. 15-4, p. 190).

15 Ask the person to grasp the trapeze.
16 Have the person flex both knees.
17 Explain that:
   a You will count "1, 2, 3."
   b The move will be on "3."
   c On "3," the person pushes against the bed with the feet if able. And the person pulls up with the trapeze.
18 Move the person to the head of the bed on the "count of 3." Shift your weight from your rear leg to your front leg (see Fig. 15-4). Your co-worker does the same.
19 Repeat steps 12 through 18 if necessary.

POST-PROCEDURE

20 Put the pillow under the person's head and shoulders. Straighten linens.
21 Position the person in good alignment. Raise the head of the bed to a level appropriate for the person.
22 Provide for comfort. (See the inside of the front cover.)
23 Place the call light and other needed items within reach.
24 Lower the bed to a safe and comfortable level. Follow the care plan.

25 Raise or lower bed rails. Follow the care plan.
26 Unscreen the person.
27 Complete a safety check of the room. (See the inside of the front cover.)
28 Practice hand hygiene.
29 Report and record your observations.

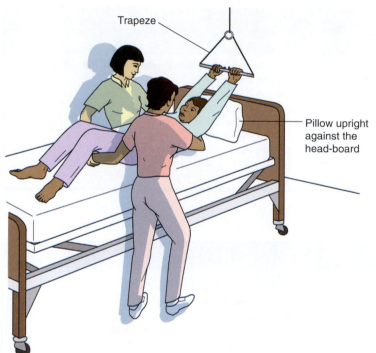

Trapeze

Pillow upright
against the
head-board

FIGURE 15-4 A person is moved up in bed by 2 nursing assistants. Each has 1 arm under the person's shoulders and the other under the thighs. They have locked arms under the person. The person grasps the trapeze and flexes the knees. The nursing assistants shift their weight from the rear leg to the front leg as the person is moved up in bed.

Moving the Person Up in Bed With an Assist Device

You use assist devices to move some persons up in bed. Such assist devices include a drawsheet (lift sheet, turning sheet), flat sheet folded in half, turning pad, slide sheet (Fig. 15-5), and large re-usable waterproof under-pad. With these devices, the person is moved more evenly. And shearing and friction are reduced.

To position the device, you must turn the person. See procedure: *Turning and Re-Positioning the Person*, p. 194. You and at least 1 co-worker:

1 Turn the person to 1 side.
2 Place the device on the bed. Open and fan-fold the device toward the person. The device is positioned from the head to above the knees or lower.
3 Tell the person that he or she will roll over a "bump." Assure the person that he or she will not fall.
4 Turn the person to the other side. The person rolls over the device.
5 Pull the device tightly. Smooth any wrinkles.
6 Roll the person onto his or her back. The person is lying on the device.

At least 2 staff members are needed to move a person with an assist device. The next procedure is used:

• Following the guidelines for moving persons in bed (see Box 15-1)
• For persons recovering from spinal cord surgery or spinal cord injuries
• For older persons
   See *Promoting Safety and Comfort: Moving the Person Up in Bed With an Assist Device.*
   See procedure: *Moving the Person Up in Bed With an Assist Device.*

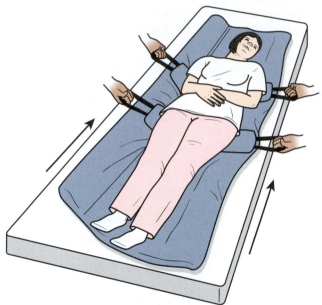

FIGURE 15-5 Slide sheet.

PROMOTING SAFETY AND COMFORT

Moving the Person Up in Bed With an Assist Device

Safety

Disposable, single-use under-pads are not strong enough to hold the person's weight during the move. Re-usable under-pads are stronger. Ask the nurse if the person's under-pad is safe as an assist device. For safety, the under-pad must:

• Be strong enough to support the person's weight.
• Extend from under the person's head to above the knees or lower.
• Be wide enough for you and other staff to get a firm grip.
   After using a slide sheet, remove it. If left in place, the person is in danger of sliding down in bed or off the bed.

Moving the Person Up in Bed With an Assist Device

QUALITY OF LIFE

- Knock before entering the person's room.
- Address the person by name.
- Introduce yourself by name and title.

- Explain the procedure before starting and during the procedure.
- Protect the person's rights during the procedure.
- Handle the person gently during the procedure.

PRE-PROCEDURE

1 Follow *Delegation Guidelines:*
  a *Preventing Work-Related Injuries,* p. 186
  b *Moving Persons in Bed,* p. 188
  See *Promoting Safety and Comfort:*
  a *Moving the Person,* p. 185
  b *Preventing Work-Related Injuries,* p. 186
  c *Moving the Person Up in Bed,* p. 189
  d *Moving the Person Up in Bed With an Assist Device*
2 Ask a co-worker to help you.

3 Obtain the needed assist device.
4 Practice hand hygiene.
5 Identify the person. Check the ID bracelet against the assignment sheet. Use 2 identifiers (Chapter 10). Also call the person by name.
6 Provide for privacy.
7 Lock (brake) the bed wheels.
8 Raise the bed for body mechanics. Bed rails are up if used.

PROCEDURE

9 Lower the head of the bed to a level appropriate for the person. It is as flat as possible.
10 Stand on 1 side of the bed. Your co-worker stands on the other side.
11 Lower the bed rails if up.
12 Remove pillows as directed by the nurse. Place a pillow upright against the head-board if the person can be without it.
13 Position the assist device.
14 Stand with a wide base of support. Point the foot near the head of the bed toward the head of the bed. Face the head of the bed.

15 Roll the sides of the assist device up close to the person. (NOTE: Omit this step if the device has handles.)
16 Grasp the rolled-up assist device firmly near the person's shoulders and hips (Fig. 15-6). Or grasp it by the handles. Support the head.
17 Bend your hips and knees.
18 Move the person up in bed on the "count of 3." Shift your weight from your rear leg to your front leg.
19 Repeat steps 14 through 18 if necessary.
20 Unroll the assist device. (NOTE: Omit this step if the device has handles.) Turn the person to remove the slide sheet if used.

POST-PROCEDURE

21 Put the pillow under the person's head and shoulders. Straighten linens.
22 Position the person in good alignment. Raise the head of the bed to a level appropriate for the person.
23 Provide for comfort. (See the inside of the front cover.)
24 Place the call light and other needed items within reach.
25 Lower the bed to a safe and comfortable level. Follow the care plan.

26 Raise or lower bed rails. Follow the care plan.
27 Unscreen the person.
28 Complete a safety check of the room. (See the inside of the front cover.)
29 Practice hand hygiene.
30 Report and record your observations.

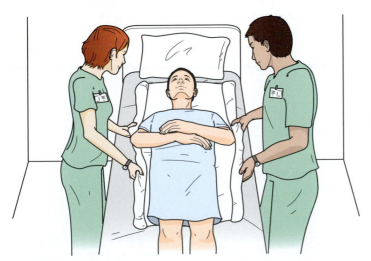

FIGURE 15-6 A drawsheet is used to move the person up in bed. It extends from the person's head to above the knees. Rolled close to the person, the drawsheet is held near the shoulders and hips.

Moving the Person to the Side of the Bed

Re-positioning and care procedures require moving the person to the side of the bed. Move the person to the side of the bed before turning. Otherwise, after turning, the person lies on the side of the bed—not in the middle.

Sometimes you have to reach over the person. During a bed bath is an example. You reach less if the person is near you.

In 1 method, the person is moved in segments (Fig. 15-7). Sometimes you can do this alone if the person is small in size. With at least 1 co-worker, a mechanical lift (Chapter 16) or an assist device is used.

- Following the guidelines for moving persons in bed (see Box 15-1)
- For older persons
- For persons with arthritis
- For persons recovering from spinal cord injuries or surgeries

Assist devices for this procedure include a drawsheet (lift sheet, turning sheet), flat sheet folded in half, turning pad, slide sheet, and large re-usable waterproof under-pad. An assist device helps prevent pain and skin damage and injury to the bones, joints, and spinal cord.

See *Promoting Safety and Comfort: Moving the Person to the Side of the Bed.*

See procedure: *Moving the Person to the Side of the Bed.*

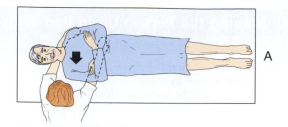

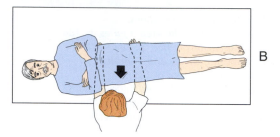

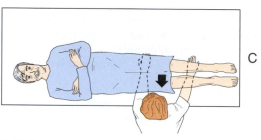

FIGURE 15-7 Moving the person to the side of the bed in segments. **A,** The upper part of the body is moved. **B,** The lower part of the body is moved. **C,** The legs and feet are moved.

PROMOTING SAFETY AND COMFORT

Moving the Person to the Side of the Bed

Safety

The person is moved to the side of the bed for tasks such as re-positioning, bedmaking, and bathing. Use the method and equipment that are best for the person. The nurse and the care plan tell you which method to use. The wrong method could cause serious injury. This is very important for persons who are very old, have arthritis, or have spinal cord involvement.

To use an assist device, you need at least 1 co-worker to help you. Depending on the person's size, more staff members may be needed.

Safety—cont'd

To use a slide sheet, place it under the person (p. 190). After moving the person, remove the device.

To move the person in segments, move the person toward you, not away from you. This helps protect you from injury.

Comfort

After moving the person to the side of the bed, position the pillow correctly. It should be under the person's head and shoulders.

Moving the Person to the Side of the Bed

QUALITY OF LIFE

- Knock before entering the person's room.
- Address the person by name.
- Introduce yourself by name and title.

- Explain the procedure before starting and during the procedure.
- Protect the person's rights during the procedure.
- Handle the person gently during the procedure.

PRE-PROCEDURE

1 Follow *Delegation Guidelines:*
  a *Preventing Work-Related Injuries,* p. 186
  b *Moving Persons in Bed,* p. 188
  See *Promoting Safety and Comfort:*
  a *Moving the Person,* p. 185
  b *Preventing Work-Related Injuries,* p. 186
  c *Moving the Person to the Side of the Bed*
2 Ask 1 or 2 co-workers to help you if using an assist device.

3 Obtain a drawsheet.
4 Practice hand hygiene.
5 Identify the person. Check the ID bracelet against the assignment sheet. Use 2 identifiers (Chapter 10). Also call the person by name.
6 Provide for privacy.
7 Lock (brake) the bed wheels.
8 Raise the bed for body mechanics. Bed rails are up if used.

PROCEDURE

9 Lower the head of the bed to a level appropriate for the person. It is as flat as possible.
10 Stand on the side of the bed to which you will move the person.
11 Lower the bed rail near you if bed rails are used. (Both bed rails are lowered for step 16.)
12 Remove pillows as directed by the nurse.
13 Cross the person's arms over the chest.
14 Stand with your feet about 12 inches apart. One foot is in front of the other. Flex your knees.
15 *Method 1—moving the person in segments:*
  a Place your arm under the person's neck and shoulders. Grasp the far shoulder.
  b Place your other arm under the mid-back.
  c Move the upper part of the person's body toward you. Rock backward and shift your weight to your rear leg (see Fig. 15-7, *A*).
  d Place 1 arm under the person's waist and 1 under the thighs.
  e Rock backward to move the lower part of the person toward you (see Fig. 15-7, *B*).
  f Repeat the procedure for the legs and feet (see Fig. 15-7, *C*). Your arms should be under the person's thighs and calves.

16 *Method 2—moving the person with a drawsheet:*
  a Position the drawsheet.
  b Roll up the drawsheet close to the person (see Fig. 15-6).
  c Grasp the rolled-up drawsheet near the person's shoulders and hips. Your co-worker does the same. Support the person's head.
  d Rock backward on the "count of 3," moving the person toward you. Your co-worker rocks backward slightly and then forward toward you while keeping the arms straight.
  e Unroll the drawsheet. Remove any wrinkles.

POST-PROCEDURE

17 Put the pillow under the person's head and shoulders. Straighten linens.
18 Position the person in good alignment.
19 Provide for comfort. (See the inside of the front cover.)
20 Place the call light and other needed items within reach.
21 Lower the bed to a safe and comfortable level. Follow the care plan.

22 Raise or lower bed rails. Follow the care plan.
23 Unscreen the person.
24 Complete a safety check of the room. (See the inside of the front cover.)
25 Practice hand hygiene.
26 Report and record your observations.

■ TURNING PERSONS

Turning persons onto their sides helps prevent complications from bedrest (Chapter 27). Procedures and care measures often require the side-lying position.

Many older persons have arthritis in their spines, hips, and knees. Less painful, logrolling (p. 196) is preferred for turning these persons.

See *Delegation Guidelines: Turning Persons.*
See *Promoting Safety and Comfort: Turning Persons.*
See procedure: *Turning and Re-Positioning the Person.*

DELEGATION GUIDELINES
Turning Persons

Before turning and re-positioning a person, you need this information from the nurse and the care plan.
- How much help the person needs
- The number of staff needed for safety
- The person's comfort level and painful body parts
- Which procedure to use
- What assist devices to use
- What supportive devices to use for positioning (Chapter 27)
- Where to place pillows
- What observations to report and record:
  - Who helped you with the procedure
  - How much help the person needed
  - How the person tolerated the procedure
  - How you positioned the person
  - Complaints of pain or discomfort
- When to report observations
- What patient or resident concerns to report at once

PROMOTING SAFETY AND COMFORT
Turning Persons

Safety

Use good body mechanics to turn a person in bed. See Chapter 14.

Position the person in good alignment. This helps prevent musculo-skeletal injuries, skin breakdown, and pressure injuries.

Do not turn a person away from you with the far bed rail down. Raise the bed rail on the side near you. Then go to the other side of the bed. Lower the bed rail if up. Turn the person toward you.

Comfort

After turning, position the person in good alignment. Use pillows as directed to support the person in the side-lying position (Chapter 14). Make sure the person's face, nose, and mouth are not covered by a pillow or other device.

Turning and Re-Positioning the Person

QUALITY OF LIFE

- Knock before entering the person's room.
- Address the person by name.
- Introduce yourself by name and title.

- Explain the procedure before starting and during the procedure.
- Protect the person's rights during the procedure.
- Handle the person gently during the procedure.

PRE-PROCEDURE

1 Follow *Delegation Guidelines:*
  a *Preventing Work-Related Injuries*, p. 186
  b *Moving Persons in Bed*, p. 188
  c *Turning Persons*
  See *Promoting Safety and Comfort:*
  a *Moving the Person*, p. 185
  b *Preventing Work-Related Injuries*, p. 186
  c *Moving the Person to the Side of the Bed*, p. 192
  d *Turning Persons*

2 Practice hand hygiene.
3 Identify the person. Check the ID bracelet against the assignment sheet. Use 2 identifiers (Chapter 10). Also call the person by name.
4 Provide for privacy.
5 Lock (brake) the bed wheels.
6 Raise the bed for body mechanics. Bed rails are up if used.

Turning and Re-Positioning the Person—cont'd

PROCEDURE

7 Lower the head of the bed to a level appropriate for the person. It is as flat as possible.
8 Stand on the side of the bed opposite to where you will turn the person.
9 Lower the bed rail.
10 Move the person to the side near you. (See procedure: *Moving the Person to the Side of the Bed*, p. 193.)
11 Cross the person's arms over the chest. Cross the leg near you over the far leg.
12 *Turning the person away from you:*
  a Stand with a wide base of support. Flex the knees.
  b Place 1 hand on the person's shoulder. Place the other on the hip near you.
  c Roll the person gently away from you toward the raised bed rail (Fig. 15-8, *A*).
  d Shift your weight from your rear leg to your front leg.

13 *Turning the person toward you:*
  a Raise the bed rail.
  b Go to the other side of the bed. Lower the bed rail.
  c Stand with a wide base of support. Flex your knees.
  d Place 1 hand on the person's shoulder. Place the other on the far hip.
  e Pull the person toward you gently (Fig. 15-8, *B*).
14 Position the person. Follow the nurse's directions and the care plan. The following are common.
  a Place a pillow under the head and neck.
  b Adjust the shoulder. The person should not be on an arm.
  c Place a small pillow under the upper hand and arm.
  d Position a pillow against the back.
  e Flex the upper knee. Position the upper leg in front of the lower leg.
  f Support the upper leg and thigh on pillows. Make sure the ankle is supported.

POST-PROCEDURE

15 Provide for comfort. (See the inside of the front cover.)
16 Place the call light and other needed items within reach.
17 Lower the bed to a safe and comfortable level. Follow the care plan.
18 Raise or lower bed rails. Follow the care plan.

19 Unscreen the person.
20 Complete a safety check of the room. (See the inside of the front cover.)
21 Practice hand hygiene.
22 Report and record your observations.

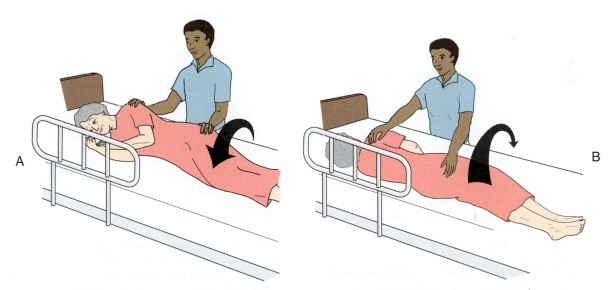

FIGURE 15-8 Turning the person. **A,** Turning the person away from you. **B,** Turning the person toward you. (*NOTE: Non-standard bed rails are used to show positioning and hand placement.*)

Logrolling

Logrolling is turning the person as a unit, in alignment, with 1 motion. The head, neck, and spine are kept straight. The procedure is used to turn:

- Older persons with arthritic spines or knees.
- Persons recovering from hip fractures.
- Persons with spinal cord injuries. The head, neck, and spine are kept straight at all times after a spinal cord injury.
- Persons recovering from spinal cord surgery. The head, neck, and spine are kept straight at all times after spinal surgery.

See *Promoting Safety and Comfort: Logrolling.*
See procedure: *Logrolling the Person.*

PROMOTING SAFETY AND COMFORT
Logrolling

Safety

For logrolling, 2 or 3 staff members are needed. If the person is tall or heavy, 3 are needed. Sometimes you use an assist device—drawsheet (lift sheet, turning sheet), turning pad, large re-usable waterproof under-pad, slide sheet.

After spinal cord injury or surgery, the head, neck, and spine are kept straight. The nurse tells you what to do step-by-step. Assist the nurse as directed.

Comfort

After spinal cord injury or surgery, the doctor orders positioning limits. Follow the nurse's directions and the care plan to position the person and use pillows.

Logrolling the Person

QUALITY OF LIFE

- Knock before entering the person's room.
- Address the person by name.
- Introduce yourself by name and title.
- Explain the procedure before starting and during the procedure.
- Protect the person's rights during the procedure.
- Handle the person gently during the procedure.

PRE-PROCEDURE

1 Follow *Delegation Guidelines:*
   a *Preventing Work-Related Injuries,* p. 186
   b *Moving Persons in Bed,* p. 188
   c *Turning Persons,* p. 194
   See *Promoting Safety and Comfort:*
   a *Moving the Person,* p. 185
   b *Preventing Work-Related Injuries,* p. 186
   c *Turning Persons,* p. 194
   d *Logrolling*

2 Ask a co-worker to help you.
3 Obtain the needed assist device.
4 Practice hand hygiene.
5 Identify the person. Check the ID bracelet against the assignment sheet. Use 2 identifiers (Chapter 10). Also call the person by name.
6 Provide for privacy.
7 Lock (brake) the bed wheels.
8 Raise the bed for body mechanics. Bed rails are up if used.

PROCEDURE

9 Make sure the bed is flat.
10 Stand on the side opposite to which you will turn the person. Your co-worker stands on the other side.
11 Lower the bed rails if used.
12 Position the assist device.
13 Move the person as a unit to the side of the bed near you. Use the assist device. (If the person has a spinal cord injury or had spinal cord surgery, assist the nurse as directed.)
14 Place the person's arms across the chest. Place a pillow between the knees.
15 Raise the bed rail if used.
16 Go to the other side.
17 Stand near the shoulders and chest. Your co-worker stands near the hips and thighs.
18 Stand with a wide base of support. One foot is in front of the other.

19 Ask the person to hold his or her body rigid.
20 Roll the person toward you (Fig. 15-9, *A*). Or use the assist device (Fig. 15-9, *B*). Turn the person as a unit.
21 Remove the slide sheet (if used).
22 Position the person in good alignment. Use pillows as directed by the nurse and care plan. The following are common (unless the spinal cord is involved).
   a Place a pillow under the head and neck if allowed.
   b Adjust the shoulder. The person should not be on an arm.
   c Place a small pillow under the upper hand and arm.
   d Position a pillow against the back.
   e Flex the upper knee. Position the upper leg in front of the lower leg.
   f Support the upper leg and thigh on pillows. Make sure the ankle is supported.

POST-PROCEDURE

23 Provide for comfort. (See the inside of the front cover.)
24 Place the call light and other needed items within reach.
25 Lower the bed to a safe and comfortable level. Follow the care plan.
26 Raise or lower bed rails. Follow the care plan.

27 Unscreen the person.
28 Complete a safety check of the room. (See the inside of the front cover.)
29 Practice hand hygiene.
30 Report and record your observations.

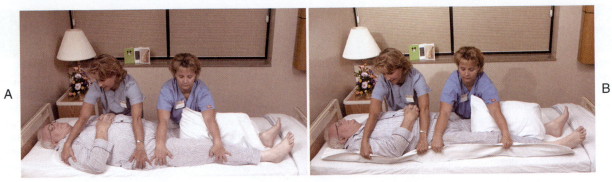

FIGURE 15-9 Logrolling. **A,** A pillow is between the person's legs. The arms are crossed on the chest. The person is on the far side of the bed. The person is turned as a unit. **B,** The assist device is used to logroll the person.

SITTING ON THE SIDE OF THE BED (DANGLING)

You will assist patients and residents to sit on the side of the bed *(dangle)*. The procedure is part of some tasks—assisting the person to stand, transferring from bed to chair, partial bath, and others. Patients and residents may become dizzy or faint when getting out of bed too fast. They may need to sit on the side of the bed for 1 to 5 minutes before walking or transferring. Or activity may increase in stages—bedrest, to dangling, to sitting in a chair, and then to walking. This is common after surgery.

While dangling the legs, the person coughs and deep breathes. He or she moves the legs back and forth in circles. This stimulates circulation.

Persons with balance and coordination problems need support. If dizziness or fainting occurs, lay the person down. Tell the nurse at once.

See *Focus on Older Persons: Dangling.*
See *Delegation Guidelines: Dangling.*
See *Promoting Safety and Comfort: Dangling,* p. 198.
See procedure: *Sitting on the Side of the Bed (Dangling),* p. 198.

FOCUS ON OLDER PERSONS

Dangling

Older persons may have circulatory changes. They may become dizzy or faint when getting up too fast. Let them sit on the side of the bed for a few minutes before standing.

DELEGATION GUIDELINES

Dangling

The nurse may ask you to help a person sit on the side of the bed. Before the dangling procedure, you need this information from the nurse and the care plan.

- Areas of weakness. For example, if the arms are weak, the person cannot hold on to the side of the mattress for support. If the left side is weak, turn the person onto the stronger right side. The person uses the right arm to help move from the lying to sitting position.
- The amount of help the person needs.
- If you need a co-worker to help you.
- If the bed is raised or in a low position. If the person will walk or transfer to a chair, the bed is in a low position safe for a transfer (Chapter 16).
- How long the person needs to sit on the side of the bed.
- What exercises are to be done while dangling.
  - Range-of-motion exercises (Chapter 27)
  - Deep-breathing and coughing exercises (Chapter 30)
- What observations to report and record:
  - Pulse and respiratory rates (Chapter 25)
  - Pale or bluish skin color *(cyanosis)*
  - Complaints of dizziness, light-headedness, or difficulty breathing
  - Who helped you with the procedure
  - How well the activity was tolerated
  - How long the person dangled
  - The amount of help needed
  - Other observations and complaints
- When to report observations.
- What patient or resident concerns to report at once.

PROMOTING SAFETY AND COMFORT
Dangling

Safety

Sitting and balance problems can occur after illness, injury, surgery, and bedrest. Some disabilities affect sitting and balance. Support the person who is sitting on the side of the bed. Have a co-worker help you. This protects the person from falling and other injuries.

As the person sits on the side of the bed, you observe the person. Lay the person down and tell the nurse at once if the person:

- Is dizzy or light-headed.
- Has an abnormal pulse or respirations.
- Has difficulty breathing.
- Has pale or bluish skin.
  Do not leave the person alone. Provide support at all times.

Comfort

Provide for warmth during the procedure. Help the person put on a robe. Or cover the shoulders and back with a bath blanket.

The person may want to perform hygiene measures while sitting on the side of the bed. Oral hygiene and washing the face and hands are examples. These measures are refreshing and stimulate circulation. Follow the nurse's directions and the care plan.

Sitting on the Side of the Bed (Dangling)

QUALITY OF LIFE

- Knock before entering the person's room.
- Address the person by name.
- Introduce yourself by name and title.

- Explain the procedure before starting and during the procedure.
- Protect the person's rights during the procedure.
- Handle the person gently during the procedure.

PRE-PROCEDURE

1 Follow *Delegation Guidelines:*
  a *Preventing Work-Related Injuries,* p. 186
  b *Dangling,* p. 197
  See *Promoting Safety and Comfort:*
  a *Moving the Person,* p. 185
  b *Preventing Work-Related Injuries,* p. 186
  c *Dangling*
2 Ask a co-worker to help you.
3 Practice hand hygiene.

4 Identify the person. Check the ID bracelet against the assignment sheet. Use 2 identifiers (Chapter 10). Also call the person by name.
5 Provide for privacy.
6 Decide which side of the bed to use.
7 Move furniture to provide moving space.
8 Lock (brake) the bed wheels.
9 Raise the bed for body mechanics. Bed rails are up if used.

Sitting on the Side of the Bed (Dangling)—cont'd

PROCEDURE

10 Lower the bed rail if up.
11 Position the person in a side-lying position facing you. The person lies on the strong side.
12 Raise the head of the bed to a sitting position.
13 Stand by the person's hips. Face the foot of the bed.
14 Stand with your feet apart. The foot near the head of the bed is in front of the other foot.
15 Slide 1 arm under the person's neck and shoulders. Grasp the far shoulder. Place your other hand over the thighs near the knees (Fig. 15-10, *A*).
16 Pivot toward the foot of the bed while moving the person's legs and feet over the side of the bed. As the legs go over the edge of the mattress, the trunk is upright (Fig. 15-10, *B*).
17 Have the person hold on to the edge of the mattress. This supports the person in the sitting position. If possible, raise a half-length bed rail (on the person's strong side) for the person to grasp. Have your co-worker support the person at all times.

18 Check the person's condition.
   • Ask how the person feels. Ask if the person feels dizzy or light-headed.
   • Check the pulse and respirations.
   • Check for difficulty breathing.
   • Note if the skin is pale or bluish in color *(cyanosis)*.
19 Reverse the procedure to return the person to bed. (Or prepare the person to walk or for a transfer to a chair or wheelchair. Lower the bed to a safe and comfortable level. The person's feet are flat on the floor.)
20 Lower the head of the bed after the person returns to bed. Help him or her move to the center of the bed.
21 Position the person in good alignment.

POST-PROCEDURE

22 Provide for comfort. (See the inside of the front cover.)
23 Place the call light and other needed items within reach.
24 Lower the bed to a safe and comfortable level. Follow the care plan.
25 Raise or lower bed rails. Follow the care plan.
26 Return furniture to its proper place.

27 Unscreen the person.
28 Complete a safety check of the room. (See the inside of the front cover.)
29 Practice hand hygiene.
30 Report and record your observations.

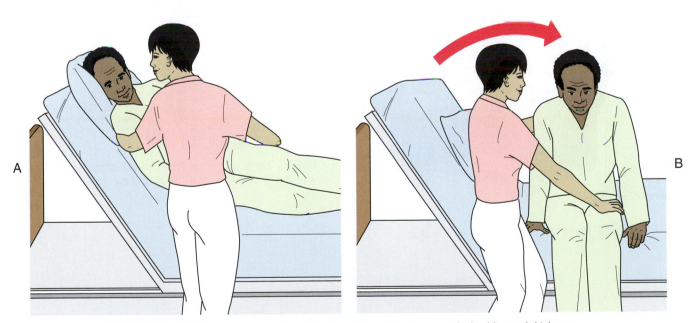

FIGURE 15-10 Helping the person sit on the side of the bed. **A,** The person's shoulders and thighs are supported. **B,** The person sits upright as the legs and feet are pulled over the edge of the bed.

RE-POSITIONING IN A CHAIR OR WHEELCHAIR

The person can slide down in a chair or wheelchair. For good alignment and safety, the person's back and buttocks must be against the back of the chair.

If the person cannot help with re-positioning, use a mechanical lift (Chapter 16). Follow the nurse's directions and the care plan for the best way to re-position a person in a chair or wheelchair. *Do not pull the person from behind the chair or wheelchair.*

If the person's chair reclines:

1 Ask a co-worker to help you.
2 Lock (brake) the wheels.
3 Recline the chair.
4 Position a friction-reducing device (drawsheet or slide sheet) under the person.
5 Grasp the device (Fig. 15-11).
6 Use the device to move the person up. See procedure: *Moving the Person Up in Bed With an Assist Device,* p. 191. Then remove the slide sheet.

Use the following method if the person is alert and cooperative. The person must be able to follow directions. And the person must have the strength to help.

1 Lock (brake) the wheelchair wheels. Remove or swing front rigging out of the way. See Chapter 16 for wheelchair safety.
2 Position the person's feet flat on the floor.
3 Apply a transfer belt (Chapter 11).
4 Position the person's arms on the armrests.
5 Stand in front of the person. Block his or her knees and feet with your knees and feet.
6 Grasp the transfer belt on each side while the person leans forward.
7 Ask the person to push with his or her feet and arms on the "count of 3."
8 Move the person back into the chair on the "count of 3" as the person pushes with his or her feet and arms (Fig. 15-12).
9 Remove the transfer belt.

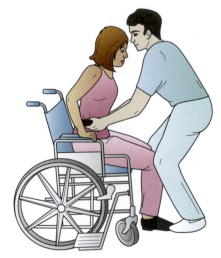

FIGURE 15-12 Re-positioning the person in a wheelchair. A transfer belt is used to move the person to the back of the chair.

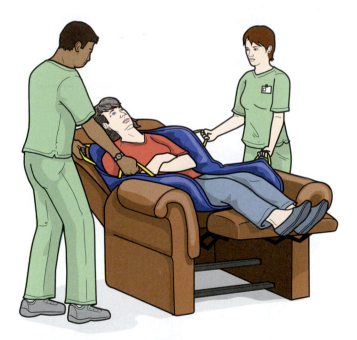

FIGURE 15-11 Re-positioning in a reclining chair.

The Person, Family, and Yourself

Personal and Professional Responsibility

Many agencies have safe handling programs. Some states have safe handling laws. The goals are to reduce the risk of injury and improve quality of care. Programs often include:

- Procedures that limit or eliminate manual lifting.
- Mechanical lifts. They can be used for many of the procedures in this chapter. See Chapter 16.
- Staff training.

When seeking a job, ask employers about safe handling programs. Ask how you can be involved in your agency's program.

Rights and Respect

How would you feel if these statements were made to you?

- "You're too heavy. I need to get help to move you."
- "I wouldn't have to move you if you would try more."
- "I'll get hurt if I try to move you."

What you say affects the person's self-worth. Do not say things that are hurtful or lower a person's dignity. Do not make the person feel useless or like a burden. Choose your words carefully. Show respect in what you say.

Independence and Social Interaction

Persons who need help moving have limited independence. They cannot turn, move in bed, or sit up alone. The person may feel embarrassed or helpless. To promote pride and independence:

- Focus on the person's abilities.
- Encourage the person.
- Let the person help as much as safely possible.
- Tell the person when you notice even small improvements. This can improve self-esteem.

Delegation and Teamwork

Moving and positioning are safer when done by 2 or more workers. This is very important when caring for bariatric persons. You may need 3, 4, or more co-workers to safely move such persons. Or special equipment may be needed. Follow the person's care plan.

Moving a person without enough help can harm you, your co-workers, and the person. Work as a team to protect yourself and others from injury.

Ethics and Laws

Before a move, you explain what you will do and what the person needs to do. Ask if there are any questions. The person may have a concern. Or the person suggests a way to make the move easier or more comfortable. Always listen. Ignoring the person is wrong. Ask the nurse if you do not know how to answer or if you are unsure how to safely move the person.

FOCUS ON PRIDE: *Application*

Most moving procedures require a team effort. How well do you work with others? What can you improve?

REVIEW QUESTIONS

Circle the BEST answer.

1 You move the person on the "count of 3" to
   a Save time
   b Distract the person from the move
   c Move the person smoothly
   d Move the person slowly

2 Good body mechanics alone will prevent injury when moving persons.
   a True
   b False

3 Before moving a person, you must know what the person is able to do.
   a True
   b False

4 Drawsheets and slide sheets are used to
   a Remove shearing
   b Reduce friction
   c Promote independence
   d Improve posture

5 To protect the person's skin when moving in bed
   a Roll the person
   b Slide the person
   c Move the mattress
   d Use a transfer belt

6 When moving persons in bed
   a The nurse tells you how to position them
   b You decide which procedure to use
   c Bed rails are used at all times
   d 3 workers are needed for safety

7 A resident with dementia needs to be moved up in bed. You should
   a Wait until the person is asleep
   b Avoid rushing
   c Move the person alone
   d Continue if the person resists the move

8 As an assist device, a drawsheet is placed so that it
   a Covers the person's body
   b Extends from the mid-back to mid-thigh level
   c Is under the head to the above the knees
   d Covers the entire mattress

9 A person needs to be moved up in bed. The person is partially able to assist. You should
   a Stand by for safety but not assist
   b Move the person up in bed by yourself
   c Tell the person not to assist to avoid injury
   d Ask for help and get a friction-reducing device

10 Before turning a person onto his or her side, you
   a Move the person to the middle of the bed
   b Move the person to the side of the bed
   c Raise the head of the bed
   d Position pillows for comfort

11 A patient with a spinal cord injury is turned with
   a The logrolling procedure
   b A transfer belt
   c A mechanical lift
   d A pillow under the head and neck

12 To assist with dangling, you need to know
   a If a transfer belt is needed
   b Where to position pillows
   c If a mechanical lift is needed
   d Which side is stronger

13 To protect the person's rights during dangling
   a Leave the room as the person dangles
   b Perform the procedure alone
   c Ask the person what procedure to use
   d Close the privacy curtain

14 A person is able to help move. To re-position the person in a wheelchair
   a Pull the person from behind
   b Unlock the wheelchair wheels
   c Position the person's feet flat on the floor
   d Position the person's arms across the chest

Answers to Chapter 15 questions are on p. 551.

FOCUS ON PRACTICE

Problem Solving

A person with right-sided weakness needs to sit on the side of the bed (dangle). Which side of the bed is best—right, left, or either? Why? The person becomes pale and dizzy while dangling. What will you do?

Transferring the Person

OBJECTIVES

- Define the key terms and key abbreviation in this chapter.
- Explain how to prevent work-related injuries during transfers.
- Identify the delegation information needed to transfer a person.
- Identify comfort and safety measures for transferring the person.
- Explain wheelchair and stretcher safety.
- Perform the procedures described in this chapter.
- Explain how to promote PRIDE in the person, the family, and yourself.

KEY TERMS

pivot To turn one's body from a set standing position

transfer How a person moves to and from a surface

KEY ABBREVIATION

ID Identification

Patients and residents are moved to and from surfaces such as beds, chairs, wheelchairs, shower chairs, commodes, toilets, and stretchers. A *transfer is how a person moves to and from a surface.* The amount of help needed and the method used vary with the person's abilities. You will assist with transfers often.

The safety measures for preventing work-related injuries and for moving persons apply to transfers (Chapters 14 and 15). So do the rules for body mechanics (Chapter 14). Protect yourself and the person from injury. Use your body and transfer devices and equipment correctly.

See *Focus on Communication: Transferring the Person.*
See *Delegation Guidelines: Transferring the Person,* p. 204.
See *Promoting Safety and Comfort: Transferring the Person,* p. 204.

FOCUS ON COMMUNICATION

Transferring the Person

Transfers can be painful for older persons and after an injury or surgery. Ask about the person's comfort.

- "Please tell me if you feel pain or discomfort."
- "Tell me to stop if you feel pain."

Before any transfer, tell the person what you and your co-workers will do. Also explain what the person needs to do. Give step-by-step instructions during the procedure.

The procedures in this chapter explain how to transfer the person on the "count of 3." You and the person or you and your co-workers move at the same time. For example:

I will help you transfer to the chair. I will count "1, 2, 3." When I say "3," push on the mattress with your hands and stand. I will steady you with the transfer belt as you stand. You will turn so your legs touch the seat's edge. Grab the chair's armrests. I will help you sit.

DELEGATION GUIDELINES
Transferring the Person

Many tasks involve transferring persons. Before doing so, you need this information from the nurse and the care plan.
- What procedure to use.
- The person's height and weight.
- The person's physical abilities. Can the person sit up, stand up, or walk without help? Does the person have strength in his or her arms and legs?
- If the person has a weak side. If yes, which side?
- If the person has problems that increase the risk of injury. Dizziness, confusion, hearing or vision problems, recent surgery, and fragile skin are examples.
- The person's ability to follow directions.
- If behavior problems are likely. Combative, agitated, uncooperative, and unpredictable behaviors are examples.
- The amount of assistance needed.
- The number of staff needed for a safe transfer.
- Any doctor's orders for transferring the person.
- What equipment to use.

PROMOTING SAFETY AND COMFORT
Transferring the Person

Safety
Many older persons have fragile bones and joints. To prevent injuries:
- Follow the rules of body mechanics and the safety measures for preventing work-related injuries (Chapter 14).
- Always have help to transfer the person.
- Use assist devices as directed by the nurse and the care plan. Examples include a wheelchair, walker or cane (Chapter 27), transfer belt (Chapter 11), stand-assist device (Fig. 16-1), and sliding board (Fig. 16-2).
- Transfer the person carefully and in good alignment.
  Decide how to transfer the person before starting the procedure. Arrange the room to allow enough space for a safe transfer. Correctly place the chair, wheelchair, or other device. Also plan to protect drainage tubes or containers connected to the person.
  Raise or lower the bed to a safe and comfortable level for the transfer. If the person will stand, the feet must be flat on the floor.

Comfort
To promote mental comfort:
- Explain what you are going to do and how the person can help.
- Screen and cover the person to protect the right to privacy.
- Reassure the person that mechanical lifts (p. 212) are safe.
  To promote physical comfort:
- Keep the person in good alignment.
- Do not pull on any part of the person's body.
- Use pillows and other positioning devices as directed by the nurse and the care plan.

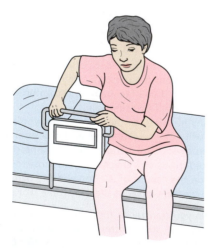

FIGURE 16-1 Stand-assist bed attachment.

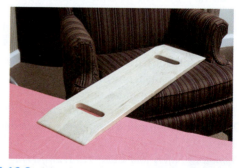

FIGURE 16-2 Sliding board for seated transfers to and from surfaces.

WHEELCHAIR AND STRETCHER SAFETY

Some people use wheelchairs (Fig. 16-3). You use the hand grips/push handles to push or pull the wheelchair. Stretchers are used to transport persons who cannot use wheelchairs.

The person can fall from the wheelchair or stretcher. Or the person can fall during transfers to and from the wheelchair or stretcher. Follow the safety measures in Box 16-1.

STAND AND PIVOT TRANSFERS

Some persons can stand and pivot. *Pivot means to turn one's body from a set standing position.* A stand and pivot transfer is used if:

- The legs are strong enough to bear some or all of the person's weight.
- The person is cooperative and can follow directions.
- The person can assist with the transfer.

See *Delegation Guidelines: Stand and Pivot Transfers*, p. 206.

See *Promoting Safety and Comfort: Stand and Pivot Transfers*, p. 206.

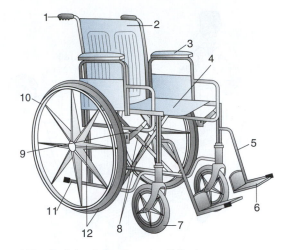

1 Hand grip/push handle	7 Caster
2 Back upholstery	8 Crossbrace
3 Armrest	9 Wheel lock/brake
4 Seat upholstery	10 Wheel and hand rim
5 Front rigging	11 Tipping lever
6 Footplate	12 Tire and wheel spokes

FIGURE 16-3 Parts of a wheelchair.

BOX 16-1 Wheelchair and Stretcher Safety

Wheelchair Safety

Maintenance

- Check the wheel locks (brakes). Make sure you can lock and unlock them.
- Check for flat or loose tires. A wheel lock will not work on a flat or loose tire.
- Make sure wheel spokes are intact. Damaged, broken, or loose spokes can interfere with moving the wheelchair or locking the wheels.
- Make sure the casters point forward. This keeps the wheelchair balanced and stable.
- Clean the wheelchair according to agency policy.
- Follow the safety measures to prevent equipment accidents (Chapter 10).

Transfers

- Lock (brake) both wheels before you transfer a person to or from the wheelchair. Make sure bed wheels are locked.
- Remove or swing front rigging out of the way for transfers to and from the wheelchair. Raise the footplates.
- Position the person's feet on the footplates before moving the chair. The feet must not touch or drag on the floor when the chair is moving.
- Do not let the person stand on the footplates.
- Do not let the footplates fall back onto the person's legs.
- Provide needed wheelchair accessories—safety belt, pouch, tray, lap-board, cushion.

Transport

- Use good body mechanics (Chapter 14).
- Follow the care plan for the number of staff needed for a safe transport. This depends on:
  - The person's weight
  - If the person is cooperative
  - If the wheelchair is motorized
- Push the chair forward to transport the person. Do not pull the chair backward unless going through a doorway or down a steep ramp or incline.

Transport—cont'd

- Ask a nurse or physical therapist to show you how to move wheelchairs up and down ramps and over curbs.
  - *Going up*—The wheelchair is pushed forward.
  - *Going down*—The wheelchair is pulled backward.
- Follow the care plan for keeping the wheels locked when not moving the wheelchair. Locking the wheels prevents the chair from moving if the person wants to move to or from the chair. (Locking the wheelchair may be viewed as a restraint. See Chapter 12.)

Stretcher Safety

- Ask 2 or more co-workers to help you transfer the person to or from the stretcher.
- Lock (brake) the stretcher wheels before the transfer.
- Fasten the safety straps when the person is properly positioned on the stretcher.
- Follow the care plan for the number of staff needed for a safe transport. As many as 4 staff members may be needed. This depends on:
  - The person's weight
  - If the person is cooperative
- Raise the side rails. Keep them up during the transport.
- Make sure the person's arms, hands, legs, and feet do not dangle through the side rail bars.
- Stand at the head of the stretcher. Your co-worker stands at the foot of the stretcher.
- Move the stretcher feet first (Fig. 16-4, p. 206). The staff member at the head of the stretcher watches the person's breathing and color during the transport.
- Do not leave the person alone.
- Use good body mechanics during the transfer and transport (Chapter 14).
- Follow the safety measures to prevent equipment accidents (Chapter 10).

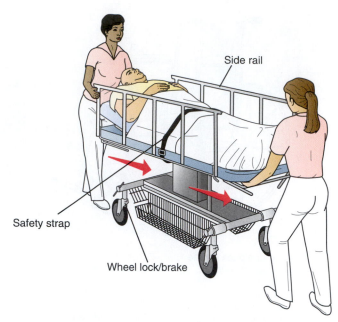

FIGURE 16-4 The stretcher is moved feet first.

Transfer Belts

Transfer belts (gait belts) are discussed in Chapter 11. They are used to:

- Support patients and residents during transfers.
- Re-position persons in chairs and wheelchairs (Chapter 15).
- Assist with ambulation (Chapter 27).

Wider belts have padded handles. They are easier to grip and allow better control should the person fall.

Bed to Chair or Wheelchair Transfers

Safety is important for chair, wheelchair, commode, and shower chair transfers. Help the person out of bed on his or her strong side. If the left side is weak and the right side is strong, get the person out of bed on the right side. In transferring, the strong side moves first. It pulls the weaker side along. Transfers from the weak side are awkward and unsafe.

See *Focus on Surveys: Bed to Chair or Wheelchair Transfers.*

See *Promoting Safety and Comfort: Bed to Chair or Wheelchair Transfers.*

See procedure: *Transferring the Person to a Chair or Wheelchair.*

Text continued on p. 210.

PROMOTING SAFETY AND COMFORT

Bed to Chair or Wheelchair Transfers

Safety

The chair, wheelchair, or other device must support the person's weight. The number of staff needed depends on the person's abilities, condition, and size. Sometimes you need a mechanical lift (p. 212).

The person must not put his or her arms around your neck. Otherwise the person can pull you forward or cause you to lose your balance. Neck, back, and other injuries are possible.

If not using a mechanical lift, use a transfer belt for chair or wheelchair transfers. It is safer for the person and you. Putting your arms around the person and grasping the shoulder blades is another method. It can cause the person discomfort. And it can be stressful for you. Use this method only if instructed to do so by the nurse and the care plan and you are comfortable doing so.

Bed and wheelchair wheels are locked for a safe transfer. After the transfer, unlock the wheelchair wheels to position

Safety—cont'd

the chair as the person prefers. Then lock the wheels or keep them unlocked according to the care plan. Locked wheels may be viewed as restraints if the person cannot unlock them to move the wheelchair (Chapter 12). However, falls and other injuries are risks if the person tries to stand when the wheels are unlocked.

Comfort

Most wheelchairs and bedside chairs have vinyl seats and backs. Vinyl holds body heat. The person becomes warm and perspires more. If the nurse allows, cover the back and seat with a folded bath blanket. This increases comfort.

Some people have wheelchair cushions or positioning devices. Ask the nurse how to use and place the devices. Also follow the manufacturer's instructions.

Transferring the Person to a Chair or Wheelchair

QUALITY OF LIFE

- Knock before entering the person's room.
- Address the person by name.
- Introduce yourself by name and title.

- Explain the procedure before starting and during the procedure.
- Protect the person's rights during the procedure.
- Handle the person gently during the procedure.

PRE-PROCEDURE

1 Follow *Delegation Guidelines:*
 a *Transferring the Person,* p. 204
 b *Stand and Pivot Transfers*
 See *Promoting Safety and Comfort:*
 a *Transfer/Gait Belts* (Chapter 11)
 b *Transferring the Person,* p. 204
 c *Stand and Pivot Transfers*
 d *Bed to Chair or Wheelchair Transfers*
2 Collect the following.
 - Wheelchair or arm chair
 - Bath blanket
 - Lap blanket (if used)
 - Robe and non-skid footwear
 - Paper or sheet
 - Transfer belt (if needed)
 - Seat cushion (if needed)

3 Practice hand hygiene.
4 Identify the person. Check the identification (ID) bracelet against the assignment sheet. Use 2 identifiers (Chapter 10). Also call the person by name.
5 Provide for privacy.
6 Decide which side of the bed to use. Move furniture for a safe transfer.

Continued

Transferring the Person to a Chair or Wheelchair—cont'd

PROCEDURE

7 Raise the wheelchair footplates. Remove or swing front rigging out of the way if possible. Position the chair or wheelchair near the bed on the person's strong side.
   a If at the head of the bed, it faces the foot of the bed.
   b If at the foot of the bed, it faces the head of the bed.
   c The armrest almost touches the bed.
8 Place a folded bath blanket or cushion on the seat (if needed).
9 Lock (brake) the wheelchair wheels. Make sure bed wheels are locked.
10 Fan-fold top linens to the foot of the bed.
11 Place the paper or sheet under the person's feet. (This protects linens from footwear.) Put footwear on the person.
12 Lower the bed to a safe and comfortable level for the person. Follow the care plan. Lock (brake) the bed wheels.
13 Help the person sit on the side of the bed (Chapter 15). His or her feet must be flat on the floor.
14 Help the person put on a robe.
15 Apply the transfer belt if needed (Chapter 11). It is applied at the waist over clothing.
16 *Method 1: using a transfer belt:*
   a Stand in front of the person.
   b Have the person hold on to the mattress.
   c Make sure the person's feet are flat on the floor.
   d Have the person lean forward.
   e Grasp the transfer belt at each side. Grasp the handles or grasp the belt from underneath. See Chapter 11.
   f Prevent the person from sliding or falling. Do 1 of the following.
      1 Brace your knees against the person's knees (Fig. 16-5). Block his or her feet with your feet.
      2 Use the knee and foot of 1 leg to block the person's weak leg or foot. Place your other foot slightly behind you for balance.
      3 Straddle your legs around the person's weak leg.
   g Explain the following.
      1 You will count "1, 2, 3."
      2 The move will be on "3."
      3 On "3," the person pushes down on the mattress and stands.
   h Ask the person to push down on the mattress and to stand on the "count of 3." Assist the person to a standing position as you straighten your knees (Fig. 16-6).

17 *Method 2: no transfer belt:* (NOTE: Use this method only if directed by the nurse and the care plan and you are comfortable doing so.)
   a Follow steps 16, a–c.
   b Place your hands under the person's arms. Your hands are around the person's shoulder blades (Fig. 16-7).
   c Have the person lean forward.
   d Prevent the person from sliding or falling. Do 1 of the following.
      1 Brace your knees against the person's knees. Block his or her feet with your feet.
      2 Use the knee and foot of 1 leg to block the person's weak leg or foot. Place your other foot slightly behind you for balance.
      3 Straddle your legs around the person's weak leg.
   e Explain the "count of 3." See step 16, g.
   f Ask the person to push down on the mattress and to stand on the "count of 3." Assist the person to a standing position as you straighten your knees.
18 Support the person in the standing position. Hold the transfer belt or keep your hands around the person's shoulder blades. Continue to prevent the person from sliding or falling.
19 Help the person pivot (turn) so he or she can grasp the far arm of the chair or wheelchair. The legs will touch the edge of the seat (Fig. 16-8).
20 Continue to help the person pivot (turn) until the other armrest is grasped.
21 Lower him or her into the chair or wheelchair as you bend your hips and knees. To assist, the person leans forward and bends the elbows and knees (Fig. 16-9).
22 Make sure the hips are to the back of the seat. Position the person in good alignment.
23 Attach the wheelchair front rigging. Position the person's feet on the footplates.
24 Cover the person's lap and legs with a lap blanket (if used). Keep the blanket off the floor and the wheels.
25 Remove the transfer belt if used.
26 Position the chair as the person prefers. Lock (brake) the wheelchair wheels according to the care plan.

POST-PROCEDURE

27 Provide for comfort. (See the inside of the front cover.)
28 Place the call light and other needed items within reach.
29 Unscreen the person.
30 Complete a safety check of the room. (See the inside of the front cover.)
31 Practice hand hygiene.
32 Report and record your observations.
33 See procedure: *Transferring the Person From a Chair or Wheelchair to Bed* (p. 210) to return the person to bed.

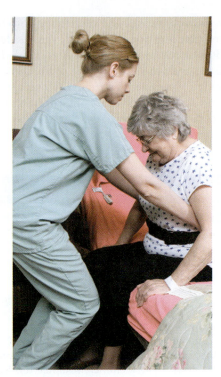

FIGURE 16-5 The person's knees are blocked by the nursing assistant's knees.

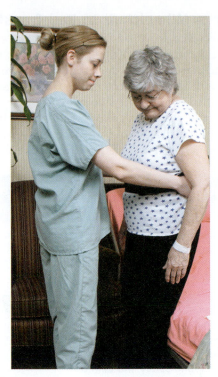

FIGURE 16-6 The person is assisted to a standing position and supported with the transfer belt.

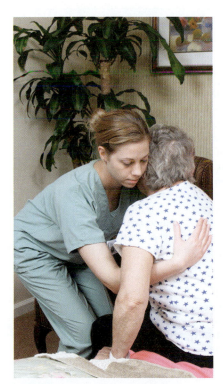

FIGURE 16-7 The person is being prepared to stand. The hands are placed under the person's arms and around the shoulder blades.

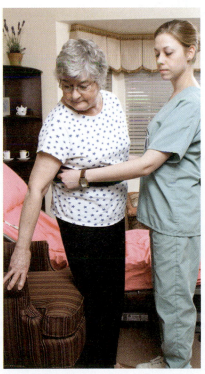

FIGURE 16-8 The person is supported as she grasps the far arm of the chair. The legs are against the chair.

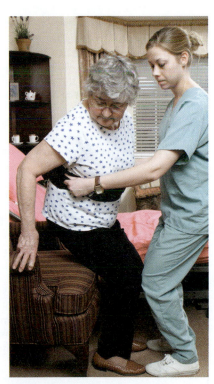

FIGURE 16-9 The person holds the armrests, leans forward, and bends the elbows and knees while being lowered into the chair.

Chair or Wheelchair to Bed Transfers

Chair or wheelchair to bed transfers have the same rules as bed to chair transfers. If the person is weak on 1 side, transfer the person so that the strong side moves first. Or position the chair or wheelchair so the person's strong side is near the bed. The strong side moves first.

For example, a resident's right side is weak. The left side is strong. To transfer out of bed, the chair was on the left side of the bed. The resident's left side (strong side) moved first. Now you will transfer the resident back to bed. With the chair on the left side of the bed, the resident's weak right side is near the bed. Moving the weak side first is not safe. Move the chair to the other side of the bed or turn the chair around. The resident's stronger left side will be near the bed. The stronger side moves first for a safe transfer.

See procedure: *Transferring the Person From a Chair or Wheelchair to Bed.*

Transferring the Person From a Chair or Wheelchair to Bed

QUALITY OF LIFE

- Knock before entering the person's room.
- Address the person by name.
- Introduce yourself by name and title.

- Explain the procedure before starting and during the procedure.
- Protect the person's rights during the procedure.
- Handle the person gently during the procedure.

PRE-PROCEDURE

1 Follow *Delegation Guidelines:*
  a *Transferring the Person,* p. 204
  b *Stand and Pivot Transfers,* p. 206
  See *Promoting Safety and Comfort:*
  a *Transfer/Gait Belts* (Chapter 11)
  b *Transferring the Person,* p. 204
  c *Stand and Pivot Transfers,* p. 206
  d *Bed to Chair or Wheelchair Transfers,* p. 207

2 Collect a transfer belt if needed.
3 Practice hand hygiene.
4 Identify the person. Check the ID bracelet against the assignment sheet. Use 2 identifiers (Chapter 10). Also call the person by name.
5 Provide for privacy.

PROCEDURE

6 Move furniture for moving space.
7 Raise the head of the bed to a sitting position. Lower the bed to a safe and comfortable level for the person. Follow the care plan. When the person transfers to the bed, the feet must be flat on the floor when sitting on the side of the bed.
8 Move the call light so it is on the strong side when the person is in bed.
9 Position the chair or wheelchair so the person's strong side is next to the bed (Fig. 16-10). Have a co-worker help you if necessary.
10 Lock (brake) the wheelchair and bed wheels.
11 Remove and fold the lap blanket.
12 Remove the person's feet from the footplates. Raise the footplates. Remove or swing front rigging out of the way. Put non-skid footwear on the person if needed.
13 Apply the transfer belt if needed.
14 Make sure the person's feet are flat on the floor.
15 Stand in front of the person.
16 Have the person hold on to the armrests. (If the nurse directs you to do so, place your arms under the person's arms. Your hands are around the shoulder blades.)
17 Have the person lean forward.
18 Grasp the transfer belt on each side if using it. Grasp underneath the belt.

19 Prevent the person from sliding or falling. Do 1 of the following.
  a Brace your knees against the person's knees. Block his or her feet with your feet.
  b Use the knee and foot of 1 leg to block the person's weak leg or foot. Place your other foot slightly behind you for balance.
  c Straddle your legs around the person's weak leg.
20 Explain the "count of 3." See procedure: *Transferring the Person to a Chair or Wheelchair,* p. 207.
21 Ask the person to push down on the armrests on the "count of 3." Assist the person into a standing position as you straighten your knees.
22 Support the person in the standing position. Hold the transfer belt or keep your hands around the shoulder blades. Continue to prevent the person from sliding or falling.
23 Help the person pivot (turn) to reach the edge of the mattress. The legs will touch the mattress.
24 Continue to help the person pivot (turn) until he or she reaches the mattress with both hands.
25 Lower him or her onto the bed as you bend your hips and knees. To assist, the person leans forward and bends the elbows and knees.
26 Remove the transfer belt.
27 Remove the robe and footwear.
28 Help the person lie down.

POST-PROCEDURE

29 Provide for comfort. (See the inside of the front cover.)
30 Place the call light and other needed items within reach.
31 Raise or lower bed rails. Follow the care plan.
32 Arrange furniture to meet the person's needs.
33 Unscreen the person.

34 Complete a safety check of the room. (See the inside of the front cover.)
35 Practice hand hygiene.
36 Report and record your observations.

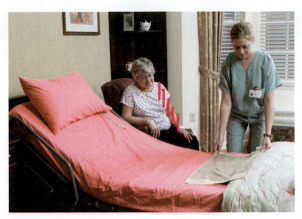

FIGURE 16-10 The chair is positioned so the person's strong side is near the bed. (*NOTE: The "weak" side is indicated by slash marks.*)

Transferring the Person To and From the Toilet

Using the bathroom for elimination promotes privacy, dignity, self-esteem, and independence. However, getting to the toilet is hard for persons who use wheelchairs. Bathrooms are often small with little room for you or a wheelchair. Therefore transfers with wheelchairs and toilets are often hard. Falls and work-related injuries are risks.

Sometimes mechanical lifts are used for toilet transfers. The following procedure can be used if the person can stand and pivot from the wheelchair to the toilet.

See *Promoting Safety and Comfort: Transferring the Person To and From the Toilet.*

See procedure: *Transferring the Person To and From the Toilet.*

PROMOTING SAFETY AND COMFORT
Transferring the Person To and From the Toilet

Safety
Make sure the person has a raised toilet seat. The toilet seat and wheelchair are at the same level.

Check the grab bars by the toilet. If loose, tell the nurse. Do not transfer the person to the toilet if grab bars are not secure.

Follow Standard Precautions and the Bloodborne Pathogen Standard. Wear gloves and practice hand hygiene as needed.

Transferring the Person To and From the Toilet

QUALITY OF LIFE

- Knock before entering the person's room.
- Address the person by name.
- Introduce yourself by name and title.

- Explain the procedure before starting and during the procedure.
- Protect the person's rights during the procedure.
- Handle the person gently during the procedure.

PRE-PROCEDURE

1 Follow *Delegation Guidelines:*
  a *Transferring the Person,* p. 204
  b *Stand and Pivot Transfers,* p. 206
  See *Promoting Safety and Comfort:*
  a *Transfer/Gait Belts* (Chapter 11)
  b *Transferring the Person,* p. 204
  c *Stand and Pivot Transfers,* p. 206
  d *Bed to Chair or Wheelchair Transfers,* p. 207
  e *Transferring the Person To and From the Toilet*

2 Practice hand hygiene.

Continued

Transferring the Person To and From the Toilet—cont'd

PROCEDURE

3 Put non-skid footwear on the person.
4 Position the wheelchair next to the toilet if there is enough room. If not, position the chair at a right angle (90-degree angle) to the toilet (Fig. 16-11). (See *Focus on Math: Fowler's Positions* in Chapter 14.) It is best if the person's strong side is near the toilet.
5 Lock (brake) the wheelchair wheels.
6 Raise the footplates. Remove or swing front rigging out of the way.
7 Apply the transfer belt.
8 Help the person unfasten clothing.
9 Use the transfer belt to help the person stand and pivot (turn) to the toilet. (See procedure: *Transferring the Person From a Chair or Wheelchair to Bed*, p. 210.) The person uses the grab bars to pivot (turn) to the toilet.
10 Support the person with the transfer belt while he or she lowers clothing. Or have the person hold on to the grab bars for support. Lower the person's clothing.
11 Use the transfer belt to lower the person onto the toilet seat. Check for proper positioning on the toilet.
12 Remove the transfer belt.
13 Tell the person you will stay nearby. Remind the person to use the call light or call for you when help is needed. Stay with the person if required by the care plan.

14 Close the bathroom door for privacy.
15 Stay near the bathroom. Complete other tasks in the person's room. Check on the person every 5 minutes.
16 Knock on the bathroom door when the person calls for you.
17 Help with wiping, perineal care (Chapter 18), flushing, and hand-washing as needed. Wear gloves and practice hand hygiene after removing the gloves.
18 Apply the transfer belt.
19 Use the transfer belt to help the person stand.
20 Help the person raise and secure clothing.
21 Use the transfer belt to transfer the person to the wheelchair. See procedure: *Transferring the Person to a Chair or Wheelchair*, p. 207.
22 Make sure the person's buttocks are to the back of the seat. Position the person in good alignment.
23 Position the person's feet on the footplates.
24 Remove the transfer belt.
25 Cover the lap and legs with a lap blanket. Keep the blanket off the floor and wheels.
26 Position the chair as the person prefers. Lock (brake) the wheelchair wheels according to the care plan.

POST-PROCEDURE

27 Provide for comfort. (See the inside of the front cover.)
28 Place the call light and other needed items within reach.
29 Unscreen the person.

30 Complete a safety check of the room. (See the inside of the front cover.)
31 Practice hand hygiene.
32 Report and record your observations.

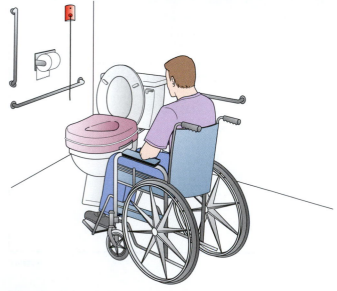

FIGURE 16-11 The wheelchair is placed at a right angle (90-degree angle) to the toilet.

MECHANICAL LIFTS

Mechanical lifts are used for persons who cannot assist with transfers. They also are used to transfer persons who are too heavy for the staff to move. Lifts are used to transfer persons to and from beds, chairs, wheelchairs, stretchers, tubs, shower chairs, toilets, commodes, whirlpools, or vehicles.

There are manual, battery-operated, and electric lifts. Some are mounted on the ceiling. Two types are common (Fig. 16-12).

- Stand-assist lifts—used for persons who require some help with transfers and can:
  - Bear some weight.
  - Follow directions.
  - Sit on the side of the bed with or without help.
  - Bend the hips, knees, and ankles.
- Full-sling mechanical lifts—used for persons who:
  - Cannot assist with transfers.
  - Are partially able or unable to bear weight.
  - Are heavy.
  - Have physical limits preventing other types of transfers.

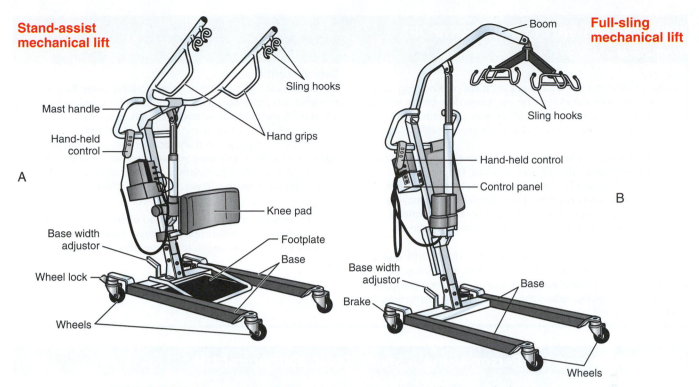

FIGURE 16-12 Mechanical lifts. **A,** Parts of a stand-assist mechanical lift. **B,** Parts of a full-sling mechanical lift.

Slings

The sling used depends on the lift type and the person's size, condition, and other needs. Slings are padded, unpadded, or made of mesh. Stand-assist slings support the upper body. Full-slings support the entire body.

- *Standard full-sling*—for normal transfers.
- *Extended length sling*—for persons with extra large thighs.
- *Bathing sling*—to transfer the person from the bed or chair into a bathtub. The sling is left in place and attached to the lift during the bath.
- *Toileting sling*—the sling bottom is open. Each person has his or her own toileting sling.
- *Amputee sling*—for the person who has had both legs amputated.
- *Bariatric sling*—for use with a bariatric lift.

The nurse and care plan tell you what sling to use. Follow agency policy and the manufacturer's instructions for handling and washing slings.

Using a Mechanical Lift

Before using a lift:
- You must be trained in its use.
- It must work.
- The sling, straps, hooks, and chains must be in good repair.
- The person's weight must not exceed the lift's capacity.
- You need enough help. At least 2 staff members are needed for most lifts. Follow agency policy and the person's care plan.

There are different types of mechanical lifts. Always follow the manufacturer's instructions. The procedures that follow are used as a guide.

See *Delegation Guidelines: Using a Mechanical Lift.*
See *Promoting Safety and Comfort: Using a Mechanical Lift,* p. 214.
See procedure: *Transferring the Person Using a Stand-Assist Mechanical Lift,* p. 214.
See procedure: *Transferring the Person Using a Full-Sling Mechanical Lift,* p. 216.

DELEGATION GUIDELINES
Using a Mechanical Lift

Before using a mechanical lift, you need this information from the nurse and the care plan.
- The person's physical abilities.
- What lift to use.
- The person's weight and the lift's weight limit. Do not exceed the lift's weight limit.
- What type and size sling to use.
- The number of staff needed for safety.

PROMOTING SAFETY AND COMFORT
Using a Mechanical Lift

Safety

Always follow the manufacturer's instructions. Knowing how to use 1 lift does not mean that you know how to use others. If you have not used a certain lift before, ask for training. Ask the nurse to help you until you are comfortable using the lift.

The lift's base widens or opens. The base closes to fit under the bed and move through narrow areas. The lift is most stable with the base in the open position. Lock the base in the wide or open position when lifting, lowering, and moving when possible. If you must narrow the base, do so briefly. Return the base to the wide or open position as soon as possible.

For many lifts, the wheels are unlocked during lifting and lowering. This allows the lift to stabilize as the person is moved. For some stand-assist lifts, the wheels are locked when lifting and lowering. Follow the manufacturer's instructions for when to lock the wheels.

Safety—cont'd

Mechanical lifts must be in good working order. Battery-powered lifts must have well-charged batteries. Tell the nurse when a lift needs repair or does not work properly.

One or 2 staff members are needed for a stand-assist mechanical lift. Follow the manufacturer's instructions and agency policy. Two staff members are needed to safely use a full-sling mechanical lift. Federal guidelines require that at least 1 staff member be 18 years of age or older.

Comfort

The person is lifted up and off the bed or chair. Falling is a common fear. For mental comfort, always explain the procedure before you begin. Also show the person how the lift works.

 ## Transferring the Person Using a Stand-Assist Mechanical Lift

QUALITY OF LIFE

- Knock before entering the person's room.
- Address the person by name.
- Introduce yourself by name and title.

- Explain the procedure before starting and during the procedure.
- Protect the person's rights during the procedure.
- Handle the person gently during the procedure.

PRE-PROCEDURE

1 Follow *Delegation Guidelines:*
  a *Transferring the Person*, p. 204
  b *Using a Mechanical Lift*, p. 213
  See *Promoting Safety and Comfort:*
  a *Transferring the Person*, p. 204
  b *Using a Mechanical Lift*
2 Ask a co-worker to help you (if needed).
3 Collect the following.
  - Stand-assist mechanical lift and sling
  - Arm chair or wheelchair
  - Footwear
  - Bath blanket or cushion
  - Lap blanket (if used)

4 Practice hand hygiene.
5 Identify the person. Check the ID bracelet against the assignment sheet. Use 2 identifiers (Chapter 10). Also call the person by name.
6 Provide for privacy.

PROCEDURE

7 Place the chair (wheelchair) at the head of the bed. It is even with the head-board and about 1 foot away from the bed. Lock (brake) the wheelchair wheels. Place a folded bath blanket or cushion in the seat if needed.
8 Assist the person to a seated position on the side of the bed. See procedure: *Sitting on the Side of the Bed (Dangling)* in Chapter 15. The person's feet are flat on the floor. Bed wheels are locked.
9 Put footwear on the person.
10 Apply the sling.
  a Position the sling at the lower back.
  b Bring the straps around to the front of the chest. The straps are positioned under the arms.
  c Secure the waist belt around the person's waist. Adjust the belt so it is snug but not tight.

11 Position the lift in front of the person.
12 Widen the lift's base.
13 Lock (brake) the lift's wheels.
14 Have the person place the feet on the footplate and the knees against the knee pad. Assist as needed. If the lift has a knee strap, secure the strap around the legs. Adjust the strap so it is snug but not tight.
15 Attach the sling to the sling hooks.
16 Have the person grasp the lift's hand grips.
17 Unlock the lift's wheels (release the brakes).
18 Raise the person slightly off the bed. Check that the sling is secure, the feet are on the footplate, and the knees are against the knee pad (Fig. 16-13, *A*). If not, lower the person and correct the problem.

Transferring the Person Using a Stand-Assist Mechanical Lift—cont'd

PROCEDURE—cont'd

19 Raise the lift until the person is clear of the bed (Fig. 16-13, *B*). Or raise the person to a standing position (Fig. 16-13, *C*). Follow the care plan.

20 Adjust the base's width to move from the bed to the chair (wheelchair) if needed. Keep the base in the wide or open position as much as possible.

21 Move the lift to the chair (wheelchair). The person's back is toward the seat.

22 Lower the person into the chair (wheelchair). Guide the person into the seat. See Figure 16-13, *D and E.*

23 Lock (brake) the lift's wheels.

24 Unhook the sling from the sling hooks.

25 Unbuckle the waist belt. Remove the sling.

26 Unlock the lift's wheels (release the brakes).

27 Have the person lift the feet off of the footplate. Assist as needed. Move the lift. Position the person's feet flat on the floor or on the wheelchair footplates.

28 Cover the lap and legs with a lap blanket (if used). Keep it off the floor.

POST-PROCEDURE

29 Provide for comfort. (See the inside of the front cover.)

30 Place the call light and other needed items within reach.

31 Unscreen the person.

32 Complete a safety check of the room. (See the inside of the front cover.)

33 Practice hand hygiene.

34 Report and record your observations.

35 Reverse the procedure to return the person to bed.

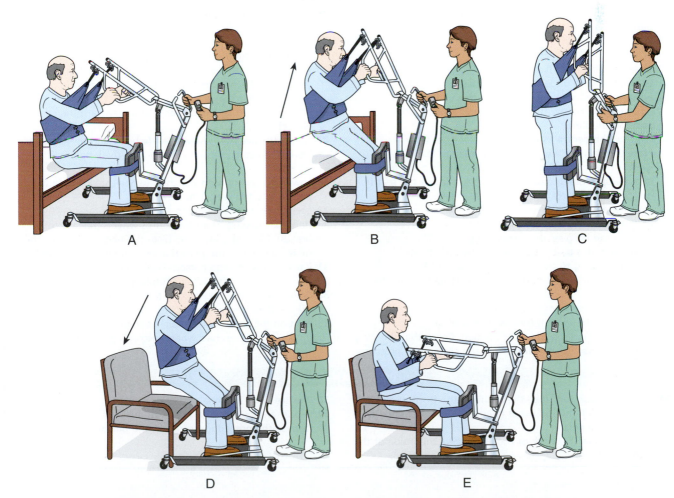

FIGURE 16-13 Using a stand-assist lift. **A,** The sling is around the person's lower back. The straps are under the arms. The waist belt is secure. Feet are on the footplate. The person holds the hand grips. **B,** The lift is raised. **C,** The person is in a standing position. **D,** The person is lowered into the chair. **E,** The person is seated. The back is against the back of the chair.

Transferring the Person Using a Full-Sling Mechanical Lift

QUALITY OF LIFE

- Knock before entering the person's room.
- Address the person by name.
- Introduce yourself by name and title.

- Explain the procedure before starting and during the procedure.
- Protect the person's rights during the procedure.
- Handle the person gently during the procedure.

PRE-PROCEDURE

1 Follow *Delegation Guidelines:*
  a *Transferring the Person,* p. 204
  b *Using a Mechanical Lift,* p. 213
  See *Promoting Safety and Comfort:*
  a *Transferring the Person,* p. 204
  b *Using a Mechanical Lift,* p. 214
2 Ask a co-worker to help you.
3 Collect the following.
  - Full-sling mechanical lift and sling
  - Arm chair or wheelchair
  - Footwear
  - Bath blanket or cushion
  - Lap blanket (if used)

4 Practice hand hygiene.
5 Identify the person. Check the ID bracelet against the assignment sheet. Use 2 identifiers (Chapter 10). Also call the person by name.
6 Provide for privacy.
7 Raise the bed for body mechanics. Bed rails are up if used.

PROCEDURE

8 Lower the head of the bed to a level appropriate for the person. It is as flat as possible.
9 Stand on 1 side of the bed. Your co-worker stands on the other side.
10 Lower the bed rails if up. Lock (brake) the bed wheels.
11 Center the sling under the person (Fig. 16-14, *A*). To position the sling, turn the person from side to side (Chapter 15). Follow the manufacturer's instructions to position the sling.
12 Position the person in the semi-Fowler's position.
13 Place the chair (wheelchair) at the head of the bed. It is even with the head-board and about 1 foot away from the bed. Place a folded bath blanket or cushion in the seat if needed. Lock (brake) the wheelchair wheels.
14 Lower the bed so it is level with the chair.
15 Raise the lift to position it over the person.
16 Position the lift over the person (Fig. 16-14, *B*).
17 Widen the lift's base. Lock (brake) the lift wheels.
18 Attach the sling to the sling hooks (Fig. 16-14, *C*).
19 Raise the head of the bed to a comfortable level for the person.
20 Cross the person's arms over the chest.
21 Unlock the lift's wheels (release the brakes).
22 Raise the person slightly from the bed. Check that the sling is secure. If not, lower the person and correct the problem.

23 Raise the lift until the person and sling are free of the bed (Fig. 16-14, *D*).
24 Have your co-worker support the person's legs as you move the lift and the person away from the bed (Fig. 16-14, *E*).
25 Adjust the base's width to move from the bed to the chair (wheelchair) if needed. Keep the base in the wide or open position as much as possible.
26 Position the lift so the person's back is toward the chair (wheelchair).
27 Adjust the position of the chair (wheelchair) as needed to lower the person into it. Lock (brake) the wheelchair wheels.
28 Lower the person into the chair (wheelchair). Guide the person into the seat (Fig. 16-14, *F*).
29 Lock (brake) the lift wheels.
30 Unhook the sling. Unlock the lift's wheels (release the brakes). Move the lift away from the person. Remove the sling from under the person unless otherwise indicated.
31 Put footwear on the person. Position the feet flat on the floor or on the wheelchair footplates.
32 Cover the lap and legs with a lap blanket (if used). Keep it off the floor and wheels.
33 Position the chair (wheelchair) as the person prefers. Lock (brake) the wheelchair wheels according to the care plan.

POST-PROCEDURE

34 Provide for comfort. (See the inside of the front cover.)
35 Place the call light and other needed items within reach.
36 Unscreen the person.
37 Complete a safety check of the room. (See the inside of the front cover.)

38 Practice hand hygiene.
39 Report and record your observations.
40 Reverse the procedure to return the person to bed.

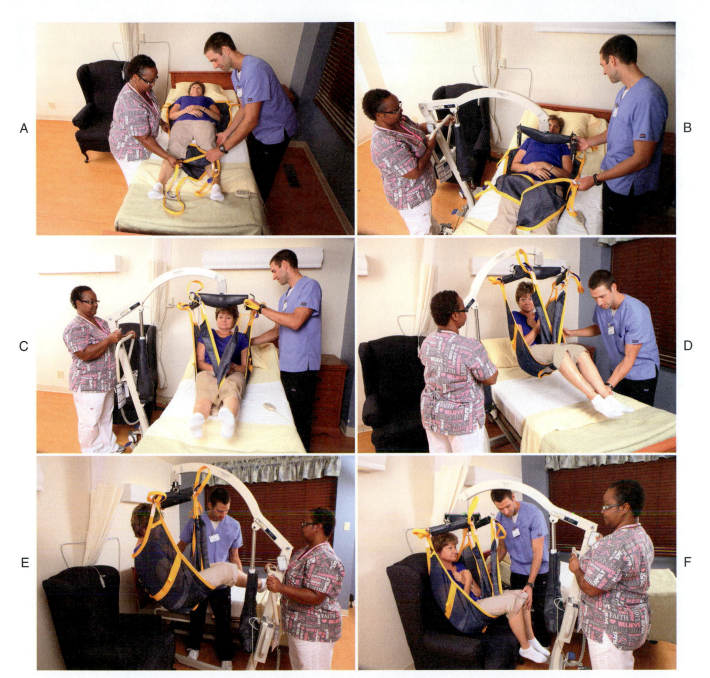

FIGURE 16-14 Using a full-sling mechanical lift. **A,** The sling is positioned under the person. **B,** The lift is over the person. **C,** The sling is attached to the lift. **D,** The lift is raised until the sling and person are off the bed. **E,** The legs are supported as the person and lift are moved away from the bed. **F,** The person is guided into a chair.

The Person, Family, and Yourself

Personal and Professional Responsibility

Before any procedure, take time to plan and prepare. Gather needed items. Organize the room and equipment for a safe transfer. Remember to:

- Lock (brake) the wheels on the bed, wheelchair, stretcher, and so on.
- Remove front rigging on a wheelchair or swing it out of the way. Raise the footplates.
- Position the chair, wheelchair, stretcher, and so on for a safe transfer.
- Adjust the bed to a safe and comfortable height.
- Make sure a mechanical lift is charged.
- Move furniture or clutter out of the way.

Planning and preparing are important for transfers. Share the plan with co-workers and the person.

Rights and Respect

Respect privacy during transfers. Close privacy curtains, doors, and window coverings. Properly cover the person. For example, a patient gown opens in the back. Apply a robe or another gown to cover the person's backside. Use a covering that is safe for transfers.

Independence and Social Interaction

How you speak to the person makes a difference. To give directions:

- Speak slowly and clearly.
- Talk loudly enough for the person to hear you.
- Speak calmly and kindly. Never yell at or insult the person.
- Face the person and use eye contact when possible.
- Give 1 direction at a time.
- Repeat directions as needed. Be patient.
- Ask if the person has questions before proceeding.

Your speech and tone must convey dignity. Show you value the person through respectful interactions.

Delegation and Teamwork

You need help to transfer a person. Your co-workers are busy. Do you ask for help? Or do you try to move the person alone?

Never be afraid to ask for help. You are not bothering a co-worker by asking for help. Ask politely and say thank you. Also, willingly help others when asked. If you cannot stop what you are doing, tell your co-worker when you can help. Then help the person when you said that you would. Work as a team for the person's safety and to protect yourself and others from injury.

Ethics and Laws

Unsafe transfers can cause injuries. To avoid injury:

- Move a person with enough help.
- Position the chair or wheelchair close to the bed.
- Use the proper equipment such as a transfer belt or mechanical lift.
- Do not pull on the person's clothing or arm, underarm, or other body part.
- Do not use broken or damaged equipment.
- Do not exceed equipment weight limits.

The right way to transfer is not always easy. Choose to give care correctly. Take pride in providing care in a way that prevents harm and promotes comfort and safety.

FOCUS ON PRIDE: *Application*

Explaining procedures improves with practice. Practice explaining a transfer from the bed to a chair using:

- A stand and pivot transfer
- A stand-assist mechanical lift
- A full-sling mechanical lift

REVIEW QUESTIONS

Circle the BEST answer.

1 To promote comfort during a transfer
   a Pull the person to a standing position
   b Explain the procedure
   c Let the person choose the procedure
   d Open the privacy curtain

2 For a safe transfer to a chair
   a Tell the person to grasp you around your neck
   b Hold the person under the underarms
   c Manually lift the person
   d Move furniture and equipment as needed

3 You are preparing to transfer a person. Which statement promotes comfort?
   a "I will move you quickly so it doesn't hurt."
   b "I can leave the door open. This will not take long."
   c "Please tell me to stop if you feel pain."
   d "This lift makes me nervous. I don't want to drop you."

4 A person uses a wheelchair. Which measure is *unsafe*?
   a The wheels are locked (braked) for transfers.
   b The chair is pulled backward to transport the person.
   c The feet are positioned on the footplates.
   d The casters point forward.

5 To use a stretcher safely
   a Unlock the wheels (release the brakes) for transfers to and from the stretcher
   b Fasten the safety straps
   c Lower the side rails during a transport
   d Move the stretcher head first

6 A stand and pivot transfer is *unsafe* for a person who
   a Is hard-of-hearing but can follow directions
   b Can bear some weight with the legs
   c Is confused and combative
   d Uses a transfer belt

7 To transfer the person to bed, a chair, or the wheelchair
   a The strong side moves first
   b The weak side moves first
   c Pillows are used for support
   d The transfer belt is removed

8 Which is *unsafe* for a stand and pivot transfer to a wheelchair?
   a The wheelchair's front rigging is removed.
   b The person's feet are flat on the floor.
   c The person is wearing non-skid footwear.
   d The wheelchair is behind you.

9 To transfer a person from a wheelchair to a toilet
   a Position the wheelchair facing the toilet
   b Remove the transfer belt when lowering clothing
   c Tell the person to hold on to the towel bar for support
   d Lock (brake) the wheelchair wheels

10 When using a mechanical lift
   a Position the lift on the person's strong side
   b Collect a sling, battery, and transfer belt
   c Compare the person's weight to the lift's weight limit
   d Allow the person to control the lift

11 For a safe transfer with a full-sling mechanical lift, at least
   a 1 worker is needed
   b 2 workers are needed
   c 3 workers are needed
   d 4 workers are needed

12 You are using a stand-assist mechanical lift. Which is *unsafe*?
   a The person is holding the lift's hand grips.
   b The person's feet are on the footplate.
   c The lift's base is narrow when lifting.
   d The person's knees are against the knee pad.

Answers to Chapter 16 questions are on p. 551.

FOCUS ON PRACTICE

Problem Solving

A resident needs to go to the bathroom right away. A full-sling mechanical lift is used for a safe transfer. You do not see another staff member nearby to help. What will you do?

OBJECTIVES

- Define the key terms and key abbreviations in this chapter.
- Explain how to maintain the person's unit.
- Describe how to control temperature, drafts, odors, noise, and lighting for the person's comfort.
- Describe the basic bed positions.
- Identify the 7 hospital bed system entrapment zones.
- Identify the persons at risk for bed entrapment.
- Explain how to use the furniture and equipment in the person's unit.

- Describe 4 ways to make beds.
- Explain how to properly handle linens.
- Explain how to assist the nurse with pain relief.
- Explain the purposes of a back massage.
- Explain how to assist the nurse with promoting sleep.
- Perform the procedures described in this chapter.
- Explain how to promote PRIDE in the person, the family, and yourself.

KEY TERMS

admission The official entry of a person into a health care setting

entrapment Getting caught, trapped, or entangled in spaces created by the bed rails, the mattress, the bed frame, the head-board, or the foot-board

Fowler's position A semi-sitting position; the head of the bed is raised between 45 and 60 degrees

full visual privacy Having the means to be completely free from public view while in bed

high-Fowler's position A semi-sitting position; the head of the bed is raised 60 to 90 degrees

insomnia A chronic condition in which the person cannot sleep or stay asleep all night

pain To ache, hurt, or be sore; discomfort

reverse Trendelenburg's position The head of the bed is raised and the foot of the bed is lowered

semi-Fowler's position The head of the bed is raised 30 degrees; or the head of the bed is raised 30 degrees and the knee portion is raised 15 degrees

sleep deprivation The amount and quality of sleep are decreased

sleepwalking The sleeping person leaves the bed and walks about

Trendelenburg's position The head of the bed is lowered and the foot of the bed is raised

KEY ABBREVIATIONS

CMS Centers for Medicare & Medicaid Services
F Fahrenheit

ID Identification

*C*omfort is a state of well-being. Many factors affect comfort. Patients, residents, and families are in a new, strange setting. You must help the person feel safe, comfortable, and secure.

NOTE: A task may require more than 1 pair of gloves. Change gloves as needed. Use careful judgment. Remember to practice hand hygiene after removing gloves.

See *Promoting Safety and Comfort: Comfort Needs.*

THE PERSON'S UNIT

The *person's unit* is the personal space, furniture, and equipment for the person in the agency (Fig. 17-1). The person's unit is designed for comfort, safety, and privacy. In nursing centers, the person's unit is as personal and home-like as possible. Always treat the person's unit with respect.

A private room is for 1 person. Semi-private rooms have 2 units. Some rooms have 3 or 4 units.

You need to keep the person's unit clean, neat, safe, and comfortable. See Box 17-1.

PROMOTING SAFETY AND COMFORT

Comfort Needs

Comfort

Admission is the official entry of a person into a health care setting. On admission to an agency, the nurse may have you orient the person and family to the area.

- Identify items in the person's unit. Explain the purpose of each.
- Explain how to use room furniture and equipment (p. 223).
  - Over-bed table
  - Call light
  - Bed, TV, and light controls
- Explain how to make phone calls. Place the phone within reach.
- Show the person the bathroom. Explain how to use the call light in the bathroom (p. 229).
- Explain visiting hours and policies.
- Explain where to find the nurses' station, lounge, chapel, dining room, and other areas.
- Identify staff—housekeeping, dietary, physical therapy, and others. Also identify students in the agency.
- Explain when meals and snacks are served.
- Give the names of nurses and nursing assistants.

Do not rush. Treat the person and family as guests. Be polite. Tell them good things about the agency. Help the person adjust to a new setting.

BOX 17-1 | Maintaining the Person's Unit

- Keep the following within the person's reach.
  - Call light (p. 228). The call light is within reach at all times.
  - Over-bed table and bedside stand.
  - Phone, TV, bed, and light controls.
  - Tissues.
- Meet the needs of persons who cannot use the call system (p. 228).
- Arrange personal items as the person prefers. They are within easy reach.
- Adjust lighting, temperature, and ventilation for the person's comfort.
- Handle equipment carefully to prevent noise.
- Explain the causes of strange noises.
- Use room deodorizers according to agency policy.
- Empty wastebaskets at least daily and when full. In some agencies, they are emptied every shift.
- Respect the person's belongings. An item may not seem important to you. Yet even a scrap of paper can have great meaning to the person.
- Do not discard any items belonging to the person.
- Do not move furniture or the person's belongings. Persons with poor vision rely on memory or feel to find items.
- Straighten bed linens and towels as often as needed.
- Complete a safety check before leaving the room. (See the inside of the front cover.)

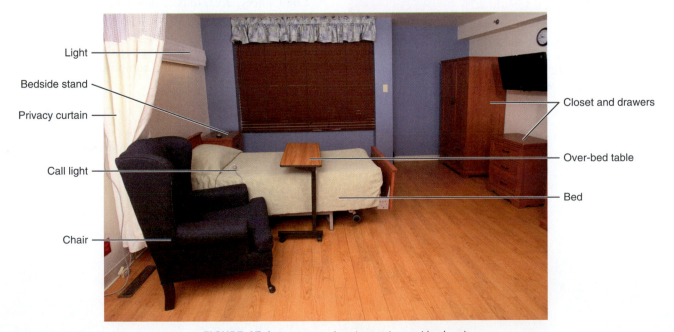

FIGURE 17-1 Furniture and equipment in a resident's unit.

COMFORT

Age, illness, and activity affect comfort. So do temperature, ventilation, noise, odors, and lighting. These factors are controlled to meet the person's needs.

See *Focus on Communication: Comfort.*

FOCUS ON COMMUNICATION

Comfort

What is comfortable for 1 person may not be comfortable for another. Ask about the person's comfort. You can say:
- "How is the temperature? Is it too hot or too cold?"
- "Is the noise level okay?"
- "Please let me know if you notice any bad odors."
- "How is the lighting? Is it too bright or too dark?"
- "Are you comfortable?"

Temperature and Ventilation

Most healthy people are comfortable with room temperatures between 68°F (Fahrenheit) and 74°F. This range may be too hot or too cold for others. Persons who are older or ill may need higher temperatures for comfort.

The Centers for Medicare & Medicaid Services (CMS) requires that nursing centers maintain a temperature of 71°F to 81°F. To protect patients and residents from cool areas and drafts:
- Have them wear enough of the correct clothing.
- Offer lap robes to those in chairs and wheelchairs. Lap robes cover the legs.
- Provide enough blankets for warmth.
- Cover them with bath blankets when giving care.
- Move them from drafty areas.

See *Focus on Older Persons: Temperature and Ventilation.*

FOCUS ON OLDER PERSONS

Temperature and Ventilation

Poor circulation and loss of the skin's fatty tissue layer occur with aging. Therefore older persons are sensitive to cold (Chapter 9). They must wear enough clothing. Many wear sweaters or jackets in warm weather. Respect the person's wishes and choices.

Odors

Odors occur in health care settings. Bowel movements and urine have embarrassing odors. So do draining wounds and vomitus. Body, breath, and smoke odors may offend others. To reduce odors:
- Empty, clean, and disinfect bedpans, urinals, commodes, and kidney basins promptly.
- Make sure toilets are flushed.
- Check incontinent persons often (Chapters 20 and 22).
- Clean persons who are wet or soiled from urine, feces, vomitus, or wound drainage.
- Change wet or soiled linens and clothing promptly.
- Keep laundry containers closed.
- Follow agency policy for wet or soiled linens and clothing.
- Dispose of incontinence and ostomy products promptly (Chapters 20 and 22).
- Provide good hygiene to prevent body and breath odors (Chapter 18).
- Use room deodorizers as needed and allowed by agency policy. Do not use sprays around persons with breathing problems. Ask the nurse if you are unsure.

Smoke odors present special problems. If you smoke, follow the agency's policy. Practice hand-washing after smoking, after handling smoking materials, and before giving care. Give careful attention to your uniform, hair, and breath because of smoke odors.

Noise

According to the CMS, a "comfortable" sound level:
- Does not interfere with a person's hearing.
- Promotes privacy when privacy is desired.
- Allows the person to take part in social activities.

Common health care sounds can be disturbing. Examples include:
- Clanging and clattering equipment, dishes, and meal trays
- Loud voices, TVs, music, and so on
- Ringing phones
- Intercom systems and call lights
- Equipment or wheels needing repair or oil
- Cleaning and housekeeping equipment

To decrease noise levels:
- Control your voice.
- Handle equipment carefully.
- Keep equipment in good working order.
- Answer phones, call lights, and intercoms promptly.

See *Focus on Communication: Noise.*
See *Focus on Older Persons: Noise.*
See *Focus on Surveys: Noise.*

Lighting

According to the CMS, comfortable lighting:
- Lessens glares.
- Lets the person control the intensity, location, and direction of light.
- Lets visually impaired persons maintain or increase independent functioning.

Glares, shadows, and dull lighting can cause falls, headaches, and eyestrain. A bright room is cheerful. Dim light is better for relaxing and rest.

Adjust window coverings and lighting to meet the person's needs. The over-bed and ceiling lights provide soft, medium, or bright lighting. Always keep light controls within the person's reach. This protects the right to personal choice.

See *Focus on Older Persons: Lighting.*

ROOM FURNITURE AND EQUIPMENT

Rooms are furnished and equipped to meet basic needs. The right to privacy is considered.

The Bed

Beds have electrical or manual controls. Beds are raised to give care and to reduce bending and reaching. A low position lets the person get out of bed with ease. The head and foot of the bed are flat or raised varying degrees.

Electric beds are common. Controls are on a side panel, bed rail, or the foot-board (Fig. 17-2, *A*, p. 224). Some controls are hand-held devices (Fig. 17-2, *B*). Patients and residents are taught to use the controls safely. They are warned not to raise the bed to the high position or to adjust the bed to harmful positions. They are told of position limits or restrictions.

Manual beds have cranks at the foot of the bed (Fig. 17-2, *C*). Pull the cranks up for use. Keep them down at all other times. Cranks in the "up" position are safety hazards. Anyone walking past may bump into them.

See *Promoting Safety and Comfort: The Bed.*

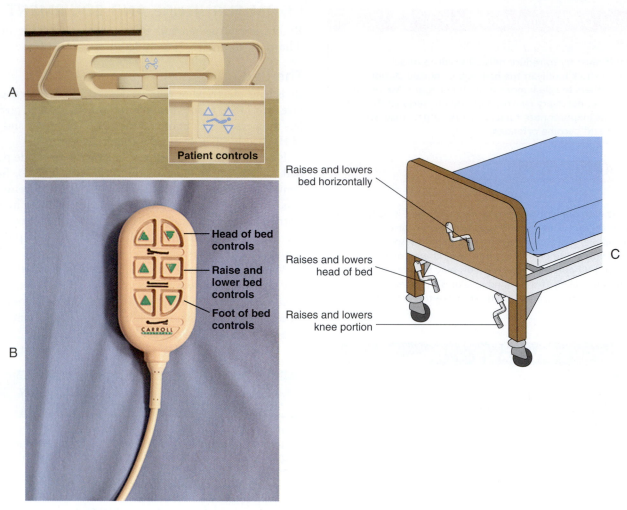

FIGURE 17-2 Bed controls. **A,** Bed controls on the bed rail. **B,** Hand-held bed control. **C,** Controls for a manually operated bed.

Bed Positions. There are 6 basic bed positions.
- *Flat* is a common sleeping position.
- *Fowler's position is a semi-sitting position. The head of the bed is raised between 45 and 60 degrees* (Fig. 17-3). See Chapter 14.
- *High-Fowler's position is a semi-sitting position. The head of the bed is raised 60 to 90 degrees* (Fig. 17-4).
- *Semi-Fowler's position means the head of the bed is raised 30 degrees* (Fig. 17-5). Some agencies define semi-Fowler's position as when *the head of the bed is raised 30 degrees and the knee portion is raised 15 degrees.* Know the definition used by your agency.
- *Trendelenburg's position means the head of the bed is lowered and the foot of the bed is raised* (Fig. 17-6). A doctor orders the position. The bed frame is tilted. Or blocks are placed under the bed legs at the foot of the bed.
- *Reverse Trendelenburg's position means the head of the bed is raised and the foot of the bed is lowered* (Fig. 17-7). A doctor orders this position. The bed frame is tilted. Or blocks are placed under the bed legs at the head of the bed.

Bed Safety. Bed safety involves the *hospital bed system*—the bed frame and its parts. The parts include the mattress, bed rails, head- and foot-boards, and bed attachments.

Hospital bed systems have 7 entrapment zones (Fig. 17-8, p. 226). ***Entrapment** means getting caught, trapped, or entangled in spaces created by the bed rails, the mattress, the bed frame, the head-board, or the foot-board.* Head, neck, or chest entrapment can cause serious injuries and death. Arm and leg entrapment also can occur. Persons at greatest risk:
- Are older.
- Are frail.
- Are confused or disoriented.
- Are restless.
- Have uncontrolled body movements.
- Have poor muscle control.
- Are small in size.
- Are restrained (Chapter 12).

Always check the person for entrapment. If a person is caught, trapped, or entangled in the bed or any of its parts, try to release the person. Also call for the nurse at once.

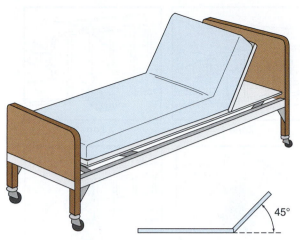

FIGURE 17-3 Fowler's position.

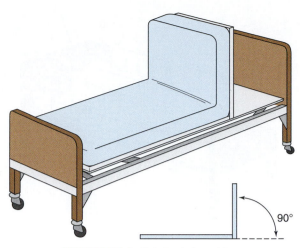

FIGURE 17-4 High-Fowler's position.

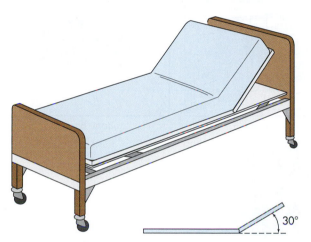

FIGURE 17-5 Semi-Fowler's position.

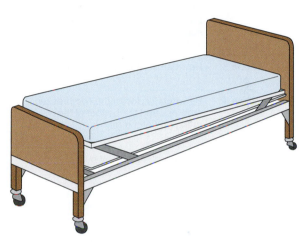

FIGURE 17-6 Trendelenburg's position.

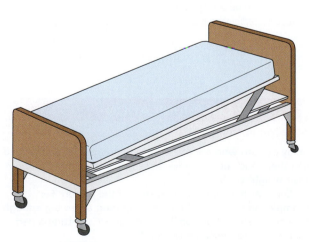

FIGURE 17-7 Reverse Trendelenburg's position.

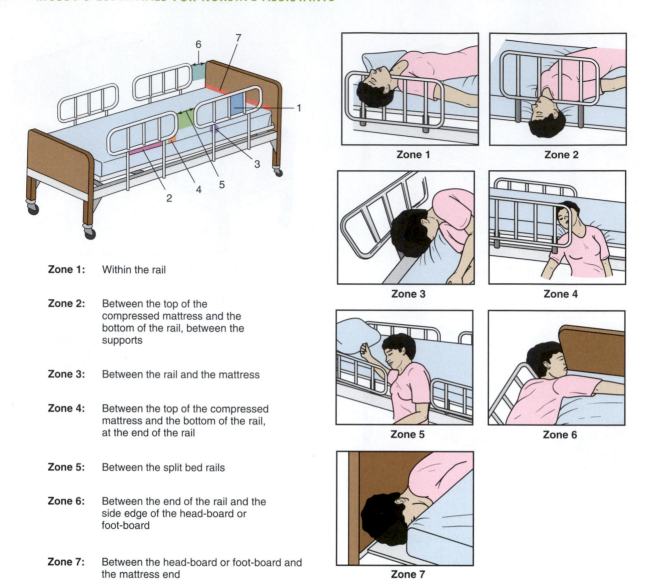

Zone 1: Within the rail

Zone 2: Between the top of the compressed mattress and the bottom of the rail, between the supports

Zone 3: Between the rail and the mattress

Zone 4: Between the top of the compressed mattress and the bottom of the rail, at the end of the rail

Zone 5: Between the split bed rails

Zone 6: Between the end of the rail and the side edge of the head-board or foot-board

Zone 7: Between the head-board or foot-board and the mattress end

FIGURE 17-8 Hospital bed system entrapment zones. (Redrawn from Food and Drug Administration: *Hospital bed system dimensional and assessment guidance to reduce entrapment,* March 10, 2006, updated June 19, 2015.)

Bariatric Beds. Bariatric beds have a weight capacity from 500 to 1000 pounds (Fig. 17-9). Bariatric beds vary depending on the model. Follow the manufacturer's instructions to use the bed safely.

See *Focus on Communication: Bariatric Beds.*

FOCUS ON COMMUNICATION

Bariatric Beds

Many persons who are obese have been insulted and judged by others. Such persons may be sensitive to comments about their weight or size.

Consider if a comment may offend the person. For example, do not say: "The nurse is getting a bed big enough for you." Instead, you can say: "The nurse is getting a bed that will be comfortable for you."

Be aware of your verbal and nonverbal communication. Your words and actions must always show dignity and respect.

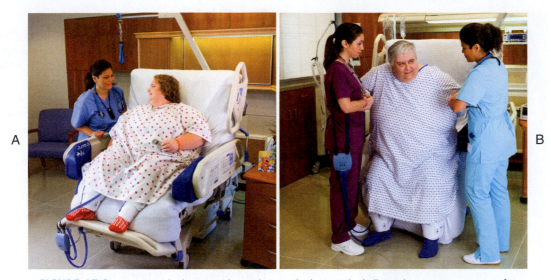

FIGURE 17-9 **A,** Bariatric bed converted to a chair. **B,** The bariatric bed allows the person to get out of bed from the chair position. (Courtesy © Hill-Rom Services, Inc. Reprinted with permission. All rights reserved.)

The Over-Bed Table

The over-bed table (see Fig. 17-1) is moved over the bed by sliding the base under the bed. The table is raised or lowered for bed or chair use. Use the handle, crank, or lever to adjust table height.

The person uses the over-bed table for meals, writing, reading, and other activities. The nursing team uses the over-bed table as a work area. Place only clean and sterile items on the table. Never place bedpans, urinals, or soiled linens on the over-bed table. Clean the table after use as a work surface. Also clean it before serving meal trays and after removing them.

The Bedside Stand

By the bed, the bedside stand has a top drawer and a lower cabinet with shelves or drawers (Fig. 17-10).
- Stand top—used for tissues, clock, photos, phone, flowers, cards, and so on.
- Top drawer—used for eyeglass case, books, kidney basin (shaped like a kidney) with oral hygiene items.
- Middle drawer or shelf—stores the wash basin with personal care items (soap, lotion, washcloth and towels, and so on).
- Bottom drawer or lower shelf—stores the bedpan, urinal, and toilet tissue.

Place only clean and sterile items on the bedside stand. Never place bedpans, urinals, or soiled linens on the top. Clean the bedside stand after use as a work surface.

Chairs

The person's unit has at least 1 chair (see Fig. 17-1). It must be comfortable, sturdy, and not move or tip during transfers. The person should be able to get in and out of the chair with ease. It should not be too low or too soft. Nursing center residents may bring chairs from home.

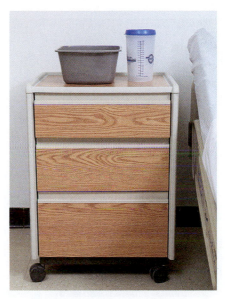

FIGURE 17-10 The bedside stand.

Privacy Curtains

Each person has the right to *full visual privacy—having the means to be completely free from public view while in bed.* The privacy curtain (see Fig. 17-1) is pulled around the bed to provide privacy. *Always pull the curtain completely around the bed before giving care.*

Privacy curtains do not block sounds or voices. Others in the room can hear sounds or talking behind the curtain.

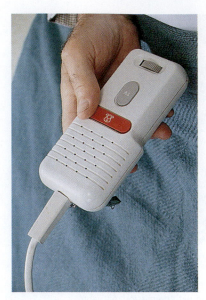

FIGURE 17-11 The call light. The call light button is pressed when help is needed. (NOTE: There are different types of call lights.)

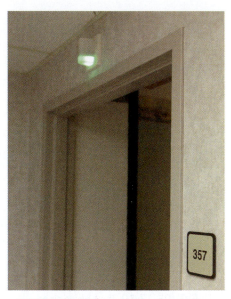

FIGURE 17-12 Light above the room door.

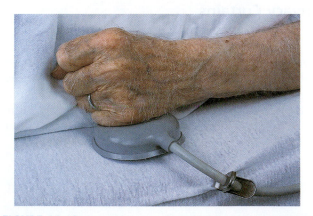

FIGURE 17-13 Call light for a person with limited hand movement.

The Call System

When in their rooms, using the toilet, or in a bathing area, patients and residents must be able to contact the staff. The call system lets the person signal for help. The call light is at the end of a long cord (Fig. 17-11). It attaches to the bed or chair with a clip. (See "The Bathroom" for call lights in bathrooms and shower and tub rooms.) *Always keep the call light within the person's reach—in the room, bathroom, and shower or tub room.*

To get help, the person presses a button on the call light device. The call light connects to a light above the room door (Fig. 17-12). The call light also connects to a computer, light panel, or intercom system at the nurses' station. These tell the staff that the person needs help.

An intercom system lets the staff talk with the person from the nurses' station. The person tells what is needed. Hard-of-hearing persons may have problems using an intercom. Remember confidentiality. When using an intercom, persons nearby can over-hear what is said.

Some call lights are turned on by tapping with a hand or fist (Fig. 17-13). They are useful for persons with limited hand movement.

Some people cannot use call lights. Examples are persons who are confused or in a coma. The care plan lists special communication measures. Check these persons often. Make sure their needs are met.

See *Focus on Communication: The Call System.*

Call System Safety. The phrase "call light" is used in this book when referring to the call system. You must:

- Keep the call light within the person's reach. Even if the person cannot use the call light, keep it within reach for use by visitors and staff. They may need to call for help.
- Place the call light on the person's strong side.
- Remind the person to signal when help is needed.
- Answer call lights promptly. For example, the person may have an urgent elimination need. Prompt bathroom use prevents embarrassing problems. You also help prevent infection, skin breakdown, pressure injuries, and falls.
- Answer bathroom and shower or tub room call lights at once.

The Bathroom

A toilet, sink, call system, and mirror are standard equipment in bathrooms. Some bathrooms have showers.

Grab bars (safety bars) are by the toilet for safety. The person uses them for support to get on and off the toilet. Some bathrooms have higher toilets or raised toilet seats. They make wheelchair transfers easier and are helpful for persons with joint problems.

Towel racks, toilet tissue, soap, paper towel dispenser, and a wastebasket are in the bathroom. They are within reach of the person.

The call light is a button or pull cord next to the toilet. The bathroom call light flashes red above the room door and at the nurses' station. To alert the staff of bathroom use, the sound at the nurses' station is different from room call lights. Someone must respond at once when a person needs help in the bathroom.

Closet and Drawer Space

Closet and drawer space are provided (see Fig. 17-1). The CMS requires that nursing centers provide each person with closet space with shelves and a clothes rack. The person must be able to reach and have free access to the closet and its contents.

Sometimes people hoard items—drugs, napkins, straws, food, sugar, salt, pepper, and so on. Hoarding can cause safety or health risks. The staff can inspect a person's closet or drawers if hoarding is suspected. The person is told of the inspection. He or she is present when it takes place.

See *Promoting Safety and Comfort: Closet and Drawer Space.*

PROMOTING SAFETY AND COMFORT
Closet and Drawer Space

Safety
Items in closets and drawers are the person's property. You need the person's permission to open or search closets or drawers.

The nurse may ask you to inspect a person's closet, drawers, or personal items. If so, the person must be present. Also have a co-worker with you as a witness. This protects you if the person claims that something was stolen or damaged.

Other Equipment

Many agencies furnish rooms with other equipment. A TV, radio, and clock provide comfort and relaxation. Many rooms have phones, a computer, and Internet access.

See *Promoting Safety and Comfort: Other Equipment.*

PROMOTING SAFETY AND COMFORT
Other Equipment

Safety
Nursing center residents are allowed personal choice in arranging items. The choices must be safe and not cause falls or other accidents. You can help the person choose the best place for personal items.

Comfort
Nursing center residents had furniture, appliances, a bathroom, and many belongings and treasures at home. Now the person lives in a new place. Leaving one's home is a hard part of growing old with poor health. The person's unit should be as home-like as possible.

Residents may bring some furniture and personal items from home. A chair, footstool, lamp, and small table are often allowed. They can bring photos, religious items, and books. Some have plants to care for.

The center is now the person's home. Help the person feel safe, secure, and comfortable. A home-like setting is important for quality of life.

BEDMAKING

Beds are made every day. Clean, dry, and wrinkle-free beds:

- Promote comfort.
- Prevent skin breakdown.
- Prevent pressure injuries (Chapter 29).

Beds are usually made in the morning after baths. Or they are made while the person is in the shower, up in the chair, or out of the room. To keep beds neat and clean:

- Change linens when they are wet, soiled, or damp.
- Straighten linens when loose or wrinkled and at bedtime.
- Check for and remove food and crumbs after meals and snacks.
- Check linens for dentures, eyeglasses, hearing aids, sharp objects, and other items.
- Follow Standard Precautions and the Bloodborne Pathogen Standard. Contact with blood, body fluids, secretions, or excretions is likely.

Types of Beds

Beds are made in these ways.

- A *closed bed* is not in use. Top linens are not folded back (Fig. 17-14). The bed is ready for a new patient or resident. In nursing centers, closed beds are made for residents who are up during the day.
- An *open bed* is ready for use. Top linens are fan-folded back so the person can get into bed. A closed bed becomes an open bed by fan-folding back the top linens (Fig. 17-15).
- An *occupied bed* is made with the person in it (Fig. 17-16).
- A *surgical bed* is made to transfer a person from a stretcher to bed (Fig. 17-17). This includes an ambulance stretcher.

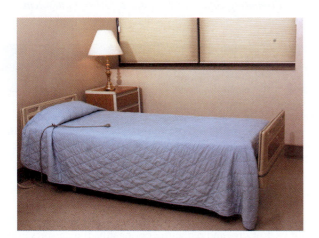

FIGURE 17-14 Closed bed.

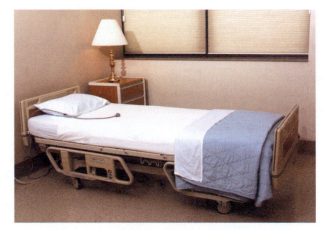

FIGURE 17-15 Open bed. Top linens are fan-folded to the foot of the bed.

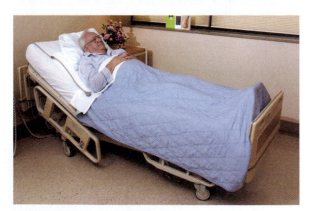

FIGURE 17-16 Occupied bed.

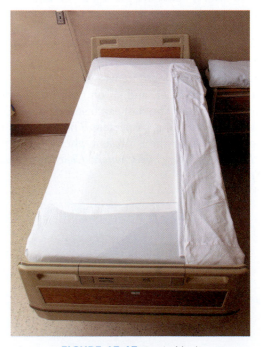

FIGURE 17-17 Surgical bed.

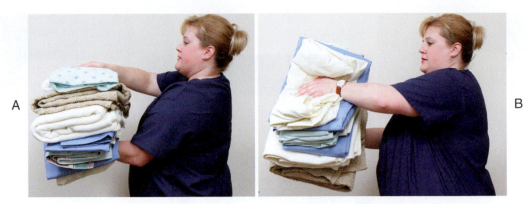

FIGURE 17-18 Collecting linens. Linens are held away from the body and uniform. Your uniform is considered *dirty*. **A,** One arm is placed over the top of the stack of linens. **B,** The stack of linens is turned onto the other arm.

Linens

Collect linens in the order you will use them. That way you avoid fumbling with linens to find the piece you need. You will use bed linens in the following order.

- Mattress pad (if needed)
- Bottom sheet (flat or fitted)
- Cotton or padded waterproof drawsheet (if needed)
- Waterproof under-pad (if needed)
- Top sheet
- Blanket
- Bedspread
- Pillowcase(s)
  You may also need:
- Bath towel(s)
- Hand towel
- Washcloth
- Gown or pajamas
- Bath blanket

Use 1 arm to hold the linens. Use your other hand to pick them up. The first item is at the bottom of the stack. To get it on top, place your arm over the stack. Then turn the stack over onto the other arm (Fig. 17-18). The first item to use is now on top. Place the clean linens on a clean surface.

Remove used linens 1 piece at a time. Roll each piece away from you. The side that touched the person is inside the roll and away from you (Fig. 17-19). Discard each piece into a laundry bag.

In hospitals, top and bottom sheets, the drawsheet, the waterproof under-pad (if used), and pillowcases are changed daily. If still clean, the mattress pad, blanket, and bedspread are re-used for the same person.

In nursing centers, linens are not changed every day. A complete linen change is usually done on the person's bath or shower day. This may be 1 or 2 times a week. Pillowcases, top and bottom sheets, and drawsheets (if used) are changed twice a week.

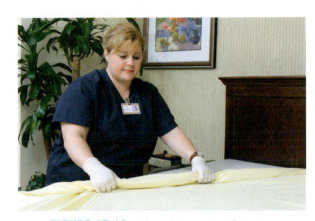

FIGURE 17-19 Roll used linens away from you.

Linens are not re-used if soiled, wet, or wrinkled. Change wet, damp, or soiled linens right away. Wear gloves and follow Standard Precautions and the Bloodborne Pathogen Standard.

See *Focus on Surveys: Linens.*

FOCUS ON **SURVEYS**

Linens

Linens may contain microbes and blood, body fluids, secretions, or excretions. You must help prevent and control the spread of infection. Surveyors will observe:

- How you transport linens.
- If you practice hand hygiene after handling soiled or used linens.
- If you double-bag linens when the outside of the laundry bag is visibly contaminated or wet.
- If you bag contaminated linens where they are used. The person's room and the shower room are examples.

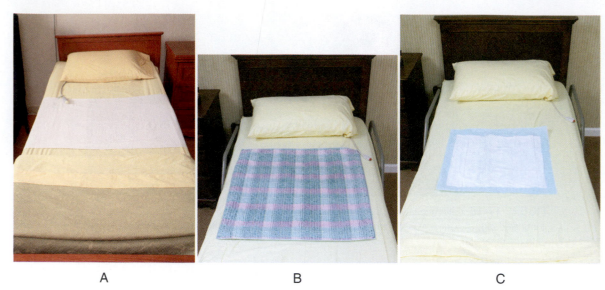

A   B   C

FIGURE 17-20 A, Cotton drawsheet. **B,** Waterproof under-pad. **C,** Disposable bed protector.

Drawsheets. A *drawsheet* is a small sheet placed over the middle of the bottom sheet. The drawsheet may have tuck tails for tucking the sheet under the mattress.
- A *cotton drawsheet* is made of cotton. It helps keep the mattress and bottom linens clean (Fig. 17-20, *A*).
- A *padded waterproof drawsheet* is a drawsheet made of an absorbent top and waterproof bottom. It protects the mattress and bottom linens from dampness and soiling. The waterproof side is placed down, away from the person. The absorbent top is up, toward the person. Disposable waterproof drawsheets are discarded when wet, soiled, or wrinkled.

Many agencies use incontinence products (Chapter 20) to keep the person and linens dry. Waterproof under-pads or disposable bed protectors also are common (Fig. 17-20, *B* and *C*).

Plastic-covered mattresses cause some persons to perspire heavily, causing discomfort. A drawsheet reduces heat retention and absorbs moisture. Drawsheets are often used as assist devices to move and transfer persons in bed (Chapters 15 and 16). If used as an assist device, do not tuck the drawsheet in at the sides.

Making Beds

Safety and medical asepsis are important for bedmaking. Follow the rules in Box 17-2.
See *Delegation Guidelines: Making Beds.*
See *Promoting Safety and Comfort: Making Beds.*

BOX 17-2	Rules for Bedmaking

- Use good body mechanics at all times (Chapter 14).
- Follow the rules in Chapters 15 and 16 to safely move and transfer the person.
- Practice medical asepsis.
- Follow Standard Precautions and the Bloodborne Pathogen Standard.
- Practice hand hygiene before handling clean linens.
- Bring only needed linens to the person's room. You cannot use extra linens for another person. Extra linens are considered contaminated. Put them with the used laundry.
- Place clean linens on a clean surface. Use the bedside chair, over-bed table, or bedside stand. Place a barrier (towel, paper towel) between the clean surface and the linens if required by agency policy.
- Do not use torn or frayed linens.
- Never shake linens. Shaking spreads microbes.
- Hold linens away from your body and uniform. Do not let used or clean linens touch your uniform.
- Never put used linens on the floor or on clean linens. Follow agency policy for used linens.
- Bag used linens in the room where they are used. Do not carry used linens un-bagged outside of the person's room.
- Keep bottom linens tucked in and wrinkle-free.
- Straighten and tighten loose sheets, blankets, and bedspreads as needed.
- Make as much of 1 side of the bed as possible before going to the other side. This saves time and energy.
- Change wet, damp, or soiled linens right away.

The Closed Bed. Closed beds are made for:
- Nursing center residents who are up for most or all of the day. Top linens are folded back at bedtime. Clean linens are used as needed.
- New patients and residents. The bed is made after the bed system (p. 224) is cleaned and disinfected. Clean linens are needed for the entire bed.
See procedure: *Making a Closed Bed.*

Text continued on p. 236.

DELEGATION GUIDELINES
Making Beds

Before making a bed, you need this information from the nurse and the care plan.

- What bed to make—closed, open, occupied, or surgical.
- If a cotton drawsheet, padded waterproof drawsheet, waterproof under-pad, or incontinence product is needed.
- If the person uses bed rails.
- The person's treatment, therapy, and activity schedules. For example, change a resident's linens after a treatment. Change another resident's bed while he or she is in physical therapy.
- Position restrictions or limits in the person's movement or activity.
- How to position the person and the positioning devices needed.
- If the bed needs to be locked into a certain position (p. 224).
- When to report observations.
- What patient or resident concerns to report at once.

PROMOTING SAFETY AND COMFORT
Making Beds

Safety
You need to raise the bed for body mechanics. The bed also is as flat as possible. If the bed is locked, unlock it. Then adjust the bed. Return the bed to the correct position when you are done. Then lock the bed.

Wear gloves to remove linens from the bed. Also follow other aspects of Standard Precautions and the Bloodborne Pathogen Standard. Linens may contain blood, body fluids, secretions, or excretions.

After making a bed, lower the bed to the correct level for the person. Follow the care plan. For an occupied bed, raise or lower bed rails according to the care plan.

Comfort
For an occupied bed, cover the person with a bath blanket before removing the top sheet. Do not leave the person uncovered. The bath blanket provides warmth and privacy.

Adjust the pillow as needed during the procedure. After the procedure, position the person as directed by the nurse and the care plan. Always make sure linens are straight and wrinkle-free.

Making a Closed Bed

QUALITY OF LIFE

- Knock before entering the person's room.
- Address the person by name.
- Introduce yourself by name and title.

- Explain the procedure before starting and during the procedure.
- Protect the person's rights during the procedure.
- Handle the person gently during the procedure.

PRE-PROCEDURE

1 Follow *Delegation Guidelines: Making Beds.* See *Promoting Safety and Comfort: Making Beds.*
2 Practice hand hygiene.
3 Collect clean linens.
   - Mattress pad (if needed)
   - Bottom sheet (flat sheet or fitted sheet)
   - Cotton drawsheet or padded waterproof drawsheet (if needed)
   - Waterproof under-pad (if needed)
   - Top sheet
   - Blanket
   - Bedspread
   - A pillowcase for each pillow
   - Bath towel
   - Hand towel
   - Washcloth
   - Gown or pajamas
   - Bath blanket
   - Gloves
   - Laundry bag
   - Paper towels (as a barrier for clean linens)
4 Place linens on a clean surface. Use the paper towels as a barrier between the clean surface and clean linens if required by agency policy.
5 Raise the bed for body mechanics. Bed rails are down.

PROCEDURE

6 Put on the gloves.
7 Remove linens. Roll each piece away from you. Place each piece in a laundry bag. (NOTE: Discard the incontinence product, disposable bed protector, and disposable drawsheet in the trash. Do not put them in the laundry bag.)
8 Clean the bed frame and mattress (if this is your job).
9 Remove and discard the gloves. Practice hand hygiene.
10 Move the mattress to the head of the bed.
11 Put the mattress pad on the mattress. It is even with the top of the mattress.

Continued

Making a Closed Bed—cont'd

PROCEDURE—cont'd

12 Place the bottom sheet on the mattress pad (Fig. 17-21). Unfold it length-wise. Place the center crease in the middle of the bed. For a flat sheet:
   a Place the lower edge even with the bottom of the mattress.
   b Place the large hem at the top and the small hem at the bottom.
   c Face hem-stitching downward, away from the person.
13 Open the sheet. Fan-fold it to the other side of the bed (Fig. 17-22).
14 Tuck the corners of a fitted sheet over the mattress at the top and then foot of the bed. For a flat sheet, tuck the top of the sheet under the mattress. The sheet is tight and smooth.
15 Make a mitered corner at the top if using a flat sheet (Fig. 17-23).
16 Place the cotton drawsheet or padded waterproof drawsheet on the bed. It is in the middle of the mattress.
   a Open and fan-fold the drawsheet to the other side of the bed.
   b Tuck the drawsheet under the mattress.
17 Go to the other side of the bed.
18 Miter the top corner of the flat bottom sheet.
19 Pull the bottom sheet tight so there are no wrinkles. Tuck in the sheet.
20 Pull the drawsheet tight so there are no wrinkles (Fig. 17-24).
21 *If using a waterproof under-pad,* place the waterproof under-pad on the bed. It is in the middle of the mattress. See Figure 17-20, *B.*
22 Go to the other side of the bed.
23 Put the top sheet on the bed.
   a Unfold it length-wise with the center crease in the middle.
   b Place the large hem even with the top of the mattress.
   c Open and fan-fold the sheet to the other side.
   d Face hem-stitching outward, away from the person.
   e Do not tuck the bottom in yet.
   f Never tuck top linens in on the sides.

24 Place the blanket on the bed.
   a Unfold it with the center crease in the middle.
   b Put the upper hem about 6 to 8 inches from the top of the mattress.
   c Open and fan-fold the blanket to the other side.
   d If steps 30 and 31 are not done, turn the top sheet down over the blanket. Hem-stitching is down, away from the person.
25 Place the bedspread on the bed.
   a Unfold it with the center crease in the middle.
   b Place the upper hem even with the top of the mattress.
   c Open and fan-fold the bedspread to the other side.
   d Make sure the bedspread facing the door is even. It covers all top linens.
26 Tuck in top linens together at the foot of the bed so they are smooth and tight. Make a mitered corner. Leave the side of the top linens untucked.
27 Go to the other side.
28 Straighten all top linens. Work from the head of the bed to the foot.
29 Tuck in top linens together at the foot of the bed. Make a mitered corner. Leave the side of the top linens untucked.
30 Turn the top hem of the bedspread under the blanket to form a cuff (Fig. 17-25).
31 Turn the top sheet down over the bedspread. Hem-stitching is down. (Steps 30 and 31 are not done in some agencies. The bedspread covers the pillow. If so, tuck the bedspread under the pillow.)
32 Put the pillowcase on the pillow (Fig. 17-26 and Fig. 17-27, p. 236). Fold extra material under the pillow at the seam end of the pillowcase.
33 Place the pillow on the bed. The open end of the pillowcase is away from the door. The seam is toward the head of the bed.

POST-PROCEDURE

34 Provide for comfort. (See the inside of the front cover.) NOTE: Omit this step if the bed is prepared for a new patient or resident.
35 Attach the call light to the bed. Or place it within the person's reach.
36 Lower the bed to a safe and comfortable level. Follow the care plan. Lock (brake) the bed wheels.

37 Put the towels, washcloth, gown or pajamas, and bath blanket in the bedside stand.
38 Complete a safety check of the room. (See the inside of the front cover.)
39 Follow agency policy for used linens.
40 Practice hand hygiene.

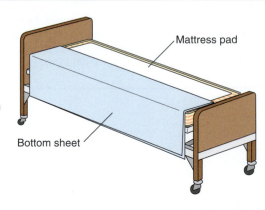

FIGURE 17-21 A flat bottom sheet is on the bed with the center crease in the middle. The lower edge of the sheet is even with the bottom of the mattress.

Mattress pad

Bottom sheet

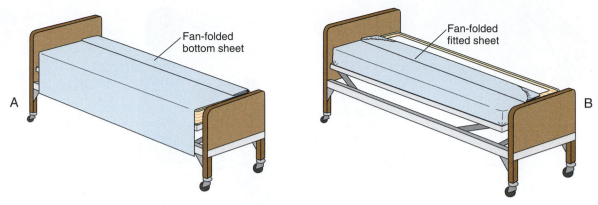

FIGURE 17-22 A, The flat bottom sheet is fan-folded to the other side of the bed. **B,** A fitted sheet is on the bed with the center crease in the middle.

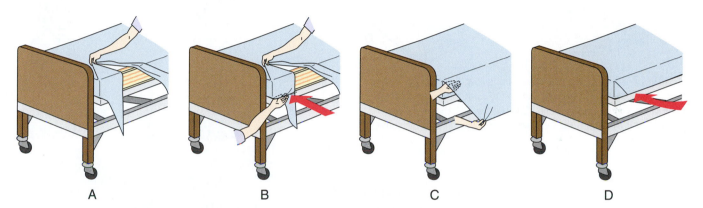

FIGURE 17-23 Making a mitered corner. **A,** The flat bottom sheet is tucked under the mattress at the head of the bed. The side of the sheet is raised onto the mattress. **B,** The remaining portion of the sheet is tucked under the mattress. **C,** The raised portion of the sheet is brought off the mattress. **D,** The entire side of the sheet is tucked under the mattress.

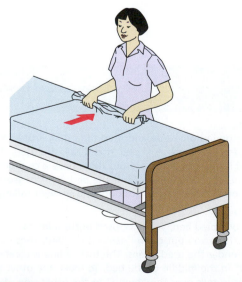

FIGURE 17-24 The drawsheet is pulled tight to remove wrinkles.

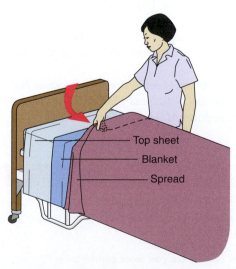

FIGURE 17-25 The top hem of the bedspread is turned under the top hem of the blanket to make a cuff.

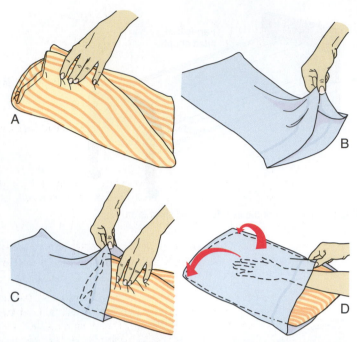

FIGURE 17-26 Putting a pillowcase on a pillow. **A,** Grasp the corners of the pillow at the seam end and form a "V" with the pillow. **B,** Open the pillowcase with your free hand. **C,** Guide the "V" end of the pillow into the pillowcase. **D,** Let the "V" end of the pillow fall into the corners of the pillowcase.

The Open Bed.

A closed bed becomes an open bed by fan-folding back the top linens. The person can get into bed with ease. Make this bed for:

- Newly admitted persons arriving by wheelchair
- Persons who are getting ready for bed
- Persons who are out of bed for a short time

The Occupied Bed.

You make an occupied bed when the person stays in bed. Keep the person in good alignment. Follow restrictions or limits in the person's movement or position.

Explain each step to the person before it is done. This is important even if the person cannot respond or is in a coma.

See *Focus on Communication: The Occupied Bed.*
See *Promoting Safety and Comfort: The Occupied Bed.*
See procedure: *Making an Occupied Bed.*

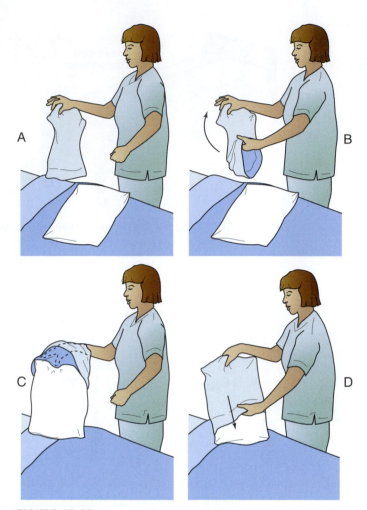

FIGURE 17-27 Putting a pillowcase on a pillow. **A,** Grasp the closed end of the pillowcase. **B,** Using your other hand, gather up the pillowcase. **C,** The pillowcase should cover your hand holding the closed end. Grasp the pillow with the hand covered by the pillowcase. **D,** Pull the pillowcase down over the pillow with your other hand.

FOCUS ON COMMUNICATION

The Occupied Bed

After making an occupied bed, ask about the person's comfort.

- "Are you comfortable?"
- "How can I make you more comfortable?"
- "Are you warm enough?"
- "Do you feel any creases or wrinkles?"
- "Can I adjust your pillow?"

After making the bed, thank the person for cooperating.

PROMOTING SAFETY AND COMFORT

The Occupied Bed

Safety

The person lies on 1 side and then the other. Protect the person from falling out of bed. If bed rails are used, the far bed rail is up. If bed rails are not used, have a co-worker help you. You work on 1 side of the bed. Your co-worker is on the other side to turn, position, and prevent falling.

Comfort

For an occupied bed, you tuck used bottom linens under the person. Then you put clean linens on the bed. These are tucked under the used linens. The tucked linens create a "bump" in the middle of the bed. To make the other side, the person rolls over the "bump" to the other side of the bed. For comfort, make the "bump" as low as possible. Do this by fan-folding used and clean bottom linens neatly and flatly.

Making an Occupied Bed

QUALITY OF LIFE

- Knock before entering the person's room.
- Address the person by name.
- Introduce yourself by name and title.

- Explain the procedure before starting and during the procedure.
- Protect the person's rights during the procedure.
- Handle the person gently during the procedure.

PRE-PROCEDURE

1 Follow *Delegation Guidelines: Making Beds,* p. 233. See *Promoting Safety and Comfort:*
   a *Making Beds,* p. 233
   b *The Occupied Bed*
2 Practice hand hygiene.
3 Collect the following.
   - Gloves
   - Laundry bag
   - Clean linens (see procedure: *Making a Closed Bed,* p. 233)
   - Paper towels (as a barrier for clean linens)

4 Place linens on a clean surface. Use the paper towels as a barrier between the clean surface and clean linens if required by agency policy.
5 Identify the person. Check the ID (identification) bracelet against the assignment sheet. Use 2 identifiers (Chapter 10). Also call the person by name.
6 Provide for privacy.
7 Remove the call light.
8 Raise the bed for body mechanics. Bed rails are up if used. Bed wheels are locked (braked).
9 Lower the head of the bed. It is as flat as possible.

PROCEDURE

10 Practice hand hygiene. Put on gloves.
11 Loosen top linens at the foot of the bed.
12 Lower the bed rail near you if up.

13 Fold and remove the bedspread (Fig. 17-28). Do the same for the blanket. Place each over the chair.

Continued

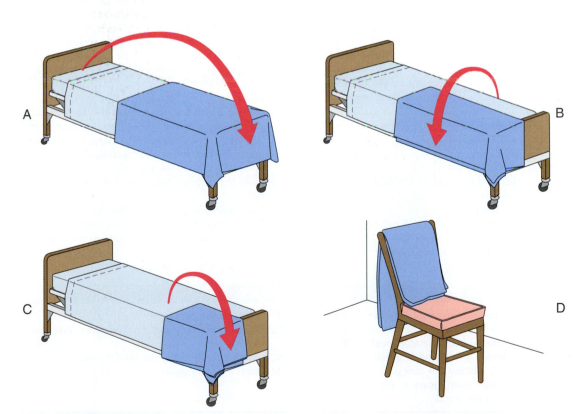

FIGURE 17-28 Folding linens for re-use. **A,** Fold the top edge of the bedspread down to the bottom edge. **B,** Fold the bedspread from the far side of the bed to the near side. **C,** Fold the top edge of the bedspread down to the bottom edge again. **D,** Place the folded bedspread over the back of the chair.

Making an Occupied Bed—cont'd

PROCEDURE—cont'd

14 Cover the person with a bath blanket from the bedside stand.
  a Unfold the bath blanket over the top sheet.
  b Have the person hold the bath blanket. If he or she cannot, tuck the top part under the person's shoulders.
  c Grasp the top sheet under the bath blanket at the shoulders. Bring the sheet down toward the foot of the bed. Remove the sheet from under the blanket (Fig. 17-29).

15 Position the person on his or her side facing away from you. Adjust the pillow for comfort.

16 Loosen bottom linens from the head to the foot of the bed.

17 Fan-fold bottom linens 1 at a time toward the person. Start with the drawsheet (Fig. 17-30). If re-using the mattress pad, do not fan-fold it.

18 Remove and discard the gloves. Practice hand hygiene. Put on clean gloves.

19 Place a clean mattress pad on the bed. Unfold it length-wise with the center crease in the middle. Fan-fold the top part toward the person. If re-using the mattress pad, straighten and smooth any wrinkles.

20 Place the bottom sheet on the mattress pad. Hem-stitching is away from the person. Unfold the sheet with the crease in the middle. For a flat sheet, the small hem is even with the bottom of the mattress. Fan-fold the top part toward the person.

21 Tuck fitted sheet corners over the mattress. For a flat sheet, make a mitered corner at the head of the bed. Tuck the sheet under the mattress from the head to the foot.

22 *If using a drawsheet* (Fig. 17-31):
  a Place the cotton drawsheet or padded waterproof drawsheet on the bed. It is in the middle of the mattress.
  b Open the drawsheet.
  c Fan-fold it toward the person.
  d Tuck in excess fabric.

23 *If using a waterproof under-pad:*
  a Place the waterproof under-pad on the bed. It is in the middle of the mattress.
  b Fan-fold it toward the person.

24 Explain to the person that he or she will roll over a "bump." Assure the person that he or she will not fall.

25 Help the person turn to the other side. Adjust the pillow for comfort.

26 Raise the bed rail. Go to the other side and lower the bed rail.

27 Loosen bottom linens. Remove 1 piece at a time. Place each piece in the laundry bag. (NOTE: Discard the disposable bed protector, incontinence product, and disposable drawsheet in the trash. Do not put them in the laundry bag.)

28 Remove and discard the gloves. Practice hand hygiene.

29 Straighten and smooth the mattress pad.

30 Pull the clean bottom sheet toward you. Tuck fitted sheet corners over the mattress. For a flat sheet, make a mitered corner at the top. Tuck the sheet under the mattress from the head to the foot of the bed.

31 Pull the drawsheet tightly toward you and tuck it in.

32 Position the person supine in the center of the bed. Adjust the pillow for comfort.

33 Put the top sheet on the bed. Unfold it length-wise with the crease in the middle. The large hem is even with the top of the mattress. Hem-stitching is on the outside.

34 Have the person hold the top sheet so you can remove the bath blanket. Or tuck the top sheet under the person's shoulders. Remove the bath blanket. Place it in the laundry bag.

35 Unfold the blanket on the bed. The crease is in the middle and it covers the person. The upper hem is 6 to 8 inches from the top of the mattress.

36 Unfold the bedspread on the bed. The center crease is in the middle and it covers the person. The top hem is even with the mattress top.

37 Turn the top hem of the bedspread under the blanket to make a cuff.

38 Bring the top sheet down over the bedspread to form a cuff.

39 Go to the foot of the bed.

40 Make a 2-inch toe pleat across the foot of the bed. The pleat is about 6 to 8 inches from the foot of the bed.

41 Lift the mattress corner with 1 arm. Tuck all top linens under the bottom of the mattress. Make a mitered corner. Leave the side of the top linens untucked.

42 Raise the bed rail. Go to the other side and lower the bed rail.

43 Straighten and smooth top linens.

44 Tuck all top linens under the bottom of the mattress. Make a mitered corner. Leave the side of the top linens untucked.

45 Change the pillowcase(s).

POST-PROCEDURE

46 Provide for comfort. (See the inside of the front cover.)

47 Place the call light and other needed items within reach.

48 Lower the bed to a safe and comfortable level. Follow the care plan. The bed wheels are locked (braked).

49 Raise or lower bed rails. Follow the care plan.

50 Put the clean towels, washcloth, gown or pajamas, and bath blanket in the bedside stand.

51 Unscreen the person.

52 Complete a safety check of the room. (See the inside of the front cover.)

53 Follow agency policy for used linens.

54 Practice hand hygiene.

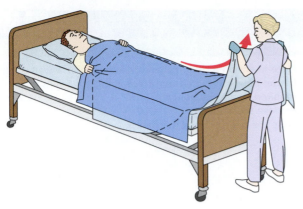

FIGURE 17-29 The person holds on to the bath blanket. The top sheet is removed from under the bath blanket. (NOTE: Bed rails are used according to the care plan.)

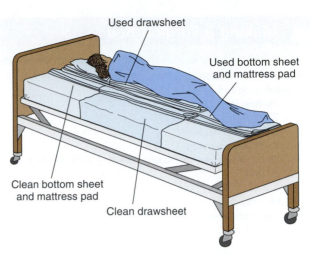

FIGURE 17-31 A clean bottom sheet and drawsheet are on the bed with both fan-folded and tucked under the person. (NOTE: Bed rails are used according to the care plan.)

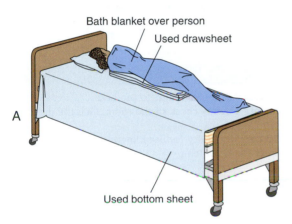
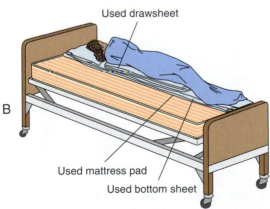

FIGURE 17-30 A, The used drawsheet is fan-folded and tucked under the person. **B,** All used bottom linens are tucked under the person. (NOTE: Bed rails are used according to the care plan.)

The Surgical Bed. The surgical bed also is called a *recovery bed* or *post-operative bed*. Top linens are folded to transfer the person from a stretcher to the bed. These beds are made for persons:

- Returning to their rooms from surgery. A complete linen change is needed.
- Who arrive at the agency by ambulance. A complete linen change is needed if the person:
  - Is a new patient or resident.
  - Is returning to the agency from the hospital.
- Who go by stretcher to treatment or therapy areas. A complete linen change is not needed.
- Using portable tubs (Chapter 18). Because of bathing, a complete linen change is needed.

See *Promoting Safety and Comfort: The Surgical Bed.*
See procedure: *Making a Surgical Bed*, p. 240.

PROMOTING SAFETY AND COMFORT

The Surgical Bed

Safety
Follow the rules for stretcher safety (Chapter 16). After the transfer, lower the bed to a safe and comfortable level for the person. Lock (brake) the bed wheels. Raise or lower bed rails according to the care plan.

Making a Surgical Bed

PRE-PROCEDURE

1 Follow *Delegation Guidelines: Making Beds,* p. 233. See *Promoting Safety and Comfort:*
   a *Making Beds,* p. 233
   b *The Surgical Bed,* p. 239
2 Practice hand hygiene.
3 Collect the following.
   • Clean linens (see procedure: *Making a Closed Bed,* p. 233)
   • Gloves
   • Laundry bag
   • Equipment requested by the nurse
   • Paper towels (as a barrier for clean linens)

4 Place linens on a clean surface. Use the paper towels as a barrier between the clean surface and clean linens if required by agency policy.
5 Remove the call light.
6 Raise the bed for body mechanics.

PROCEDURE

7 Remove and place all linens in the laundry bag. Wear gloves. Practice hand hygiene after removing and discarding them.
8 Make a closed bed (see procedure: *Making a Closed Bed,* p. 233). Do not tuck top linens under the mattress.
9 Fold all top linens at the foot of the bed back onto the bed. The fold is even with the edge of the mattress (Fig. 17-32, *A*).

10 Know on which side of the bed the stretcher will be placed. Fan-fold linens length-wise to the other side of the bed (Fig. 17-32, *B*).
11 Put a pillowcase on each pillow.
12 Place the pillow(s) on a clean surface.

POST-PROCEDURE

13 Leave the bed in its highest position.
14 Leave both bed rails down.
15 Put the clean towels, washcloth, gown or pajamas, and bath blanket in the bedside stand.
16 Move furniture away from the bed. Allow room for the stretcher and the staff.

17 Do not attach the call light to the bed.
18 Complete a safety check of the room. (See the inside of the front cover.)
19 Follow agency policy for used linens.
20 Practice hand hygiene.

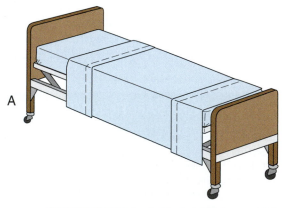 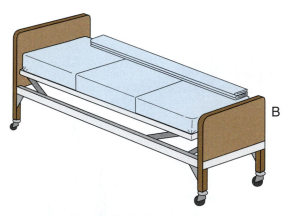

FIGURE 17-32 Surgical bed. **A,** The bottom of the top linens is folded back onto the bed. The fold is even with the bottom edge of the mattress. **B,** Top linens are fan-folded length-wise to the side of the bed. (NOTE: Bed rails are used according to the care plan.)

PAIN RELIEF

***Pain** or discomfort means to ache, hurt, or be sore.* Pain is subjective (Chapter 6). That is, you cannot see, hear, touch, or smell pain or discomfort. You must rely on what the person says.

The nurse uses the nursing process to promote comfort and relieve pain. See Chapter 25 for the types, signs, and symptoms of pain. Report the person's complaints and your observations. The person's care plan may include the measures in Box 17-3.

See *Focus on Communication: Pain Relief.*
See *Focus on Surveys: Pain Relief.*

<table>
<tr><td>

BOX 17-3 Comfort and Pain-Relief Measures

- Position the person in good alignment. Use pillows for support.
- Keep bed linens tight and wrinkle-free.
- Make sure the person is not lying on tubes.
- Assist with elimination needs.
- Adjust the room temperature to meet the person's needs.
- Provide blankets for warmth and to prevent chilling.
- Use correct moving and turning procedures.
- Wait 30 minutes after pain-relief drugs are given to give care or start activities.
- Give a back massage (p. 242).
- Provide soft music to distract the person.
- Talk softly and gently.
- Use touch to provide comfort.
- Allow family and friends at the bedside as requested by the person.
- Avoid sudden or jarring movements of the bed or chair.
- Handle the person gently.
- Practice safety measures if the person takes strong pain-relief drugs or sedatives.
  - Keep the bed in a low position that is safe and comfortable for the person. Follow the care plan.
  - Raise bed rails as directed. Follow the care plan.
  - Check on the person every 10 to 15 minutes.
  - Provide help when the person needs to get up and when he or she is up and about.
- Apply warm or cold applications as directed by the nurse (Chapter 28).
- Provide a calm, quiet, darkened setting.

</td></tr>
</table>

FOCUS ON COMMUNICATION

Pain Relief

Communicating about pain promotes comfort. You can say:
- "I want you to be comfortable. Please tell me if you are having pain."
- "I'll tell the nurse about your pain."

If a person complains of pain, the person has pain. You must rely on what the person tells you. Promptly report any complaints of pain to the nurse.

FOCUS ON SURVEYS

Pain Relief

Pain interferes with well-being—function, mobility, mood, sleep, and quality of life. The agency must:
- Recognize when a person has pain.
- Identify when pain might occur.
- Evaluate pain and its causes.
- Manage or prevent pain.

You may be the first to notice signs and symptoms of pain. You must recognize and report a change in the person's behavior and function.

You follow the care plan for pain-relief measures. Therefore a surveyor may ask you about pain. Examples are:
- What are the signs and symptoms of pain?
- How do you ask a person to rate the intensity of pain?
- What factors can cause pain or make it worse?
- When and how do you report observations about pain?
- How do you assist the nurse with pain-relief measures?

Factors Affecting Pain

Many factors affect reactions to pain.

- *Past experience.* The severity of pain, its cause, how long it lasted, and if relief occurred all affect the current response to pain. Knowing what to expect can help or hinder the person's response. Some people have not had pain. When it occurs, pain can cause fear and anxiety. They can make pain worse.
- *Anxiety.* Anxiety relates to feelings of fear, dread, worry, and concern. The person is uneasy and tense. Pain and anxiety are related. Pain can cause anxiety. Anxiety worsens pain. Reducing anxiety helps lessen pain.
- *Rest and sleep.* Rest and sleep restore energy and reduce body demands. Without needed rest and sleep, thinking and coping with daily life are affected. Pain seems worse. When unable to sleep, the person has time to think about pain.
- *Attention.* Thinking about pain makes it seem worse. Pain may be all that the person thinks about. Even mild pain can seem worse if it is the person's main focus.
- *Personal and family duties.* Often pain is ignored when there are children to care for. Some people work with pain. Others deny pain, fearing a serious illness. Illness can interfere with a job, school, or caring for family members.
- *The value or meaning of pain.* To some people, pain is a sign of weakness. It may mean a serious illness with painful tests and treatments. Sometimes pain brings pleasure. The pain of childbirth is an example. For some persons, pain is used to avoid certain people or things. The pain is useful. Some people like to be doted on and pampered. The person values and wants the attention.
- *Support from others.* Dealing with pain is often easier when family and friends offer comfort and support. The use of touch by a valued person is comforting. Just being nearby also helps. With no family or friends, some people deal with pain alone. Being alone can increase anxiety.
- *Culture.* Culture affects pain responses. Non-English-speaking persons may have problems describing pain in English. The agency uses interpreters to communicate with the person. See *Caring About Culture: Pain Reactions*, p. 242.
- *Illness.* Some diseases affect pain sensations. Central nervous system disorders are examples. The person may not feel pain. Or it may be severe.
- *Age.* See *Focus on Older Persons: Factors Affecting Pain*, p. 242.

CARING ABOUT CULTURE

Pain Reactions

Some people of *Mexico* and the *Philippines* may appear stoic in reaction to pain. (*Stoic* means *to show no reaction to joy, sorrow, pleasure, or pain.*) In the *Philippines*, some people view pain as the will of God and believe that God will give strength to bear the pain.

In *Vietnam*, pain may be severe before some people request pain-relief measures. In *China*, showing emotion may be viewed as a weakness of character. If so, pain is often suppressed.

(NOTE: Each person is unique. A person may not follow all of the beliefs and practices of his or her culture. Follow the care plan.)

Modified from D'Avanzo CE: *Pocket guide to cultural health assessment*, ed 4, St Louis, 2008, Mosby.

FOCUS ON OLDER PERSONS

Factors Affecting Pain

Some older persons have many painful health problems. Chronic (long-term) pain may mask new pain. Or new pain is ignored. They may think it relates to a known problem. Or pain is denied or ignored because of what it may mean.

Thinking and reasoning are affected in some older persons. Some cannot tell you about pain. Behavior changes may signal pain. Increased confusion, grimacing, restlessness, and loss of appetite are examples. A person who normally moans and groans may become quiet and withdraw. A friendly and outgoing person may become agitated and aggressive. One who is nonverbal and quiet may become restless and cry easily.

Always report behavior changes. All persons have the right to correct pain management. The nurse does a pain assessment when behavior changes.

The Back Massage

The back massage (back rub) can promote comfort and help relieve pain. It relaxes muscles and stimulates circulation. Good times for back massages are after re-positioning, after baths or showers, and with evening care. Back massages last 3 to 5 minutes. Observe the skin before the massage. Look for breaks in the skin, bruises, reddened areas, and other signs of skin breakdown.

Lotion reduces friction during the massage and keeps the skin soft. Warm the lotion before applying it. Do 1 of the following.

- Rub some lotion between your hands.
- Place the bottle in the bath water.
- Hold the bottle under warm water.

Use firm strokes. Also keep your hands in contact with the person's skin. After the massage, apply lotion to the elbows, knees, and heels. Those bony areas are at risk for skin breakdown.

See *Delegation Guidelines: The Back Massage.*
See *Promoting Safety and Comfort: The Back Massage.*
See procedure: *Giving a Back Massage.*

DELEGATION GUIDELINES

The Back Massage

Before giving a back massage, you need this information from the nurse and the care plan.

- If the person can have a back massage (see *Promoting Safety and Comfort: The Back Massage*).
- How to position the person.
- If the person has position limits. If yes, what are they?
- When to give a back massage.
- If the person needs back massages often for comfort and to relax.
- What observations to report and record:
  - Breaks in the skin
  - Bruising
  - Reddened areas
  - Signs of skin breakdown
- When to report observations.
- What patient or resident concerns to report at once.

PROMOTING SAFETY AND COMFORT

The Back Massage

Safety
Back massages can harm persons with certain heart diseases, back injuries and surgeries, skin diseases, and lung disorders. Check with the nurse and the care plan before giving back massages.

Do not massage reddened bony areas. Reddened areas signal skin breakdown and pressure injuries. Massage can cause more tissue damage.

Wear gloves if the person's skin is not intact. Do not massage areas of non-intact skin. Always follow Standard Precautions and the Bloodborne Pathogen Standard.

Comfort
The prone position is best for a massage. The side-lying position is often used. Older and disabled persons usually find the side-lying position more comfortable.

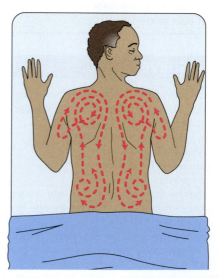

FIGURE 17-33 The person is in the prone position for a back massage. Stroke upward from the lower back to the shoulders, down over the upper arms, back up the upper arms, across the shoulders, and down to the lower back.

Giving a Back Massage

QUALITY OF LIFE

- Knock before entering the person's room.
- Address the person by name.
- Introduce yourself by name and title.

- Explain the procedure before starting and during the procedure.
- Protect the person's rights during the procedure.
- Handle the person gently during the procedure.

PRE-PROCEDURE

1 Follow *Delegation Guidelines: The Back Massage.* See *Promoting Safety and Comfort: The Back Massage.*
2 Practice hand hygiene.
3 Identify the person. Check the ID bracelet against the assignment sheet. Use 2 identifiers (Chapter 10). Also call the person by name.

4 Collect the following.
   - Bath blanket
   - Bath towel
   - Lotion
5 Provide for privacy.
6 Raise the bed for body mechanics. Bed rails are up if used.

PROCEDURE

7 Lower the bed rail near you if up.
8 Position the person in the prone or side-lying position. The back is toward you.
9 Cover the person with a bath blanket. Expose the back, shoulders, and upper arms.
10 Lay the towel on the bed along the back. Do this if the person is in a side-lying position.
11 Warm the lotion.
12 Explain that the lotion may feel cool and wet.
13 Apply lotion to the lower back area.
14 Stroke up from the lower back to the shoulders. Then stroke down over the upper arms. Stroke up the upper arms, across the shoulders, and down the back (Fig. 17-33). Use firm strokes. Keep your hands in contact with the person's skin.
15 Repeat step 14 for at least 3 minutes.

16 Knead the back (Fig. 17-34).
   a Grasp the skin between your thumb and fingers.
   b Knead half of the back. Start at the lower back and move up to the shoulder. Then knead down from the shoulder to the lower back.
   c Repeat on the other half of the back.
17 Apply lotion to bony areas. Use circular motions with the tips of your index and middle fingers. (*Do not massage reddened bony areas.*)
18 Use fast movements to stimulate. Use slow movements to relax the person.
19 Stroke with long, firm movements to end the massage. Tell the person when you are finishing.
20 Straighten and secure clothing or sleepwear.
21 Cover the person. Remove the towel and bath blanket.

POST-PROCEDURE

22 Provide for comfort. (See the inside of the front cover.)
23 Place the call light and other needed items within reach.
24 Lower the bed to a safe and comfortable level. Follow the care plan.
25 Raise or lower bed rails. Follow the care plan.
26 Return lotion to its proper place.

27 Unscreen the person.
28 Complete a safety check of the room. (See the inside of the front cover.)
29 Follow agency policy for used linens.
30 Practice hand hygiene.
31 Report and record your observations.

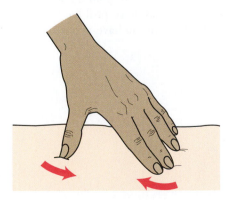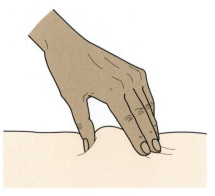

FIGURE 17-34 Knead by picking up tissue between the thumb and fingers.

SLEEP

Sleep is a basic need. The mind and body rest. The body saves energy. Body functions slow. Vital signs (temperature, pulse, respirations, and blood pressure) are lower than when awake. Tissue healing and repair occur. Sleep lowers stress, tension, and anxiety. It refreshes and renews the person. The person regains energy and mental alertness. The person thinks and functions better after sleep.

Measures are planned to promote sleep (Box 17-4). Follow the care plan.

See *Focus on Older Persons: Sleep.*

BOX 17-4	Promoting Sleep

- Plan care for uninterrupted rest.
- Avoid physical activity before bedtime.
- Encourage the person to avoid business or family matters before bedtime.
- Allow a flexible bedtime. Bedtime is when the person is tired, not a certain time.
- Provide a comfortable room temperature.
- Let the person take a warm bath or shower.
- Provide a bedtime snack.
- Avoid caffeine (coffee, tea, colas, chocolate).
- Avoid alcoholic beverages.
- Have the person urinate before going to bed.
- Make sure incontinent persons are clean and dry.
- Follow bedtime routines.
- Have the person wear loose-fitting sleepwear.
- Provide for extra warmth (blankets, socks) as needed.
- Make sure linens are clean, dry, and wrinkle-free.
- Position the person in good alignment and in a comfortable position.
- Support body parts as ordered.
- Give a back massage.
- Provide measures to relieve pain.
- Let the person read, listen to music, or watch TV.
- Assist with relaxation exercises as ordered.
- Sit and talk with the person.
- Reduce noise.
- Darken the room—close window coverings and the privacy curtain. Shut off or dim lights.
- Dim lights in hallways and the nursing unit.

Factors Affecting Sleep

Many factors affect the amount and quality of sleep.

- *Age.* Sleep needs vary for each age-group. The amount needed decreases with age.
- *Illness.* Illness increases the need for sleep. Pain, nausea, vomiting, coughing, difficulty breathing, diarrhea, frequent voiding, and itching can interfere with sleep. So can treatments and therapies and being awakened for treatments or drugs. Care devices can cause uncomfortable positions.
- *Nutrition.* Foods with caffeine (chocolate, coffee, tea, or colas) prevent sleep. Caffeine is a stimulant and prevents sleep. The protein *tryptophan* tends to help sleep. It is found in protein sources—milk, cheese, red meat, fish, poultry, and peanuts.
- *Exercise.* Exercise causes the release of substances into the bloodstream that stimulate the body. Exercise is avoided 2 hours before bedtime.
- *Environment.* People adjust to their usual sleep settings. They get used to the bed, pillows, noises, lighting, and a sleeping partner. Any change in the usual setting can affect sleep.
- *Drugs and other substances.* Sleeping pills promote sleep. Drugs for anxiety, depression, and pain may cause sleep. Alcohol interferes with sleep. Some drugs contain caffeine. The side effects of some drugs cause frequent voiding and nightmares.
- *Emotional problems.* Fear, worry, depression, and anxiety affect sleep. People may have problems falling asleep or they awaken often. Some have problems getting back to sleep.

Sleep Disorders

Sleep disorders involve repeated sleep problems. The amount and quality of sleep are affected. Physical and behavioral problems may result.

- *Insomnia is a chronic condition in which the person cannot sleep or stay asleep all night.* There are 3 forms of insomnia.
  - Cannot fall asleep
  - Cannot stay asleep
  - Early awakening and cannot fall back asleep
- *Sleep deprivation means the amount and quality of sleep are decreased.* Sleep is interrupted.
- *Sleepwalking is when the person leaves the bed and walks about.* The person is not aware of sleepwalking and has no memory of the event. The event lasts 3 to 4 minutes or longer. Protect the person from injury. Falling is a risk. Guide sleepwalkers back to bed. They startle easily. Awaken them gently.

FOCUS ON P R I D E
The Person, Family, and Yourself

P ersonal and Professional Responsibility

Loud talking and laughter can disturb patients, residents, and visitors. They may think the staff is not working. Or they may think the staff is talking about or laughing at them. They may become anxious, uncomfortable, or angry.

Do your part to reduce noise. Politely remind others to speak softly. Take pride in providing a quiet and comfortable setting.

R ights and Respect

Nursing center residents have the right to a home-like setting. Residents often bring bedspreads, blankets, quilts, and so on from home. The items have meaning and value. For example, an afghan brought from home may comfort a resident.

Protect personal items from loss and damage. Handle the person's belongings with care and respect.

I ndependence and Social Interaction

Allow personal choice when possible. What is best for you may not be best for the person. For example, you plan to make beds after residents are done with breakfast. However, some residents want their beds made while at breakfast.

Ask about the person's preferences. Consider such preferences when planning your day and managing your time. The more choices are allowed, the greater the person's sense of control and independence.

D elegation and Teamwork

Agencies have different ways of handling used linens. Some have containers in each room. Others have carts in the hallways. The carts are emptied as needed. Some agencies have a room where used linens are placed. Others have chutes.

When handling used linens:

- Wear gloves.
- Follow agency policy for used linens.
- Do not over-fill the bag or container. The person emptying the bag or cart may be injured.
- Work as a team. Some units assign a person to empty linen containers. Linens must not over-flow carts. If you see a full cart, empty it. Do so without complaining. The person assigned the task may be busy. If no one is assigned the task, work together to complete it.
- Clean up after yourself. If you fill a cart, empty it. If you place an item in a cart that will cause an odor, empty it.
- Place used linens in the correct location. Do not place used linens in a room or cart where they do not belong. If chutes are used, use the correct chute. Other chutes in the area may be for trash.

E thics and Laws

This chapter focused on how objects and surroundings in the person's unit affect comfort and well-being. You are a part of that setting. You must help the person feel safe, secure, and comfortable.

Your words and actions are heard and seen by others. Bad conduct reduces quality of care and reflects poorly on you. You can lose your job and the ability to work as a nursing assistant. Always provide care in a way that promotes comfort, safety, and quality of life.

FOCUS ON PRIDE: *Application*

Family and visitors often provide comfort. How will you welcome the person's visitors? How will you show you value them and their time with the person?

REVIEW QUESTIONS

*Circle **T** if the statement is TRUE or **F** if it is FALSE.*

1. **T F** You can adjust the person's room temperature for your comfort.

2. **T F** The call light is placed on the person's strong side.

3. **T F** You can look through a person's closet and drawers.

4. **T F** Top linens are fan-folded to the foot of the bed for an open bed.

5. **T F** A cotton drawsheet is used with a padded waterproof drawsheet.

6. **T F** Changes in usual behavior may signal pain.

7. **T F** A person's culture may affect how he or she reacts to pain.

8. **T F** A back massage relaxes muscles and stimulates circulation.

9. **T F** Persons with dementia usually sleep well at night.

Circle the BEST answer.

10. To protect a person from drafts
    a. Adjust the room temperature to 70°F
    b. Provide a bath blanket during a bed bath
    c. Dress the person in light-weight clothing
    d. Position the person near a fan

11. To prevent odors
    a. Place flowers in the room
    b. Empty commodes at the end of your shift
    c. Keep laundry containers open
    d. Clean persons who are wet or soiled

12. To control noise
    a. Answer phones after the third ring
    b. Use the intercom system when possible
    c. Handle equipment carefully
    d. Talk with others in the hallway

13. The head of the bed is raised 30 degrees. This is called
    a. Fowler's position
    b. Semi-Fowler's position
    c. Trendelenburg's position
    d. Reverse Trendelenburg's position

14. Bed safety involves
    a. Monitoring older and confused persons closely for entrapment
    b. Removing the entrapment zones from the bed
    c. Leaving the bed in the raised position
    d. Restraining persons at risk for entrapment

15. Call lights are answered
    a. When you have time
    b. At the end of your shift
    c. Promptly
    d. When you are near the person's room

16. When handling linens
    a. Put used linens on the floor
    b. Hold linens away from your body and uniform
    c. Shake linens to unfold them
    d. Take extra linens to another person's room

17. A resident is out of bed most of the day. Which bed should you make?
    a. A closed bed
    b. An open bed
    c. An occupied bed
    d. A surgical bed

18. A complete linen change is done when
    a. The bottom linens are wet or soiled
    b. The bed is made for a new person
    c. The person will transfer from a stretcher to a bed
    d. Linens are loose or wrinkled

19. When making an occupied bed
    a. Explain that the person will roll over a "bump" of linens
    b. Wear the same gloves throughout the procedure
    c. Lower the far bed rail if working alone
    d. Fan-fold top linens to the foot of the bed

20. The nurse gave a person a drug for pain relief. When should you give scheduled care?
    a. Before the drug is given
    b. Right after the drug is given
    c. 30 minutes after the drug is given
    d. The next day

21. A drug was given for pain relief. To promote safety
    a. Keep the bed in the raised position
    b. Quickly change positions to avoid dizziness
    c. Check on the person every hour
    d. Provide help if the person needs to get up

22. Which measure promotes comfort and pain relief?
    a. Providing a blanket
    b. Speaking loudly
    c. Keeping the lights on in the room
    d. Asking about comfort every 5 minutes

23. When giving a back massage
    a. Massage for 15 to 20 minutes
    b. Warm the lotion before applying it
    c. Massage reddened areas
    d. Position the person in Fowler's position

24. Which prevents sleep?
    a. Cheese
    b. Chocolate
    c. Milk
    d. Beef

25. Which measure before bedtime promotes sleep?
    a. Having the person urinate
    b. Having the person walk
    c. Providing hot tea
    d. Leaving the hallway light on

Answers to Chapter 17 questions are on p. 551.

FOCUS ON PRACTICE

Problem Solving

Since your shift began an hour ago, a resident has called for help 10 times. You just left the room and are helping another resident. The call light is used again. What do you do?

The resident uses the call light more often at night, after family visits, and when not checked on regularly. How might this information be helpful for the nurse in care planning?

Hygiene Needs

OBJECTIVES

- Define the key terms and key abbreviations in this chapter.
- Explain why personal hygiene is important.
- Identify the observations related to hygiene needs.
- Describe the care given before and after breakfast, after lunch, and in the evening.
- Explain the purposes of oral hygiene.
- Describe the safety measures for giving mouth care to unconscious persons.
- Explain how to care for dentures.
- Describe the rules for bathing.
- Identify safety measures for tub baths and showers.
- Explain the purposes of perineal care.
- Perform the procedures described in this chapter.
- Explain how to promote PRIDE in the person, the family, and yourself.

KEY TERMS

aspiration Breathing fluid, food, vomitus, or an object into the lungs
circumcised The fold of skin (foreskin) covering the glans of the penis was surgically removed
denture An artificial tooth or a set of artificial teeth

oral hygiene Mouth care
perineal care Cleaning the genital and anal areas; pericare
uncircumcised The male has foreskin covering the head of the penis

KEY ABBREVIATIONS

C Centigrade
F Fahrenheit

ID Identification

The skin defends the body against disease. Intact skin prevents microbes from entering the body and causing an infection. Likewise, mucous membranes of the mouth, genital area, and anus must be clean and intact. Besides cleansing, hygiene measures prevent body and breath odors. They also are relaxing and increase circulation.

Culture and personal choice affect hygiene. (See *Caring About Culture: Personal Hygiene.*) The person's care preferences are part of the care plan.

See *Focus on Communication: Hygiene Needs*, p. 248.
See *Focus on Older Persons: Hygiene Needs*, p. 248.
See *Promoting Safety and Comfort: Hygiene Needs*, p. 248.

CARING ABOUT CULTURE

Personal Hygiene

Personal hygiene is very important to *East Indian Hindus*. For religious duty, at least 1 bath a day is required. Some believe bathing after a meal is harmful. Another belief is that a cold bath prevents a blood disease. Some believe that eye injuries can occur if bath water is too hot. Hot water can be added to cold water. However, cold water is not added to hot water for a bath. After bathing, the body is carefully dried with a towel.

(NOTE: *Each person is unique. A person may not follow all of the beliefs and practices of his or her culture. Follow the care plan.*)

Modified from Giger JN: *Transcultural nursing: assessment and intervention*, ed 6, St Louis, 2013, Mosby.

FOCUS ON COMMUNICATION

Hygiene Needs

During hygiene procedures, the person must be warm enough. You can ask:

- "Is the water warm enough?" "Is it too hot?" "Is it too cold?"
- "Are you warm enough?"
- "Do you need another bath blanket?"
- "Is the water starting to cool?"
- "Is the room warm enough?"

FOCUS ON OLDER PERSONS

Hygiene Needs

Some older persons resist hygiene efforts. Illness, disability, dementia, and personal choice are common reasons. Follow the care plan. Also see Chapter 35.

Bending and reaching are hard for older and disabled persons. Some have weak hand grips. They cannot hold soap or a washcloth. Adaptive (assistive) devices for hygiene promote independence (Fig. 18-1). Let the person do as much as safely possible.

PROMOTING SAFETY AND COMFORT

Hygiene Needs

Safety

Hygiene measures often involve exposing and touching private areas—breasts, perineum, rectum. Sexual abuse has occurred in health care settings. The person may feel threatened or is actually being abused. He or she needs to call for help. Keep the call light within the person's reach at all times. And always act in a professional manner.

You make observations while assisting with hygiene needs. The *Delegation Guidelines* in this chapter list the observations to report and record. Also report the following at once.

- Bleeding
- Signs of skin breakdown
- Discharge from the vagina, urinary tract, or rectum
- Unusual odors
- Changes from prior observations

NOTE: *A task may require more than 1 pair of gloves. Change gloves as needed. Use careful judgment. Remember to practice hand hygiene after removing gloves.*

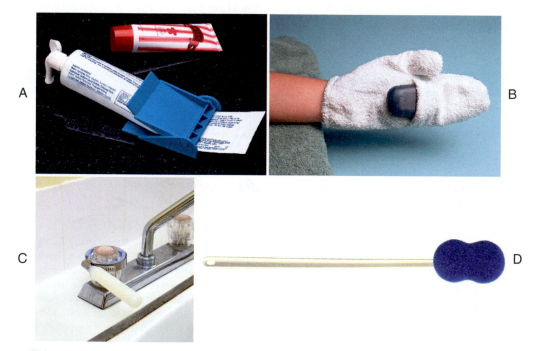

FIGURE 18-1 Adaptive (assistive) devices for hygiene. **A,** Tube squeezer for toothpaste. **B,** The wash mitt holds a bar of soap. **C,** A tap turner makes round knobs easy to turn. **D,** A long-handled sponge is used for hard-to-reach body parts. (Courtesy ElderStore, Alpharetta, Ga.)

DAILY CARE

Most people have hygiene routines and habits. For example, teeth are brushed and the face and hands washed after sleep. These and other hygiene measures are often done before and after meals and at bedtime.

Routine care is given during the day and evening (Box 18-1). You also assist with hygiene as needed. Always protect the right to privacy and to personal choice.

BOX 18-1 Daily Care

Before Breakfast (Early Morning Care or AM Care)
- Prepare persons for breakfast or morning tests.
- Assist with elimination.
- Clean incontinent persons.
- Change wet or soiled linens and garments.
- Assist with face- and hand-washing and oral hygiene.
- Assist with dressing and hair care.
- Assist with eyeglasses or contact lenses, hearing aids, and other needed devices.
- Position patients and residents for breakfast—dining room, bedside chair, or in bed.
- Make beds and straighten units.

After Breakfast (Morning Care)
- Assist with elimination.
- Clean incontinent persons.
- Change wet or soiled linens and garments.
- Assist with face- and hand-washing, oral hygiene, bathing, and perineal care.
- Provide back massages and other comfort measures (Chapter 17).
- Assist with hair care, shaving, dressing, and undressing.
- Assist with range-of-motion exercises and ambulation.
- Clean eyeglasses.
- Make beds and straighten rooms.

Afternoon Care
- Prepare persons for naps, visitors, or activity programs.
- Assist with elimination.
- Clean incontinent persons.
- Change wet or soiled linens and garments.
- Assist with face- and hand-washing, oral hygiene, and hair care.
- Assist with range-of-motion exercises and ambulation.
- Straighten beds and units.

Evening Care (PM Care)
- Prepare persons for sleep.
- Assist with elimination.
- Clean incontinent persons.
- Change wet or soiled linens and garments.
- Assist with face- and hand-washing and oral hygiene.
- Provide back massages and other comfort measures (Chapter 17).
- Help persons change into sleepwear.
- Store eyeglasses or contact lenses, hearing aids, and other devices.
- Straighten beds and units.

ORAL HYGIENE

Oral hygiene (mouth care):
- Keeps the mouth and teeth clean.
- Prevents mouth odors and infections.
- Increases comfort.
- Makes food taste better.
- Reduces the risk for *cavities (dental caries)* and *periodontal disease (gum disease, pyorrhea).*

The nurse assesses the person's need for mouth care. Illness, disease, and some drugs often cause:
- A bad taste in the mouth
- A whitish coating in the mouth and on the tongue
- Redness and swelling in the mouth and on the tongue
- Dry mouth—common from oxygen, smoking, decreased fluid intake, and anxiety

See *Delegation Guidelines: Oral Hygiene.*
See *Promoting Safety and Comfort: Oral Hygiene.*

DELEGATION GUIDELINES
Oral Hygiene

To assist with oral hygiene, you need this information from the nurse and the care plan.
- The type of oral hygiene to give. See procedures:
  - *Brushing and Flossing the Person's Teeth,* p. 250
  - *Providing Mouth Care for the Unconscious Person,* p. 253
  - *Providing Denture Care,* p. 254
- If flossing is needed.
- If you apply lubricant to the lips. If yes, what lubricant to use.
- How often to give oral hygiene.
- How much help the person needs.
- What observations to report and record:
  - Dry, cracked, swollen, or blistered lips
  - Mouth or breath odor
  - Redness, swelling, irritation, sores, or white patches in the mouth or on the tongue
  - Bleeding, swelling, or redness of the gums
  - Loose teeth
  - Rough, sharp, or chipped areas on dentures
- When to report observations.
- What patient or resident concerns to report at once.

PROMOTING SAFETY AND COMFORT
Oral Hygiene

Safety
Follow Standard Precautions and the Bloodborne Pathogen Standard. You may have contact with the person's mucous membranes. Gums may bleed during mouth care. Also, the mouth has many microbes. Pathogens spread through sexual contact may be in the mouths of some persons.

Brush gently and carefully. Brushing hard can cause the gums to bleed. Inserting the toothbrush too far can stimulate the gag reflex.

Comfort
Assist with oral hygiene after sleep, after meals, and at bedtime. Many people practice oral hygiene before meals. Some persons need mouth care every 2 hours or more often.

Flossing

Dental floss is a soft thread for cleaning between the teeth. Flossing:

- Removes *plaque* (a thin film that sticks to teeth) from areas brushing cannot reach
- Removes food from between the teeth

Usually done after brushing, it can be done at other times. Some people floss after meals. If done once a day, the best time to floss is at bedtime or when there is time to floss thoroughly. You need to floss for persons who cannot do so themselves.

Brushing and Flossing Teeth

Many people perform oral hygiene themselves. Others need help gathering and setting up oral hygiene equipment. You perform oral hygiene for persons who:

- Are very weak.
- Cannot move or use their arms.
- Are too confused to brush their teeth.
  See procedure: *Brushing and Flossing the Person's Teeth*.

Brushing and Flossing the Person's Teeth

QUALITY OF LIFE

- Knock before entering the person's room.
- Address the person by name.
- Introduce yourself by name and title.

- Explain the procedure before starting and during the procedure.
- Protect the person's rights during the procedure.
- Handle the person gently during the procedure.

PRE-PROCEDURE

1 Follow *Delegation Guidelines: Oral Hygiene*, p. 249. See *Promoting Safety and Comfort:*
  a *Hygiene Needs*, p. 248
  b *Oral Hygiene*, p. 249
2 Practice hand hygiene.
3 Collect the following.
- Toothbrush with soft bristles
- Toothpaste
- Mouthwash (or solution noted on the care plan)
- Dental floss (if used)
- Water cup with cool water
- Straw

- Kidney basin
- Hand towel
- Paper towels
- Gloves

4 Place the paper towels on the over-bed table. Arrange items on top of them.
5 Identify the person. Check the ID (identification) bracelet against the assignment sheet. Use 2 identifiers (Chapter 10). Also call the person by name.
6 Provide for privacy.
7 Raise the bed for body mechanics. Bed rails are up if used.

PROCEDURE

8 Lower the bed rail near you if up.
9 Assist the person to a sitting position or to a side-lying position near you. (NOTE: Some state competency tests require that the person is at a 75- to 90-degree angle.)
10 Place the towel across the chest.
11 Adjust the over-bed table so you can reach it with ease.
12 Practice hand hygiene. Put on the gloves.
13 Hold the toothbrush over the kidney basin. Pour some water over the brush.
14 Apply toothpaste to the toothbrush.
15 Brush the teeth gently (Fig. 18-2). Brush the inner, outer, and chewing surfaces of upper and lower teeth.
16 Brush the tongue gently. Also gently brush the roof of the mouth, inside of the cheeks, and gums.
17 Let the person rinse the mouth with water. Hold the kidney basin under the chin (Fig. 18-3). Repeat this step as needed.

18 Floss the person's teeth (optional).
  a Break off an 18-inch piece of floss from the dispenser.
  b Hold the floss between the middle fingers of each hand (Fig. 18-4, *A*).
  c Stretch the floss with your thumbs. Hold the floss between your thumbs and index fingers.
  d Start at the upper back tooth on the right side. Work around to the left side.
  e Rub gently against the side of the tooth. Use up-and-down motions (Fig. 18-4, *B*). Do not jerk or snap the floss against the tooth. Work from the top of the crown to the gum line.
  f Move to a new section of floss after every second tooth.
  g Floss the lower teeth. Use gentle up-and-down motions as for the upper teeth. Start on the right side. Work around to the left side.
19 Let the person use mouthwash or other solution. Hold the kidney basin under the chin.
20 Wipe the person's mouth. Remove the towel.
21 Remove and discard the gloves. Practice hand hygiene.

Brushing and Flossing the Person's Teeth—cont'd

POST-PROCEDURE

22 Provide for comfort. (See the inside of the front cover.)
23 Place the call light and other needed items within reach.
24 Lower the bed to a safe and comfortable level. Follow the care plan.
25 Raise or lower bed rails. Follow the care plan.
26 Rinse the toothbrush. Clean, rinse, and dry equipment. Use clean, dry paper towels for drying. Return the toothbrush and equipment to their proper place. Wear gloves.

27 Wipe off the over-bed table with the paper towels. Discard the paper towels.
28 Unscreen the person.
29 Complete a safety check of the room. (See the inside of the front cover.)
30 Follow agency policy for used linens.
31 Remove and discard the gloves. Practice hand hygiene.
32 Report and record your observations.

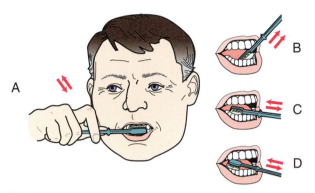

FIGURE 18-2 Brushing teeth. **A,** The brush is held at a 45-degree angle to the gums. Teeth are brushed with short strokes. **B,** The brush is at a 45-degree angle against the inside of the front teeth. Teeth are brushed from the gum to the crown of the tooth with short strokes. **C,** The brush is held horizontally against the inner surfaces of the teeth. The teeth are brushed back and forth. **D,** The brush is positioned on the chewing surfaces of the teeth. The teeth are brushed back and forth.

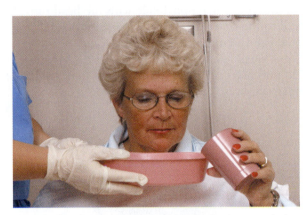

FIGURE 18-3 The kidney basin is held under the person's chin.

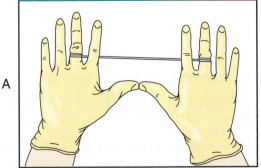
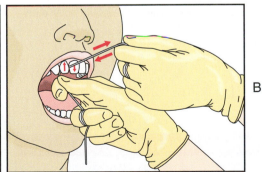

FIGURE 18-4 Flossing. **A,** Floss is wrapped around the middle fingers. **B,** Floss is moved in up-and-down motions between the teeth. Floss is moved up and down from the crown to the gum line.

Mouth Care for the Unconscious Person

Unconscious persons cannot eat or drink. Some breathe with their mouths open. Many receive oxygen. These factors cause mouth dryness. They also cause crusting on the tongue and mucous membranes. Oral hygiene keeps the mouth clean and moist. It also helps prevent infection.

The care plan tells you what cleaning agent to use. Use sponge swabs to apply the cleaning agent. Apply a lubricant (check the care plan) to the lips after cleaning. It prevents cracking of the lips.

Unconscious persons usually cannot swallow. Protect them from choking and aspiration. *Aspiration is breathing fluid, food, vomitus, or an object into the lungs.* It can cause pneumonia and death. To prevent aspiration:

- Position the person on 1 side with the head turned well to the side (Fig. 18-5). In this position, excess fluid can run out of the mouth.
- Use a small amount of fluid to clean the mouth.
- Do not insert dentures. Unconscious persons do not wear dentures.

Keep the person's mouth open with a plastic tongue depressor (Fig. 18-6). Do not use your fingers. The person can bite down on them. The bite breaks the skin and creates a portal of entry for microbes. Infection is a risk.

Mouth care is given at least every 2 hours. Follow the nurse's directions and the care plan.

See *Focus on Communication: Mouth Care for the Unconscious Person.*

See *Promoting Safety and Comfort: Mouth Care for the Unconscious Person.*

See procedure: *Providing Mouth Care for the Unconscious Person.*

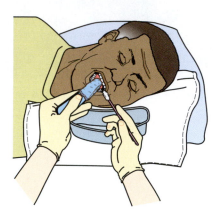

FIGURE 18-5 The unconscious person's head is turned well to the side to prevent aspiration. A plastic tongue depressor keeps the mouth open while cleaning the mouth with swabs.

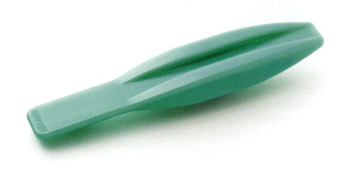

FIGURE 18-6 Plastic tongue depressor. (© American Diagnostic Corp., 2017.)

Providing Mouth Care for the Unconscious Person

QUALITY OF LIFE

- Knock before entering the person's room.
- Address the person by name.
- Introduce yourself by name and title.

- Explain the procedure before starting and during the procedure.
- Protect the person's rights during the procedure.
- Handle the person gently during the procedure.

PRE-PROCEDURE

1 Follow *Delegation Guidelines: Oral Hygiene*, p. 249. See *Promoting Safety and Comfort:*
   a *Hygiene Needs*, p. 248
   b *Oral Hygiene*, p. 249
   c *Mouth Care for the Unconscious Person*
2 Practice hand hygiene.
3 Collect the following.
   - Cleaning agent (check the care plan)
   - Sponge swabs
   - Plastic tongue depressor
   - Water cup with cool water
   - Hand towel

- Kidney basin
- Lip lubricant
- Paper towels
- Gloves

4 Place the paper towels on the over-bed table. Arrange items on top of them.
5 Identify the person. Check the ID bracelet against the assignment sheet. Use 2 identifiers (Chapter 10). Also call the person by name.
6 Provide for privacy.
7 Raise the bed for body mechanics. Bed rails are up if used.

PROCEDURE

8 Lower the bed rail near you.
9 Position the person in a side-lying position near you. Turn his or her head well to the side.
10 Place the towel under the person's face.
11 Put on the gloves.
12 Place the kidney basin under the chin.
13 Separate the upper and lower teeth. Use the plastic tongue depressor. Be gentle. Never use force. If you have problems, ask the nurse for help.
14 Moisten the sponge swabs with the cleaning agent. Squeeze out excess cleaning agent.

15 Clean the mouth.
   a Clean the chewing and inner surfaces of the teeth.
   b Clean the gums and outer surfaces of the teeth.
   c Swab the roof of the mouth, inside of the cheeks, and the lips.
   d Swab the tongue.
   e Moisten and squeeze out a clean swab. Swab the mouth to rinse.
   f Place used swabs in the kidney basin.
16 Remove the kidney basin and supplies.
17 Wipe the person's mouth. Remove the towel.
18 Apply lubricant to the lips.
19 Remove and discard the gloves. Practice hand hygiene.

POST-PROCEDURE

20 Provide for comfort. (See the inside of the front cover.)
21 Place the call light and other needed items within reach.
22 Lower the bed to a safe and comfortable level. Follow the care plan.
23 Raise or lower bed rails. Follow the care plan.
24 Clean, rinse, dry, and return equipment to its proper place. Use clean, dry paper towels for drying. Discard disposable items. (Wear gloves.)
25 Wipe off the over-bed table with paper towels. Discard the paper towels.

26 Unscreen the person.
27 Complete a safety check of the room. (See the inside of the front cover.)
28 Tell the person that you are leaving the room. Tell him or her when you will return.
29 Follow agency policy for used linens.
30 Remove and discard the gloves. Practice hand hygiene.
31 Report and record your observations.

Denture Care

A *denture* is an artificial tooth or a set of artificial teeth (Fig. 18-7). Often called *false teeth*, dentures replace missing teeth.

- *Full dentures.* Dentures replace all of the upper or lower teeth.
- *Partial dentures.* The person has some teeth. The partial denture replaces the missing teeth.

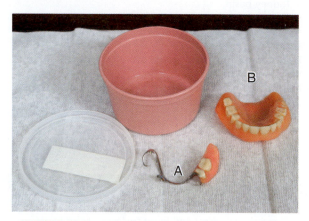

FIGURE 18-7 Dentures. **A,** Partial denture. **B,** Full denture.

Mouth care is given and dentures cleaned as often as natural teeth. Dentures are slippery when wet. They easily break or chip if dropped onto a hard surface (floor, sink, counter). Hold them firmly when removing or inserting them. During cleaning, firmly hold them over a sink filled half-way with water. Line the sink with a towel. This prevents the dentures from falling onto a hard surface.

Use only denture cleaning products to avoid damaging dentures. The manufacturer's instructions tell how to use the cleaning agent and what water temperature to use.

Hot water causes dentures to lose their shape (warp). If not worn after cleaning, store dentures in a container with cool or warm water or a denture soaking solution. Otherwise they can dry out and warp.

Dentures are usually removed at bedtime. Some people soak their dentures over-night in a denture cleaning solution. Others soak them in water. Rinse the dentures before they are inserted.

Some people do not wear their dentures. Others wear dentures for eating and remove them after meals. Remind patients and residents not to wrap dentures in tissues or napkins. Otherwise, they are easily discarded.

See *Promoting Safety and Comfort: Denture Care.*
See procedure: *Providing Denture Care.*

PROMOTING SAFETY AND COMFORT
Denture Care

Safety

Dentures are the person's property. They are costly. Handle them very carefully. Label the denture cup with the person's name and room and bed number. Report lost or damaged dentures at once. Losing or damaging dentures is negligent conduct.

Never carry dentures in your hands. Always use a denture cup or kidney basin. You could easily drop the dentures if holding them.

Dentures are rinsed under running water. Do not rinse dentures in the water used to fill the sink. The sink is contaminated.

Comfort

Many people do not like being seen without their dentures. Privacy is important. Allow privacy when the person cleans dentures. If you clean dentures, return them to the person as quickly as possible.

Persons with partial dentures have some teeth. They need to brush and floss natural teeth. See procedure: *Brushing and Flossing the Person's Teeth*, p. 250.

Providing Denture Care

QUALITY OF LIFE

- Knock before entering the person's room.
- Address the person by name.
- Introduce yourself by name and title.

- Explain the procedure before starting and during the procedure.
- Protect the person's rights during the procedure.
- Handle the person gently during the procedure.

Providing Denture Care—cont'd

PRE-PROCEDURE

1 Follow *Delegation Guidelines: Oral Hygiene*, p. 249. See *Promoting Safety and Comfort:*
   a *Hygiene Needs*, p. 248
   b *Oral Hygiene*, p. 249
   c *Denture Care*
2 Practice hand hygiene.
3 Collect the following.
   - Denture brush or toothbrush (for cleaning dentures)
   - Denture cup labeled with the person's name and room and bed number
   - Denture cleaning agent
   - Soft-bristled toothbrush or sponge swabs (for oral hygiene)
   - Toothpaste
   - Water cup with cool water
   - Straw
   - Mouthwash (or other noted solution)
   - Kidney basin
   - 2 hand towels
   - Gauze squares
   - Paper towels
   - Gloves

4 Place the paper towels on the over-bed table. Arrange items on top of them.
5 Identify the person. Check the ID bracelet against the assignment sheet. Use 2 identifiers (Chapter 10). Also call the person by name.
6 Provide for privacy.

PROCEDURE

7 Line the bottom of the sink with a towel. Do not use paper towels. Fill the sink half-way with water.
8 Raise the bed for body mechanics.
9 Lower the bed rail near you if up.
10 Practice hand hygiene. Put on the gloves.
11 Place a towel over the person's chest.
12 Have the person remove the dentures. Carefully place them in the kidney basin.
13 Remove the dentures if the person cannot do so. Use gauze squares for a good grip on the slippery dentures.
   a Grasp the upper denture with your thumb and index finger (Fig. 18-8, p. 256). Move it up and down slightly to break the seal. Gently remove the denture. Place it in the kidney basin.
   b Grasp and remove the lower denture with your thumb and index finger. Turn it slightly and lift it out of the person's mouth. Place it in the kidney basin.
14 Follow the care plan for raising bed rails.
15 Take the kidney basin, denture cup, denture brush, and denture cleaning agent to the sink.
16 Rinse the denture cup and lid.
17 Rinse each denture under cool or warm running water. Follow agency policy for water temperature.
18 Return dentures to the kidney basin.
19 Apply the denture cleaning agent to the brush.
20 Brush the dentures as in Figure 18-9, p. 256. Brush the inner, outer, and chewing surfaces and all surfaces that touch the gums.
21 Rinse the dentures under running water. Use warm or cool water as directed by the cleaning agent manufacturer.

22 Place dentures in the denture cup. Cover the dentures with cool or warm water. Follow agency policy for water temperature.
23 Clean the kidney basin.
24 Take the denture cup and kidney basin to the over-bed table.
25 Lower the bed rail if up.
26 Position the person for oral hygiene.
27 Clean the person's gums and tongue. Brush any natural teeth. Use toothpaste and the toothbrush (or sponge swabs).
28 Have the person use mouthwash (or noted solution). Hold the kidney basin under the chin.
29 Have the person insert the dentures. Insert them if the person cannot.
   a Hold the upper denture firmly with your thumb and index finger. Raise the upper lip with the other hand. Insert the denture. Gently press on the denture with your index finger to make sure it is in place.
   b Hold the lower denture with your thumb and index finger. Pull the lower lip down slightly. Insert the denture. Gently press down on it to make sure it is in place.
30 Place the denture cup with the dentures in the top drawer of the bedside stand if the dentures are not worn. The dentures must be in water or in a denture soaking solution.
31 Wipe the person's mouth. Remove the towel.
32 Remove and discard the gloves. Practice hand hygiene.

POST-PROCEDURE

33 Assist with hand-washing.
34 Provide for comfort. (See the inside of the front cover.)
35 Place the call light and other needed items within reach.
36 Lower the bed to a safe and comfortable level. Follow the care plan.
37 Raise or lower bed rails. Follow the care plan.
38 Remove the towel from the sink. Drain the sink.
39 Rinse the brushes. Empty and rinse the denture cup. Clean, rinse, and dry equipment. Use clean, dry paper towels for drying. Return the brushes and equipment to their proper place. Discard disposable items. Wear gloves for this step.

40 Wipe off the over-bed table with paper towels. Discard the paper towels.
41 Unscreen the person.
42 Complete a safety check of the room. (See the inside of the front cover.)
43 Follow agency policy for used linens.
44 Remove and discard the gloves. Practice hand hygiene.
45 Report and record your observations.

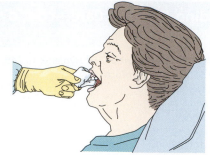

FIGURE 18-8 Remove the upper denture by grasping it with the thumb and index finger of 1 hand. Use a piece of gauze to grasp the denture.

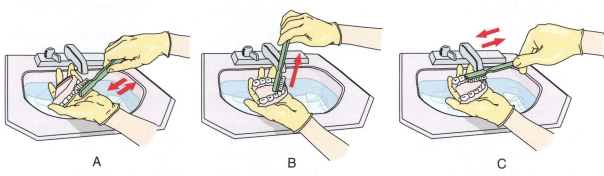

A   B   C

FIGURE 18-9 Cleaning dentures. **A,** Brush the outer surfaces of the denture with back-and-forth motions. (Note that the denture is held over the sink. The sink is lined with a towel and filled half-way with water.) **B,** Position the brush vertically to clean the inner surfaces of the denture. Use upward strokes. **C,** Brush the chewing surfaces with back-and-forth motions.

BATHING

Bathing cleans the skin. It also cleans the mucous membranes of the genital and anal areas. Microbes, dead skin, perspiration, and excess oils are removed. A bath is refreshing and relaxing. Circulation is stimulated and body parts exercised. Observations are made and you have time to talk to the person.

Complete or partial bed baths, tub baths, or showers are given. The method depends on the person's condition, self-care abilities, and personal choice. In hospitals, bathing is common after breakfast. In nursing centers, bathing is usually before or after breakfast or after the evening meal. The person's choice of bath time is respected when possible.

Bathing frequency is a personal matter. Some people bathe daily. Others bathe 1 or 2 times a week. Personal choice, weather, activity, and illness affect bathing. Other illnesses and dry skin may limit bathing to every 2 or 3 days.

The rules for bed baths, showers, and tub baths are listed in Box 18-2.

See *Focus on Communication: Hygiene Needs,* p. 248.
See *Focus on Older Persons: Bathing.*
See *Delegation Guidelines: Bathing.*
See *Promoting Safety and Comfort: Bathing,* p. 258.

BOX 18-2	Rules for Bathing

- Follow the care plan for bathing method and skin care products.
- Allow personal choice when possible.
- Follow Standard Precautions and the Bloodborne Pathogen Standard.
- Collect needed items before the procedure.
- Remove hearing aids before bathing. Water will damage hearing aids.
- Provide for privacy. Screen the person. Close doors and window coverings—drapes, shades, blinds, shutters, and so on.
- Assist with elimination. Bathing stimulates the need to urinate. Comfort and relaxation increase if the person urinates first.
- Cover the person for warmth and privacy.
- Reduce drafts. Close doors and windows.
- Protect the person from falling.
- Use good body mechanics at all times.
- Follow the rules to safely move and transfer the person (Chapters 15 and 16).
- Know what water temperature to use. See *Delegation Guidelines: Bathing.*
- Keep bar soap in the soap dish between latherings. This prevents soapy water. It also prevents slipping and falls in showers and tubs.
- Wash from the cleanest areas to the dirtiest areas.
- Encourage the person to help as much as is safely possible.
- Rinse the skin thoroughly. You must remove all soap.
- Pat dry the skin to avoid irritating or breaking the skin. Do not rub the skin.
- Dry well under the breasts, between skin folds, in the perineal area, and between the toes.
- Bathe skin when urine or feces are present. This prevents skin breakdown and odors.

FOCUS ON OLDER PERSONS

Bathing

Dry skin occurs with aging. Soap also dries the skin. Dry skin is easily damaged. Therefore older persons need a complete bed bath, tub bath, or shower only twice a week. Partial baths are taken on the other days. Some bathe daily but not with soap. Thorough rinsing is needed for soap. Lotions and oils help keep the skin soft.

Bathing procedures can threaten persons with dementia. They do not understand what is happening or why. They may fear harm or danger. Confusion can increase. Some may resist care and become agitated and combative. They may shout at you and cry out for help. Remain calm, patient, and soothing.

The person may be calmer and less confused or agitated during a certain time of day. Bathing is scheduled for calm times.

Persons with dementia may respond well to a *towel bath*. An over-sized towel covers the body from the neck to the feet. The towel is wet with a solution that does not need rinsing—water and cleaning, skin-softening, and drying agents. The drying agent lets the skin dry fast.

The nurse decides the best bathing procedure for the person. The rules in Box 18-2 apply. The care plan also includes measures to help the person through the bath. For example:

- Use terms such as "cleaned up" or "washed" rather than "shower" or "bath."
- Complete pre-procedure activities. For example, ready supplies and linens. Have everything you need.
- Provide for warmth. Prevent drafts. Have extra towels and a robe nearby.
- Provide good lighting.
- Play soft music to help the person relax.
- Provide for safety.
  - Use a hand-held shower nozzle.
  - Have the person use a shower chair or shower bench.
  - Do not use bath oil. It can make the tub or shower slippery. And it may cause a urinary tract infection.
  - Do not leave the person alone in the tub or shower.
- Draw bath water ahead of time. Test the water temperature and adjust as needed.
- Tell the person what you are doing step-by-step. Use clear, simple statements.
- Let the person help as much as possible. For example, give the person a washcloth. Ask him or her to wash the arms. If the person does not know what to do, let the person hold the washcloth if safe to do so.
- Put a towel over the shoulders or lap (tub bath or shower). This helps the person feel less exposed.
- Do not rush the person.
- Use a calm, pleasant voice.
- Distract the person if needed.
- Calm the person.
- Handle the person gently.
- Try a partial bath if a shower or tub bath agitates the person.
- Try the bath later if the person continues to resist care.

DELEGATION GUIDELINES

Bathing

To assist with bathing, you need this information from the nurse and the care plan.

- What bath to give—complete bed bath, partial bath, tub bath, shower, or towel bath.
- How much help the person needs.
- The person's activity or position limits.
- What water temperature to use. Bath water cools rapidly. Heat is lost to the bath basin, over-bed table, washcloth, and your hands. Therefore water temperature for complete bed baths and partial bed baths is usually between 110°F and 115°F (Fahrenheit) (43.3°C and 46.1°C [centigrade]) for adults. Older persons have fragile skin. They need lower water temperatures.
- What skin care products to use and what the person prefers.
- What observations to report and record:
  - The color of the skin, lips, nail beds, and sclera (whites of the eyes)
  - If the skin appears pale, gray-ish, yellow (*jaundice*—Chapter 33), or bluish (*cyanotic*)
  - The location and description of rashes
  - Skin texture—smooth, rough, scaly, flaky, dry, moist
  - *Diaphoresis*—profuse (excessive) sweating
  - Bruises or open skin areas
  - Pale, reddened, or discolored areas, particularly over bony parts
  - Drainage or bleeding from wounds or body openings
  - Swelling of the feet and legs
  - Corns or calluses on the feet
  - Skin temperature (cold, cool, warm, hot)
  - Complaints of pain or discomfort
- When to report observations.
- What patient or resident concerns to report at once.

PROMOTING SAFETY AND COMFORT
Bathing

Safety

Hot water can burn the skin. Measure water temperature according to agency policy. If unsure if the water is too hot, ask the nurse to check it.

Protect the person from drafts, falls, and other injuries. Practice the safety and comfort measures in Chapters 10, 11, and 17.

Use good body mechanics to protect yourself from injury (Chapter 14). For the procedure that follows, you work on 1 side of the bed. To avoid straining and reaching, move the person to the side of the bed near you. Or wash 1 side of the body and then move to the other side to finish the bath. If room space allows, wash the side of the body near you (eyes and face, arm, hand, chest, abdomen, leg, foot). Then move the over-bed table with equipment and supplies to the other side of the bed. Finish the bath (arm, hand, leg, foot, back, and perineal care) on that side.

Apply powder with caution. Do not use powders near persons with respiratory disorders. Inhaling powder can irritate the airway and lungs. Before using powder, check with the nurse and the care plan. To safely apply powder:

- Turn away from the person.
- Sprinkle a small amount onto your hand or a cloth. Do not shake or sprinkle powder onto the person.
- Apply the powder in a thin layer.
- Make sure powder does not get on the floor. Powder is slippery and can cause falls.

Safety—cont'd

You make beds after baths. After making the bed, lower the bed to a safe and comfortable level for the person. Follow the care plan. For an occupied bed, raise or lower bed rails according to the care plan. Make sure the bed wheels are locked.

Protect the person and yourself from infection. During baths and bedmaking, contact with blood, body fluids, secretions, or excretions is likely. Follow Standard Precautions and the Bloodborne Pathogen Standard.

Comfort

Before bathing, let the person meet elimination needs (Chapters 20 and 22). Bathing stimulates the need to urinate. Comfort is greater when the bladder is empty. Also, bathing is not interrupted.

Oral hygiene is common before or after bathing. Allow personal choice and follow the person's care plan.

Provide for warmth. Cover the person with a bath blanket. Make sure the water is warm enough. Cool water causes chilling.

If the person prefers, remove sleepwear after washing the eyes, face, ears, and neck. Removing sleepwear at this time helps the person feel less exposed and provides more mental comfort with the bath.

If the person is able, let him or her wash the genital area. This promotes privacy and helps prevent embarrassment. See "Perineal Care," p. 266.

The Complete Bed Bath

For a complete bed bath, you wash the person's entire body in bed. Bed baths are usually needed by persons who are:

- Unconscious
- Paralyzed
- In casts or traction
- Weak from illness or surgery

A bed bath is new to some people. Some are embarrassed to have their bodies seen. Some fear exposure. Explain how you give the bath. Also explain how you cover the body for privacy.

See procedure: *Giving a Complete Bed Bath.*

Text continued on p. 262.

Giving a Complete Bed Bath

QUALITY OF LIFE

- Knock before entering the person's room.
- Address the person by name.
- Introduce yourself by name and title.

- Explain the procedure before starting and during the procedure.
- Protect the person's rights during the procedure.
- Handle the person gently during the procedure.

PRE-PROCEDURE

1 Follow *Delegation Guidelines: Bathing,* p. 257. See *Promoting Safety and Comfort:*
   a *Hygiene Needs,* p. 248
   b *Bathing*
2 Practice hand hygiene.
3 Identify the person. Check the ID bracelet against the assignment sheet. Use 2 identifiers (Chapter 10). Also call the person by name.
4 Collect clean linens. (See procedure: *Making a Closed Bed* in Chapter 17.) Place linens on a clean surface.
5 Collect the following.
   - Wash basin
   - Soap
   - Water thermometer
   - Orangewood stick or nail file

- Washcloth (and at least 4 washcloths for perineal care, p. 266)
- 2 bath towels and 2 hand towels
- Bath blanket
- Clothing or sleepwear
- Lotion and powder
- Deodorant or antiperspirant
- Brush and comb
- Other grooming items as requested
- Paper towels
- Gloves
6 Cover the over-bed table with paper towels. Arrange items on the over-bed table. Adjust the height as needed.
7 Provide for privacy.
8 Raise the bed for body mechanics. Bed rails are up if used. Lower the bed rail near you if up.

PROCEDURE

9 Practice hand hygiene. Put on gloves.
10 Remove the sleepwear. Do not expose the person. Follow agency policy for used sleepwear.
11 Cover the person with a bath blanket. Remove top linens (see procedure: *Making an Occupied Bed* in Chapter 17).
12 Lower the head of the bed. It is as flat as possible. The person has a least 1 pillow.
13 Fill the wash basin ⅔ (two-thirds) full with water. Raise the bed rail before leaving the bedside. Follow the care plan for water temperature. Water temperature is usually 110°F to 115°F (43.3°C to 46.1°C) for adults. Measure water temperature. Use the water thermometer. Or dip your elbow or inner wrist into the basin to test the water.
14 Lower the bed rail near you if up.

15 Have the person check the water temperature. Adjust the water temperature as needed. Raise the bed rail before leaving the bedside. Lower it when you return.
16 Place the basin on the over-bed table.
17 Place a hand towel over the person's chest.
18 Make a mitt with the washcloth (Fig. 18-10). Use a mitt for the entire bath.
19 Have the person close the eyes. Wash the eyelids and around the eyes with water. Do not use soap.
   a Clean the far eye. Gently wipe from the inner to the outer aspect of the eye with a corner of the mitt (Fig. 18-11).
   b Clean around the eye near you. Use a clean part of the washcloth for each stroke.

Continued

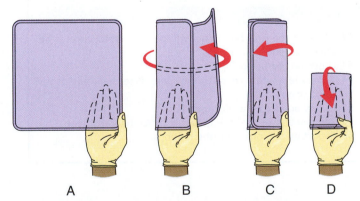

FIGURE 18-10 Making a mitted washcloth. **A,** Grasp the near side of the washcloth with your thumb. **B,** Bring the washcloth around and behind your hand. **C,** Fold the side of the washcloth over your palm as you grasp it with your thumb. **D,** Fold the top of the washcloth down and tuck it under next to your palm.

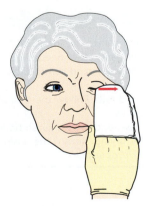

FIGURE 18-11 Wash the eyes with a mitted washcloth. Wipe from the inner to the outer aspect of the eye.

Giving a Complete Bed Bath—cont'd

PROCEDURE—cont'd

20 Ask if the person wants soap to wash the face.
21 Wash the face, ears, and neck. Rinse and pat dry with the towel on the chest.
22 Help the person move to the side of the bed near you.
23 Expose the far arm. Place a bath towel length-wise under the arm. Apply soap to the washcloth.
24 Support the arm with your palm under the person's elbow. His or her forearm rests on your forearm.
25 Wash the arm, shoulder, and underarm. Use long, firm strokes (Fig. 18-12). Rinse and pat dry.
26 Place the basin on the towel. Put the person's hand into the water (Fig. 18-13). Wash the hand well. Clean under the fingernails with an orangewood stick or nail file.
27 Have the person exercise the hand and fingers.
28 Remove the basin. Dry the hand well. Cover the arm with the bath blanket.
29 Repeat steps 23 to 28 for the near arm.
30 Place a bath towel over the chest cross-wise. Hold the towel in place. Pull the bath blanket from under the towel to the waist. Apply soap to the washcloth.
31 Lift the towel slightly and wash the chest (Fig. 18-14). Do not expose the person. Rinse and pat dry, especially under the breasts.
32 Move the towel length-wise over the chest and abdomen. Do not expose the person. Pull the bath blanket down to the pubic area. Apply soap to the washcloth.
33 Lift the towel slightly and wash the abdomen (Fig. 18-15). Rinse and pat dry.
34 Pull the bath blanket up to the shoulders. Cover both arms. Remove the towel.
35 Change soapy or cool water. Measure bath water temperature as in step 13. If bed rails are used, raise the bed rail near you before leaving the bedside. Lower it when you return.
36 Uncover the far leg. Do not expose the genital area. Place a towel length-wise under the foot and leg. Apply soap to a washcloth.
37 Bend the knee and support the leg with your arm. Wash it with long, firm strokes. Rinse and pat dry.
38 Place the basin on the towel near the foot.
39 Lift the leg slightly. Slide the basin under the foot.

40 Place the foot in the basin (Fig. 18-16). Use an orangewood stick or nail file to clean under the toenails if necessary. If the person cannot bend the knees:
  a Wash the foot. Carefully separate the toes. Rinse and pat dry.
  b Clean under the toenails with an orangewood stick or nail file if necessary.
41 Remove the basin. Dry the leg and foot. Apply lotion to the foot if directed by the nurse and care plan. Cover the leg with the bath blanket. Remove the towel.
42 Repeat steps 36 to 41 for the near leg.
43 Change the water. Measure water temperature as in step 13. Raise the bed rail near you before leaving the bedside. Lower it when you return.
44 Turn the person onto the side away from you. The person is covered with the bath blanket.
45 Uncover the back and buttocks. Do not expose the person. Place a towel length-wise on the bed along the back. Apply soap to a washcloth.
46 Wash the back. Work from the back of the neck to the lower end of the buttocks. Use long, firm, continuous strokes (Fig. 18-17). Rinse and dry well.
47 Turn the person onto his or her back.
48 Change water for perineal care (p. 266). See step 14 in procedure: *Giving Female Perineal Care* (p. 268) for water temperature. (Some state competency tests also require changing gloves and hand hygiene at this time.) Raise the bed rail near you before leaving the bedside. Lower it when you return.
49 Allow the person to perform perineal care if able. Provide perineal care if the person cannot do so (p. 266). At least 4 washcloths are used. (Practice hand hygiene and wear gloves for perineal care.)
50 Remove and discard the gloves. Practice hand hygiene.
51 Give a back massage (Chapter 17).
52 Apply lotion, powder, and deodorant or antiperspirant as requested. See *Promoting Safety and Comfort: Bathing,* p. 258.
53 Put clean garments on the person (Chapter 19).
54 Comb and brush the person's hair (Chapter 19).
55 Make the bed.

POST-PROCEDURE

56 Provide for comfort. (See the inside of the front cover.)
57 Place the call light and other needed items within reach.
58 Lower the bed to a safe and comfortable level. Follow the care plan.
59 Raise or lower bed rails. Follow the care plan.
60 Put on clean gloves.
61 Empty, clean, rinse, and dry the wash basin. Use clean, dry paper towels for drying. Return the basin and other supplies to their proper place.

62 Wipe off the over-bed table with paper towels. Discard the paper towels.
63 Unscreen the person.
64 Complete a safety check of the room. (See the inside of the front cover.)
65 Follow agency policy for used linens.
66 Remove and discard the gloves. Practice hand hygiene.
67 Report and record your observations.

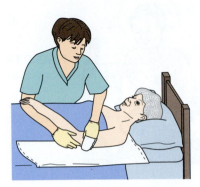

FIGURE 18-12 The arm is washed with firm, long strokes using a mitted washcloth. (NOTE: Bed rails are used according to the care plan.)

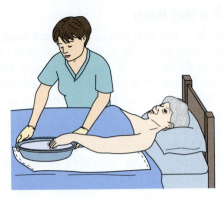

FIGURE 18-13 The hand is washed by placing the wash basin on the bed. (NOTE: Bed rails are used according to the care plan.)

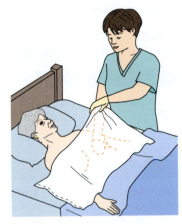

FIGURE 18-14 The breasts are not exposed during the bath. A bath towel is placed horizontally over the chest area. The towel is lifted slightly to reach under and wash the breasts and chest.

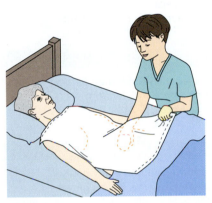

FIGURE 18-15 The bath towel is turned so that it is vertical to cover the breasts and abdomen. The towel is lifted slightly to bathe the abdomen. The bath blanket covers the pubic area.

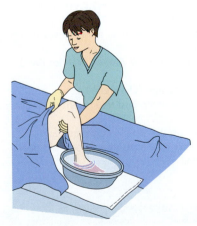

FIGURE 18-16 The foot is washed by placing it in the wash basin on the bed.

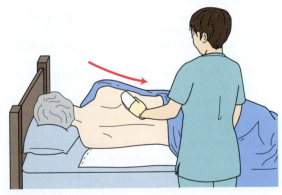

FIGURE 18-17 The back is washed with long, firm, continuous strokes. Note that the person is in a side-lying position. A towel is placed length-wise on the bed to protect the linens from water. (NOTE: Bed rails are used according to the care plan.)

The Partial Bath

For a *partial bath*, the face, hands, underarms, back, buttocks, and perineal area are washed. Bathing prevents odors and discomfort in those areas. Some persons can wash in bed or at the sink. You assist as needed. Most need help washing the back. You give partial baths to persons who cannot bathe themselves.

The rules for bathing apply (see Box 18-2). So do the complete bed bath considerations.

See procedure: *Assisting With the Partial Bath*.

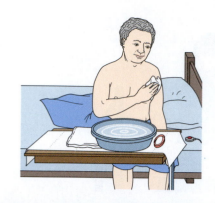

FIGURE 18-18 The person is bathing himself while sitting on the side of the bed. Needed equipment is within reach.

Assisting With the Partial Bath

QUALITY OF LIFE

- Knock before entering the person's room.
- Address the person by name.
- Introduce yourself by name and title.

- Explain the procedure before starting and during the procedure.
- Protect the person's rights during the procedure.
- Handle the person gently during the procedure.

PRE-PROCEDURE

1 Follow *Delegation Guidelines: Bathing*, p. 257. See *Promoting Safety and Comfort*:
   a *Hygiene Needs*, p. 248
   b *Bathing*, p. 258

2 Follow steps 2 through 7 in procedure: *Giving a Complete Bed Bath*, p. 259.

PROCEDURE

3 Make sure the bed is in a low position.
4 Practice hand hygiene. Put on gloves.
5 Cover the person with a bath blanket. Remove top linens.
6 Fill the wash basin ⅔ (two-thirds) full with water. Water temperature is usually 110°F to 115°F (43.3°C to 46.1°C) or as directed by the nurse. Measure water temperature with the water thermometer. Or test bath water by dipping your elbow or inner wrist into the basin.
7 Have the person check the water temperature. Adjust the water temperature as needed.
8 Place the basin on the over-bed table.
9 Position the person in Fowler's position. Or assist him or her to sit at the bedside.
10 Adjust the over-bed table so the person can reach the basin and supplies.
11 Help the person undress. Use the bath blanket for privacy and warmth.
12 Have the person wash easy-to-reach body parts (Fig. 18-18). Explain that you will wash the back and areas the person cannot reach.
13 Place the call light within reach. Have the person signal when help is needed or bathing is complete.

14 Remove and discard the gloves. Practice hand hygiene. Then leave the room.
15 Return when the call light is on. Knock before entering. Practice hand hygiene.
16 Change the bath water. Measure bath water temperature as in step 6.
17 Raise the bed for body mechanics. The far bed rail is up if used.
18 Ask what was washed. Put on gloves. Wash and dry areas the person could not reach. The face, hands, underarms, back, buttocks, and perineal area are washed for the partial bath.
19 Remove and discard the gloves. Practice hand hygiene.
20 Give a back massage (Chapter 17).
21 Apply lotion, powder, and deodorant or antiperspirant as requested.
22 Help the person put on clean garments.
23 Assist with hair care and other grooming needs.
24 Make the bed.

POST-PROCEDURE

25 Provide for comfort. (See the inside of the front cover.)
26 Place the call light and other needed items within reach.
27 Lower the bed to a safe and comfortable level. Follow the care plan.
28 Raise or lower bed rails. Follow the care plan.
29 Put on clean gloves.
30 Empty, clean, rinse, and dry the bath basin. Use clean, dry paper towels for drying. Return the basin and supplies to their proper place.

31 Wipe off the over-bed table with the paper towels. Discard the paper towels.
32 Unscreen the person.
33 Complete a safety check of the room. (See the inside of the front cover.)
34 Follow agency policy for used linens.
35 Remove and discard the gloves. Practice hand hygiene.
36 Report and record your observations.

Tub Baths and Showers

Some people like tub baths. Others like showers. Falls, burns, and chilling from water are risks. Safety is important (Box 18-3). The measures in Box 18-2 also apply. Also follow the nurse's directions and the care plan.

Tub Baths.   Tub baths are relaxing. A tub bath can make a person feel faint, weak, or tired. These are great risks for persons who were on bedrest. A tub bath lasts no longer than 20 minutes.

To get in and out of the tub, the person may use:
- A tub with a side entry door (Fig. 18-19).
- Bathing lift. The device transports and lifts the person into the tub (Fig. 18-20).
- Mechanical lift (Chapter 16).

Whirlpool tubs have a cleansing action. You wash the upper body. Carefully wash under the breasts and between skin folds. Also wash the perineal area. Pat dry the person with towels after the bath.

BOX 18-3	Tub Bath and Shower Safety

- Clean, disinfect, and dry the tub or shower before and after use.
- Dry the tub or shower room floor.
- Make sure hand rails, grab bars (safety bars), hydraulic lifts, and other safety aids are in working order.
- Place a bath mat in the tub or on the shower floor. This is not needed if there are non-skid strips or a non-skid surface.
- Provide for warmth and privacy. This includes during transport to and from the shower or tub room.
- Place the call light and other needed items within reach.
- Show the person how to use the call light in the shower or tub room.
- Have the person use grab bars (safety bars) to get in and out of the tub. Towel bars are not used for support.
- Follow the safety measures for wheelchairs when using wheeled shower chairs. See Chapter 16.
- Know what water temperature to use (usually 105°F/40.5°C).
- Turn cold water on first, then hot water. Turn hot water off first, then cold water.
- Adjust water temperature and pressure to prevent chilling or burns. Do this before the person gets into the shower.
- Direct water away from the person to adjust the water temperature and pressure.

- Fill the tub before the person gets into it. For a tub with a side entry door, fill the tub with the person in it. Follow the manufacturer's instructions. Closely check water temperature as the tub fills.
- Measure water temperature. For showers and tub baths, use the digital display. Or you use a water thermometer for a tub bath.
- Keep the water spray directed toward the person during the shower. This helps keep him or her warm. (NOTE: Do not direct the water spray toward the face. This can frighten the person.)
- Keep bar soap in the soap dish between latherings. This helps prevent slipping and falls in showers and tubs. It also prevents soapy tub water.
- Avoid bath oils. They make tub and shower surfaces slippery.
- Do not leave weak or unsteady persons unattended.
- Stay within hearing distance if the person can be left alone. Wait outside the shower curtain or door. You must be nearby if the person calls for you or has an accident.
- Drain the tub before the person gets out of the tub. Turn off the shower before the person gets out of the shower. Cover him or her to provide privacy and prevent chilling.

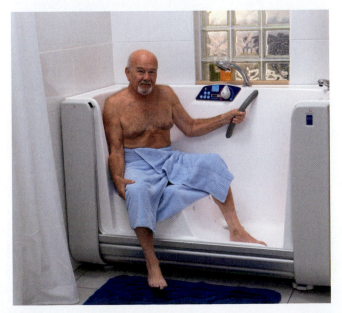

FIGURE 18-19 Tub with a side entry door. (Courtesy ARJOHUNTLEIGH, Addison, Ill., 800-307-2756.)

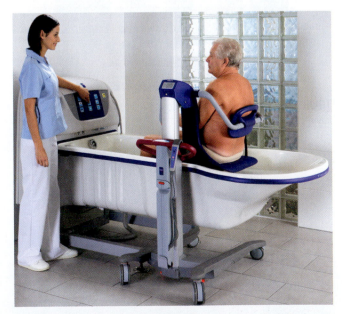

FIGURE 18-20 The lift lowers the person into the tub. (Courtesy ARJOHUNTLEIGH, Addison, Ill., 800-307-2756.)

Showers.   Some people can stand during a shower. Grab bars (safety bars) are used for support. Showers have non-skid surfaces. If not, a bath mat is used. Weak or unsteady persons use:

- *Shower chairs.* Water drains through an opening (Fig. 18-21). You use the chair to transport the person to and from the shower. Lock (brake) the wheels during the shower to prevent the chair from moving.
- *Shower stalls or cabinets.* The person walks into the device or is wheeled to the cabinet in a wheelchair (Fig. 18-22). Use the hand-held nozzle for the shower.
- *Shower trolleys (portable tubs).* The person has a shower lying down (Fig. 18-23). Lower the sides to transfer the person from the bed to the trolley. Then raise the side rails to transport the person to the tub or shower room. Use the hand-held nozzle to give the shower.

Some shower rooms have 2 or more stations. Provide for privacy. Properly screen and cover the person. Also close doors and shower curtains.

See *Delegation Guidelines: Tub Baths and Showers.*

See *Promoting Safety and Comfort: Tub Baths and Showers.*

See procedure: *Assisting With a Tub Bath or Shower.*

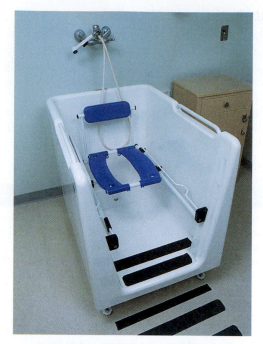

FIGURE 18-22   A shower cabinet.

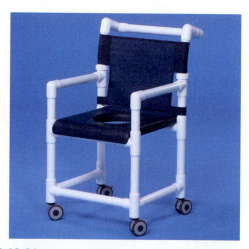

FIGURE 18-21   A shower chair. (Courtesy Innovative Products Unlimited, Niles, Mich.)

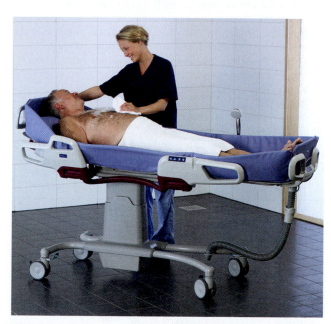

FIGURE 18-23   Shower trolley. The sides are lowered for transfers into and out of the trolley. (Courtesy ARJOHUNTLEIGH, Addison, Ill., 800-307-2756.)

DELEGATION GUIDELINES
Tub Baths and Showers

Before assisting with a tub bath or shower, you need this information from the nurse and the care plan:

- If the person takes a tub bath or shower
- What water temperature to use (usually 105°F/40.5°C)
- What equipment is needed—bathing lift, mechanical lift, shower chair, shower cabinet, shower trolley, and so on
- How much help the person needs
- If the person can bathe himself or herself
- What observations to report and record:
  - Dizziness
  - Light-headedness
  - See *Delegation Guidelines: Bathing*, p. 257
- When to report observations
- What patient or resident concerns to report at once

PROMOTING SAFETY AND COMFORT
Tub Baths and Showers

Safety

Some persons are very weak. At least 2 staff are needed for safe tub baths and showers. If the person is heavy, 3 or more staff may be needed.

The person may use a tub with a side entry door, a shower chair, a shower trolley, or other device. Follow the manufacturer's instructions.

Protect the person from falls, chilling, and burns. Follow the safety measures in Chapters 10 and 11. Remember to measure water temperature.

Clean, disinfect, and dry the tub or shower before and after use. This prevents the spread of microbes and infection.

Comfort

Warmth and privacy promote comfort during tub baths and showers.

- Make sure the tub or shower room is warm.
- Provide for privacy. Close the room door, screen the person, and close window coverings.
- Make sure the water is warm enough for the person.
- Have the person remove clothing or robe and footwear just before getting into the tub or shower. Do not have the person exposed longer than necessary.
- Leave the room if the person can be left alone. Stay within hearing distance.

Assisting With a Tub Bath or Shower

QUALITY OF LIFE

- Knock before entering the person's room.
- Address the person by name.
- Introduce yourself by name and title.

- Explain the procedure before starting and during the procedure.
- Protect the person's rights during the procedure.
- Handle the person gently during the procedure.

PRE-PROCEDURE

1 Follow *Delegation Guidelines:*
   a *Bathing*, p. 257
   b *Tub Baths and Showers*
   See *Promoting Safety and Comfort:*
   a *Hygiene Needs*, p. 248
   b *Bathing*, p. 258
   c *Tub Baths and Showers*
2 Reserve the tub or shower room.
3 Practice hand hygiene.
4 Identify the person. Check the ID bracelet against the assignment sheet. Use 2 identifiers (Chapter 10). Also call the person by name.

5 Collect the following.
- Washcloth and 2 bath towels
- Bath blanket
- Soap
- Water thermometer (for a tub bath)
- Clothing or sleepwear
- Grooming items as requested
- Robe and non-skid footwear
- Rubber bath mat if needed
- Disposable bath mat
- Gloves
- Wheelchair, shower chair, and so on as needed

PROCEDURE

6 Place items in the tub or shower room. Use the space provided or a chair.
7 Clean, disinfect, and dry the tub or shower. Use clean, dry paper towels for drying. Wear gloves for this step. Practice hand hygiene after removing and discarding the gloves.
8 Place a rubber bath mat in the tub or on the shower floor. Do not block the drain.
9 Place the disposable bath mat on the floor in front of the tub or shower.

10 Put the OCCUPIED sign on the door.
11 Return to the person's room. Provide for privacy. Practice hand hygiene.
12 Help the person sit on the side of the bed.
13 Help the person put on a robe and non-skid footwear. Or the person can leave on clothing.
14 Assist or transport the person to the tub or shower room.
15 Have the person sit on a chair if he or she walked to the tub or shower room.

Continued

Assisting With a Tub Bath or Shower—cont'd

PROCEDURE—cont'd

16 Provide for privacy.
17 *For a tub bath:*
  a Fill the tub half-way with warm water (usually 105°F/40.5°C). Follow the care plan for water temperature.
  b Measure water temperature. Use the water thermometer or check the digital display.
  c Have the person check the water temperature. Adjust the water temperature as needed.
18 *For a shower:*
  a Turn on the shower.
  b Adjust water temperature and pressure. Check the digital display. Water temperature is usually 105°F/40.5°C.
  c Have the person check the water temperature. Adjust the water temperature as needed.
19 Help the person undress and remove footwear.
20 Help the person into the tub or shower. Position the shower chair and lock (brake) the wheels.
21 Assist with washing as necessary. Wear gloves.
22 Have the person use the call light when done or when help is needed. Remind the person that a tub bath lasts no longer than 20 minutes.

23 Place a towel across the chair.
24 Leave the room if the person can bathe alone. If not, stay in the room or nearby. Remove and discard the gloves and practice hand hygiene if you will leave the room.
25 Check the person at least every 5 minutes.
26 Return when the person signals for you. Knock before entering. Practice hand hygiene.
27 Turn off the shower or drain the tub. Cover the person with the bath blanket while the tub drains.
28 Help the person out of the shower or tub and onto the chair.
29 Help the person dry off. Pat gently. Dry well under the breasts, between skin folds, in the perineal area, and between the toes.
30 Apply lotion, powder, and deodorant or antiperspirant as requested.
31 Help the person dress and put on footwear.
32 Help the person return to the room. Provide for privacy.
33 Assist the person to a chair or into bed.
34 Provide a back massage if the person returns to bed (Chapter 17).
35 Assist with hair care and other grooming needs.

POST-PROCEDURE

36 Provide for comfort. (See the inside of the front cover.)
37 Place the call light and other needed items within reach.
38 Raise or lower bed rails. Follow the care plan.
39 Unscreen the person.
40 Complete a safety check of the room. (See the inside of the front cover.)
41 Clean, disinfect, and dry the tub or shower. Dry the tub or shower room floor. Remove soiled linens. Wear gloves.

42 Discard disposable items. Put the UNOCCUPIED sign on the door. Return supplies to their proper place.
43 Follow agency policy for used linens.
44 Remove and discard the gloves. Practice hand hygiene.
45 Report and record your observations.

PERINEAL CARE

Perineal care (pericare) involves cleaning the genital and anal areas. These areas provide a warm, moist, and dark place for microbes to grow. Cleaning prevents infection and odors and promotes comfort.

Perineal care is done daily during the bath. It also is done when the area is soiled with urine or feces. Perineal care is very important for persons who:

- Have urinary catheters (Chapter 21).
- Have had rectal or genital surgery.
- Are menstruating (Chapter 8).
- Are incontinent of urine or feces (Chapters 20 and 22).
- Are uncircumcised (Fig. 18-24). Being *circumcised means that the fold of skin (foreskin) covering the glans of the penis was surgically removed.* Being *uncircumcised means that the male has foreskin covering the head of the penis.*

The person does perineal care if able. Otherwise, the nursing staff does so. This procedure embarrasses many people and staff, especially when it involves the other sex.

Perineal and *perineum* are not common terms. Most people understand *privates, private parts, crotch, genitals,* or *the area between your legs.* Use terms the person understands and that sound professional. Do not use slang or vulgar terms.

Work from the cleanest area to the dirtiest. This is commonly called from *front to back* or *top to bottom.* The urethral area (front or top) is the cleanest. The anal area (back or bottom) is the dirtiest. Therefore clean from the urethra to the anal area. This prevents spreading bacteria from the anal area to the vagina and urinary system.

The perineal area is delicate and easily injured. Use warm water, not hot. Use washcloths, towelettes, cotton balls, or swabs according to agency policy. Rinse thoroughly. Pat dry after rinsing. This reduces moisture and promotes comfort.

See *Focus on Communication: Perineal Care.*
See *Delegation Guidelines: Perineal Care.*
See *Promoting Safety and Comfort: Perineal Care.*
See procedure: *Giving Female Perineal Care, p. 268.*
See procedure: *Giving Male Perineal Care, p. 270.*

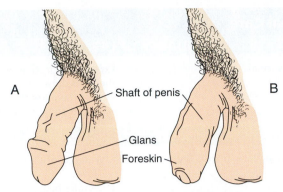

FIGURE 18-24 A, Circumcised male. **B,** Uncircumcised male.

Giving Female Perineal Care

QUALITY OF LIFE

- Knock before entering the person's room.
- Address the person by name.
- Introduce yourself by name and title.

- Explain the procedure before starting and during the procedure.
- Protect the person's rights during the procedure.
- Handle the person gently during the procedure.

PRE-PROCEDURE

1 Follow *Delegation Guidelines: Perineal Care*, p. 267. See *Promoting Safety and Comfort:*
  a *Hygiene Needs*, p. 248
  b *Perineal Care*, p. 267
2 Practice hand hygiene.
3 Collect the following.
  - Soap or other cleansing agent as directed
  - At least 4 washcloths
  - Bath towel
  - Bath blanket
  - Water thermometer
  - Wash basin

  - Waterproof under-pad
  - Gloves
  - Laundry bag
  - Paper towels
4 Cover the over-bed table with paper towels. Arrange items on top of them.
5 Identify the person. Check the ID bracelet against the assignment sheet. Use 2 identifiers (Chapter 10). Also call the person by name.
6 Provide for privacy.
7 Raise the bed for body mechanics. Bed rails are up if used.

PROCEDURE

8 Lower the bed rail near you if up.
9 Practice hand hygiene. Put on gloves.
10 Cover the person with a bath blanket. Move top linens to the foot of the bed.
11 Position the person on the back.
12 Drape the person as in Figure 18-25.
13 Raise the bed rail if used.
14 Fill the wash basin. Water temperature is usually 105°F to 109°F (40.5°C to 42.7°C). Follow the care plan for water temperature. Measure water temperature according to agency policy.
15 Have the person check the water temperature. Adjust the water temperature as needed. Raise the bed rail before leaving the bedside. Lower it when you return.
16 Place the basin on the over-bed table.
17 Lower the bed rail if up.
18 Help the person flex her knees and spread her legs. Or help her spread her legs as much as possible with the knees straight.
19 Fold the corner of the bath blanket between her legs onto her abdomen.

20 Place a waterproof under-pad under her buttocks. Remove any wet or soiled incontinence products.
21 Remove and discard the gloves. Practice hand hygiene. Put on clean gloves.
22 Wet the washcloths.
23 Squeeze out water from a washcloth. Make a mitted washcloth. Apply soap. (Squeeze out water every time you change washcloths. Do not place used washcloths back in the basin. Put used washcloths in the laundry bag.)
24 Clean the perineum. Change washcloths as needed.
  a Separate the labia.
  b Clean 1 side of the labia. Clean downward from front to back (top to bottom) with 1 stroke (Fig. 18-26, A). Use 1 part of a washcloth.
  c Clean the other side of the labia. Clean downward from front to back (top to bottom) with 1 stroke (Fig. 18-26, B). Use a clean part of a washcloth.
  d Clean the vaginal area. Clean downward from front to back (top to bottom) with 1 stroke (Fig. 18-26, C). Use a clean part of a washcloth.

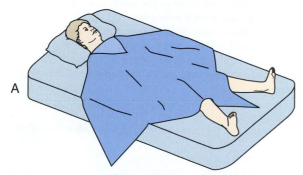
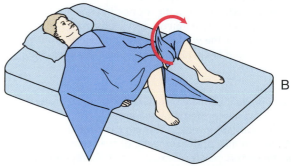

FIGURE 18-25 Draping for perineal care. **A,** Position the bath blanket like a diamond: 1 corner is at the neck, there is a corner at each side, and 1 corner is between the legs. **B,** Wrap the blanket around a leg by bringing the corner around the leg and over the top. Tuck the corner under the hip. Repeat for the other leg.

Giving Female Perineal Care—cont'd

PROCEDURE—cont'd

25 Rinse the perineum with a clean washcloth. Change washcloths as needed.
  a Separate the labia.
  b Rinse 1 side of the labia. Rinse downward from front to back (top to bottom) with 1 stroke. Use 1 part of a washcloth.
  c Rinse the other side of the labia. Rinse downward from front to back (top to bottom) with 1 stroke. Use a clean part of a washcloth.
  d Rinse the vaginal area. Rinse downward from front to back (top to bottom) with 1 stroke. Use a clean part of a washcloth.
26 Pat dry the perineal area with the towel. Dry from front to back (top to bottom).
27 Fold the blanket back between her legs.
28 Help the person lower her legs and turn onto her side away from you.
29 Apply soap to a clean mitted washcloth.

30 Clean and rinse the rectal area.
  a Clean from the vagina to the anus with 1 stroke (Fig. 18-27). Use 1 part of the washcloth.
  b Repeat steps 29 and 30-a until the area is clean. Use a clean part of the washcloth for each stroke. Change washcloths as needed.
  c Rinse the rectal area with a clean washcloth. Rinse from the vagina to the anus. Repeat as necessary. Use a clean part of the washcloth for each stroke. Change washcloths as needed.
31 Pat dry the rectal area with the towel. Dry from the vagina to the anus.
32 Remove the waterproof under-pad.
33 Remove and discard the gloves. Practice hand hygiene. Put on clean gloves.
34 Provide clean and dry linens and incontinence products as needed.
35 Position the person on her back.

POST-PROCEDURE

36 Cover the person. Remove the bath blanket.
37 Provide for comfort. (See the inside of the front cover.)
38 Place the call light and other needed items within reach.
39 Lower the bed to a safe and comfortable level. Follow the care plan.
40 Raise or lower bed rails. Follow the care plan.
41 Empty, clean, rinse, and dry the wash basin. Use clean, dry paper towels for drying.
42 Return the basin and supplies to their proper place.

43 Wipe off the over-bed table with the paper towels. Discard the paper towels.
44 Unscreen the person.
45 Complete a safety check of the room. (See the inside of the front cover.)
46 Follow agency policy for used linens.
47 Remove and discard the gloves. Practice hand hygiene.
48 Report and record your observations.

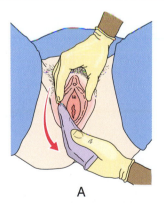 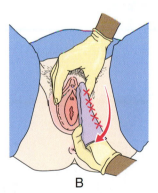 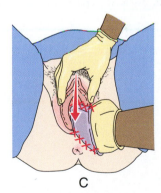

A   B   C

FIGURE 18-26 Cleaning the perineum. **A,** Separate the labia with 1 hand. Use a mitted washcloth to clean 1 side of the labia with a downward stroke. **B,** Clean the other side of the labia with a clean part of the washcloth. Use a downward stroke. **C,** Clean the vaginal area with a clean part of the washcloth. Use a downward stroke. (NOTE: Used areas of the washcloth are marked with Xs.)

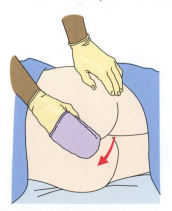

FIGURE 18-27 Clean the rectal area by wiping from the vagina to the anus. The side-lying position allows thorough cleaning of the anal area.

Giving Male Perineal Care

QUALITY OF LIFE

- Knock before entering the person's room.
- Address the person by name.
- Introduce yourself by name and title.

- Explain the procedure before starting and during the procedure.
- Protect the person's rights during the procedure.
- Handle the person gently during the procedure.

PROCEDURE

1 Follow steps 1 through 17 in procedure: *Giving Female Perineal Care, p. 268*. Drape the person as in Figure 18-25.
2 Fold the corner of the bath blanket between the legs onto the person's abdomen.
3 Place a waterproof under-pad under the buttocks. Remove any wet or soiled incontinence products.
4 Remove and discard the gloves. Practice hand hygiene. Put on clean gloves.
5 Wet the washcloths.
6 Squeeze out water from a washcloth. Make a mitted washcloth. Apply soap. (Squeeze out water every time you change washcloths. Do not place used washcloths back in the basin. Put used washcloths in the laundry bag.)
7 Retract the foreskin if the person is uncircumcised (Fig. 18-28).
8 Grasp the penis.
9 Clean the tip. Use a circular motion. Start at the meatus and work outward (Fig. 18-29, A). Repeat as needed. Use a clean part of the washcloth each time.
10 Rinse the tip with another washcloth. Use the same circular motion.
11 Return the foreskin to its natural position immediately after rinsing.
12 Clean the shaft of the penis. Use firm downward strokes (Fig. 18-29, B). Use a clean part of a washcloth for each stroke.

13 Rinse the shaft. Use the same downward motion as in step 12. Use a clean part of a washcloth for each stroke.
14 Help the person flex his knees and spread his legs. Or help him spread his legs as much as possible with his knees straight.
15 Clean the scrotum. Use a clean part of a washcloth.
16 Rinse the scrotum. Use a clean part of a washcloth. Observe for redness and irritation of the skin folds.
17 Pat dry the penis and the scrotum. Use the towel.
18 Fold the bath blanket back between his legs.
19 Help him lower his legs and turn onto his side away from you.
20 Clean the rectal area. Clean from the scrotum (front or top) to the anus (back or bottom). (See procedure: *Giving Female Perineal Care, p. 268*). Rinse and dry well.
21 Remove the waterproof under-pad.
22 Remove and discard the gloves. Practice hand hygiene. Put on clean gloves.
23 Provide clean and dry linens and incontinence products.
24 Position the person on his back.
25 Follow steps 36 through 48 in procedure: *Giving Female Perineal Care, p. 269*.

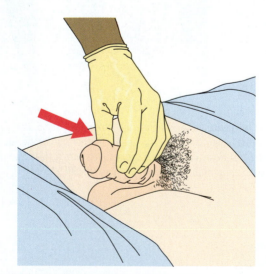

FIGURE 18-28 Pull back the foreskin of the uncircumcised male for perineal care. Return it to the normal position immediately after cleaning and rinsing.

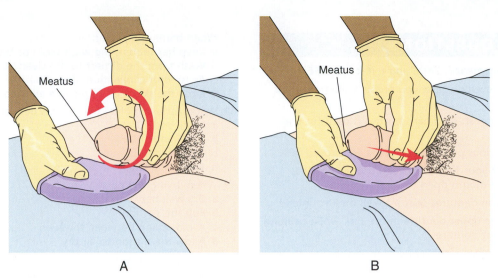

FIGURE 18-29 Cleaning the penis. **A,** Clean the tip with a circular motion starting at the meatus. **B,** Clean the shaft with downward strokes.

FOCUS ON P R I D E

The Person, Family, and Yourself

Personal and Professional Responsibility

Patients and residents depend on you for hygiene needs. You are responsible for maintaining or improving the person's quality of life, health, and safety. To do so:
- Follow the guidelines and procedures in this chapter.
- Focus on the "Quality of Life" section at the beginning of each procedure.
- View the person as an individual with unique needs. Ask about the person's needs and preferences.

Take pride in giving care that helps the person's over-all well-being.

Rights and Respect

Patients and residents have the right to choose schedules and routines. They also have the right to refuse care. Some persons refuse if it does not meet their preferences. For example:
- A resident refuses a shower because he or she prefers a bath.
- A patient prefers to bathe at night, not in the morning.
- A male resident prefers care by a male nursing assistant, not a female.

Refusing care for these reasons does not mean the person refuses to be clean. The person may accept if preferences are met. Tell the nurse of any refusal. Adjust as needed to respect the person's preferences.

Independence and Social Interaction

Hygiene is a personal matter. Allow personal choice for such matters as bath time, products used, and what to wear. Encourage the person to do as much self-care as safely possible. Doing so promotes independence and improves self-esteem.

Delegation and Teamwork

Some agencies have commercial warmers for bath blankets. If a warmer is getting low, fill it. Otherwise, staff find an empty warmer. A co-worker has to fill it and wait for a blanket to heat up.

Avoid having the attitude that "someone else can do it." This shows poor teamwork and work ethics. Take pride in being a helpful and courteous team member.

Ethics and Laws

You will perform some tasks often. Bathing and other personal hygiene measures are examples. Over time, some staff become less careful with routine tasks. They may forget about dangers. Or they think that nothing bad will happen. This is very unsafe.

Always be careful. Harm can result from routine care measures. Follow the safety measures in this chapter at all times.

FOCUS ON PRIDE: *Application*

The care measures in this chapter are private and personal. At first, you may feel embarrassed. This improves with practice and experience. What concerns do you have about the procedures in this chapter? How will you stay calm and professional and ease the person's worries?

REVIEW QUESTIONS

Circle T if the statement is TRUE and F if it is FALSE.

1 **T F** During evening care, you prepare the person for sleep.

2 **T F** A toothbrush with hard bristles is used for oral hygiene.

3 **T F** Unconscious persons are supine for mouth care.

4 **T F** You use your fingers to keep the unconscious person's mouth open for oral hygiene.

5 **T F** You clean dentures over a towel on a counter.

6 **T F** Place the upper denture in the sink while cleaning the lower denture.

7 **T F** A person has a partial denture. Natural teeth are brushed.

8 **T F** To wash the eye, wash from the inner to the outer aspect.

9 **T F** A tub bath lasts 30 minutes.

10 **T F** Washcloths are rinsed and re-used during perineal care.

11 **T F** Foreskin is returned to its normal position immediately after rinsing.

Circle the BEST answer.

12 When assisting with daily care, you
   a Clean an incontinent person as often as needed
   b Give early morning care after breakfast
   c Follow your own routines and habits
   d Change soiled linens in the afternoon

13 You perform oral hygiene to
   a Prevent aspiration
   b Remove excess oils and perspiration
   c Prevent mouth odors and infection
   d Remove cavities

14 When is the best time to floss?
   a In the morning
   b Before a meal
   c Before brushing
   d At bedtime

15 Which must you report to the nurse?
   a Clean skin
   b Moist and intact lips
   c A bruise on the arm
   d Food between the teeth

16 To apply powder
   a Turn the person toward you
   b Sprinkle a small amount onto your hand
   c Apply a thick layer of powder
   d Shake the powder onto the person

17 When bathing a person
   a Keep bar soap in the wash basin or tub
   b Wash from the dirtiest to the cleanest area
   c Assist with elimination after a bath
   d Rinse the skin well to remove all soap

18 Water for a complete bed bath is between
   a 100°F and 104°F
   b 105°F and 109°F
   c 110°F and 115°F
   d 120°F and 125°F

19 When drying the person
   a Dry well between skin folds
   b Rub the skin dry
   c Avoid drying between the toes
   d Allow the person to air dry

20 When assisting with a shower in a shower room
   a Direct the water spray at the person's face
   b Allow a weak person to stand if you provide support
   c Go to the person's room to make the bed during the shower
   d Clean, disinfect, and dry the shower before and after use

21 Water temperature for perineal care is between
   a 100°F and 104°F
   b 105°F and 109°F
   c 110°F and 115°F
   d 120°F and 125°F

22 These statements are about perineal care. Which is *true*?
   a Do not explain the procedure to avoid embarrassment.
   b The person does perineal care if able.
   c Clean from the back (bottom) to the front (top).
   d Draping the person is not needed.

Answers to Chapter 18 questions are on p. 552.

FOCUS ON PRACTICE

Problem Solving

You are helping a nursing assistant give perineal care. The nursing assistant does not wear gloves and does not use a clean part of the washcloth for each stroke. How can you correct the situation?

Grooming Needs

OBJECTIVES

- Define the key terms and key abbreviations in this chapter.
- Explain why grooming is important.
- Explain how to safely provide grooming measures—hair care, shaving, nail and foot care, and changing garments.
- Perform the procedures described in this chapter.
- Explain how to promote PRIDE in the person, the family, and yourself.

KEY TERMS

alopecia Hair loss
dandruff Excessive amounts of dry, white flakes from the scalp
hirsutism Excessive body hair
lice See "pediculosis"

pediculosis Infestation with wingless insects that feed on blood; lice
scabies A skin disorder caused by a female mite

KEY ABBREVIATIONS

C	Centigrade	ID	Identification
F	Fahrenheit	IV	Intravenous

Hair care, shaving, nail and foot care, and clean garments prevent infection and promote comfort. Such measures affect love, belonging, and self-esteem needs.

The person performs grooming measures to the extent possible. This promotes independence and quality of life. The person may use adaptive (assistive) devices (Fig. 19-1).

See *Focus on Surveys: Grooming Needs.*

NOTE: *A task may require more than 1 pair of gloves. Change gloves as needed. Use careful judgment. Remember to practice hand hygiene after removing gloves.*

FOCUS ON SURVEYS

Grooming Needs

Grooming promotes self-esteem and self-worth. Therefore surveyors will observe if patients and residents:

- Are groomed according to their wishes.
- Have hair combed and styled.
- Have beards shaved or trimmed.
- Are dressed in their own clothes.
- Are wearing the correct clothing for the time of day.
- Can reach grooming supplies.

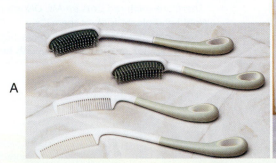
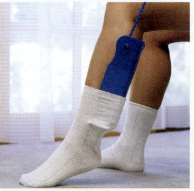

FIGURE 19-1 Grooming aids. **A,** Long-handled combs and brushes for hair care. **B,** A sock assist to pull on socks and stockings. (Courtesy North Coast Medical Inc., Morgan Hill, Calif.)

HAIR CARE

The look and feel of hair affect mental well-being. The nursing process reflects the person's culture, personal choice, skin and scalp conditions, health history, and self-care ability. You assist with hair care as needed.

Beauty and barber shops are common in nursing centers. Residents can have shampoos, hair-cuts, and hair styled.

Skin and Scalp Conditions

Skin and scalp conditions include:

*   *Alopecia means hair loss.* Hair loss may be complete or partial. A result of heredity, male pattern baldness occurs with aging. Hair thins in some women with aging. Cancer treatments (radiation therapy to the head and chemotherapy) may cause alopecia in all age-groups.
*   *Hirsutism is excessive body hair.* It can occur in men, women, and children. Causes are heredity and abnormal amounts of male hormones.
*   *Dandruff is the excessive amount of dry, white flakes from the scalp.* Itching is common. Sometimes eyebrows and ear canals are involved.
*   *Pediculosis (lice) is the infestation with wingless insects that feed on blood* (Fig. 19-2). *Infestation* means *being in or on a host.* Lice attach their eggs (*nits*) to hair shafts. After hatching, they bite the scalp or skin to feed on blood. About the size of a sesame seed, adult lice are tan to gray-ish white in color. Lice easily spread to others through clothing, head coverings, furniture, beds, towels, bed linens, and sexual contact and by sharing combs and brushes. Lice are treated with medicated shampoos, lotions, and creams specific for lice. Thorough bathing is needed. So is washing clothing and linens in hot water. Lice bites cause severe itching.
    *   *Pediculosis capitis* ("head lice") is the infestation of the scalp (*capitis*) with lice.
    *   *Pediculosis pubis* ("crabs") is the infestation of the pubic (*pubis*) hair with lice.
    *   *Pediculosis corporis* is the infestation of the body (*corporis*) with lice.
*   *Scabies is a skin disorder caused by a female mite* (Fig. 19-3). A *mite* is a very small spider-like organism. The female mite burrows into the skin and lays eggs. After hatching, the females produce more eggs. Infested with mites, the person has a rash and intense itching. Common sites are between the fingers, the wrists, underarm areas, thighs, and genital area. Other sites include the breasts, waist, and buttocks. Highly contagious, scabies is transmitted to others by close contact. Special creams are ordered to kill the mites. The person's room is cleaned. Clothing and linens are washed in hot water.

See *Focus on Communication: Skin and Scalp Conditions.*

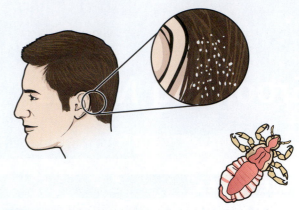

FIGURE 19-2 Head lice. (Redrawn from Medline Plus: *Head lice.* Bethesda, Md., National Institutes of Health.)

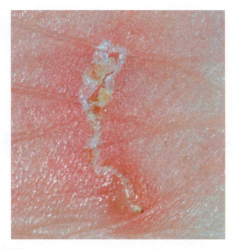

FIGURE 19-3 Scabies. (From Marks JG, Miller JJ: *Lookingbill & Marks' principles of dermatology,* ed 4, St Louis, 2006, Saunders.)

FOCUS ON COMMUNICATION

Skin and Scalp Conditions

Some skin or scalp conditions may alarm you. Remain professional. Do not say things that may embarrass the person.

Report an abnormal skin or scalp condition. Describe what you saw as best as you can. For example:

*   "There are small red dots on Mr. Olson's right underarm. Would you please look at them?"
*   "I saw some small white specks in Ms. Smith's hair. Would you please look at them before I wash her hair?"

Brushing and Combing Hair

Brushing and combing hair are part of early morning care, morning care, and afternoon care. Some people also do so at bedtime. Provide hair care when needed and before visitors arrive.

Encourage patients and residents to do their own hair care. The person chooses how to brush, comb, and style hair. Assist as needed.

Daily brushing and combing prevent tangled and matted hair. So does braiding. You need the person's consent to braid hair. *Never cut the person's hair.*

Special measures are needed for curly, coarse, and dry hair. The person may have certain hair care practices and products. They are part of the care plan. Also, let the person guide you when giving hair care.

See *Caring about Culture: Brushing and Combing Hair.*
See *Delegation Guidelines: Brushing and Combing Hair.*
See *Promoting Safety and Comfort: Brushing and Combing Hair.*
See procedure: *Brushing and Combing Hair,* p. 276.

CARING ABOUT CULTURE
Brushing and Combing Hair

Small braids (cornrows) are common in some cultural groups. The braids are left intact for shampooing. To undo these braids, the nurse obtains the person's consent.

(NOTE: Each person is unique. A person may not follow all of the beliefs and practices of his or her culture. Follow the care plan.)

DELEGATION GUIDELINES
Brushing and Combing Hair

To brush and comb hair, you need this information from the nurse and the care plan.
- How much help the person needs
- What to do for matted or tangled hair
- What to do for curly, coarse, or dry hair
- What hair care products to use
- The person's preferences and routine hair care measures
- What observations to report and record:
  - Scalp sores
  - Flaking
  - Itching
  - Rash
  - Hair falling out in patches; patches of hair loss
  - Very dry or very oily hair
  - Matted or tangled hair
  - The presence of nits or lice
    - Nits (lice eggs attached to hair shafts)—oval and yellow to white in color
    - Lice—about the size of a sesame seed and gray-ish white in color
    - Itching
    - Complaints of a tickling feeling or something moving in the hair
    - Irritability
    - Sores on the head or body caused by scratching
    - Rash
- When to report observations
- What patient or resident concerns to report at once

PROMOTING SAFETY AND COMFORT
Brushing and Combing Hair

Safety
Sharp brush bristles can injure the scalp. So can a comb with sharp or broken teeth. Report concerns about the person's brush or comb.

Wear gloves if the person has scalp sores. Follow Standard Precautions and the Bloodborne Pathogen Standard.

Comfort
Place a towel across the person's back and shoulders to protect garments from falling hair. For the person in bed, give hair care before changing linens and the pillowcase. If after a linen change, place a towel across the pillow to collect falling hair.

Brushing and Combing Hair

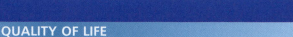

QUALITY OF LIFE

- Knock before entering the person's room.
- Address the person by name.
- Introduce yourself by name and title.

- Explain the procedure before starting and during the procedure.
- Protect the person's rights during the procedure.
- Handle the person gently during the procedure.

PRE-PROCEDURE

1 Follow *Delegation Guidelines: Brushing and Combing Hair,* p. 275. See *Promoting Safety and Comfort: Brushing and Combing Hair,* p. 275.
2 Practice hand hygiene.
3 Identify the person. Check the ID (identification) bracelet against the assignment sheet. Use 2 identifiers (Chapter 10). Also call the person by name.

4 Ask the person how to style hair.
5 Collect the following.
- Comb and brush
- Bath towel
- Other hair care items as requested
6 Arrange items on the bedside stand.
7 Provide for privacy.

PROCEDURE

8 Lower the bed rail if up.
9 Position the person.
   a *In a chair*—Help the person to the chair. The person puts on a robe and non-skid footwear when up.
   b *In bed*—Raise the bed for body mechanics. Bed rails are up if used. Lower the bed rail near you. Assist the person to a semi-Fowler's position if allowed.
10 Place a towel across the back and shoulders or across the pillow.
11 Have the person remove eyeglasses. Put them in the eyeglass case. Put the case inside the bedside stand.
12 *Brush and comb hair that is not matted or tangled.*
   a Use the comb to part the hair.
      1 Part hair down the middle into 2 sides (Fig. 19-4, *A*).
      2 Divide 1 side into 2 smaller sections (Fig. 19-4, *B*).

   b Brush 1 of the small sections of hair. Start at the scalp and brush toward the hair ends (Fig. 19-5). Do the same for the other small section of hair. If the person prefers, brush long hair starting at the hair ends.
   c Repeat steps 12, a(2) and b for the other side.
13 *Brush or comb matted or tangled hair.*
   a Take a small section of hair near the ends.
   b Comb or brush through to the hair ends.
   c Add small sections of hair as you work up to the scalp.
   d Comb or brush through each longer section to the hair ends.
14 Style the hair as the person prefers.
15 Remove the towel.
16 Let the person put on the eyeglasses.

POST-PROCEDURE

17 Provide for comfort. (See the inside of the front cover.)
18 Place the call light and other needed items within reach.
19 Lower the bed to a safe and comfortable level. Follow the care plan.
20 Raise or lower bed rails. Follow the care plan.
21 Remove hair from the brush or comb. Clean, rinse, dry, and return hair care items to their proper place. Use clean, dry paper towels for drying. Wear gloves for this step. Remove and discard the gloves. Practice hand hygiene.

22 Unscreen the person.
23 Complete a safety check of the room. (See the inside of the front cover.)
24 Follow agency policy for used linens.
25 Practice hand hygiene.

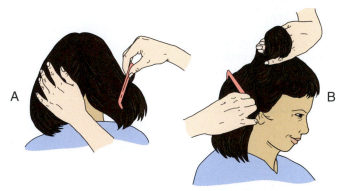

FIGURE 19-4 Parting hair. **A,** Part hair down the middle. Divide it into 2 sides. **B,** Then part 1 side into 2 smaller sections.

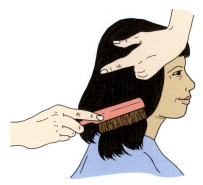

FIGURE 19-5 Brush hair by starting at the scalp. Brush down to the hair ends.

Shampooing

People shampoo 1, 2, or 3 times a week or daily. Factors affecting frequency include hair and scalp condition, hairstyle, and personal choice.

In nursing centers, shampoos are done on bath days. If done by a hairdresser or barber, do not shampoo hair. Provide a shower cap for the bath or shower.

The shampoo method depends on the person's condition, safety factors, and personal choice. The nurse tells you what method to use.

- *Shampoo during the shower or tub bath.* Use a hand-held nozzle for persons in shower chairs or taking tub baths. Direct a spray of water at the hair.
- *Shampoo at the sink.* The person sits or lies facing away from the sink. A folded towel placed over the sink edge protects the neck. The person's head is tilted back over the sink edge (Fig. 19-6). Use a water pitcher or hand-held nozzle to wet and rinse the hair.
- *Shampoo in bed.* The person's head and shoulders are at the edge of the bed if possible. A shampoo tray under the head protects the linens and mattress from water. The tray drains into a basin on a chair by the bed (Fig. 19-7). Use a water pitcher to wet and rinse the hair.

Dry and style hair as soon as possible after the shampoo. Women may want hair curled or rolled up before drying. Check with the nurse before doing so.

See *Focus on Older Persons: Shampooing.*
See *Delegation Guidelines: Shampooing.*
See *Promoting Safety and Comfort: Shampooing,* p. 278.
See procedure: *Shampooing the Person's Hair,* p. 278.

See *Promoting Safety and Comfort: Shampooing,* p. 278.
See procedure: *Shampooing the Person's Hair,* p. 278.

FOCUS ON OLDER PERSONS

Shampooing

Oil gland secretion decreases with aging. Therefore older persons have dry hair. They may shampoo less often than younger adults do.

DELEGATION GUIDELINES

Shampooing

To shampoo a person, you need this information from the nurse and the care plan.

- When to shampoo the person's hair
- What method to use
- What shampoo and conditioner to use
- How to use and store medicated products
- The person's position restrictions or limits
- What water temperature to use—usually 105°F (Fahrenheit) (40.5°C [centigrade])
- If hair is curled or rolled up before drying
- What observations to report and record:
  - Scalp sores
  - Flaking
  - Itching
  - The presence of nits or lice (p. 274)
  - Hair falling out in patches; patches of hair loss
  - Very dry or very oily hair
  - Matted or tangled hair
  - How the person tolerated the procedure
- When to report observations
- What patient or resident concerns to report at once

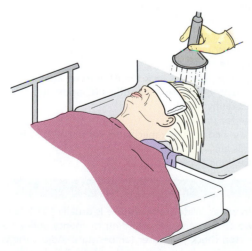

FIGURE 19-6 Shampooing with the person on a stretcher. The stretcher is in front of the sink.

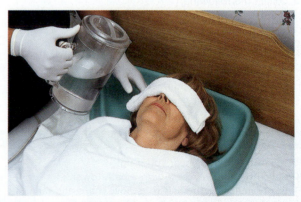

FIGURE 19-7 A shampoo tray for a person in bed. The tray is directed to the side of the bed so water drains into a collecting basin.

PROMOTING SAFETY AND COMFORT
Shampooing

Safety

Remove hearing aids before shampooing. Water will damage hearing aids.

Wear gloves if the person has scalp sores. Follow Standard Precautions and the Bloodborne Pathogen Standard.

Keep shampoo away from and out of the eyes. Have the person hold a washcloth over the eyes. To rinse, cup your hand at the person's forehead. This keeps soapy water from running down the forehead and into the eyes.

For a shampoo on a stretcher at a sink, see Chapter 16 for stretcher safety. Lock (brake) the wheels and use the safety straps and side rails. Keep the far side rail raised during the procedure.

Some people shampoo themselves during a tub bath or shower. Place an extra towel, shampoo, and hair conditioner within the person's reach. Assist as needed.

Comfort

For a shampoo during the tub bath or shower, the person tips the head back to keep shampoo and water out of the eyes. Support the back of the head with 1 hand. Shampoo with your other hand. Some persons cannot tip their heads back. They lean forward and hold a folded washcloth over the eyes. Support the forehead with 1 hand as you shampoo with the other. Make sure that the person can breathe easily.

Many people have limited range of motion in their necks. They are not shampooed at the sink or on a stretcher.

Shampooing the Person's Hair

QUALITY OF LIFE

- Knock before entering the person's room.
- Address the person by name.
- Introduce yourself by name and title.

- Explain the procedure before starting and during the procedure.
- Protect the person's rights during the procedure.
- Handle the person gently during the procedure.

PRE-PROCEDURE

1 Follow *Delegation Guidelines: Shampooing*, p. 277. See *Promoting Safety and Comfort: Shampooing.*
2 Practice hand hygiene.
3 Collect the following.
   - 2 bath towels
   - Washcloth
   - Shampoo
   - Hair conditioner (if requested)
   - Water thermometer
   - Pitcher or hand-held nozzle (if needed)
   - Shampoo tray (if needed)
   - Basin or pan (if needed)

- Waterproof pad (if needed)
- Gloves (if needed)
- Comb and brush
- Hair dryer
4 Arrange items nearby.
5 Identify the person. Check the ID bracelet against the assignment sheet. Use 2 identifiers (Chapter 10). Also call the person by name.
6 Provide for privacy.
7 Raise the bed for body mechanics for a shampoo in bed. Bed rails are up if used.
8 Practice hand hygiene.

PROCEDURE

9 Lower the bed rail near you if up.
10 Cover the person's chest with a bath towel.
11 Brush and comb the hair to remove snarls and tangles.
12 Position the person for the method used. For a shampoo in bed:
   a Lower the head of the bed and remove the pillow.
   b Place the waterproof pad and shampoo tray under the head and shoulders.
   c Support the head and neck with a folded towel if necessary.
13 Raise the bed rail if used.

14 Obtain water. Water temperature is usually 105°F (40.5°C). Test water temperature according to agency policy. Have the person check the water temperature. Adjust the water temperature as needed. Raise the bed rail before leaving the bedside.
15 Lower the bed rail near you if up.
16 Put on gloves (if needed).
17 Have the person hold a washcloth over the eyes. It should not cover the nose and mouth. (NOTE: A damp washcloth is easier to hold. It will not slip. However, your agency may require a dry washcloth.)

Shampooing the Person's Hair—cont'd

PROCEDURE—cont'd

18 Use the water pitcher or nozzle to wet the hair. Ask the person about the water temperature and adjust as needed.
19 Apply a small amount of shampoo.
20 Work up a lather with both hands. Start at the hairline. Work toward the back of the head.
21 Massage the scalp with your fingertips. Do not scratch the scalp with your fingernails.
22 Rinse the hair until the water runs clear.
23 Repeat steps 19 through 22.
24 Apply conditioner. Follow directions on the container.
25 Squeeze water from the hair.

26 Cover the hair with a bath towel.
27 Remove the shampoo tray, basin, and waterproof pad.
28 Dry the person's face with the towel on the chest.
29 Help the person raise the head if appropriate. For the person in bed, raise the head of the bed.
30 Rub the hair and scalp with the towel. Rub gently. Use the second towel if the first one is wet.
31 Comb the hair to remove snarls and tangles.
32 Dry and style hair.
33 Remove and discard the gloves (if used). Practice hand hygiene.

POST-PROCEDURE

34 Provide for comfort. (See the inside of the front cover.)
35 Place the call light and other needed items within reach.
36 Lower the bed to a safe and comfortable level. Follow the care plan.
37 Raise or lower bed rails. Follow the care plan.
38 Unscreen the person.
39 Complete a safety check of the room. (See the inside of the front cover.)

40 Clean the brush and comb. Clean, rinse, dry, and return equipment to its proper place. Use clean, dry paper towels for drying. Wear gloves for this step. Discard disposable items. Remove and discard the gloves.
41 Follow agency policy for used linens.
42 Practice hand hygiene.
43 Report and record your observations.

Shampoo Caps. Commercial shampoo caps have a cleaning agent that does not need rinsing. Some include a conditioner. To use a shampoo cap:

- Warm the package in a microwave oven or commercial warmer. Follow the manufacturer's instructions for microwave settings and warming times.
- Check the temperature. The cap should be warm. Do not use a cap that is too hot.
- Apply the cap to the person's head.
- Massage the cap gently. Follow the manufacturer's instructions for how long to massage—usually 1 to 3 minutes. Longer hair may require more time.
- Remove the cap. You do not need to rinse the hair. Dry the hair with a towel if needed.
- Comb and dry the hair.

▮ SHAVING

Facial shaving is common among men. Many women shave their legs and underarms. Some women have facial hair. Hair removal methods include shaving, waxing, hair removal products, plucking, and threading. See Box 19-1 for shaving rules.

Safety razors or electric shavers are used (Fig. 19-8, p. 280). Some persons have their own electric shavers. If the agency's shaver is used, clean it before and after use. To brush out whiskers or hair, follow the manufacturer's instructions. Also follow agency procedures.

BOX 19-1   Rules for Shaving

- Use electric shavers for persons taking anticoagulant drugs (p. 280). Never use safety razors.
- Protect bed linens. Place a towel under the part to be shaved. Or place a towel across the person's chest and shoulders to protect clothing.
- Soften facial hair before shaving. Apply a warm, moist washcloth or towel to the face for a few minutes. Then pat dry the face and apply talcum powder if using an electric shaver.
- Lather the area with shaving cream or soap and water if using a safety razor.
- Encourage the person to do as much as safely possible.
- Hold the skin taut as needed.
- Shave in the correct direction.
  - *Shaving the face with a safety razor*—shave in the direction of hair growth.
  - *Shaving the underarms with a safety razor*—shave in the direction of hair growth.
  - *Shaving the legs with a safety razor*—shave up from the ankles. This is against hair growth.
  - *Using an electric shaver*—shave against the direction of hair growth. For a rotary-type shaver, move the shaver in small circles over the face. (NOTE: Some state competency tests require shaving in the direction of hair growth. Follow the manufacturer's instructions and the rules in your state and agency.)
- Do not cut, nick, or irritate the skin.
- Rinse the skin thoroughly.
- Apply direct pressure to nicks or cuts (Chapter 36).
- Report nicks, cuts, or irritation at once.

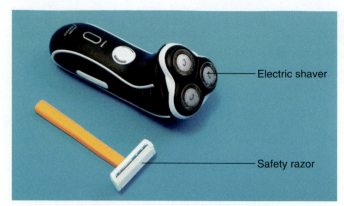

FIGURE 19-8 Electric shaver and safety razor.

Safety razors (blade razors) have razor blades. They can cause nicks and cuts. Do not use safety razors on persons with healing problems or on those taking anticoagulant drugs. An *anticoagulant* is a drug that prevents or slows down *(anti)* blood clotting *(coagulate)*. Bleeding occurs easily and is hard to stop. A nick or cut can cause serious bleeding. Electric shavers are used.

See *Focus on Older Persons: Shaving.*
See *Delegation Guidelines: Shaving.*
See *Promoting Safety and Comfort: Shaving.*
See procedure: *Shaving the Person's Face With a Safety Razor.*

Shaving the Person's Face With a Safety Razor

QUALITY OF LIFE

- Knock before entering the person's room.
- Address the person by name.
- Introduce yourself by name and title.

- Explain the procedure before starting and during the procedure.
- Protect the person's rights during the procedure.
- Handle the person gently during the procedure.

PRE-PROCEDURE

1 Follow *Delegation Guidelines: Shaving.* See *Promoting Safety and Comfort: Shaving.*
2 Practice hand hygiene.
3 Collect the following.
   - Wash basin
   - Bath towel
   - Hand towel
   - Washcloth
   - Safety razor
   - Mirror
   - Shaving cream, soap, or lotion
   - Shaving brush
   - After-shave or lotion
   - Tissues or paper towels
   - Gloves

4 Arrange paper towels and supplies on the over-bed table.
5 Identify the person. Check the ID bracelet against the assignment sheet. Use 2 identifiers (Chapter 10). Also call the person by name.
6 Provide for privacy.
7 Raise the bed for body mechanics. Bed rails are up if used.

PROCEDURE

8 Fill the wash basin with warm water.
9 Place the basin on the over-bed table.
10 Lower the bed rail near you if up.
11 Practice hand hygiene. Put on gloves.
12 Assist the person to semi-Fowler's position if allowed or to the supine position.
13 Adjust lighting to clearly see the person's face.
14 Place the towel over the person's chest and shoulders.
15 Adjust the over-bed table for easy reach.
16 Tighten the razor blade to the shaver if necessary.
17 Wash the person's face. Do not dry.
18 Wet the washcloth or towel. Wring it out.
19 Apply the washcloth or towel to the face for a few minutes.

20 Apply shaving cream with your hands. Or use a shaving brush to apply lather.
21 Hold the skin taut with 1 hand.
22 Shave in the direction of hair growth. Use shorter strokes around the chin and lips (Fig. 19-9).
23 Rinse the razor often. Wipe it with tissues or paper towels.
24 Apply direct pressure to any bleeding areas (Chapter 36).
25 Wash off any remaining shaving cream or soap. Pat dry with a towel.
26 Apply after-shave or lotion if requested. (If there are nicks or cuts, do not apply after-shave or lotion.)
27 Remove and discard the towel and gloves. Practice hand hygiene.

POST-PROCEDURE

28 Provide for comfort. (See the inside of the front cover.)
29 Place the call light and other needed items within reach.
30 Lower the bed to a safe and comfortable level. Follow the care plan.
31 Raise or lower bed rails. Follow the care plan.
32 Clean, rinse, dry, and return equipment and supplies to their proper place. Use clean, dry paper towels for drying. Discard the razor blade or disposable razor into the sharps container. Discard other disposable items. Wear gloves.

33 Wipe off the over-bed table with clean, dry paper towels. Discard the paper towels.
34 Unscreen the person.
35 Complete a safety check of the room. (See the inside of the front cover.)
36 Follow agency policy for used linens.
37 Remove and discard the gloves. Practice hand hygiene.
38 Report nicks, cuts, irritation, or bleeding to the nurse at once. Also report and record other observations.

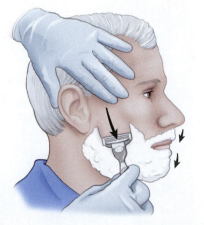

FIGURE 19-9 Shave the face in the direction of hair growth. Use long strokes on the larger areas of the face. Use short strokes around the chin and lips.

Caring for Mustaches and Beards

Mustaches and beards need daily care. Food and mouth and nose drainage can collect in the whiskers. Daily washing and combing are needed. Ask the person how to groom his mustache or beard. *Never shave or trim a mustache or beard.*

Shaving Legs and Underarms

Many women shave their legs and underarms. This practice varies among cultures. To shave legs and underarms:
- Follow the rules in Box 19-1.
- Collect shaving items with bath items.
- Shave after bathing while the skin is soft.
- Use soap and water, shaving cream, or lotion for the lather. Follow the care plan.
- Use the kidney basin to rinse the razor. Do not use bath water.

◾ NAIL AND FOOT CARE

Nail and foot care prevents infection, injury, and odors. Hangnails, ingrown nails (nails that grow in at the side), and nails torn away from the skin cause skin breaks. These breaks are portals of entry for microbes. Long or broken nails can scratch skin and snag clothing.

Dirty feet, socks, or stockings harbor microbes and cause odors. Shoes and socks provide a warm, moist place for microbes to grow. Injuries occur from stubbing toes, stepping on sharp objects, or being stepped on. Poorly fitting shoes cause blisters.

Poor circulation prolongs healing. Diabetes and vascular diseases cause poor circulation. Foot injuries or infections are very serious for older persons and those with circulatory disorders.

Nails are easier to trim and clean right after soaking or bathing. Use nail clippers to cut fingernails. *Never use scissors.* Use extreme caution to prevent damage to nearby tissues.

Trimming and clipping toenails can easily cause injuries. *Some agencies do not let nursing assistants cut or trim toenails. Follow agency policy.*

See *Delegation Guidelines: Nail and Foot Care.*
See *Promoting Safety and Comfort: Nail and Foot Care.*
See procedure: *Giving Nail and Foot Care.*

DELEGATION GUIDELINES
Nail and Foot Care

To give nail and foot care, you need this information from the nurse and the care plan.
- What water temperature to use
- How long to soak fingernails (usually 5 to 10 minutes)
- How long to soak feet (usually 15 to 20 minutes)
- If nails should be filed but not trimmed
- What observations to report and record:
  - Dry, reddened, irritated, or callused areas
  - Breaks in the skin
  - Corns (Chapter 28) on top of and between the toes
  - Blisters
  - Very thick nails
  - Loose nails
- When to report observations
- What patient or resident concerns to report at once

PROMOTING SAFETY AND COMFORT
Nail and Foot Care

Safety

To cut fingernails, use nail clippers. Clip the fingernails straight across (Fig. 19-10). Then file the nails.

Some states and agencies do not let nursing assistants cut and trim toenails. A nurse or podiatrist (foot [*pod*] doctor) cuts toenails and provides foot care for the following persons. *You do not cut or trim the fingernails or toenails for persons who:*
- Have diabetes
- Have poor circulation
- Take drugs that affect blood clotting
- Have nail fungus (Chapter 28), very thick nails, or ingrown nails

Check between the toes for cracks and sores. If not treated, a serious infection could occur.

The feet are easily burned. Persons with decreased sensation or circulatory problems may not feel hot temperatures.

After soaking, apply lotion or petroleum jelly to the feet. This can cause slippery feet. Help the person put on non-skid footwear before you transfer the person or let the person walk.

Breaks in the skin and bleeding can occur. Follow Standard Precautions and the Bloodborne Pathogen Standard.

Comfort

Sometimes you just trim the fingernails. Sometimes you just give foot care. To do both, the person sits at the over-bed table (Fig. 19-11). Provide for warmth and comfort.

Provide for your comfort during nail and foot care. Sit in front of the over-bed table to clean and trim fingernails. For foot care, rest the person's lower leg and foot on your lap. Or position the feet on the floor and kneel on the floor. Lay a towel across your lap or put a bath mat on the floor to protect your uniform. Use good body mechanics. Always support the person's foot and ankle during foot care.

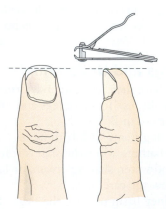

FIGURE 19-10 Clip fingernails straight across. Use nail clippers.

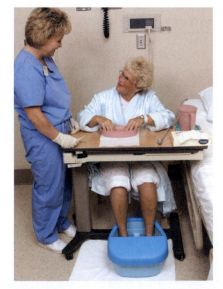

FIGURE 19-11 Nail and foot care. The feet soak in a whirlpool foot bath. The fingers soak in a kidney basin.

Giving Nail and Foot Care

QUALITY OF LIFE

- Knock before entering the person's room.
- Address the person by name.
- Introduce yourself by name and title.

- Explain the procedure before starting and during the procedure.
- Protect the person's rights during the procedure.
- Handle the person gently during the procedure.

PRE-PROCEDURE

1 Follow *Delegation Guidelines: Nail and Foot Care.* See *Promoting Safety and Comfort: Nail and Foot Care.*
2 Practice hand hygiene.
3 Collect the following.
   - Wash basin or whirlpool foot bath
   - Soap
   - Water thermometer
   - Bath towel
   - Hand towel
   - Washcloth
   - Kidney basin
   - Nail clippers
   - Orangewood stick
   - Emery board or nail file
   - Lotion for the hands
   - Lotion or petroleum jelly for the feet
   - Paper towels
   - Bath mat
   - Gloves
4 Arrange paper towels and other items on the over-bed table.
5 Identify the person. Check the ID bracelet against the assignment sheet. Use 2 identifiers (Chapter 10). Also call the person by name.
6 Provide for privacy.
7 Assist the person to the bedside chair. Remove footwear and socks or stockings. Place the call light and other needed items within reach.

PROCEDURE

8 Place the bath mat under the feet.
9 Fill the wash basin or whirlpool foot bath ⅔ (two-thirds) full with water. The nurse tells you what water temperature to use. (Measure water temperature with a water thermometer. Or test it by dipping your elbow or inner wrist into the basin. Follow agency policy.) Have the person check the water temperature and adjust as needed.
10 Place the basin or foot bath on the bath mat.
11 Put on gloves.
12 Help the person put his or her bare feet into the water. Both feet are covered by water.
13 Adjust the over-bed table in front of the person.
14 Fill the kidney basin ⅔ (two-thirds) full with water. See step 9 for water temperature.
15 Place the kidney basin on the over-bed table.
16 Place the person's fingers into the basin. Position the arms for comfort (see Fig. 19-11).
17 Let the fingers soak for 5 to 10 minutes. Let the feet soak for 15 to 20 minutes. Re-warm water as needed.
18 Remove the kidney basin.
19 Dry the hands and between the fingers thoroughly.
20 Clean under the fingernails with the orangewood stick. Wipe the orangewood stick with a towel after each nail.
21 Push cuticles back gently with the orangewood stick or a washcloth (Fig. 19-12, p. 284).

22 Clip fingernails straight across with the nail clippers (see Fig. 19-10).
23 File and shape nails with an emery board or nail file. Nails are smooth with no rough edges. Check each nail for smoothness. File as needed.
24 Apply lotion to the hands. Warm the lotion first.
25 Move the over-bed table to the side.
26 Remove and discard the gloves. Practice hand hygiene. Put on clean gloves. (NOTE: Some state competency tests require clean gloves for foot care.)
27 Lift a foot out of the water. Support the foot and ankle with 1 hand. With your other hand, wash the foot and between the toes with soap and a washcloth. Return the foot to the water to rinse the foot and between the toes.
28 Repeat step 27 for the other foot.
29 Remove the feet from the water. Dry thoroughly, especially between the toes. Support the foot and ankle as needed.
30 Apply lotion or petroleum jelly to the tops, soles, and heels of the feet. Do not apply between the toes. Warm lotion or petroleum jelly first. Remove excess lotion or petroleum jelly with a towel. Support the foot and ankle as needed.
31 Remove and discard the gloves. Practice hand hygiene.
32 Help the person put on non-skid footwear.

POST-PROCEDURE

33 Provide for comfort. (See the inside of the front cover.)
34 Place the call light and other needed items within reach.
35 Raise or lower bed rails. Follow the care plan.
36 Clean, rinse, dry, and return equipment and supplies to their proper place. Use clean, dry paper towels for drying. Discard disposable items. Wear gloves.

37 Unscreen the person.
38 Complete a safety check of the room. (See the inside of the front cover.)
39 Follow agency policy for used linens.
40 Remove and discard the gloves. Practice hand hygiene.
41 Report and record your observations.

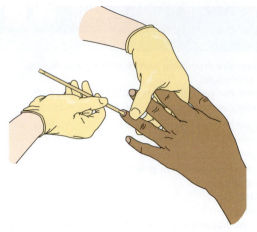

FIGURE 19-12 Push the cuticle back with an orangewood stick.

CHANGING GARMENTS

Hospital patients wear patient gowns or other sleepwear. Nursing center residents wear street clothes during the day and sleepwear at bedtime. Garments are changed:
- After bathing
- When wet or soiled
- On admission and discharge

Dressing and Undressing

Some persons dress and undress themselves. Others need help. Personal choice is a resident right. Let the person choose what to wear. To assist with dressing and undressing, follow the rules in Box 19-2.

See *Focus on Communication: Dressing and Undressing.*
See *Focus on Older Persons: Dressing and Undressing.*
See *Delegation Guidelines: Dressing and Undressing.*
See *Promoting Safety and Comfort: Dressing and Undressing.*
See procedure: *Undressing the Person.*
See procedure: *Dressing the Person, p. 287.*

Text continued on p. 289.

BOX 19-2	Rules for Dressing and Undressing

- Provide for privacy. Do not expose the person.
- Encourage the person to do as much as possible.
- Let the person choose what to wear. Have the person choose the right under-garments.
- Make sure garments and footwear are the correct size.
- Remove clothing from the strong or "good" side first. This is often called the *unaffected side.*
- Put clothing on the weak side first. This is often called the *affected side.*
- Support the arm or leg to remove or put on a garment.
- Move and handle the body gently. Do not force a joint beyond its range of motion or to the point of pain. See Chapter 27.

FOCUS ON COMMUNICATION
Dressing and Undressing

Promote personal choice and independence when assisting with dressing and undressing. You can ask:
- "What would you like to wear today?"
- "There's a concert today. Do you want to wear something special?"
- "Can I help you with those buttons?"
- "Do you need help with that zipper?"

FOCUS ON OLDER PERSONS
Dressing and Undressing

Persons with dementia may not want to change clothes. Or they may not know how. For example, a person tries to put slacks over his or her head. Or summer shorts are worn in the winter. The Alzheimer's Disease Education and Referral Center (ADEAR) suggests the following.
- Try to assist with dressing at the same time each day. Dressing becomes part of the daily routine.
- Let the person dress to the extent possible. Allow extra time. Do not rush the person.
- Let the person choose from 2 or 3 outfits. The family may buy several of the same outfit. Dressing is easier if the person insists on wearing the same thing.
- Choose comfortable, easy to get on and off clothes. Garments with elastic waistbands and Velcro closures are examples. There are no zippers, buttons, hooks, snaps, or other closures.
- Stack clothes in the order they are put on. The person sees 1 item at a time. For example, an under-garment is put on first. The item is on top of the stack.
- Give clear, simple, and step-by-step directions.

DELEGATION GUIDELINES
Dressing and Undressing

To assist with dressing and undressing, you need this information from the nurse and the care plan.
- How much help the person needs
- Which side is the person's strong side
- If certain garments are needed
- What observations to report and record:
  - How much help was given
  - How the person tolerated the procedure
  - Complaints by the person
  - Changes in the person's behavior
- When to report observations
- What patient or resident concerns to report at once

PROMOTING SAFETY AND COMFORT
Dressing and Undressing

Safety

To assist with dressing and undressing, you turn the person from side to side. If the person uses bed rails, raise the far bed rail. If bed rails are not used, ask a co-worker to help turn and position the person. This protects the person from falling.

Undressing the Person

QUALITY OF LIFE

- Knock before entering the person's room.
- Address the person by name.
- Introduce yourself by name and title.

- Explain the procedure before starting and during the procedure.
- Protect the person's rights during the procedure.
- Handle the person gently during the procedure.

PRE-PROCEDURE

1 Follow *Delegation Guidelines: Dressing and Undressing.* See *Promoting Safety and Comfort: Dressing and Undressing.*
2 Ask a co-worker to help turn and position the person if needed.
3 Practice hand hygiene.
4 Collect a bath blanket and clothing requested by the person.
5 Identify the person. Check the ID bracelet against the assignment sheet. Use 2 identifiers (Chapter 10). Also call the person by name.

6 Provide for privacy.
7 Raise the bed for body mechanics. Bed rails are up if used.
8 Lower the bed rail on the person's weak side.
9 Position him or her supine.
10 Cover the person with a bath blanket. Fan-fold linens to the foot of the bed.

PROCEDURE

11 Remove garments that open in back.
   a Raise the head and shoulders. Or turn the person onto the side away from you.
   b Undo buttons, zippers, ties, or snaps.
   c Bring the sides of the garment to the sides of the person (Fig. 19-13, p. 286). For a side-lying position, tuck the far side of the garment under the person. Fold the near side onto the chest (Fig. 19-14, p. 286).
   d Position the person supine.
   e Slide the garment off the shoulder on the strong side. Remove it from the arm (Fig. 19-15, p. 286).
   f Remove the garment from the weak side.
12 Remove garments that open in the front.
   a Undo buttons, zippers, ties, or snaps.
   b Slide the garment off the shoulder and arm on the strong side.
   c Help the person sit up or raise the head and shoulders. Bring the garment to the weak side (Fig. 19-16, p. 286).
   d Lower the head and shoulders. Remove the garment from the weak side.
   e If you cannot raise the head and shoulders:
      1 Turn the person toward you. Tuck the removed part of the garment under the person.
      2 Turn the person onto the side away from you.
      3 Pull the side of the garment out from under the person. Make sure he or she will not lie on it when supine.
      4 Return the person to the supine position.
      5 Remove the garment from the weak side.

13 Remove pullover garments.
   a Undo buttons, zippers, ties, or snaps.
   b Remove the garment from the strong side.
   c Raise the head and shoulders. Or turn the person onto the side away from you. Bring the garment up to the neck (Fig. 19-17, p. 286).
   d Bring the garment over the head.
   e Remove the garment from the weak side.
   f Position the person in the supine position.
14 Remove pants or slacks.
   a Remove footwear and socks.
   b Position the person supine.
   c Undo buttons, zippers, ties, snaps, or buckles.
   d Remove the belt.
   e Have the person lift the buttocks off the bed. Slide the pants down over the hips and buttocks (Fig. 19-18, p. 286). Have the person lower the hips and buttocks.
   f If the person cannot raise the hips off the bed:
      1 Turn the person toward you.
      2 Slide the pants off the hip and buttocks on the strong side (Fig. 19-19, p. 287).
      3 Turn the person away from you.
      4 Slide the pants off the hip and buttocks on the weak side (Fig. 19-20, p. 287).
   g Slide the pants down the legs and over the feet.
15 Dress the person. See procedure: *Dressing the Person,* p. 287.

POST-PROCEDURE

16 Provide for comfort. (See the inside of the front cover.)
17 Place the call light and other needed items within reach.
18 Lower the bed to a safe and comfortable level. Follow the care plan.
19 Raise or lower bed rails. Follow the care plan.
20 Unscreen the person.

21 Complete a safety check of the room. (See the inside of the front cover.)
22 Follow agency policy for removed clothing.
23 Practice hand hygiene.
24 Report and record your observations.

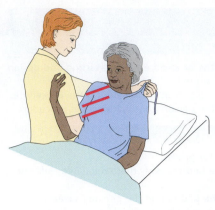

FIGURE 19-13 The sides of the garment are brought from the back to the sides of the person. (NOTE: *The "weak" side is indicated by slash marks.*)

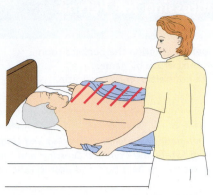

FIGURE 19-14 A garment that opens in the back is removed from the person in the side-lying position. The far side of the garment is tucked under the person. The near side is folded onto the person's chest. (NOTE: *The "weak" side is indicated by slash marks.*)

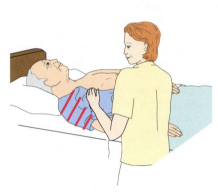

FIGURE 19-15 The garment is removed from the strong side first. (NOTE: *The "weak" side is indicated by slash marks.*)

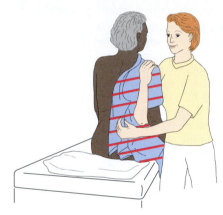

FIGURE 19-16 A front-opening garment is removed with the person's head and shoulders raised. The garment is removed from the strong side first. Then it is brought around the back to the weak side. (NOTE: *The "weak" side is indicated by slash marks.*)

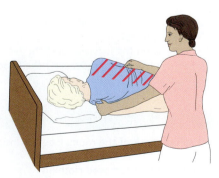

FIGURE 19-17 A pullover garment is removed from the strong side first. Then the garment is brought up to the person's neck so that it can be removed from the weak side. (NOTE: *The "weak" side is indicated by slash marks.*)

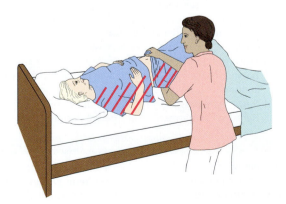

FIGURE 19-18 The person lifts the hips and buttocks to remove the pants. The pants are slid down over the hips and buttocks. (NOTE: *The "weak" side is indicated by slash marks.*)

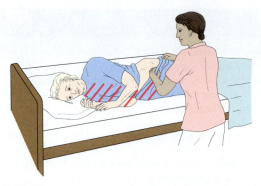

FIGURE 19-19 Pants are removed in the side-lying position. They are removed from the strong side first. They are slid over the hip and buttock. (NOTE: *The "weak" side is indicated by slash marks.*)

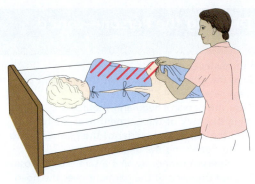

FIGURE 19-20 The person is turned onto the strong side. The pants are removed from the weak side. (NOTE: *The "weak" side is indicated by slash marks.*)

Dressing the Person

QUALITY OF LIFE

- Knock before entering the person's room.
- Address the person by name.
- Introduce yourself by name and title.

- Explain the procedure before starting and during the procedure.
- Protect the person's rights during the procedure.
- Handle the person gently during the procedure.

PRE-PROCEDURE

1 Follow *Delegation Guidelines: Dressing and Undressing,* p. 284. See *Promoting Safety and Comfort: Dressing and Undressing,* p. 284.
2 Ask a co-worker to help turn and position the person if needed.
3 Practice hand hygiene.
4 Ask what the person would like to wear.
5 Get a bath blanket and clothing requested by the person.
6 Identify the person. Check the ID bracelet against the assignment sheet. Use 2 identifiers (Chapter 10). Also call the person by name.

7 Provide for privacy.
8 Raise the bed for body mechanics. Bed rails are up if used.
9 Lower the bed rail (if up) on the person's weak side.
10 Position the person supine.
11 Cover the person with a bath blanket. Fan-fold linens to the foot of the bed.
12 Undress the person. See procedure: *Undressing the Person,* p. 285.

PROCEDURE

13 Put on garments that open in the back.
  a Slide the garment onto the arm and shoulder of the weak side.
  b Slide the garment onto the arm and shoulder of the strong side.
  c Raise the person's head and shoulders.
  d Bring the sides to the back.
  e If you cannot raise the person's head and shoulders:
    1 Turn the person toward you.
    2 Bring 1 side of the garment to the person's back (Fig. 19-21, *A,* p. 288).
    3 Turn the person away from you.
    4 Bring the other side to the person's back (Fig. 19-21, *B,* p. 288).
  f Fasten buttons, zippers, ties, snaps, or other closures.
  g Position the person supine.

14 Put on garments that open in the front.
  a Slide the garment onto the arm and shoulder on the weak side.
  b Raise the head and shoulders. Bring the side of the garment around to the back. Lower the person down. Slide the garment onto the arm and shoulder of the strong arm.
  c If the person cannot raise the head and shoulders:
    1 Turn the person away from you.
    2 Tuck the garment under him or her.
    3 Turn the person toward you.
    4 Pull the garment out from under him or her.
    5 Turn the person back to the supine position.
    6 Slide the garment over the arm and shoulder of the strong arm.
  d Fasten buttons, zippers, ties, snaps, or other closures.

Continued

Dressing the Person—cont'd

PROCEDURE—cont'd

15 Put on pullover garments.
  a Slide the arm and shoulder of the garment onto the weak side (Fig. 19-22, A).
  b Raise the person's head and shoulders.
  c Bring the neck of the garment over the head.
  d Slide the arm and shoulder of the garment onto the strong side. Bring the garment down.
  e If the person cannot assume a semi-sitting position:
    1 Bring the neck of the garment over the head.
    2 Slide the arm and shoulder of the garment onto the strong side (Fig. 19-22, B).
    3 Turn the person onto the strong side.
    4 Pull the garment down on the person's weak side.
    5 Turn the person onto the weak side.
    6 Pull the garment down on the person's strong side.
  f Position the person supine.

16 Put on pants or slacks:
  a Slide the pants over the feet and up the legs.
  b Have the person raise the hips and buttocks off the bed.
  c Bring the pants up over the buttock and hip on the weak side.
  d Pull the pants over the buttock and hip on the strong side.
  e If the person cannot raise the hips and buttocks:
    1 Turn the person onto the strong side.
    2 Pull the pants over the buttock and hip on the weak side.
    3 Turn the person onto the weak side.
    4 Pull the pants over the buttock and hip on the strong side.
    5 Position the person supine.
  f Fasten buttons, zippers, ties, snaps, a belt buckle, or other closures.
17 Put socks and non-skid footwear on the person. Socks are up all the way and smooth.
18 Help the person get out of bed. If the person stays in bed, cover the person. Remove the bath blanket.

POST-PROCEDURE

19 Provide for comfort. (See the inside of the front cover.)
20 Place the call light and other needed items within reach.
21 Lower the bed to a safe and comfortable level. Follow the care plan.
22 Raise or lower bed rails. Follow the care plan.
23 Unscreen the person.

24 Complete a safety check of the room. (See the inside of the front cover.)
25 Follow agency policy for removed clothing.
26 Practice hand hygiene.
27 Report and record your observations.

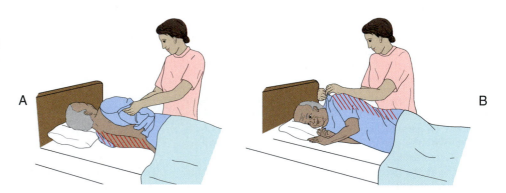

FIGURE 19-21 Applying garments that open in the back. **A,** The side-lying position can be used to put on garments that open in the back. Turn the person toward you after the garment is put on the arms. The side of the garment is brought to the person's back. **B,** Then turn the person away from you. The other side of the garment is brought to the back and fastened. (NOTE: *The "weak" side is indicated by slash marks.*)

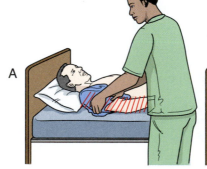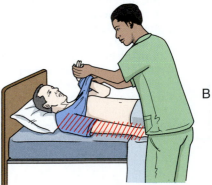

FIGURE 19-22 Applying pullover garments. **A,** The garment is applied to the weak side first. **B,** The garment is brought up over the head. The garment's arm and shoulder are slid onto the strong side. (NOTE: *The "weak" side is indicated by slash marks.*)

Changing Patient Gowns

Patient gowns are designed for comfort and to allow treatment. IV (intravenous [Chapter 24]) therapy gowns open along the sleeve and close with ties, snaps, or Velcro. Sometimes standard gowns are used for IV therapy.

For injury or paralysis, remove the gown from the strong arm first. Support the weak arm while removing the gown. Put the clean gown on the weak arm first and then on the strong arm.

See *Delegation Guidelines: Changing Patient Gowns.*
See *Promoting Safety and Comfort: Changing Patient Gowns.*
See procedure: *Changing a Standard Patient Gown on a Person With an IV.*

DELEGATION GUIDELINES

Changing Patient Gowns

Before changing a gown, you need this information from the nurse and the care plan.
- Which arm has the IV
- If the person has an IV pump (see *Promoting Safety and Comfort: Changing Patient Gowns*)

PROMOTING SAFETY AND COMFORT

Changing Patient Gowns

Safety

IV pumps control the *flow rate*—how fast fluid enters a vein. For an IV pump and a standard gown, do not use the following procedure. The nurse handles the arm with the IV.

To change a gown, you move the IV bag. Moving the IV bag can change the IV flow rate. Always ask the nurse to check the flow rate after you change a gown.

Do not disconnect or remove any part of the IV set-up.

Comfort

Some gowns tie at the upper back. The back and buttocks are exposed when the person stands. Cover the person for warmth and privacy. A robe or a second gown worn backwards will cover the back and buttocks. Other gowns over-lap in the back and tie at the side. These gowns provide more privacy. When tied at the side, uncomfortable bows and knots at the back are avoided.

Changing a Standard Patient Gown on a Person With an IV

QUALITY OF LIFE

- Knock before entering the person's room.
- Address the person by name.
- Introduce yourself by name and title.

- Explain the procedure before starting and during the procedure.
- Protect the person's rights during the procedure.
- Handle the person gently during the procedure.

PRE-PROCEDURE

1 Follow *Delegation Guidelines: Changing Patient Gowns.* See *Promoting Safety and Comfort: Changing Patient Gowns.*
2 Practice hand hygiene.
3 Get a clean gown and bath blanket.

4 Identify the person. Check the ID bracelet against the assignment sheet. Use 2 identifiers (Chapter 10). Also call the person by name.
5 Provide for privacy.
6 Raise the bed for body mechanics. Bed rails are up if used.

Continued

Changing a Standard Patient Gown on a Person With an IV—cont'd

PROCEDURE

7 Lower the bed rail near you (if up).
8 Cover the person with the bath blanket. Fan-fold linens to the foot of the bed.
9 Untie the gown. Free parts that the person is lying on.
10 Remove the gown from the arm with *no IV.*
11 Gather up the sleeve of the arm *with the IV.* Slide it over the IV site and tubing. Remove the arm and hand from the sleeve (Fig. 19-23, *A*).
12 Keep the sleeve gathered. Slide your arm along the tubing to the bag (Fig. 19-23, *B*).
13 Remove the bag from the pole. Slide the bag and tubing through the sleeve (Fig. 19-23, *C*). Do not pull on the tubing. Keep the bag above the person.

14 Hang the IV bag on the pole.
15 Gather the sleeve of the clean gown that will go on the arm with the IV.
16 Remove the bag from the pole. Slip the sleeve over the bag at the shoulder part of the gown (Fig. 19-23, *D*). Hang the bag.
17 Slide the gathered sleeve over the tubing, hand, arm, and IV site. Then slide it onto the shoulder.
18 Put the other side of the gown on the person. Fasten the gown.
19 Cover the person. Remove the bath blanket.

POST-PROCEDURE

20 Provide for comfort. (See the inside of the front cover.)
21 Place the call light and other needed items within reach.
22 Lower the bed to a safe and comfortable level. Follow the care plan.
23 Raise or lower bed rails. Follow the care plan.
24 Unscreen the person.

25 Complete a safety check of the room. (See the inside of the front cover.)
26 Follow agency policy for used linens.
27 Practice hand hygiene.
28 Ask the nurse to check the flow rate.
29 Report and record your observations.

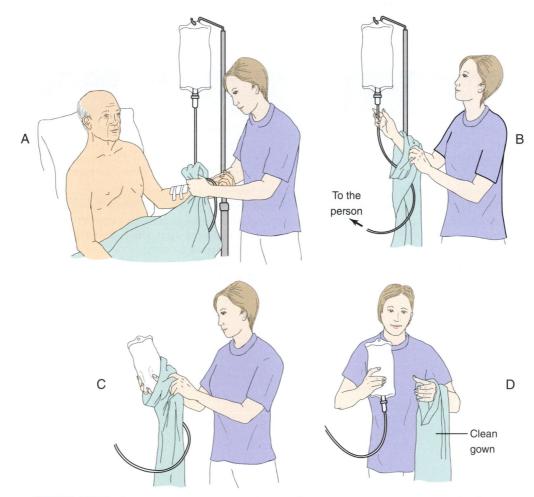

FIGURE 19-23 Changing a gown. **A,** Remove the gown from the arm with no IV. Gather up the sleeve on the arm with the IV. Slip it over the IV site and tubing, and remove it from the arm and hand. **B,** Slip the gathered sleeve along the IV tubing to the bag. **C,** Remove the IV bag from the pole and pass it through the sleeve. **D,** Slip the gathered sleeve of the clean gown over the IV bag at the shoulder part of the gown.

Personal and Professional Responsibility

Grooming promotes comfort, self-esteem, and body image. Clean hair, nails, and garments help mental well-being. So does a clean-shaven face or a well-groomed beard or mustache.

Your attitude is reflected in how you give care. To show value for the person's self-esteem and comfort:

- Be pleasant. Talk with the person.
- Ask about preferences. Allow personal choice.
- Avoid seeming rushed. Let the person know that you have time for him or her.
- Avoid thinking of care measures as tasks to complete. You are caring for a *person*. Show that you care about the person's needs and feelings.
- Do a good job. Be thorough and careful.
- Clean up after yourself. Leave the person's setting neat and orderly.

Focus on your appearance. Patients, residents, and families notice when others are not well groomed. If not groomed well, they may question the quality of care you provide. Have a professional appearance.

Rights and Respect

Grooming preferences vary. Ask what the person prefers. For example, ask what he or she would like to wear. Or ask how to style hair. Follow the person's grooming routines when possible.

You may not like the person's hair-style, clothing choices, or personal care products. Do not judge the person by your standards or impose your choices on the person. Respect the right to choose. Assist with grooming in a way that improves the person's self-esteem.

Independence and Social Interaction

Some family members want to help with grooming. For example, they want to style the person's hair. Or they want to apply lotion to the person's hands and feet.

With the person's permission, allow family members to assist with grooming as much as safely possible. This promotes social interaction. It also involves the family in the person's care.

Delegation and Teamwork

Grooming takes time. You, the person, the nurse, and other team members work together to plan and organize care. For example, a resident had a stroke. Breakfast is at 0800, speech therapy is at 0930, and family visits during lunch. The resident prefers to comb hair, shave, and change clothes after breakfast but before visitors arrive. You plan to assist the resident with grooming after breakfast and before speech therapy.

Grooming is important. Do not neglect grooming because of a busy schedule. Plan to meet the person's needs at a time best for the person and the team.

Ethics and Laws

Patients and residents have the right to be free from mistreatment and restraint (Chapter 2). Never force a care measure on a person. If a person resists or refuses care, stop. Do not proceed. Politely ask the person for the reason. Tell the nurse. You, the nurse, and the person can discuss a solution.

Special care measures are needed for persons with confusion or dementia who resist care. See Chapter 35. Patience, kindness, and problem solving are needed. A co-worker or family member may give care. Or care is given at a different time. Provide care in a way that protects the person's rights and shows dignity and respect.

FOCUS ON PRIDE: *Application*

The family may notice when grooming differs from usual. The family may tell you what they expect. Why are their comments important? How can you show that you value their input?

Circle T if the statement is TRUE and F if it is FALSE.

1 **T F** Mustaches are trimmed weekly.

2 **T F** Feet are soaked for 5 to 10 minutes.

3 **T F** Fingernails are clipped straight across.

4 **T F** Clothing is removed from the weak side first.

5 **T F** A person has poor circulation in the legs and feet. You can trim the person's toenails.

Circle the BEST answer.

6 A person with alopecia has
   a Excessive body hair
   b Dry, white flakes from the scalp
   c An infestation with lice
   d Hair loss

7 Which prevents hair from matting and tangling?
   a Bedrest
   b Daily brushing and combing
   c Daily shampooing
   d Cutting hair

8 A person's hair is *not* matted or tangled. When brushing hair, start at
   a The forehead and brush backward
   b The hair ends
   c The scalp
   d The back of the neck and brush forward

9 Brushing keeps the hair
   a Soft and shiny
   b Clean
   c Free of lice
   d Long

10 A person requests a shampoo. You should
   a Shampoo hair during the person's shower
   b Shampoo hair at the sink
   c Shampoo the person in bed
   d Follow the care plan

11 When shaving a person's face with a safety razor
   a Discard the razor in the wastebasket when done
   b Shave against the direction of hair growth
   c Hold the skin taut
   d Shave when the skin is dry

12 A person is nicked during shaving. Your *first* action is to
   a Wash your hands
   b Apply direct pressure
   c Tell the nurse
   d Apply a bandage

13 Fingernails are cut with
   a An emery board
   b Scissors
   c A nail file
   d Nail clippers

14 Garments are applied
   a To the weak side first
   b To the strong side first
   c To either the weak or the strong side first
   d In the same way they are removed

15 When changing the gown on a person with an IV
   a Keep the IV bag below the person's arm
   b Stop the IV pump to change the gown
   c Have the nurse check the flow rate afterward
   d Disconnect the IV to change the gown

Answers to Chapter 19 questions are on p. 552.

FOCUS ON PRACTICE

Problem Solving

A resident with dementia has long fingernails. Some are broken and have rough edges. As you begin nail care, the resident resists by pulling away and yelling at you. What do you do? Why is nail care important for this resident? How might you provide care safely?

Urinary Needs

OBJECTIVES

- Define the key terms and key abbreviations in this chapter.
- Describe the rules for normal urination.
- Describe normal urine.
- Identify the observations to report to the nurse.
- Describe urinary incontinence and the care required.

- Describe bladder training methods.
- Perform the procedures described in this chapter.
- Explain how to promote PRIDE in the person, the family, and yourself.

KEY TERMS

dysuria Painful or difficult *(dys)* urination *(uria);* burning on urination

functional incontinence The person has bladder control but cannot use the toilet in time

hematuria Blood *(hemat)* in the urine *(uria)*

mixed incontinence The combination of stress incontinence and urge incontinence

nocturia Frequent urination *(uria)* at night *(noc)*

oliguria Scant amount *(olig)* of urine *(uria);* less than 500 mL in 24 hours

over-flow incontinence Small amounts of urine leak from a full bladder

polyuria Abnormally large amounts *(poly)* of urine *(uria)*

reflex incontinence Urine is lost at predictable intervals when a specific amount of urine is in the bladder

stress incontinence When urine leaks during exercise and certain movements that cause pressure on the bladder

transient incontinence Temporary or occasional incontinence that is reversed when the cause is treated

urge incontinence The loss of urine in response to a sudden, urgent need to void; the person cannot get to a toilet in time; over-active bladder

urinary frequency Voiding at frequent intervals

urinary incontinence The involuntary loss or leakage of urine

urinary retention Not being able to completely empty the bladder

urinary urgency The need to void at once

urination The process of emptying urine from the bladder; voiding

voiding See "urination"

KEY ABBREVIATIONS

BM Bowel movement
mL Milliliter

UTI Urinary tract infection

Eliminating waste is a physical need. The urinary system removes waste products from the blood. It also maintains the body's water and electrolyte balance.

See *Promoting Safety and Comfort: Urinary Needs.*

PROMOTING SAFETY AND COMFORT

Urinary Needs

Safety

Urinary elimination measures often involve exposing and touching private areas—the perineum and rectum. Sexual abuse has occurred in health care settings. The person may feel threatened or is actually being abused. He or she needs to call for help. Keep the call light within the person's reach at all times. Always act in a professional manner.

Urine may contain blood and microbes. Microbes can live and grow in bedpans, urinals, commodes, and urinary drainage bags (Chapter 21). Follow Standard Precautions and the Bloodborne Pathogen Standard (Chapter 13) to handle urinary devices and their contents. This includes incontinence products. Thoroughly clean and disinfect bedpans, urinals, and commodes after use. Remember to practice hand hygiene.

Each person is given his or her own bedpan or urinal. Some states and agencies require labeling the devices with the person's name and room and bed number. Equipment is not shared among patients and residents.

NOTE: A task may require more than 1 pair of gloves. Change gloves as needed. Use careful judgment. Remember to practice hand hygiene after removing gloves.

NORMAL URINATION

The healthy adult produces about 1500 mL (milliliters) or 3 pints of urine a day. Many factors affect urine production—age, disease, the amount and kinds of fluid ingested, salt, body temperature, perspiration (sweating), and some drugs. Some substances increase urine production—coffee, tea, alcohol, and some drugs. A diet high in salt and some drugs cause the body to retain water. When water is retained, less urine is produced.

Urination (voiding) means the process of emptying urine from the bladder. The amount of fluid intake, habits, and available toilet facilities affect frequency. So do activity, work, and illness. People usually void at bedtime, after sleep, and before meals. Some void more often.

Some persons need help getting to the bathroom. Others use bedpans, urinals, or commodes. Follow the rules in Box 20-1 and the person's care plan.

See *Focus on Communication: Normal Urination.*

BOX 20-1 Rules for Normal Urination

- Practice medical asepsis.
- Follow Standard Precautions and the Bloodborne Pathogen Standard.
- Provide fluids as the nurse and care plan direct.
- Follow the person's voiding routines and habits. Check with the nurse and the care plan.
- Help the person to the bathroom upon request. Or provide the commode, bedpan, or urinal. The need to void may be urgent.
- Help the person assume a normal position for voiding if possible. Women sit or squat. Men stand.
- Warm the bedpan or urinal.
- Cover the person for warmth and privacy.
- Provide for privacy. Pull the privacy curtain around the bed, close room and bathroom doors, and close window coverings. Leave the room if the person can be alone.
- Tell the person that running water, flushing the toilet, or playing music can mask voiding sounds. Voiding with others nearby embarrasses some people.
- Stay nearby if the person is weak or unsteady.
- Place the call light and toilet tissue within reach.
- Allow enough time. Do not rush the person.
- Promote relaxation. Some people like to read.
- Run water in a sink if the person cannot start the urine stream. Or place the person's fingers in warm water.
- Provide perineal care as needed (Chapter 18).
- Assist with hand-washing after voiding. Provide a wash basin, soap, washcloth, and towel.
- Assist the person to the bathroom or offer the bedpan, urinal, or commode at regular times. Some people are embarrassed or are too weak to ask for help.

FOCUS ON COMMUNICATION

Normal Urination

Patients and residents may not use the terms "voiding" or "urinating." The person may not understand what you are saying. Do not ask: "Do you need to void?" or "Do you need to urinate?" Instead, you can ask these questions.

- "Do you need to use the bathroom?"
- "Do you need to use the bedpan (urinal)?"
- "Do you need to pass urine?"
- "Do you need to pass water?"
- "Do you need to pee?"

The word "pee" may offend some persons. Choose words the person understands and uses. Follow the care plan.

Observations

Normal urine is pale yellow, straw-colored, or amber (Fig. 20-1). It is clear with no particles. A faint odor is normal. Observe urine for color, clarity, odor, amount (output), particles, and blood.

Ask the nurse to observe urine that looks or smells abnormal. Report these problems.

- *Dysuria—painful or difficult* (dys) *urination* (uria); *burning on urination*
- *Hematuria—blood* (hemat) *in the urine* (uria)
- *Nocturia—frequent urination* (uria) *at night* (noc)
- *Oliguria—scant amount* (olig) *of urine* (uria); *less than 500 mL in 24 hours*
- *Polyuria—abnormally large amounts* (poly) *of urine* (uria)
- *Urinary frequency—voiding at frequent intervals*
- *Urinary incontinence—the involuntary loss or leakage of urine*
- *Urinary retention—not being able to completely empty the bladder*
- *Urinary urgency—the need to void at once*

Bedpans

Bedpans are used when the person cannot be out of bed. Women use bedpans for voiding and bowel movements (BMs). Men use them for BMs.

The *standard bedpan* is shown in Figure 20-2, *A*. The wide rim goes under the buttocks. A *fracture pan* has a thin rim. It is only about ½-inch deep at one end (Fig. 20-2, *B*). The smaller end (flat end) goes under the buttocks (Fig. 20-3). Fracture pans are used:

- By persons with casts
- By persons in traction
- By persons with limited back motion
- By older persons with osteoporosis (fragile bones) or arthritis (Chapter 33)
- After spinal cord injury or surgery
- After a hip fracture or hip replacement surgery
  See *Delegation Guidelines: Bedpans*, p. 296.
  See *Promoting Safety and Comfort: Bedpans*, p. 296.
  See procedure: *Giving the Bedpan*, p. 296.

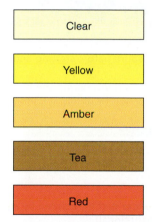

| Clear |
| Yellow |
| Amber |
| Tea |
| Red |

FIGURE 20-1 Color chart for urine. (Redrawn from Weldon, Inc., Fort Worth, Tex.)

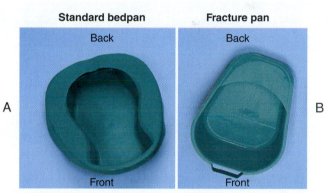

FIGURE 20-2 Bedpans. **A,** Standard bedpan. **B,** Fracture pan.

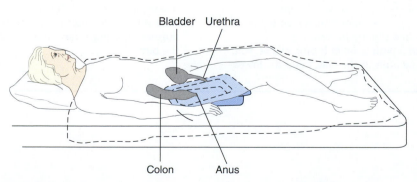

FIGURE 20-3 A person positioned on a fracture pan. The small end (flat end) is under the buttocks.

DELEGATION GUIDELINES

Bedpans

To assist with a bedpan, you need this information from the nurse and the care plan.

- What bedpan to use—standard bedpan or fracture pan
- Position or activity limits
- If you can leave the room or if you need to stay with the person
- If the nurse will observe the results before you flush the contents
- What observations to report and record:
  - Urine color, clarity, and odor
  - Amount
  - Presence of particles
  - Blood in the urine
  - Cloudy urine
  - Complaints of urgency, burning, dysuria, or other problems
  - For bowel movements, see Chapter 22
- When to report observations
- What patient or resident concerns to report at once

PROMOTING SAFETY AND COMFORT

Bedpans

Safety

Remember to raise the bed as needed for good body mechanics. Lower the bed before leaving the room. Raise or lower the bed rails according to the care plan.

Comfort

Most bedpans are plastic. Metal bedpans are often cold. Warm metal bedpans with warm water and dry them before use. Use clean, dry paper towels for drying.

The person must not sit on a bedpan for a long time. Bedpans are uncomfortable. They can lead to pressure injuries (Chapter 29).

Giving the Bedpan

QUALITY OF LIFE

- Knock before entering the person's room.
- Address the person by name.
- Introduce yourself by name and title.

- Explain the procedure before starting and during the procedure.
- Protect the person's rights during the procedure.
- Handle the person gently during the procedure.

PRE-PROCEDURE

1 Follow *Delegation Guidelines: Bedpans.* See *Promoting Safety and Comfort:*
   a *Urinary Needs,* p. 294
   b *Bedpans*
2 Provide for privacy.
3 Practice hand hygiene.
4 Put on gloves.

5 Collect the following.
   - Bedpan
   - Bedpan cover
   - Toilet tissue
   - Waterproof under-pad (if required by agency policy)
   - Bath blanket (optional)
6 Arrange equipment on the chair or bed.

PROCEDURE

7 Raise the bed for body mechanics (if the person's needs are not urgent). Lower the bed rail near you (if up).
8 Lower the head of the bed. Position the person supine. Or raise the head of the bed slightly for comfort.
9 Cover the person with a bath blanket if time allows. Fold the top linens and gown out of the way. Keep the lower body covered.

10 Have the person flex the knees and raise the buttocks. He or she pushes against the mattress with the feet.
11 Slide your hand under the lower back. Help raise the buttocks. If using a waterproof under-pad, place it under the buttocks.

Giving the Bedpan—cont'd

PROCEDURE—cont'd

12 Slide the bedpan under the person (Fig. 20-4). Make sure the bedpan is centered under the person.
13 If the person cannot assist in getting on the bedpan:
   a Place the waterproof under-pad under the buttocks if using one.
   b Turn the person onto the side away from you.
   c Place the bedpan firmly against the buttocks (Fig. 20-5, p. 298).
   d Hold the bedpan securely. Turn the person onto his or her back.
   e Make sure the bedpan is centered under the person.
14 Cover the person.
15 Raise the head of the bed so the person is in a sitting position (Fowler's position) for a standard bedpan. (NOTE: Some state competency tests require removing gloves and hand-washing before raising the head of the bed.)
16 Make sure the person is correctly positioned on the bedpan (Fig. 20-6, p. 298).
17 Raise the bed rail if used. Lower the bed.
18 Place the toilet tissue and call light within reach. (NOTE: For some state competency tests you ask the person to use hand wipes for hand hygiene after wiping with toilet tissue.)
19 Ask the person to signal when done or when help is needed. (Stay with the person if necessary. Be respectful. Provide as much privacy as possible.)
20 Remove and discard the gloves. Practice hand hygiene.
21 Leave the room and close the door.
22 Return when the person signals. Or check on the person every 5 minutes. Knock before entering.

23 Practice hand hygiene. Put on gloves.
24 Raise the bed for body mechanics. Lower the bed rail (if used) and lower the head of the bed.
25 Have the person raise the buttocks. Remove the bedpan. Or hold the bedpan and turn the person onto the side away from you.
26 Clean the genital area if the person cannot do so.
   a Clean from the meatus (front or top) to the anus (back or bottom) with toilet tissue. Use fresh tissue for each wipe.
   b Provide perineal care if needed (Chapter 18).
   c Remove and discard the waterproof under-pad (if used).
27 Cover the bedpan. Take it to the bathroom. Raise the bed rail (if used) before leaving the bedside.
28 Note the color, amount (output), and character of urine or feces. See "Measuring Intake and Output" in Chapter 24.
29 Empty the bedpan contents into the toilet and flush.
30 Rinse the bedpan. Pour the rinse into the toilet and flush.
31 Clean the bedpan with a disinfectant. Pour disinfectant into the toilet and flush. Dry the bedpan with clean, dry paper towels.
32 Return the bedpan and clean cover to the bedside stand.
33 Remove and discard the gloves. Practice hand hygiene and put on clean gloves.
34 Help the person with hand-washing.
35 Remove and discard the gloves. Practice hand hygiene.
36 Cover the person with the top linens. Remove the bath blanket (if used).

POST-PROCEDURE

37 Provide for comfort. (See the inside of the front cover.)
38 Place the call light and other needed items within reach.
39 Lower the bed to a safe and comfortable level. Follow the care plan.
40 Raise or lower bed rails. Follow the care plan.
41 Unscreen the person.

42 Complete a safety check of the room. (See the inside of the front cover.)
43 Follow agency policy for used linens.
44 Practice hand hygiene.
45 Report and record your observations.

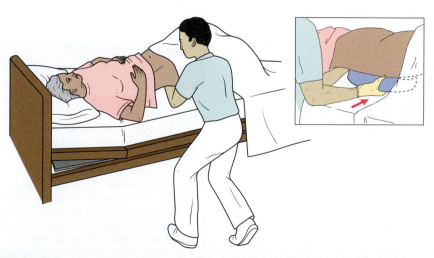

FIGURE 20-4 The person raises the buttocks off the bed with help. The bedpan is slid under the person.

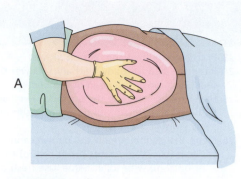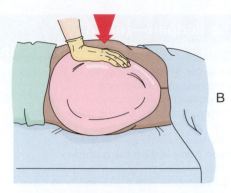

FIGURE 20-5 Giving a bedpan. **A,** Position the person on the side away from you. Place the bedpan firmly against the buttocks. **B,** Push downward on the bedpan and toward the person.

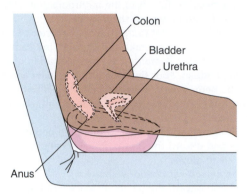

FIGURE 20-6 The person is positioned on the bedpan so the urethra and anus are directly over the opening.

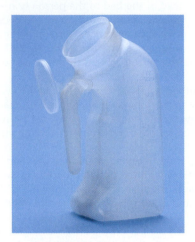

FIGURE 20-7 Male urinal.

Urinals

Men use urinals to void (Fig. 20-7). Urinals have caps and hook-type handles. The urinal hooks to the bed rail within the man's reach. He stands to use the urinal if possible. Or he sits on the side of the bed or lies in bed to use it. Some men need support when standing.

After voiding, he closes the urinal cap. This prevents urine spills. Remind men to hang urinals on bed rails and to signal after using them. Remind them not to place urinals on over-bed tables and bedside stands. These surfaces must not be contaminated with urine.

Some beds do not have bed rails. Follow agency policy for where to place urinals.

See *Focus on Communication: Urinals.*
See *Delegation Guidelines: Urinals.*
See *Promoting Safety and Comfort: Urinals.*
See procedure: *Giving the Urinal.*

PROMOTING SAFETY AND COMFORT

Urinals

Safety

Empty urinals promptly to prevent odors and the spread of microbes. A filled urinal spills easily, causing hazards. Also, it is an unpleasant sight and causes odor. Urinals are cleaned and disinfected like bedpans.

Comfort

For some men, you may need to place the penis in the urinal. This may embarrass the person and you. Act in a professional manner.

Giving the Urinal

QUALITY OF LIFE

- Knock before entering the person's room.
- Address the person by name.
- Introduce yourself by name and title.

- Explain the procedure before starting and during the procedure.
- Protect the person's rights during the procedure.
- Handle the person gently during the procedure.

PRE-PROCEDURE

1 Follow *Delegation Guidelines: Urinals.* See *Promoting Safety and Comfort:*
  a *Urinary Needs,* p. 294
  b *Urinals*
2 Provide for privacy.
3 Determine if the man will stand, sit, or lie in bed.

4 Practice hand hygiene.
5 Put on gloves.
6 Collect the following.
  - Urinal
  - Non-skid footwear for standing

PROCEDURE

7 *Using the urinal in bed:*
  a Give him the urinal.
  b Remind him to tilt the bottom down to prevent spills.
8 *Standing to use the urinal:*
  a Help him sit on the side of the bed.
  b Put non-skid footwear on him.
  c Help him stand. Provide support if he is unsteady.
  d Give him the urinal.
9 *Positioning the urinal (in bed or standing):*
  a Help the person stand (step 8) if he will stand.
  b Position the urinal.
  c Place the penis in the urinal if he cannot do so.
  d Cover him for privacy.
10 Place the call light within reach. Ask him to signal when done or when help is needed.
11 Provide for privacy.
12 Remove and discard the gloves. Practice hand hygiene.

13 Leave the room and close the door.
14 Return when he signals for you. Or check on him every 5 minutes. Knock before entering.
15 Practice hand hygiene. Put on gloves.
16 Close the urinal cap. Take it to the bathroom.
17 Note the color, amount (output), and clarity of urine.
18 Empty the urinal into the toilet and flush.
19 Rinse the urinal with cold water. Pour rinse into the toilet and flush.
20 Clean the urinal with a disinfectant. Pour disinfectant into the toilet and flush. Dry the urinal with clean, dry paper towels.
21 Return the urinal to its proper place.
22 Remove and discard the gloves. Practice hand hygiene and put on clean gloves.
23 Assist with hand-washing.
24 Remove and discard the gloves. Practice hand hygiene.

POST-PROCEDURE

25 Provide for comfort. (See the inside of the front cover.)
26 Place the call light and other needed items within reach.
27 Raise or lower bed rails. Follow the care plan.
28 Unscreen him.
29 Complete a safety check of the room. (See the inside of the front cover.)

30 Follow agency policy for used linens.
31 Practice hand hygiene.
32 Report and record your observations.

Commodes

A commode (bedside commode) is a chair or wheelchair with an opening for a container (Fig. 20-8). Persons unable to walk to the bathroom often use commodes. The commode allows a normal position for elimination. The commode arms and back provide support and help prevent falls.

Some commodes, with the containers removed, are placed over toilets. The person uses the commode arms for support to sit and stand. And the commode serves as a higher toilet seat. If the commode has wheels, lock the wheels after properly positioning the commode over the toilet.

See *Delegation Guidelines: Commodes.*
See *Promoting Safety and Comfort: Commodes.*
See procedure: *Helping the Person to the Commode.*

DELEGATION GUIDELINES
Commodes

You need this information from the nurse and care plan when assisting with commode use.
- If the commode is used at the bedside or over the toilet
- How much help the person needs
- If you can leave the room or if you need to stay with the person
- If the nurse needs to observe urine or BMs before you flush the contents
- What observations to report and record (see *Delegation Guidelines: Bedpans*, p. 296)
- When to report observations
- What patient or resident concerns to report at once

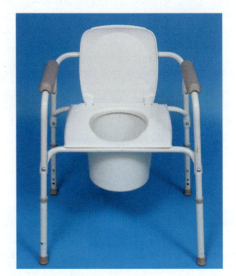

FIGURE 20-8 The commode has a toilet seat with a container. The container slides out from under the seat for emptying or to use the commode over the toilet.

PROMOTING SAFETY AND COMFORT
Commodes

Safety
You will transfer the person to and from the commode. Practice safe transfer procedures (Chapter 16). Use the transfer belt and lock the wheels. Remove the transfer belt after the transfer. See "Transfer/Gait Belts" in Chapter 11.

Each person is given his or her own commode. The commode is not shared among patients and residents. When no longer needed, the commode is returned to the supply department for disinfection.

Comfort
After transfer to the commode, cover the person's lap and legs with a bath blanket. This promotes warmth and privacy.

Helping the Person to the Commode

QUALITY OF LIFE

- Knock before entering the person's room.
- Address the person by name.
- Introduce yourself by name and title.

- Explain the procedure before starting and during the procedure.
- Protect the person's rights during the procedure.
- Handle the person gently during the procedure.

PRE-PROCEDURE

1 Follow *Delegation Guidelines: Commodes.* See *Promoting Safety and Comfort:*
   a *Urinary Needs,* p. 294
   b *Commodes*
2 Provide for privacy.
3 Practice hand hygiene.
4 Put on gloves.

5 Collect the following.
   - Commode
   - Toilet tissue
   - Bath blanket
   - Transfer belt
   - Robe and non-skid footwear

PROCEDURE

6 Place the commode next to the bed.
7 Help the person sit on the side of the bed. Lower the bed rail if used.
8 Help the person put on a robe and non-skid footwear.
9 Apply the transfer belt.
10 Assist the person to the commode. Use the transfer belt.
11 Remove the transfer belt. Cover the person with a bath blanket for warmth.
12 Place the toilet tissue and call light within reach.
13 Ask the person to signal when done or when help is needed. (Stay with the person if necessary. Be respectful. Provide as much privacy as possible.)
14 Remove and discard the gloves. Practice hand hygiene.
15 Leave the room. Close the door.
16 Return when the person signals. Or check on the person every 5 minutes. Knock before entering.
17 Practice hand hygiene. Put on the gloves.
18 Help the person clean the genital area as needed. Remove and discard the gloves. Practice hand hygiene.

19 Apply the transfer belt. Help the person back to bed using the transfer belt. Remove the transfer belt, robe, and footwear. Raise the bed rail if used.
20 Put on clean gloves. Remove and cover the commode container.
21 Take the container to the bathroom.
22 Observe urine and feces for color, amount (output), and character.
23 Empty the contents into the toilet and flush.
24 Rinse the container. Pour the rinse into the toilet and flush.
25 Clean and disinfect the container. Pour disinfectant into the toilet and flush. Dry the container with clean, dry paper towels.
26 Return the container to the commode. Close the lid. Clean other parts of the commode if necessary.
27 Return supplies to their proper place.
28 Remove and discard the gloves. Practice hand hygiene and put on clean gloves.
29 Assist with hand-washing.
30 Remove and discard the gloves. Practice hand hygiene.

POST-PROCEDURE

31 Provide for comfort. (See the inside of the front cover.)
32 Place the call light and other needed items within reach.
33 Raise or lower bed rails. Follow the care plan.
34 Unscreen the person.
35 Complete a safety check of the room. (See the inside of the front cover.)

36 Follow agency policy for used linens.
37 Practice hand hygiene.
38 Report and record your observations.

URINARY INCONTINENCE

Urinary incontinence is the involuntary loss or leakage of urine. Incontinence is not a normal part of aging. However, older persons are at risk because of urinary tract changes, medical and surgical conditions, and drug therapy.

Types of Incontinence

Incontinence may be temporary or permanent. Common types of incontinence are:

- *Stress incontinence. Urine leaks during exercise and certain movements that cause pressure on the bladder.* Urine loss is small. Often called *dribbling*, it occurs with laughing, sneezing, coughing, lifting, or other activities.
- *Urge incontinence (over-active bladder). Urine is lost in response to a sudden, urgent need to void. The person cannot get to a toilet in time.* Urinary frequency, urinary urgency, and night-time voiding are common.
- *Mixed incontinence. The person has a combination of stress incontinence and urge incontinence.* Many older women have this type.
- *Over-flow incontinence. Small amounts of urine leak from a full bladder.* The person feels like the bladder is not empty. The person dribbles and may have a weak urine stream.
- *Functional incontinence. The person has bladder control but cannot use the toilet in time.* Immobility, restraints, unanswered call lights, no call light within reach, and difficulty removing clothing are causes. Not knowing where to find the bathroom, confusion, and disorientation are other causes.
- *Reflex incontinence. Urine is lost at predictable intervals when a specific amount of urine is in the bladder.* The person does not feel the need to void. Nervous system disorders and injuries are common causes.
- *Transient incontinence. This refers to temporary or occasional incontinence that is reversed when the cause is treated. (Transient means for a short time.)*

Incontinence may result from a physical illness or drugs. Some causes can be reversed. Others cannot. If incontinence is a new problem, tell the nurse at once.

Managing Incontinence

The goals of managing incontinence are to:
- Prevent urinary tract infections (UTIs).
- Restore as much bladder function as possible.

Incontinence is embarrassing. Garments are wet and odors develop. The person is uncomfortable. Skin irritation, infection, and pressure injuries are risks. Falling is a risk when trying to get to the bathroom quickly. Pride, dignity, and self-esteem are affected. Social isolation, loss of independence, and depression are common. Quality of life suffers.

The person's care plan may include some of the measures listed in Box 20-2. *Good skin care and dry garments and linens are essential.* Promoting normal urinary elimination prevents incontinence in some people (see Box 20-1). Others need bladder training (p. 307). Sometimes catheters are needed (Chapter 21).

Incontinence is linked to abuse, mistreatment, and neglect. Frequent care is needed. The person may wet again right after skin care and changing wet garments and linens. Remember, incontinence is beyond the person's control. It is not something the person chooses to do. Be patient. The person's needs are great. If feeling short-tempered, talk to the nurse. The person has the right to be free from abuse, mistreatment, and neglect. Kindness, empathy, understanding, and patience are needed.

See *Focus on Older Persons: Managing Incontinence.*
See *Focus on Surveys: Managing Incontinence.*

BOX 20-2 Urinary Incontinence—Nursing Measures

- Record the person's voidings—times and amount (output). This includes incontinent times and successful use of the toilet, commode, bedpan, or urinal.
- Answer call lights promptly. The need to void may be urgent.
- Promote normal urinary elimination (see Box 20-1).
- Promote normal bowel elimination (Chapter 22).
- Assist with elimination after sleep, before and after meals, and at bedtime.
- Follow the person's bladder training program (p. 307).
- Provide a clear path to the bathroom.
- Have the person wear easy-to-remove clothing. Incontinence can occur while dealing with buttons, zippers, other closures, and under-garments.
- Encourage pelvic muscle exercises as instructed by the nurse.
- Check the person often to make sure he or she is clean and dry.
- Help prevent UTIs.
  - Promote fluid intake as the nurse directs.
  - Have the person wear cotton underwear.
  - Keep the perineal area clean and dry.
  - Clean from front to back (top to bottom) during perineal care (Chapter 18).
- Decrease fluid intake at bedtime.
- Provide good skin care.
- Apply a barrier cream or moisturizer (cream, lotion, paste) to the skin or perineum as directed by the nurse. The application prevents irritation and skin damage.
- Provide dry garments and linens.
- Observe for signs of skin breakdown (Chapters 28 and 29).
- Use incontinence products as the nurse directs. Follow the manufacturer's instructions.
- Do not leave urinals in place to catch urine for men who are incontinent.
- Keep the perineal area clean and dry (Chapter 18).
  - Protect the person and dry garments and linens from the wet incontinence product.
  - Remove wet incontinence products, garments, and linens.
  - Expose only the perineal area.
  - Use soap and water or a no-rinse incontinence cleanser (perineal rinse). Follow the care plan. For soap and water, use a safe and comfortable water temperature.
  - Dry the perineal area and buttocks.
  - Apply a clean, dry incontinence product and clean, dry garments and linens.
- Follow Standard Precautions and the Bloodborne Pathogen Standard.

FOCUS ON OLDER PERSONS

Managing Incontinence

Complications from incontinence pose serious problems for older persons. These include falls, pressure injuries, and UTIs. Long hospital or long-term care stays are often necessary.

Persons with dementia may void in the wrong places. Trash cans, planters, heating vents, and closets are examples. Some persons throw incontinence products on the floor or in the toilet. Others resist staff efforts to keep them clean and dry.

Provide safe care. The care plan lists needed measures. The care plan may include measures recommended by the Alzheimer's Disease Education and Referral Center (ADEAR).

- Follow the person's bathroom routine. For example, take the person to the bathroom every 2 to 3 hours during the day. Do not wait for the person to ask.
- Observe for signs of needing to void. Restlessness and pulling at clothes are examples. Respond quickly.
- Stay calm when the person is incontinent. Reassure the person if he or she becomes upset.
- Report incontinence. Report the time, what the person was doing, and other observations. An incontinence pattern may emerge. If so, measures are planned to prevent the problem.
- Prevent incontinence during sleep. Limit the type and amount of fluids in the evening. Follow the care plan.
- Plan ahead for the person leaving the agency. Have the person wear easy-to-remove clothing. Pack extra clothing, incontinence products, and hygiene supplies. Know where to find restrooms.

You may need a co-worker's help to keep the person clean and dry. If you have questions, ask the nurse for help.

Remember, everyone has the right to privacy and safe care. They also have the right to be treated with dignity.

FOCUS ON SURVEYS

Managing Incontinence

Surveyors observe how incontinence is prevented, improved, or managed. They observe if staff:
- Follow the person's care plan.
- Keep call lights within reach.
- Answer call lights promptly.
- Provide a clear path to the bathroom.
- Provide good lighting for voiding.
- Assist with bedpans, urinals, and commodes as needed.
- Assist the person to the bathroom as needed.
- Respond appropriately when incontinence occurs.
- Protect the person's dignity when incontinence occurs.
- Check incontinent persons often.
- Change wet incontinence products and clothing promptly.
- Prevent prolonged exposure of the skin to urine.
- Provide hygiene measures to prevent skin breakdown.

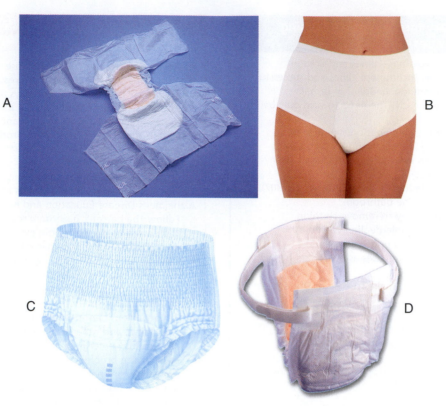

FIGURE 20-9 Disposable incontinence products. **A,** Complete incontinence brief. **B,** Pad and under-garment. **C,** Pull-on underwear. **D,** Belted under-garment. (**B,** Courtesy Hartmann USA, Inc., Rock Hill, S.C. **C,** Courtesy Hartmann Inc., Heidenheim, Germany. **D,** Courtesy Principle Business Enterprises, Dunbridge, Ohio.)

Applying Incontinence Products

Incontinence products help keep the person dry. They usually have 2 layers and a waterproof back. Fluid passes through the top layer. It is absorbed by the bottom layer.

Common incontinence products are shown in Figure 20-9. The nurse helps the person select products for his or her needs. To use them, follow the manufacturer's instructions and agency procedures.

See *Focus on Communication: Applying Incontinence Products.*

See *Delegation Guidelines: Applying Incontinence Products.*

See *Promoting Safety and Comfort: Applying Incontinence Products.*

See procedure: *Applying an Incontinence Brief.*

DELEGATION GUIDELINES

Applying Incontinence Products

To apply an incontinence product, you need this information from the nurse and the care plan.
- What product to use.
- What size to use.
- If you need to apply a barrier cream. If yes, what cream to use.
- What observations to report and record:
  - Complaints of pain, burning, irritation, or the need to void
  - Signs and symptoms of skin breakdown:
    - Redness, irritation, blisters
    - Complaints of pain, burning, tingling, or itching
  - The amount of urine—small, moderate, large
  - Urine color
  - Blood in the urine
  - Leakage
  - A poor product fit
- When to report observations.
- What patient or resident concerns to report at once.

PROMOTING SAFETY AND COMFORT
Applying Incontinence Products

Safety

To safely apply an incontinence product, follow the manufacturer's instructions. The guidelines in Box 20-3 will help prevent:

- Leakage
- Skin irritation, skin damage, and pressure injuries
- Tearing of the product
   Remove the soiled incontinence product from front to back (top to bottom). Apply the new product from front to back (top to bottom). This prevents spreading bacteria from the anal area to the urinary system.

Comfort

For comfort, use the correct size. If the product is too large, urine can leak. If too small, the product will cause discomfort from being too tight.

BOX 20-3	Applying Incontinence Products

- Follow the manufacturer's instructions.
- Use the correct size. The nurse tells you what size to use.
- Note the front and back of the product.
- Center the product in the perineal area.
- Position the man's penis downward.
- Check for proper placement. The product should be in the creases between the thighs and the perineal area (groin area). It should fit the shape of the body.
- Note the amount of urine (small, moderate, large). Also note how often you change the product. An extended wear product may be needed for large amounts of urine or diarrhea (Chapter 22).
- Do not let the plastic backing touch the person's skin.
- Provide perineal care after each incontinent episode.
- Do not use the product as a turning or lift sheet.
- Attach the tabs correctly. Some products will tear if you try to unfasten the tape or change the tape's position.
  - Attach the lower tape first. Stretch the tape and attach it at a slightly upward angle. Do so for both sides.
  - Attach the upper tape after the lower tape is fastened. Stretch the tape and attach it in a horizontal manner. Do so for both sides.

Applying an Incontinence Brief

QUALITY OF LIFE

- Knock before entering the person's room.
- Address the person by name.
- Introduce yourself by name and title.

- Explain the procedure before starting and during the procedure.
- Protect the person's rights during the procedure.
- Handle the person gently during the procedure.

PRE-PROCEDURE

1. Follow *Delegation Guidelines: Applying Incontinence Products.* See *Promoting Safety and Comfort:*
   a. *Urinary Needs,* p. 294
   b. *Applying Incontinence Products*
2. Practice hand hygiene.
3. Collect the following.
   - Incontinence brief
   - Barrier cream or moisturizer as directed by the nurse
   - Cleanser
   - Items for perineal care (Chapter 18)
   - Waterproof under-pad
   - Paper towels
   - Trash bag
   - Gloves

4. Cover the over-bed table with paper towels. Arrange items on top of them.
5. Identify the person. Check the ID (identification) bracelet against the assignment sheet. Use 2 identifiers (Chapter 10). Also call the person by name.
6. Mark the date, time, and your initials on the new product. Follow agency policy.
7. Provide for privacy.
8. Fill the wash basin. Water temperature is usually 105°F to 109°F (Fahrenheit) (40.5°C to 42.7°C [centigrade]). Measure water temperature according to agency policy. Have the person check the water temperature and adjust as needed.
9. Raise the bed for body mechanics. Bed rails are up if used.

PROCEDURE

10. Lower the head of the bed. The bed is as flat as possible.
11. Lower the bed rail near you if up.
12. Practice hand hygiene. Put on the gloves.
13. Cover the person with a bath blanket. Lower top linens to the foot of the bed. Lower the pants or slacks.
14. Place a waterproof under-pad under the buttocks. Have the person raise the buttocks off the bed. Or turn the person from side to side.

15. Loosen the tabs on each side of the used brief.
16. Turn the person onto the side away from you.
17. Remove the brief from front to back (top to bottom). Observe the urine as you roll the product up (Fig. 20-10, *A*, p. 306).
18. Place the used brief in the trash bag. Set the bag aside.
19. Perform perineal care (Chapter 18) wearing clean gloves. Apply the barrier cream or moisturizer.

Continued

Applying an Incontinence Brief—cont'd

PROCEDURE—cont'd

20 Remove and discard the gloves. Practice hand hygiene. Put on clean gloves.
21 Open the new brief. Fold it in half length-wise along the center (Fig. 20-10, B).
22 Insert the brief between the legs from front to back (top to bottom) (Fig. 20-10, C).
23 Unfold and spread the back panel (Fig. 20-10, D).
24 Center the brief in the perineal area.
25 Turn the person onto his or her back.
26 Unfold and spread the front panel. Provide a "cup" shape in the perineal area. For a man, position the penis downward.
27 Make sure the brief is positioned high in the groin folds. The brief fits the shape of the body.

28 Secure the brief (Fig. 20-10, E).
  a Pull the lower tape tab forward on the side near you. Attach it at a slightly upward angle. Do the same for the other side.
  b Pull the upper tape tab forward on the side near you. Attach it in a horizontal manner. Do the same for the other side.
29 Smooth out all wrinkles and folds.
30 Ask about comfort. Ask if the product feels too loose or too tight. Check for wrinkles or creases. Make sure the product does not rub or irritate the groin. Adjust the product as needed.
31 Remove and discard the gloves. Practice hand hygiene.
32 Raise or put on pants or slacks.

POST-PROCEDURE

33 Provide for comfort. (See the inside of the front cover.)
34 Place the call light and other needed items within reach.
35 Lower the bed to a safe and comfortable level. Follow the care plan.
36 Raise or lower bed rails. Follow the care plan.
37 Unscreen the person.
38 Practice hand hygiene. Put on clean gloves.
39 Estimate the amount of urine in the used brief: small, moderate, large. Open the product to observe for urine color and blood.

40 Clean, rinse, dry, and return the wash basin and other equipment. Use clean, dry paper towels for drying. Return items to their proper place.
41 Remove and discard the gloves. Practice hand hygiene.
42 Complete a safety check of the room. (See the inside of the front cover.)
43 Follow agency policy for used linens.
44 Practice hand hygiene.
45 Report and record your observations.

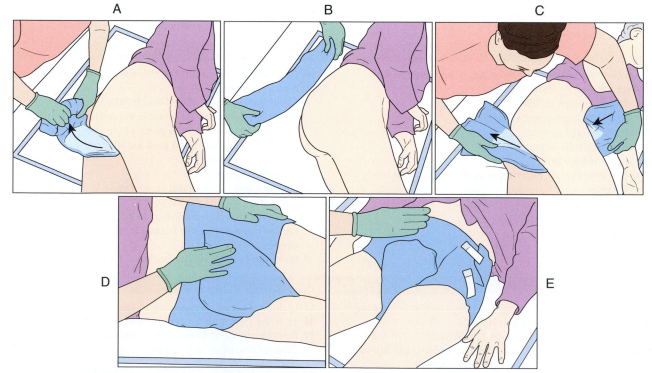

FIGURE 20-10 Applying an incontinence brief. **A,** The used brief is removed from front to back (top to bottom). **B,** The new brief is opened length-wise. **C,** The new brief is inserted length-wise between the legs from front to back (top to bottom). **D,** The back panel is spread open. **E,** The lower tape tab is attached at a slightly upward angle. The upper tape tab is attached in a horizontal manner.

BLADDER TRAINING

Bladder training may help with urinary incontinence. Some persons need bladder training after catheter removal (Chapter 21). Control of urination is the goal. Bladder control promotes comfort and quality of life. It also increases self-esteem.

Bladder training methods are:
- *Bladder re-training (bladder rehabilitation).* The person needs to:
  - Resist or ignore the strong desire to urinate.
  - Postpone or delay voiding.
  - Urinate following a schedule rather than the urge to void.

  The time between voidings increases as bladder re-training progresses.
- *Prompted voiding.* The person voids at scheduled times. The person learns to:
  - Recognize when the bladder is full.
  - Recognize the need to void.
  - Ask for help.
  - Respond when prompted to void.
- *Habit training/scheduled voiding.* Voiding is scheduled at regular times to match the person's voiding habits. This is usually every 2 to 4 hours while awake. The person does not delay or resist voiding. Timed-voiding follows the person's usual voiding patterns.
- *Catheter clamping.* The catheter is clamped to prevent urine flow from the bladder (Chapter 21). See Figure 20-11. It is usually clamped for 1 hour at first. Over time, it is clamped for 3 to 4 hours. Urine drains when the catheter is unclamped. After catheter removal, voiding is encouraged every 3 to 4 hours or as directed by the care plan.

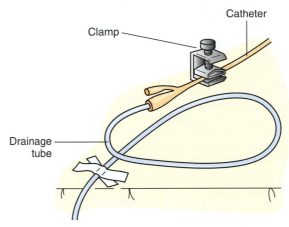

FIGURE 20-11 The clamped catheter prevents urine from draining out of the bladder. The clamp is applied directly to the catheter, not to the drainage tube.

REVIEW QUESTIONS

Circle the BEST answer.

1 Which is abnormal?
   a Clear, amber urine
   b Urine with a faint odor
   c Cloudy urine with particles
   d Urine output of 1500 mL in 24 hours

2 Which prevents normal elimination?
   a Helping the person assume a normal position for voiding
   b Providing privacy
   c Helping the person to the bathroom as soon as requested
   d Staying with the person who uses a bedpan

3 Which definition is *correct*?
   a Dysuria means painful or difficult urination.
   b Oliguria means a large amount of urine.
   c Urinary retention means the need to void at once.
   d Urinary incontinence means the inability to void.

4 The person using a standard bedpan is in
   a Fowler's position
   b The supine position
   c The prone position
   d The side-lying position

5 To use a fracture pan
   a The person is in Fowler's position
   b The smaller end (flat end) is under the buttocks
   c The nurse must position the pan
   d The pan can be left in place for a long time

6 After using the urinal, the man should
   a Put it on the bedside stand
   b Use the call light
   c Put it on the over-bed table
   d Empty it

7 After a person uses a commode, you should
   a Empty, clean, and disinfect the commode
   b Return the commode to the supply area
   c Get a new container
   d Get a new commode

8 Urinary incontinence
   a Is always permanent
   b Requires bladder training
   c Is a normal part of aging
   d Requires good skin care

9 Which is a cause of functional incontinence?
   a A nervous system disorder
   b Sneezing
   c Unanswered call light
   d UTI

10 When applying an incontinence product
   a Let the plastic backing touch the person's skin
   b Remove the old product from back to front
   c Apply the new product from front to back
   d Use the product to turn and position the person

11 The goal of bladder training is to
   a Control the amount voided daily
   b Promote voiding at times best for staff
   c Allow the person to walk to the bathroom
   d Gain control of urination

12 A person learns to ignore the urge to void. This type of bladder training is called
   a Bladder re-training
   b Prompted voiding
   c Habit training
   d Scheduled voiding

Answers to Chapter 20 questions are on p. 552.

FOCUS ON PRACTICE

Problem Solving

You assist a patient onto the commode. The person is unsteady and cannot be left alone. The person says: "I can't go if you stand here." What do you do? How will you provide privacy and safe care?

Urinary Catheters

OBJECTIVES

- Define the key terms and key abbreviations in this chapter.
- Explain why urinary catheters are used.
- Describe 2 types of urinary catheters.
- Explain the purpose and rules for catheter care.
- Describe 2 urine drainage systems.

- Explain how to re-connect a catheter and drainage tubing.
- Explain how to apply a condom catheter.
- Perform the procedures described in this chapter.
- Explain how to promote PRIDE in the person, the family, and yourself.

KEY TERMS

catheter A tube used to drain or inject fluid through a body opening
catheterization The process of inserting a catheter
condom catheter A soft sheath that slides over the penis and is used to drain urine

indwelling catheter A catheter left in the bladder so urine drains constantly into a drainage bag; retention or Foley catheter
straight catheter A catheter that drains the bladder and then is removed

KEY ABBREVIATIONS

BM Bowel movement
IV Intravenous

mL Milliliter
UTI Urinary tract infection

A *catheter is a tube used to drain or inject fluid through a body opening.* Inserted through the urethra into the bladder, a urinary catheter drains urine. *Catheterization is the process of inserting a catheter.* With proper training and supervision, some states and agencies let nursing assistants insert and remove urinary catheters.

See *Focus on Surveys: Urinary Catheters.*

See *Promoting Safety and Comfort: Urinary Catheters,* p. 310.

FOCUS ON SURVEYS

Urinary Catheters

Surveys are done to check the quality of treatments and services. The surveyor may ask you about:
- Your understanding of the person's bladder management
- Your training about handling catheters, catheter tubing, drainage bags, catheter care, urinary tract infections (UTIs), catheter-related injuries, dislodgment, and skin breakdown
- What observations to report, when to report them, and to whom you should report

  Answer questions the best you can. If you do not know an answer, tell the surveyor who you would ask or where you would find the answer.

PURPOSES AND TYPES OF CATHETERS

These types of catheters are common.

- A *straight catheter drains the bladder and then is removed.*
- An *indwelling catheter (retention or Foley catheter) is left in the bladder. Urine drains constantly into a drainage bag.* A balloon by the tip is inflated with sterile water after the catheter is inserted. The balloon prevents the catheter from coming out of the bladder (Fig. 21-1). Tubing connects the catheter to a urine drainage bag. See Figure 21-2.

Catheters create a risk for UTIs. However, they are used:

- To keep the bladder empty before, during, and after surgery.
- To promote comfort. Some people cannot use the bedpan, urinal, commode, or toilet. For them, catheters can promote comfort and prevent incontinence.
- To protect wounds and pressure injuries from contact with urine.
- For hourly urine output measurements.
- To collect sterile urine specimens.
- To measure the amount of urine in the bladder after the person voids (*residual urine*).

Catheters do not treat the cause of incontinence. They are a last resort for incontinence.

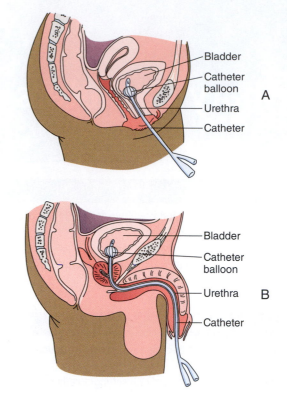

FIGURE 21-1 Indwelling catheter. **A,** Indwelling catheter in the female bladder. The inflated balloon at the tip prevents the catheter from slipping out through the urethra. **B,** Indwelling catheter with the balloon inflated in the male bladder.

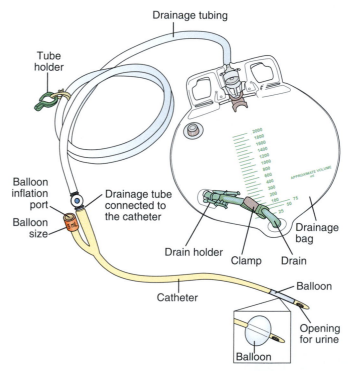

FIGURE 21-2 Parts of an indwelling catheter and urine drainage system.

CATHETER CARE

You will care for persons with indwelling catheters. The risk of UTI is high. Follow the rules in Box 21-1 to promote safety and comfort.

See *Delegation Guidelines: Catheter Care*, p. 312.
See *Promoting Safety and Comfort: Catheter Care*, p. 312.
See procedure: *Giving Catheter Care*, p. 313.

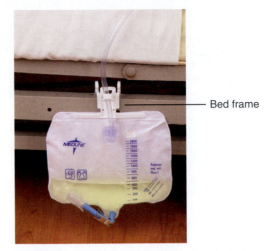

FIGURE 21-3 Urine drainage bag secured to the bed frame.

BOX 21-1   Indwelling Catheter Care

Preventing Infection
- Follow the rules of medical asepsis.
- Follow Standard Precautions and the Bloodborne Pathogen Standard.
- Encourage fluid intake as directed by the nurse and care plan.

The Drainage System
- Allow urine to flow freely through the catheter and drainage tube. Tubing should not have kinks. The person should not lie on the tubing.
- Keep the catheter connected to the drainage tube. Follow the measures on p. 314 if the catheter and drainage tube are disconnected.
- Keep the drainage tube and bag below the bladder. This prevents urine from flowing backward into the bladder. For a bed or chair transfer, keep the drainage bag lower than the bladder. Secure the drainage bag to the bed frame or chair after the transfer. See Figure 21-3.
- Move the drainage bag to the other side of the bed for turning and re-positioning on the other side.
- Hang the bag from the bed frame, lower part of the chair or wheelchair, or lower part of the IV (intravenous) pole.
- *Do not hang the drainage bag on a bed rail.* The bag is higher than the bladder when the bed rail is raised.
- Position tubing so it will not get tangled in the wheelchair wheels.
- Hold the bag lower than the bladder when the person walks.
- Do not let the drainage bag touch or rest on the floor. This can contaminate the system.
- Position drainage tubing in a straight line or coil it on the bed. Secure it to the bottom linens (Fig. 21-4, p. 312). Follow the nurse's directions and agency policy. Use a clip, bed sheet clamp, tape, or other device as the nurse directs. Tubing must not loop below the drainage bag.

The Catheter
- Secure the catheter as the nurse directs.
  - Females: to the thigh (see Fig. 21-4, *A*).
  - Males:
    - To the abdomen (see Fig. 21-4, *B*). This site is common for long-term catheter use. The drainage bag remains below the bladder. Drainage is not affected.
    - To the thigh (see Fig. 21-4, *C*).

The Catheter—cont'd
- Use a tube holder, tape, leg band, or other device to secure the catheter to the thigh or abdomen. The nurse tells you what to use. Securing the catheter prevents excess movement and friction at the insertion site (meatus). Catheter movement and friction can damage the meatus.
- Check for leaks. Check the connections to the drainage tube and the drainage bag. Report any leaks at once.
- Provide perineal care and catheter care according to the care plan—daily, twice a day, after bowel movements (BMs), or when vaginal discharge is present. (See procedure: *Giving Catheter Care*, p. 313.)

Measuring Urine (Output)
- Empty the drainage bag and measure urine:
  - At the end of the shift
  - To change to and from a leg bag and a standard drainage bag (p. 316)
  - When the bag is becoming full
- Report an increase or decrease in urine amount.
- Provide a measuring container for each person. This prevents the spread of microbes from 1 person to another.
- Do not let the drain on the drainage bag touch any surface.
- See procedure: *Emptying a Urine Drainage Bag*, p. 315.

Observations
- Report complaints at once—pain, burning, the need to void, or irritation. Also report the color, clarity, and odor of urine and the presence of particles or blood.
- Observe for signs and symptoms of a UTI. Report the following at once.
  - Fever.
  - Chills.
  - Flank pain or tenderness. The flank area is in the back between the ribs and the hip.
  - Change in the urine—blood, foul smell, particles, cloudiness, *oliguria* (scant amount of urine).
  - Change in mental or functional status—confusion, decreased appetite, falls, decreased activity, tiredness, and so on.
- Urine leakage around the catheter.

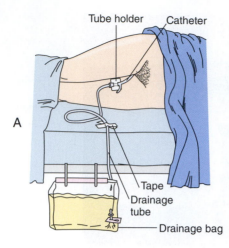

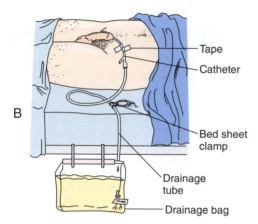

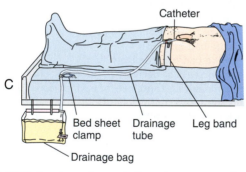

FIGURE 21-4 Securing catheters. **A,** The catheter is secured to the woman's thigh with a tube holder. The drainage tube is coiled on the bed and secured to bottom linens with tape. **B,** The catheter is secured to the man's abdomen with tape. Drainage tubing is secured to bottom linens with a bed sheet clamp. **C,** The catheter is secured to the man's thigh with a leg band. Drainage tubing is in a straight line and secured to bottom linens with a bed sheet clamp. The drainage bag is at the foot of the bed.

DELEGATION GUIDELINES
Catheter Care

When delegated catheter care, you need this information from the nurse and the care plan.

- When to give catheter care—daily, twice a day, after BMs, or because of vaginal discharge
- What water temperature to use for perineal care
- Where to secure the catheter—thigh or abdomen
- How to secure the catheter—tube holder, tape, leg band, or other device
- How to position the drainage tubing—straight line or coiled on the bed
- How to secure drainage tubing—clip, bed sheet clamp, tape, or other device
- What observations to report and record:
  - Complaints of pain, burning, irritation, or the need to void (report at once)
  - Crusting, abnormal drainage, or secretions
  - The color, clarity, and odor of urine
  - Particles in the urine
  - Blood in the urine (report at once)
  - Cloudy urine
  - Urine leaking at the insertion site
  - Drainage system leaks
- When to report observations
- What patient or resident concerns to report at once

PROMOTING SAFETY AND COMFORT
Catheter Care

Safety

In some agencies, perineal care (Chapter 18) is sufficient hygiene for indwelling catheters. The procedure that follows is not used. Follow agency policy and the care plan when a person has a catheter.

Comfort

The catheter must not pull at the insertion site. This causes discomfort and irritation. Hold the catheter securely during catheter care. Then properly secure the catheter. Make sure the tubing is not under the person. Besides blocking urine flow, lying on the tubing is uncomfortable. It can also cause skin breakdown. To promote comfort, see Box 21-1.

Giving Catheter Care

QUALITY OF LIFE

- Knock before entering the person's room.
- Address the person by name.
- Introduce yourself by name and title.

- Explain the procedure before starting and during the procedure.
- Protect the person's rights during the procedure.
- Handle the person gently during the procedure.

PRE-PROCEDURE

1 Follow *Delegation Guidelines:*
   a *Perineal Care* (Chapter 18)
   b *Catheter Care*
   See *Promoting Safety and Comfort:*
   a *Perineal Care* (Chapter 18)
   b *Urinary Catheters,* p. 310
   c *Catheter Care*
2 Practice hand hygiene.
3 Collect the following.
   - Items for perineal care (Chapter 18)
   - Gloves
   - Bath blanket

4 Cover the over-bed table with paper towels. Arrange items on top of them.
5 Identify the person. Check the ID (identification) bracelet against the assignment sheet. Use 2 identifiers (Chapter 10). Also call the person by name.
6 Provide for privacy.
7 Fill the wash basin. Water temperature is about 105°F to 109°F (Fahrenheit) (40.5°C to 42.7°C [centigrade]). Measure water temperature according to agency policy. Have the person check the water temperature and adjust as needed.
8 Raise the bed for body mechanics. Bed rails are up if used.
9 Lower the bed rail near you if up.

PROCEDURE

10 Practice hand hygiene. Put on the gloves.
11 Cover the person with a bath blanket. Fan-fold top linens to the foot of the bed.
12 Position and drape the person for perineal care (Chapter 18).
13 Fold back the bath blanket to expose the perineal area.
14 Have the person flex the knees and raise the buttocks off the bed. Place the waterproof under-pad under the buttocks. Have the person lower the buttocks.
15 Check the drainage tubing. Make sure it is not kinked and that urine can flow freely.
16 Separate the labia (female). In an uncircumcised male, retract the foreskin (Chapter 18). Check for crusts, abnormal drainage, or secretions.
17 Give perineal care (Chapter 18). Keep the foreskin of the uncircumcised male retracted until step 25.
18 Apply soap to a clean, wet washcloth.
19 Hold the catheter at the meatus. Do so for steps 20 through 24.
20 Wash around the catheter at the meatus. Use a circular motion (Fig. 21-5, A, p. 314). (NOTE: Complete this step if required by agency policy or your state's competency test.)
21 Clean the catheter from the meatus down the catheter at least 4 inches (Fig. 21-5, B, p. 314). Clean downward, away from the meatus with 1 stroke. Do not tug or pull on the catheter. Repeat as needed with a clean area of the washcloth. Use a clean washcloth if needed.

22 Rinse around the catheter at the meatus with a clean washcloth. (NOTE: Complete this step if required by agency policy or your state's competency test.)
23 Rinse the catheter from the meatus down the catheter at least 4 inches. Rinse downward, away from the meatus with 1 stroke. Do not tug or pull on the catheter. Repeat as needed with a clean area of the washcloth. Use a clean washcloth if needed.
24 Pat dry the areas washed. Dry from the meatus down the catheter at least 4 inches. Do not tug or pull on the catheter.
25 Return the foreskin (uncircumcised male) to its natural position.
26 Pat dry the perineal area. Dry from front to back (top to bottom).
27 Secure the catheter. Position the tubing in a straight line or coiled on the bed. Follow the nurse's directions. Secure the tubing to the bottom linens (see Fig. 21-4).
28 Remove the waterproof under-pad.
29 Cover the person. Remove the bath blanket.
30 Remove and discard the gloves. Practice hand hygiene.

POST-PROCEDURE

31 Provide for comfort. (See the inside of the front cover.)
32 Place the call light and other needed items within reach.
33 Lower the bed to a safe and comfortable level. Follow the care plan.
34 Raise or lower bed rails. Follow the care plan.
35 Clean, rinse, dry, and return equipment to its proper place. Use clean, dry paper towels for drying. Discard disposable items. (Wear gloves for this step.)

36 Unscreen the person.
37 Complete a safety check of the room. (See the inside of the front cover.)
38 Follow agency policy for used linens.
39 Remove and discard the gloves. Practice hand hygiene.
40 Report and record your observations.

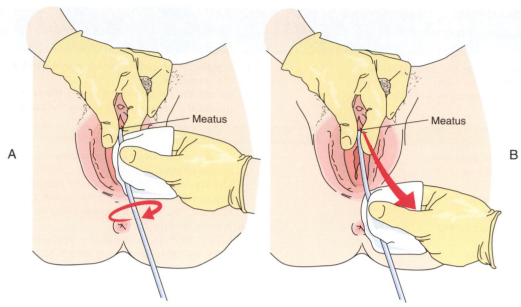

FIGURE 21-5 Cleaning the catheter. **A,** Clean the catheter with a circular motion at the meatus. **B,** Start at the meatus and clean downward at least 4 inches.

URINE DRAINAGE SYSTEMS

A closed drainage system is used for indwelling catheters. Only urine should enter the system. The urinary system is sterile. Infection can occur if microbes enter the drainage system. The microbes travel up the tubing or catheter into the bladder and kidneys. A UTI can threaten health and life. See Box 21-1 to prevent infection and for proper care of the drainage system.

There are 2 types of urine drainage bags.

- *Standard drainage bags* usually hold at least 2000 mL (milliliters) of urine (see Fig. 21-3).
- *Leg bags* attach to the thigh or calf with elastic bands or Velcro (p. 316). Leg bags hold less than 1000 mL of urine.

Drainage systems can become disconnected. If that happens, tell the nurse at once. Do not touch the ends of the catheter or tubing. Box 21-2 describes how to re-connect the catheter and tubing.

See *Delegation Guidelines: Urine Drainage Systems.*
See *Promoting Safety and Comfort: Urine Drainage Systems.*
See procedure: *Emptying a Urine Drainage Bag.*

BOX 21-2	Re-Connecting a Catheter and Drainage Tube

1 Practice hand hygiene. Put on gloves.
2 Wipe the end of the drainage tube with an antiseptic wipe.
3 Wipe the end of the catheter with another antiseptic wipe.
4 Do not put the ends down. Do not touch the ends after you clean them.
5 Connect the drainage tubing to the catheter.
6 Discard the wipes into a biohazard bag.
7 Remove the gloves. Practice hand hygiene.

DELEGATION GUIDELINES
Urine Drainage Systems

Delegated tasks may involve urine drainage systems. If so, you need this information from the nurse and the care plan.

- When to empty the urine drainage bag
- If the person uses a leg bag
- What leg bag straps to use—elastic or Velcro
- When to switch a standard drainage bag and leg bag
- If you should clean or discard the drainage bag
- What observations to report and record:
  - The amount of urine measured (Chapter 24)
  - The color, clarity, and odor of urine
  - Particles in the urine
  - Blood in the urine
  - Cloudy urine
  - Complaints of pain, burning, irritation, or the need to urinate
  - Drainage system leaks
- When to report observations
- What patient or resident concerns to report at once

PROMOTING SAFETY AND COMFORT
Urine Drainage Systems

Safety
Leg bags hold less urine than standard drainage bags. Check leg bags often. Empty the leg bag if it is becoming half full. Measure, report, and record the amount of urine.

Comfort
Urine in a drainage bag embarrasses some people. Visitors can see the urine. To promote mental comfort, have visitors sit on the side away from the drainage bag. Try to empty the bag before visitors arrive. Measure, report, and record the amount of urine.

Some agencies have drainage bag holders. The drainage bag is placed inside the holder. Urine is hidden.

Emptying a Urine Drainage Bag

QUALITY OF LIFE

- Knock before entering the person's room.
- Address the person by name.
- Introduce yourself by name and title.

- Explain the procedure before starting and during the procedure.
- Protect the person's rights during the procedure.
- Handle the person gently during the procedure.

PRE-PROCEDURE

1 Follow *Delegation Guidelines: Urine Drainage Systems.* See *Promoting Safety and Comfort:*
   a *Urinary Catheters,* p. 310
   b *Urine Drainage Systems*
2 Collect the following.
   - Graduate (measuring container)
   - Gloves
   - Paper towels
   - Antiseptic wipes

3 Practice hand hygiene.
4 Identify the person. Check the ID bracelet against the assignment sheet. Use 2 identifiers (Chapter 10). Also call the person by name.
5 Provide for privacy.

PROCEDURE

6 Put on the gloves.
7 Place a paper towel on the floor. Place the graduate on top of it.
8 Place the graduate under the drainage bag.
9 Open the clamp on the drain.
10 Let all urine drain into the graduate. The drain does not touch the graduate (Fig. 21-6).
11 Clean the end of the drain with an antiseptic wipe.
12 Clamp and position the drain in the holder (Fig. 21-7).
13 Measure urine. See procedure: *Measuring Intake and Output* in Chapter 24.

14 Remove and discard the paper towel.
15 Empty the graduate into the toilet and flush.
16 Rinse the graduate. Empty the rinse into the toilet and flush.
17 Clean, disinfect, and dry the graduate. Use clean, dry paper towels for drying.
18 Return the graduate to its proper place.
19 Remove and discard the gloves. Practice hand hygiene.
20 Record the time and amount of urine on the intake and output (I&O) record (Chapter 24).

POST-PROCEDURE

21 Provide for comfort. (See the inside of the front cover.)
22 Place the call light and other needed items within reach.
23 Unscreen the person.

24 Complete a safety check of the room. (See the inside of the front cover.)
25 Report and record the amount of urine and other observations.

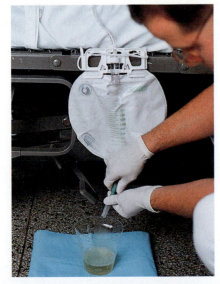

FIGURE 21-6 The clamp on the drainage bag is opened. The drain is directed into the graduate. The drain does not touch the inside of the graduate. (From Potter PA, Perry AG, Stockert PA, Hall, AM: *Fundamentals of nursing,* ed 9, St Louis, 2017, Elsevier.)

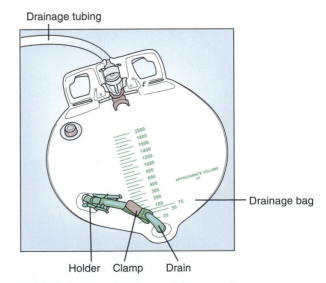

FIGURE 21-7 The clamp is closed and positioned in the holder on the drainage bag.

Condom Catheters

Condom catheters are often used for incontinent men. They also are called *external catheters*, *Texas catheters*, and *urinary sheaths*. A **condom catheter** *is a soft sheath that slides over the penis and is used to drain urine.* Tubing connects the condom catheter to the drainage bag. Many men prefer leg bags (Fig. 21-8).

Condom catheters are changed daily after perineal care. To apply a condom catheter, follow the manufacturer's instructions. Thoroughly wash the penis with soap and water. Dry it before applying the catheter.

Some condom catheters are self-adhering. Adhesive inside the catheter adheres to the penis. Other catheters are secured with elastic tape. Use the elastic tape packaged with the catheter. *Apply the tape in a spiral.* This allows blood flow to the penis. *Only use elastic tape. Adhesive and other tapes do not expand. Never use such tapes to secure condom catheters. Blood flow to the penis is cut off, injuring the penis.*

See *Delegation Guidelines: Condom Catheters.*
See *Promoting Safety and Comfort: Condom Catheters.*
See procedure: *Applying a Condom Catheter.*

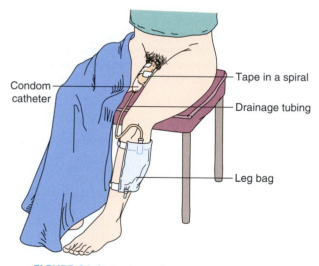

FIGURE 21-8 Condom catheter attached to a leg bag.

Condom catheter
Tape in a spiral
Drainage tubing
Leg bag

Applying a Condom Catheter

QUALITY OF LIFE

- Knock before entering the person's room.
- Address the person by name.
- Introduce yourself by name and title.

- Explain the procedure before starting and during the procedure.
- Protect the person's rights during the procedure.
- Handle the person gently during the procedure.

PRE-PROCEDURE

1 Follow *Delegation Guidelines:*
  a *Perineal Care* (Chapter 18)
  b *Condom Catheters*
  See *Promoting Safety and Comfort:*
  a *Perineal Care* (Chapter 18)
  b *Urinary Catheters*, p. 310
  c *Condom Catheters*
2 Practice hand hygiene.
3 Collect the following.
  - Condom catheter
  - Elastic tape (if needed)
  - Standard drainage bag or leg bag
  - Cap for the drainage bag
  - Basin of warm water (See procedure: *Giving Male Perineal Care* in Chapter 18.)

  - Soap
  - Towel and washcloths
  - Bath blanket
  - Gloves
  - Waterproof under-pad
  - Paper towels
4 Cover the over-bed table with paper towels. Arrange items on top of them.
5 Identify the person. Check the ID bracelet against the assignment sheet. Use 2 identifiers (Chapter 10). Also call the person by name.
6 Provide for privacy.
7 Raise the bed for body mechanics. Bed rails are up if used.

PROCEDURE

8 Lower the bed rail near you if up.
9 Practice hand hygiene. Put on the gloves.
10 Cover the person with a bath blanket. Lower top linens to the knees.
11 Have the person raise his buttocks off the bed. Or turn him onto his side away from you.
12 Slide the waterproof under-pad under his buttocks.
13 Have him lower the buttocks. Or turn him onto his back.
14 Secure the standard drainage bag to the bed frame. Or have a leg bag ready. Close the drain.
15 Expose the genital area.
16 Remove the condom catheter.
  a Remove the tape. Roll the sheath off the penis.
  b Disconnect the drainage tubing from the condom. Cap the drainage tube.
  c Discard the tape and condom.
17 Provide perineal care (Chapter 18). Observe the penis for reddened areas, skin breakdown, and irritation.

18 Remove and discard the gloves. Practice hand hygiene. Put on clean gloves.
19 Remove the protective backing from the condom. This exposes the adhesive strip.
20 Hold the penis firmly. Roll the condom onto the penis. Leave a 1-inch space between the penis and the end of the catheter (Fig. 21-9, p. 318).
21 Secure the condom.
  a *Self-adhering condom:* press the condom to the penis.
  b *Condom secured with elastic tape:* apply elastic tape in a spiral. See Figure 21-9. Do not apply tape completely around the penis.
22 Make sure the penis tip does not touch the condom. Make sure the condom is not twisted.
23 Connect the condom to the drainage tubing. Secure excess tubing on the bed. Or attach a leg bag.
24 Remove the waterproof under-pad and gloves. Discard them. Practice hand hygiene.
25 Cover the person. Remove the bath blanket.

POST-PROCEDURE

26 Provide for comfort. (See the inside of the front cover.)
27 Place the call light and other needed items within reach.
28 Lower the bed to a safe and comfortable level. Follow the care plan.
29 Raise or lower bed rails. Follow the care plan.
30 Unscreen the person.
31 Practice hand hygiene. Put on clean gloves.
32 Measure and record the amount of urine in the bag. Clean or discard the drainage bag.

33 Clean, rinse, dry, and return the wash basin and other equipment. Use clean, dry paper towels for drying. Return items to their proper place.
34 Remove and discard the gloves. Practice hand hygiene.
35 Complete a safety check of the room. (See the inside of the front cover.)
36 Report and record your observations.

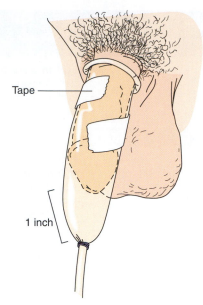

Tape

1 inch

FIGURE 21-9 A condom catheter applied to the penis. A 1-inch space is between the penis and the end of the catheter. Elastic tape is applied in a *spiral* to secure the condom catheter to the penis.

FOCUS ON P R I D E
The Person, Family, and Yourself

Personal and Professional Responsibility
With urinary catheters, the risk of UTIs is high. How you give care can decrease the risk of UTI. Do you:
- Prevent urine from flowing back into the bladder when moving the drainage bag?
- Use a clean area of the washcloth for each stroke during catheter care?
- Keep the drain from touching the graduate or other surface?
- Use a clean, separate graduate to empty each person's drainage bag?

UTIs can be very serious. They can threaten life in older persons. Give care in a way that promotes quality of life, health, and safety. Be careful when handling and caring for catheters. Your care makes a difference.

Rights and Respect
Respect the right to privacy. Simple actions make a difference. For example, knock before entering a room. Before any procedure, explain how you will provide privacy. This is very important for procedures that involve exposing and touching private areas.

Independence and Social Interaction
Urinary catheters are short-term or long-term. Some persons manage their own catheters. The nurse teaches the person to provide catheter care. You:
- Give encouragement. Be kind, patient, and professional.
- Reinforce the nurse's instructions.
- Tell the nurse if the person has questions or if you think more teaching is needed.

Delegation and Teamwork
Tasks become more complex as more care equipment is needed. For example, you are to turn and re-position a resident with a urinary catheter. As you move the drainage bag to the other side of the bed you must:
- Keep the catheter and drainage tube free of kinks.
- Keep the drainage bag below bladder level.
- Make sure the person is not lying on the drainage tube.
- Avoid resting the bag on the floor.

As you study, think of how care equipment and the person's needs affect delegated tasks.

Ethics and Laws
Some states and agencies allow nursing assistants to remove urinary catheters. Others do not. With more training, some allow nursing assistants to insert catheters. Follow state and agency rules. *Never* perform a task outside your role limits.

FOCUS ON PRIDE: Application
How might needing a urinary catheter affect the person mentally? How can you promote mental comfort?

REVIEW QUESTIONS

Circle the BEST answer.

1 Urinary catheters are used
   a To prevent urinary tract infections
   b To treat the cause of incontinence
   c To keep the bladder empty for surgery
   d For staff convenience with incontinent persons

2 A person has a catheter. Which is *safe?*
   a Keeping the drainage bag above the bladder level
   b Taping a leak at the connection site
   c Attaching the drainage bag to the bed rail
   d Removing a kink from the drainage tubing

3 A person has a catheter. Which is *correct?*
   a Report pain, burning, or irritation at once.
   b Allow the tubing to hang below the drainage bag.
   c Empty the drainage bag once daily.
   d Use the same graduate for all persons.

4 A person has a catheter. You are going to turn the person from the left to the right side. What should you do with the drainage bag?
   a Move it to the right side.
   b Keep it on the left side.
   c Hang it from an IV pole.
   d Remove it.

5 To secure a catheter on a female
   a Tape it to her lower abdomen
   b Use a safety pin to secure it to her gown
   c Secure it to her thigh with tape or a tube holder
   d Secure it to the bottom linens with a bed sheet clamp

6 For catheter care
   a Clean from the drainage tube connection up the catheter at least 4 inches
   b Clean from the meatus down the catheter at least 4 inches
   c Pull on the catheter to make sure it is secure
   d Clamp the catheter to prevent leaking

7 Which statement about drainage systems is *true?*
   a A leg bag holds about 2000 mL.
   b A standard drainage bag holds less than a leg bag.
   c A closed drainage system means the drain cannot be opened.
   d Microbes in the drainage system can cause a UTI.

8 A drainage system becomes disconnected. You need
   a A new drainage bag and paper towels
   b A sterile cap and catheter plug
   c Gloves and an antiseptic wipe
   d A waterproof under-pad and a catheter clamp

9 When emptying a standard drainage bag
   a Do not let the drain touch the graduate
   b Gloves are not needed
   c Clamp the catheter
   d Clean the end of the catheter with an antiseptic wipe

10 For a condom catheter, you apply elastic tape
   a Completely around the penis
   b To the thigh
   c To the abdomen
   d In a spiral

Answers to Chapter 21 questions are on p. 552.

FOCUS ON PRACTICE

Problem Solving

A patient with a urinary catheter tells you: "I feel like I have to pee, and I feel pressure down there." The patient points to the lower abdomen. There is no urine in the drainage bag. Is this normal? What do you do?

Bowel Needs

OBJECTIVES

- Define the key terms and key abbreviations in this chapter.
- Describe normal defecation and the observations to report.
- Identify the factors affecting bowel elimination.
- Explain how to promote comfort and safety during defecation.
- Describe the common bowel elimination problems.
- Describe bowel training.

- Explain why enemas are given.
- Describe the common enema solutions.
- Describe the rules for giving enemas.
- Describe how to care for a person with an ostomy.
- Perform the procedure described in this chapter.
- Explain how to promote PRIDE in the person, the family, and yourself.

KEY TERMS

colostomy A surgically created opening (*stomy*) between the colon (*colo*) and the body's surface
constipation The passage of a hard, dry stool
defecation The process of excreting feces from the rectum through the anus; a bowel movement
diarrhea The frequent passage of liquid stools
enema The introduction of fluid into the rectum and lower colon
fecal impaction The prolonged retention and buildup of feces in the rectum
fecal incontinence The inability to control the passage of feces and gas through the anus
feces The semi-solid mass of waste products in the colon that is expelled through the anus; stool or stools

flatulence The excessive formation of gas or air in the stomach and intestines
flatus Gas or air passed through the anus
ileostomy A surgically created opening (*stomy*) between the ileum (small intestine [*ileo*]) and the body's surface
ostomy A surgically created opening that connects an internal organ to the body's surface; see "colostomy" and "ileostomy"
stoma A surgically created opening seen on the body's surface; see "colostomy" and "ileostomy"
stool Excreted feces
suppository A cone-shaped, solid drug that is inserted into a body opening; it melts at body temperature

KEY ABBREVIATIONS

BM	Bowel movement	mL	Milliliter
C. diff	*Clostridium difficile*	oz	Ounce
GI	Gastro-intestinal		

Bowel elimination is a basic physical need. Wastes are excreted from the gastro-intestinal (GI) system (Chapter 8). You assist patients and residents to meet elimination needs.

See *Delegation Guidelines: Bowel Needs.*
See *Promoting Safety and Comfort: Bowel Needs.*

DELEGATION GUIDELINES
Bowel Needs

Your state and agency may not allow you to perform the procedure and some of the care measures in this chapter. Before performing a procedure, make sure that:
- Your state allows you to perform the procedure.
- The procedure is in your job description.
- You have the necessary education and training.
- You review the procedure with a nurse.
- A nurse is available to answer questions and to supervise you.

PROMOTING SAFETY AND COMFORT

Bowel Needs

Safety

Assisting with bowel needs may involve exposing and touching the rectum, a private area. And you may have to give perineal care. Sexual abuse has occurred in health care settings. The person may feel threatened or is actually being abused. He or she needs to call for help. Always keep the call light within the person's reach. And always act in a professional manner.

Contact with feces is likely when assisting with bowel needs. Feces contain microbes and may contain blood. Follow Standard Precautions and the Bloodborne Pathogen Standard (Chapter 13).

NOTE: A task may require more than 1 pair of gloves. Change gloves as needed. Use careful judgment. Remember to practice hand hygiene after removing gloves.

NORMAL BOWEL ELIMINATION

Some people have a bowel movement (BM) every day. Others do so every 2 to 3 days. Some people have 2 or 3 BMs a day. Many people have a BM after breakfast. Others do so in the evening.

To assist with bowel elimination, you need to know these terms.

- *Defecation (bowel movement) is the process of excreting feces from the rectum through the anus.*
- *Feces (stool or stools) refers to the semi-solid mass of waste products in the colon that is expelled through the anus.*
- *Stool refers to excreted feces.*

Observations

Stools are normally brown. Bleeding in the stomach and small intestine causes black or tarry stools. Bleeding in the lower colon and rectum causes red-colored stools. So do beets, tomato juice or soup, red Jell-O, and foods with red food coloring. Green vegetables can cause green stools. Diseases and infection can cause clay-colored or white, pale, orange-colored, or green-colored stools and stools with mucus. Figure 22-1 shows a color chart for stools.

Stools are normally soft, formed, moist, and shaped like the rectum. They have a normal odor.

Carefully observe stools. Ask the nurse to observe abnormal stools. Report and record the following.

- Color (see Fig. 22-1)
- Amount
- Presence of mucus
- Signs of bleeding
- Odor
- Shape and consistency (Fig. 22-2)
- The time the person had a BM
- Frequency of BMs
- Complaints of pain or discomfort
  See *Focus on Communication: Observations,* p. 322.

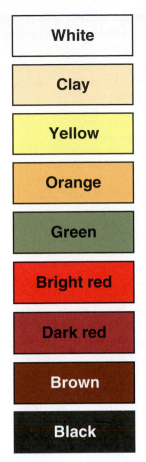

FIGURE 22-1 Color chart for stools.

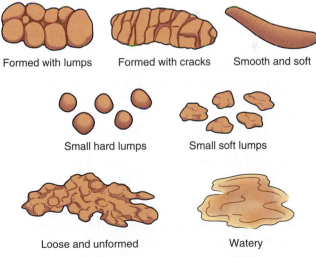

Formed with lumps   Formed with cracks   Smooth and soft

Small hard lumps   Small soft lumps

Loose and unformed   Watery

FIGURE 22-2 Stool shapes and consistencies.

FACTORS AFFECTING BMs

These factors affect bowel needs. Normal, regular elimination is a goal of the nursing process.

- *Privacy.* Lack of privacy can prevent a BM despite the urge. Odors and sounds are embarrassing. Some people ignore the urge when people are present.
- *Habits.* After breakfast is a common time for BMs. A BM is easier when relaxed, not tense. To relax, some people drink a hot beverage, read, or take a walk.
- *Diet—high-fiber foods.* High-fiber foods leave a residue, creating bulk to prevent constipation. Fruits, vegetables, and whole-grain cereals and breads are high in fiber. These foods may be hard to chew with missing teeth or poorly fitting dentures. Sometimes bran is added to cereal, prunes, or prune juice.
- *Diet—other foods.* Milk and milk products can cause constipation or diarrhea. Chocolate and other foods cause similar reactions. Spicy foods can irritate the intestines, causing frequent BMs or diarrhea. Gas-forming foods stimulate peristalsis, aiding BMs. Such foods include onions, beans, cabbage, cauliflower, radishes, and cucumbers.
- *Fluids.* Feces contain water. Stool consistency depends on how much water is absorbed by the colon. Feces harden and dry when large amounts of water are absorbed or from poor fluid intake. Hard, dry feces move slowly through the colon. Constipation can occur. Drinking 6 to 8 glasses of water daily promotes normal BMs. Warm fluids—coffee, tea, hot cider, warm water—increase peristalsis.
- *Activity.* Exercise and activity maintain muscle tone and stimulate peristalsis.
- *Drugs.* Drugs can prevent constipation or control diarrhea. Other drugs have diarrhea or constipation as side effects.
- *Disability.* Some people have a BM whenever feces enter the rectum. They have no control. A bowel training program is needed (p. 324).
- *Aging.* Age affects bowel elimination.
See *Focus on Older Persons: Factors Affecting BMs.*

Safety and Comfort

The care plan has measures to meet bowel needs. It may involve diet, fluids, and exercise. The measures in Box 22-1 promote safety and comfort.

See *Focus on Communication: Safety and Comfort.*

COMMON PROBLEMS

Common problems include constipation, fecal impaction, diarrhea, fecal incontinence, and flatulence.

Constipation

Constipation is the passage of a hard, dry stool. The person strains to have a BM. Stools are large or marble-sized. Large stools cause pain as they pass through the anus. Constipation occurs when feces move slowly through the bowel. This allows more time for water absorption. Common causes of constipation include:

- A low-fiber diet
- Ignoring the urge to have a BM
- Decreased fluid intake
- Inactivity
- Drugs
- Aging
- Certain diseases

Diet changes, fluids, and activity prevent or relieve constipation. The doctor may order 1 or more of the following.

- Stool softeners—drugs that soften feces
- Laxatives—drugs that promote bowel elimination
- Suppositories
- Enemas (p. 325)

Fecal Impaction

A *fecal impaction is the prolonged retention and buildup of feces in the rectum.* Feces are hard or putty-like. Fecal impaction results from un-relieved constipation. The person cannot have a BM. More water is absorbed from the already hard feces. Liquid feces pass around the hardened fecal mass in the rectum and seep from the anus.

Signs and symptoms of fecal impaction include:

- Trying many times to have a BM
- Abdominal discomfort
- Abdominal distention (swelling)
- Nausea
- Cramping
- Rectal pain
- Poor appetite (especially older persons)
- Confusion (especially older persons)
- Fever (especially older persons)

Diarrhea

Diarrhea is the frequent passage of liquid stools. Feces move through the intestines rapidly. This reduces the time for fluid absorption. The need for a BM is urgent. Some people cannot get to a bathroom in time. Abdominal cramping, nausea, and vomiting may occur. Dehydration is a risk from fluid loss (Chapter 24).

Causes of diarrhea include infections, some drugs, irritating foods, and microbes in food and water. Diet and drugs are ordered to reduce peristalsis. You need to:

- Assist with elimination needs promptly.
- Dispose of stools promptly. This prevents odors and the spread of microbes.
- Give good skin care. Liquid stools irritate the skin. So does frequent wiping with toilet tissue. Skin breakdown and pressure injuries are risks.

Microbes can cause diarrhea. Preventing the spread of infection is important. Always follow Standard Precautions and the Bloodborne Pathogen Standard when in contact with stools.

See *Focus on Older Persons: Diarrhea.*
See *Promoting Safety and Comfort: Diarrhea.*

FOCUS ON OLDER PERSONS

Diarrhea

Older persons are at risk for dehydration. The amount of body water decreases with aging. Many diseases common in older persons affect body fluids. So do many drugs. Report signs of diarrhea at once. Ask the nurse to observe the stool. Death is a risk when dehydration is not recognized and treated.

PROMOTING SAFETY AND COMFORT

Diarrhea

Safety

Clostridium difficile (C. difficile) is a microbe that causes diarrhea and intestinal infections. Commonly called *C. diff,* it can cause death. Persons at risk are older, are ill, or have prolonged use of antibiotics. Signs and symptoms include:

- Watery diarrhea
- Fever
- Loss of appetite
- Nausea
- Abdominal pain or tenderness

The microbe is found in feces. A person becomes infected by touching items or surfaces contaminated with feces and when touching his or her mouth or mucous membranes. *C. diff* can be found on bed linens, bed rails, toilets, bathroom fixtures, sinks, care supplies and equipment, walker handles, cart handles, bedside and over-bed tables, phones, TV remotes, and so on. You can spread the microbe if your contaminated hands or gloves:

- Touch a person
- Contaminate surfaces

Contact precautions are required (Chapter 13). Practice good hand hygiene. Alcohol-based hand sanitizers are not as effective against *C. difficile* as soap and water. Wash your hands with soap and water. Care items and surfaces are disinfected with a bleach solution. Also follow Standard Precautions and the Bloodborne Pathogen Standard.

Fecal Incontinence

Fecal incontinence is the inability to control the passage of feces and gas through the anus. Causes include:

- Intestinal diseases.
- Nervous system diseases and injuries.
- Fecal impaction or diarrhea.
- Some drugs.
- Chronic illness.
- Aging.
- Mental health disorders or dementia (Chapters 34 and 35). The person may not recognize the need for or the act of having a BM.
- Unanswered call lights.
- Not getting to the bathroom in time. The person may have mobility problems or may walk slowly. The bathroom may be too far away or in use.
- Problems removing clothes.
- Not finding the bathroom in a new setting.

Fecal incontinence has emotional effects. Frustration, embarrassment, anger, and humiliation are common. The person may need:

- Bowel training
- Help with elimination after meals and every 2 to 3 hours
- Incontinence products to keep garments and linens clean
- Good skin care

See *Focus on Older Persons: Fecal Incontinence.*

FOCUS ON OLDER PERSONS

Fecal Incontinence

Persons with dementia may smear feces on themselves, furniture, and walls. Some are not aware of having BMs. Some resist care. Follow the care plan. The measures for urinary incontinence (Chapter 20) may be part of the care plan. Be patient. Ask for help from co-workers. Talk to the nurse if you have problems keeping the person clean.

Flatulence

Gas and air are normally in the stomach and intestines. They are expelled through the mouth (burping, belching, eructating) and anus. *Gas or air passed through the anus is called* **flatus.** *Flatulence is the excessive formation of gas or air in the stomach and intestines.* Causes include:

- Swallowing air while eating and drinking
- Bacterial action in the intestines
- Gas-forming foods (p. 322)
- Constipation
- Bowel and abdominal surgeries
- Drugs that decrease peristalsis

If flatus is not expelled, the intestines swell or enlarge (distend) from the pressure of gases. Abdominal cramping or pain, shortness of breath, and a swollen abdomen occur. *Bloating* is a common complaint. Exercise, walking, moving in bed, and the left side-lying position often expel flatus. Doctors may order enemas and drugs to relieve flatulence.

BOWEL TRAINING

Bowel training has 2 goals.

- To gain control of BMs.
- To develop a regular pattern of elimination. Fecal impaction, constipation, and fecal incontinence are prevented.

Meals, especially breakfast, stimulate the urge for a BM. The person's usual time for a BM is noted on the care plan. So is toilet, commode, or bedpan use. Offer help with elimination at the times noted. The care plan includes a high-fiber diet, increased fluids, warm fluids, activity, and privacy. The nurse tells you about a person's bowel training program.

The doctor may order a suppository to stimulate a BM. A **suppository** *is a cone-shaped, solid drug that is inserted into a body opening. It melts at body temperature.* A nurse inserts a rectal suppository into the rectum (Fig. 22-3). A BM occurs about 30 minutes later.

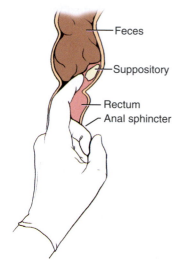

Feces
Suppository
Rectum
Anal sphincter

FIGURE 22-3 The suppository is inserted along the rectal wall. (Modified from deWit SC, O'Neill P: *Fundamental concepts and skills for nursing,* ed 4, Philadelphia, 2014, Saunders.)

ENEMAS

An *enema is the introduction of fluid into the rectum and lower colon.* Doctors order enemas to:

- Remove feces.
- Relieve constipation, fecal impaction, or flatulence.
- Clean the bowel of feces before certain surgeries and diagnostic procedures.

Safety and comfort measures for bowel elimination are practiced when giving enemas (see Box 22-1).

The doctor orders the enema solution. The solution depends on the enema's purpose—cleansing, constipation, fecal impaction, or flatulence.

- *Tap water enema*—is obtained from a faucet.
- *Saline enema*—a solution of salt and water. For adults, 1 or 2 teaspoons of table salt is added to 500 to 1000 mL (milliliters) of tap water.
- *Soapsuds enema (SSE)*—for adults, 3 to 5 mL of castile soap is added to 500 to 1000 mL of tap water.
- *Small-volume enema*—the adult size has about 120 mL (4 ounces [oz]) of solution.
- *Oil-retention enema*—has mineral, olive, or cottonseed oil. The adult size has about 120 mL (4 oz) of solution.

See *Promoting Safety and Comfort: Enemas.*

PROMOTING SAFETY AND COMFORT

Enemas

Safety

Enemas are usually safe procedures. Many people give themselves enemas at home. However, enemas are dangerous for older persons and those with certain heart and kidney diseases.

Comfort

The nurse may ask you to assist with enemas. Or you may be asked to give a small-volume enema. Before an enema, make sure that the bathroom is ready for use. If the person will use the commode or bedpan, have the device ready. Always keep a bedpan nearby in case the enema solution and stools are expelled. You promote mental comfort when the person knows the bathroom, commode, or bedpan is ready for use.

The person should retain the solution as long as possible. Provide for a comfortable Sims' or left side-lying position. When comfortable, it is easier to tolerate the procedure.

To prevent cramping:

- Use the correct water temperature. Cool water causes cramping.
- Give the solution slowly.

The Cleansing Enema

Cleansing enemas clean the bowel of feces and flatus. They relieve constipation and fecal impaction. They are given before certain surgeries and diagnostic procedures.

The doctor orders a tap water, saline, or soapsuds enema. An *enemas until clear* order means that enemas are given until the return solution is clear and free of stools. Agency policy may allow repeating enemas 2 or 3 times. You may be asked to assist the nurse with cleansing enemas.

The Small-Volume Enema

Small-volume enemas irritate and distend the rectum. This causes a BM. They are ordered for constipation or when the bowel does not need complete cleansing.

These enemas are ready to give. This solution is usually given at room temperature. To give the enema, squeeze and roll up the plastic container from the bottom. Do not release pressure on the bottle. Otherwise, solution is drawn from the rectum back into the bottle. Follow the rules for giving a small-volume enema in Box 22-2.

See *Delegation Guidelines: The Small-Volume Enema.*

See procedure: *Giving a Small-Volume Enema,* p. 326.

BOX 22-2   Giving a Small-Volume Enema

- Have the person void first. This increases comfort during the procedure.
- Give the amount of solution ordered.
- Position the person as the nurse directs. The Sims' or left side-lying position is preferred.
- Stop insertion if you feel resistance, the person complains of pain, or bleeding occurs.
- Have the person retain the solution until he or she needs to have a BM. This usually takes 5 to 10 minutes.
- Keep the person in the Sims' or left side-lying position to help retain the enema. Cover the person for warmth.
- Make sure the bathroom will be vacant when the person needs to have a BM. Make sure that another person will not use the bathroom. If the person uses the bedpan or commode, have the device ready.
- Ask the nurse to observe the enema results.

DELEGATION GUIDELINES

The Small-Volume Enema

If giving an enema to an adult is delegated to you, make sure the conditions in *Delegation Guidelines: Bowel Needs* (p. 320) are met. If those conditions are met, you need this information from the nurse.

- When to give the enema
- What position to use—Sims' or left side-lying position
- How far to insert the enema tip—usually 2 inches for adults
- How long the person should try to retain the solution
- What observations to report and record:
  - The amount of solution given
  - Bleeding or resistance when inserting the enema tip
  - How long the person retained the enema solution
  - Color, amount, consistency, shape, and odor of stools
  - Complaints of cramping, pain, or discomfort
  - Complaints of nausea or weakness
  - How the person tolerated the procedure
- When to report observations
- What patient or resident concerns to report at once

Giving a Small-Volume Enema

QUALITY OF LIFE

- Knock before entering the person's room.
- Address the person by name.
- Introduce yourself by name and title.

- Explain the procedure before starting and during the procedure.
- Protect the person's rights during the procedure.
- Handle the person gently during the procedure.

PRE-PROCEDURE

1 Follow *Delegation Guidelines:*
   a *Bowel Needs,* p. 320
   b *The Small-Volume Enema,* p. 325
   See *Promoting Safety and Comfort:*
   a *Bowel Needs,* p. 321
   b *Enemas,* p. 325
2 Practice hand hygiene.
3 Collect the following before going to the person's room.
   - Small-volume enema
   - Waterproof under-pad
   - Gloves
4 Arrange items in the person's room.
5 Practice hand hygiene.

6 Identify the person. Check the ID (identification) bracelet against the assignment sheet. Use 2 identifiers (Chapter 10). Also call the person by name.
7 Put on gloves.
8 Collect the following.
   - Commode or bedpan
   - Toilet tissue
   - Robe and non-skid footwear
   - Bath blanket
9 Remove and discard the gloves. Practice hand hygiene. Put on clean gloves.
10 Provide for privacy.
11 Raise the bed for body mechanics. Bed rails are up if used.

PROCEDURE

12 Lower the bed rail near you if up.
13 Cover the person with a bath blanket. Fan-fold top linens to the foot of the bed.
14 Position the person in the Sims' or left side-lying position.
15 Place the waterproof under-pad under the buttocks.
16 Expose the anal area.
17 Position the bedpan by the person.
18 Remove the cap from the enema tip.
19 Separate the buttocks to see the anus.
20 Ask the person to take a deep breath through the mouth.
21 Insert the enema tip 2 inches into the adult's rectum (Fig. 22-4). Do this as the person exhales. Insert the tip gently. Stop if the person complains of pain, you feel resistance, or bleeding occurs.
22 Squeeze and roll up the container gently. Release pressure on the bottle after you remove the tip from the rectum.
23 Put the container into the box, tip first. Discard the container and box.
24 Assist the person to the bathroom or commode when he or she has the urge to have a BM. The person wears a robe and non-skid footwear when up. The bed is at a low level that is safe and comfortable. Or help the person onto the bedpan and raise the head of the bed. Raise or lower bed rails according to the care plan.

25 Place the call light and toilet tissue within reach. Remind the person not to flush the toilet.
26 Discard disposable items.
27 Remove and discard the gloves. Practice hand hygiene.
28 Leave the room if the person can be left alone.
29 Return when the person signals. Or check on the person every 5 minutes. Knock before entering the room or bathroom.
30 Practice hand hygiene. Put on gloves.
31 Lower the bed rail if up.
32 Observe enema results for amount, color, consistency, shape, and odor. Call the nurse to observe the results.
33 Provide perineal care as needed.
34 Remove the waterproof under-pad.
35 Empty, rinse, clean, disinfect, and dry equipment. Use clean, dry paper towels for drying. Flush the toilet after the nurse observes the results.
36 Return equipment to its proper place.
37 Remove and discard the gloves. Practice hand hygiene.
38 Assist with hand-washing. Wear gloves for this step. Practice hand hygiene after removing and discarding the gloves.
39 Cover the person. Remove the bath blanket.

POST-PROCEDURE

40 Provide for comfort. (See the inside of the front cover.)
41 Place the call light and other needed items within reach.
42 Lower the bed to a safe and comfortable level. Follow the care plan.
43 Raise or lower bed rails. Follow the care plan.
44 Unscreen the person.

45 Complete a safety check of the room. (See the inside of the front cover.)
46 Follow agency policy for used linens and used supplies.
47 Practice hand hygiene.
48 Report and record your observations.

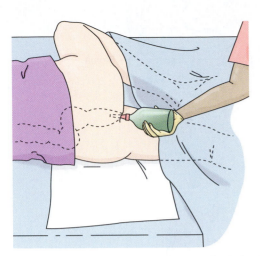

FIGURE 22-4 The small-volume enema tip is inserted 2 inches into the rectum.

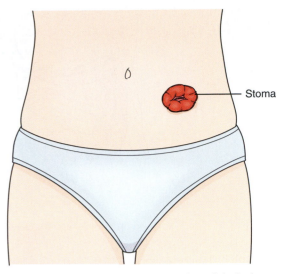

FIGURE 22-5 A stoma on the surface of the body.

The Oil-Retention Enema

Oil-retention enemas relieve constipation and fecal impaction. The oil softens feces and lubricates the rectum so feces pass with ease. The oil is retained for 30 minutes to 1 to 3 hours. Most oil-retention enemas are ready-to-use.

Giving an oil-retention enema is like giving a small-volume enema. After giving an oil-retention enema:

- Leave the person in the Sims' or left side-lying position. Cover the person for warmth.
- Urge the person to retain the enema for the time ordered.
- Place extra waterproof under-pads on the bed if needed.
- Check the person often while he or she retains the enema.
  See *Promoting Safety and Comfort: The Oil-Retention Enema.*

THE PERSON WITH AN OSTOMY

Sometimes part of the intestines is removed surgically. Cancer, bowel disease, and trauma (stab or bullet wounds) are common reasons. An ostomy is sometimes necessary. An *ostomy is a surgically created opening that connects an internal organ to the body's surface. The surgically created opening seen on the body's surface is called a* **stoma** (Fig. 22-5). An ostomy pouch is worn over the stoma to collect stools and flatus.

Colostomy

A *colostomy is a surgically created opening* (stomy) *between the colon (colo) and the body's surface.* Part of the colon is brought out onto the body's surface and a stoma is made. Feces and flatus pass through the stoma instead of the anus.

With a permanent colostomy, the diseased part of the colon is removed. A temporary colostomy gives the diseased or injured bowel time to heal. After healing, the bowel is surgically re-connected.

The colostomy site depends on the site of disease or injury (Fig. 22-6, p. 328). Stool consistency—liquid to formed—depends on the colostomy site. The more colon remaining to absorb water, the more solid and formed the stool. If the colostomy is near the end of the colon, stools are formed.

Stools irritate the skin. Skin care prevents skin breakdown around the stoma. The skin is washed and dried. Then a skin barrier is applied around the stoma. It prevents stools from having contact with the skin. The skin barrier is part of the pouch or a separate device.

Ileostomy

An *ileostomy is a surgically created opening* (stomy) *between the ileum (small intestine [ileo]) and the body's surface.* Part of the ileum is brought out onto the body's surface and a stoma is made. The entire colon is removed (Fig. 22-7, p. 328).

Liquid stools drain constantly from an ileostomy. Water is not absorbed because the colon was removed. Feces in the small intestine contain digestive juices that are very irritating to the skin. The ostomy pouch must fit well. Stools must not touch the skin. Good skin care is required.

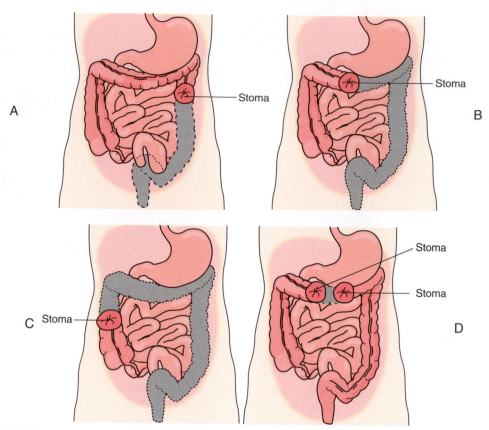

FIGURE 22-6 Colostomy sites. *Shading* shows the part of the bowel surgically removed. **A,** Sigmoid or descending colostomy. **B,** Transverse colostomy. **C,** Ascending colostomy. **D,** Double-barrel colostomy has 2 stomas. One allows for the excretion of feces. The other is for drugs to help the bowel heal. This type is usually temporary.

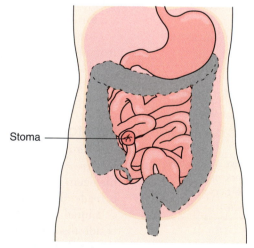

FIGURE 22-7 An ileostomy. The entire large intestine is removed. *Shading* shows the part of the bowel surgically removed.

Ostomy Pouches

A plastic ostomy pouch with an adhesive back is applied to the skin. Some pouches are secured to ostomy belts (Fig. 22-8).

A drain at the bottom of the pouch closes with a clip, clamp, or wire closure. The drain is opened to empty the pouch. The pouch is emptied when stools are present. It is opened when it balloons or bulges to release flatus. The drain is wiped with toilet tissue before closing.

The pouch is changed every 2 to 7 days and when it leaks. Frequent pouch changes can damage the skin.

Odors are prevented by:

- Using odor-free pouches.
- Performing good hygiene.
- Emptying the pouch.
- Avoiding gas-forming foods.
- Putting deodorants into the pouch. The nurse tells you what to use.

The person wears normal clothes. Tight garments can prevent feces from entering the pouch. Also, bulging from stools and flatus can be seen with tight clothes.

Peristalsis increases after eating and drinking. Therefore stomas are usually quiet after sleep. That is, expelling feces is less likely at this time. If the person showers or bathes with the pouch off, it is best done before breakfast. Showers and baths are delayed for 1 to 2 hours after applying a new pouch. This gives adhesive time to seal to the skin.

Do not flush pouches down the toilet. Follow agency policy for disposal.

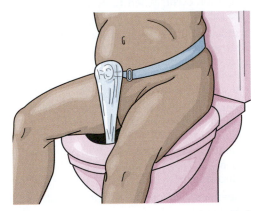

FIGURE 22-8 The ostomy pouch is secured to an ostomy belt. The pouch is emptied by directing it into the toilet and opening the end.

FOCUS ON **P R I D E**

The Person, Family, and Yourself

Personal and Professional Responsibility
You must know the legal limits of your role. Some states and agencies allow nursing assistants to insert some types of suppositories. For example, you may be allowed to insert suppositories in persons who use them for constipation. You cannot give a suppository for fever or vomiting. Know what you can and cannot do. Never perform a task beyond the legal limits of your role.

Rights and Respect
Bowel elimination is a private act. Illness, disease, surgery, and aging can affect this private act. Some persons are embarrassed to have a BM in a strange setting. To promote comfort and privacy:

- Ask others to leave the room.
- Close doors, privacy curtains, and window coverings.
- Turn on water or music to mask sounds.
- Cover the person.
- Allow enough time. Place the call light nearby and ask the person to call if help is needed.
- Knock before entering the room. Tell the person who you are. Ask if you can enter before opening the door completely.
- Use an agency-approved spray for odors.

Independence and Social Interaction
Some persons have had ostomies for a long time. They may have special routines or care measures. Do not react to things that seem odd to you. When you assist, ask what they prefer. Listen to their requests. Follow their choices in ostomy care. To promote independence, allow personal choice and control as much as safely possible.

Delegation and Teamwork
The nurse may delegate a task that you have not done before. Giving an enema is an example. Never attempt a task that you are not comfortable doing. Make sure your state and agency allow you to perform the procedure. If those conditions are met, you can politely say: "I'm sorry, but I have not done that task before. I am not comfortable doing it on my own. Would you please show me how it is done?" Take pride in making the right choice to tell the nurse about your delegation concerns.

Ethics and Laws
All persons must be protected from abuse, mistreatment, and neglect. Examples include:

- Leaving a person sitting or lying in urine or feces
- Leaving a person on a toilet, commode, or bedpan for a long time
- Telling a person to void or have a BM in bed

Federal and state laws require the reporting and investigating of abuse, mistreatment, and neglect. If found guilty you will lose your job. The offense is noted on your registry. You cannot work in a nursing center or on a skilled care nursing unit in a hospital. Protect yourself from being accused. Check patients or residents often. Be careful and focused. Always treat the person with dignity.

FOCUS ON PRIDE: *Application*

You are asked to do an unfamiliar task. Do you seek help? Do you try to do it alone? Does asking for help bother you?

Supervision is part of the nurse's role in delegation. The nurse needs to know your comfort level with tasks. Never be ashamed to ask for supervision.

REVIEW QUESTIONS

Circle the BEST answer.

1 Which is *true*?
   a A person must have a BM every day.
   b Stools are normally brown, soft, and formed.
   c Diarrhea occurs when feces move slowly through the bowel.
   d Constipation occurs when feces move quickly through the bowel.

2 Which should you ask the nurse to observe?
   a A black and tarry stool
   b The person's first BM of the day
   c Stool with an odor
   d Liquid stool from an ileostomy

3 The prolonged retention and buildup of feces in the rectum is called
   a Constipation
   b Fecal impaction
   c Diarrhea
   d Fecal incontinence

4 These measures promote normal BMs. Which is outside your role limits?
   a Provide oral fluids according to the care plan.
   b Assist with activity according to the care plan.
   c Give drugs to control diarrhea.
   d Provide privacy for bowel elimination.

5 A person has *C. difficile*. You should
   a Disinfect care items with soap and water
   b Use an alcohol-based hand sanitizer for hand hygiene
   c Wear a gown and gloves
   d Refuse to care for the person

6 Bowel training is aimed at
   a Bowel control and regular elimination
   b Ostomy control
   c Promoting toilet use
   d Preventing bleeding

7 Your state and agency allow you to insert rectal suppositories. You insert a suppository
   a Into the feces
   b Into the stoma
   c Along the rectal wall
   d With an enema tube

8 Which is used for a cleansing enema?
   a Mineral, olive, or cottonseed oil
   b A suppository
   c A 120 mL bottle of solution
   d Tap water, saline, or a soapsuds enema

9 When giving an enema
   a Use a cool solution
   b Give the solution slowly
   c Have the person void after giving the enema
   d Place the person in the supine position

10 A small-volume enema is retained
   a For 2 minutes
   b At least 10 to 20 minutes
   c At least 30 minutes
   d Until the urge to have a BM is felt

11 Which care measure for an ostomy should you question?
   a Use deodorant in the pouch.
   b Perform good skin care around the stoma.
   c Change the pouch daily.
   d Apply a skin barrier around the stoma.

12 An ostomy pouch is usually emptied
   a Every 4 to 6 hours
   b When it is full
   c Every 2 to 7 days
   d When stools are present

Answers to Chapter 22 questions are on p. 552.

FOCUS ON PRACTICE

Problem Solving

You respond to a resident's call light. The resident needs to have a BM urgently. The bathroom is occupied by the roommate. What do you do?

Nutrition Needs

OBJECTIVES

- Define the key terms and key abbreviations in this chapter.
- Explain the purpose and use of the MyPlate symbol.
- Describe the functions and sources of nutrients.
- Describe the factors that affect eating and nutrition.
- Describe OBRA requirements for serving food.
- Describe the special diets and between-meal snacks.
- Identify the signs, symptoms, and precautions for aspiration and regurgitation.

- Explain how to assist with measuring food intake.
- Explain how to assist with nutrition needs.
- Explain how to assist with enteral nutrition.
- Perform the procedures described in this chapter.
- Explain how to promote PRIDE in the person, the family, and yourself.

KEY TERMS

anorexia The loss of appetite
aspiration Breathing fluid, food, vomitus, or an object into the lungs
calorie The fuel or energy value of food
dysphagia Difficulty (dys) swallowing (phagia)
enteral nutrition Giving nutrients into the gastro-intestinal (GI) tract (enteral) through a feeding tube

gavage The process of giving a tube feeding
nutrient A substance that is ingested, digested, absorbed, and used by the body
nutrition The processes involved in the ingestion, digestion, absorption, and use of food and fluids by the body
regurgitation The backward flow of stomach contents into the mouth

KEY ABBREVIATIONS

GI	Gastro-intestinal		NPO	Nothing per mouth
ID	Identification		OBRA	Omnibus Budget Reconciliation Act of 1987
mg	Milligram		oz	Ounce
NG	Naso-gastric		USDA	United States Department of Agriculture

Food is a basic need. The person's diet affects physical and mental well-being and function. A poor diet and poor eating habits:
- Increase the risk for disease and infection.
- Cause chronic illnesses to become worse.
- Cause healing problems.
- Increase the risk for accidents and injuries.

You help meet nutritional needs by preparing patients and residents for meals and serving meal trays. When necessary, you may need to feed a person.

NOTE: *A task may require more than 1 pair of gloves. Change gloves as needed. Use careful judgment. Remember to practice hand hygiene after removing gloves.*

See *Focus on Surveys: Nutrition Needs.*

FOCUS ON SURVEYS

Nutrition Needs

The health team develops a care plan to meet nutritional needs. Surveyors may ask you:
- How food and fluid intake (Chapter 24) are observed and reported.
- How eating ability is observed and reported.
- About the measures to prevent or meet changes in nutritional needs. Snacks and frequent meals are examples.
- About the goals for nutrition in the care plan.

BASIC NUTRITION

Nutrition is the processes involved in the ingestion, digestion, absorption, and use of food and fluids by the body. Good nutrition is needed for growth, healing, and body functions. A *nutrient is a substance that is ingested, digested, absorbed, and used by the body.* Nutrients are grouped into fats, proteins, carbohydrates, vitamins, minerals, and water (p. 334).

Fats, proteins, and carbohydrates provide fuel for energy. A *calorie is the fuel or energy value of food.*

- 1 gram of fat—9 calories
- 1 gram of protein—4 calories
- 1 gram of carbohydrate—4 calories

MyPlate

The MyPlate symbol (Fig. 23-1) encourages healthy eating from 5 food groups. Issued by the United States Department of Agriculture (USDA), MyPlate promotes wise food choices by:

- Balancing calories
  - Eating less
  - Avoiding over-sized portions
- Increasing certain foods
  - Making half of your plate fruits and vegetables
  - Making at least half of your grains whole grains
  - Drinking fat-free or low-fat (1%) milk
- Reducing certain foods
  - Choosing low-sodium foods
  - Drinking water instead of sugary drinks

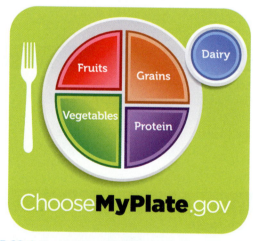

FIGURE 23-1 The MyPlate symbol. (Courtesy U.S. Department of Agriculture, Center for Nutrition and Policy Promotion, 2011.)

Physical Activity. The USDA recommends that adults do at least 1 of the following weekly.

- 2 hours and 30 minutes of moderate physical activity
- 1 hour and 15 minutes of vigorous physical activity

See Box 23-1 for examples of moderate and vigorous activities.

Physical activity at least 3 days a week is best. Each activity should last at least 10 minutes. Adults also should do strengthening activities at least 2 days a week. Push-ups, sit-ups, and weight-lifting are examples.

BOX 23-1 Physical Activities

Moderate Physical Activities
- Walking briskly (about 3½ miles per hour)
- Bicycling (less than 10 miles per hour)
- Gardening (raking, trimming bushes)
- Dancing
- Golf (walking and carrying clubs)
- Water aerobics
- Canoeing
- Tennis (doubles)

Vigorous Physical Activities
- Running and jogging (5 miles per hour)
- Walking very fast (4½ miles per hour)
- Bicycling (more than 10 miles per hour)
- Heavy yard work (chopping wood)
- Swimming (freestyle laps)
- Aerobics
- Basketball (competitive)
- Tennis (singles)

Modified from U.S. Department of Agriculture: *What is physical activity?* June 10, 2015.

Food Groups

The 5 food groups are:

- Grains group
- Vegetable group
- Fruit group
- Dairy group
- Protein foods group

The amount needed from each food group depends on age, sex, and physical activity. See Table 23-1 for sources, daily servings, serving sizes, and health benefits.

TABLE 23-1	Food Groups	
Sources	**Daily Servings and Serving Sizes**	**Health Benefits**
Grains • Grains are foods made from wheat, rice, oats, cornmeal, barley, or other cereal grains. Bread, pasta, oatmeal, breakfast cereals, tortillas, and grits are examples. • *Whole grains* have the entire grain kernel. Whole-wheat flour, bulgur (cracked wheat), oatmeal, whole cornmeal, and brown rice are examples. • *Refined grains* are processed to remove the grain kernel. White flour, white bread, and white rice are examples. They have less dietary fiber than whole grains.	**Daily Servings** • Adult women: 5 to 6 ounces (oz); at least 3 oz from whole grains • Adult men: 6 to 8 oz; at least 3 to 4 oz from whole grains **Serving Sizes** • 1 oz = 1 slice of bread • 1 oz = 1 cup breakfast cereal • 1 oz = ½ cup cooked rice, cereal, or pasta	• Reduce the risk of heart disease. • May prevent constipation. • May help with weight management. • May prevent certain birth defects. • Contain dietary fiber, several B vitamins (thiamin, riboflavin, niacin, folate [folic acid]), and minerals (iron, magnesium, and selenium).
Vegetables • Vegetables can be raw, cooked, fresh, frozen, canned, dried, or juiced. • *Dark green vegetables*—broccoli, collard greens, dark green leafy lettuce, kale, mustard greens, romaine lettuce, spinach, turnip greens, watercress. • *Red and orange vegetables*—acorn, butternut, and hubbard squashes; carrots; pumpkin; red peppers; sweet potatoes; tomatoes; tomato juice. • *Beans and peas*—black beans, black-eyed peas, garbanzo beans (chickpeas), kidney beans, pinto beans, soybeans, split peas. • *Starchy vegetables*—corn, green peas, potatoes. • *Other vegetables*—bean sprouts, cabbage, cauliflower, celery, cucumbers, green beans, green peppers, iceberg (head) lettuce, mushrooms, onions, summer squash, zucchini.	**Daily Servings** • Adult women: 2 to 2½ cups • Adult men: 2½ to 3 cups **Serving Sizes** • 1 cup = 1 cup raw or cooked vegetables or vegetable juice • 1 cup = 2 cups raw leafy greens	• May reduce the risk for stroke, high blood pressure, heart disease, and type 2 diabetes. • May protect against certain cancers—mouth, stomach, colon-rectum. • May reduce the risk of kidney stones. • May reduce the risk of bone loss. • May help lower calorie intake. Most vegetables are low in fat and calories. • Contain no *cholesterol* (a soft, waxy substance found in the bloodstream and all body cells). • May prevent certain birth defects. • Contain potassium, dietary fiber, folate (folic acid), and vitamins A and C.
Fruits • Any fruit or 100% fruit juice counts as part of the fruit group. • Fruits may be fresh, frozen, canned, or dried. • Avoid fruits canned in syrup. Syrup contains added sugar. Choose fruits canned in 100% fruit juice or water.	**Daily Servings** • Adult women: 1½ to 2 cups • Adult men: 2 cups **Serving Sizes** • 1 cup = 1 cup fruit • 1 cup = 1 cup fruit juice • 1 cup = ½ cup dried fruit	• May reduce the risk for stroke, heart disease and heart attack, high blood pressure, obesity, and type 2 diabetes. • May protect against certain cancers. • May reduce the risk of kidney stones. • May reduce the risk of bone loss. • May help prevent constipation. • May prevent certain birth defects. • May help lower fat and calorie intake. Most fruits are low in fat and calories. • Contain no cholesterol. • Are low in sodium. • Contain potassium, dietary fiber, vitamin C, and folate (folic acid).
Dairy • All fluid milk products are part of the dairy group. So are many foods made from milk. Yogurt and cheese are examples. • Low-fat or fat-free choices are best. • Cream, cream cheese, and butter are not in this group.	**Daily Servings** • Adult women: 3 cups • Adult men: 3 cups **Serving Sizes** • 1 cup = 1 cup milk or yogurt • 1 cup = 1½ oz natural cheese • 1 cup = 2 oz processed cheese	• Helps build and maintain bone mass. This may reduce the risk of osteoporosis. • May reduce the risk of cardiovascular disease, type 2 diabetes, and high blood pressure. • Contains calcium, potassium, and vitamin D.

Continued

TABLE 23-1 Food Groups—cont'd		
Sources	**Daily Servings and Serving Sizes**	**Health Benefits**

Protein Foods
• All foods made from meat, poultry, seafood, eggs, processed soy products, nuts, and seeds are protein foods.
• Beans and peas are in this group and the vegetable group.
• For healthy choices, remember:
  • Choose lean or low-fat meat and poultry. Regular ground beef (75% to 80% lean) and chicken with skin are higher in fat.
  • Avoid fat for cooking. Fried chicken and eggs fried in butter are examples.
  • Salmon, trout, and herring may reduce heart disease risk.
  • Liver and other organ meats are high in cholesterol.
  • Egg yolks are high in cholesterol. Egg whites are cholesterol-free.
  • Processed meats (ham, sausage, hot dogs, luncheon and deli meats) have added sodium (salt).
	Daily Servings
	• Adult women: 5 to 5½ oz
	• Adult men: 5½ to 6½ oz
	
	Serving Sizes
	• 1 oz = 1 oz lean meat, poultry, or fish
	• 1 oz = 1 egg
	• 1 oz = 1 tablespoon peanut butter
	• 1 oz = ¼ cup cooked dry beans
	• 1 oz = ½ oz nuts or seeds
		• Contain protein, B vitamins (niacin, thiamin, riboflavin, and B_6), vitamin E, iron, zinc, and magnesium.
		• Many proteins are high in fat and cholesterol. Heart disease is a risk. However, this group provides nutrients needed for health and body maintenance.

Modified from U.S. Department of Agriculture: MyPlate, January 2016.

Oils

Oils are fats that are liquid at room temperature. Vegetable oils for cooking include canola oil, corn oil, and olive oil. Oils come from plants and fish. Because they have nutrients, the USDA includes oils in food patterns. However, *oils are not a food group.*

Adult women are allowed 5 to 6 teaspoons daily. Adult men can have 6 to 7 teaspoons daily. Some foods are high in oil—nuts, olives, some fish, and avocados.

When making oil choices, remember:
• Oils are high in calories.
• The best oil choices come from fish, nuts, and vegetables.
• Some foods are mainly oil. Mayonnaise, some salad dressings, and soft margarine are examples.
• Oils from plant sources do not contain cholesterol.
• *Solid fats* are solid at room temperature. Solid fats include butter, milk fat, beef fat (tallow, suet), chicken fat, pork fat (lard), stick margarine, and shortening.
• Oils and solid fats have about 120 calories in each tablespoon.
• Enough oil is usually consumed daily from nuts, fish, cooking oil, and salad dressings.

Nutrients

No food or food group has every essential nutrient. A well-balanced diet ensures an adequate intake of these essential nutrients.
• *Protein*—the most important nutrient, it is needed for tissue growth and repair. Sources include meat, fish, poultry, eggs, milk and milk products, cereals, beans, peas, and nuts.
• *Carbohydrates*—provide energy and fiber for bowel elimination. Sources are fruits, vegetables, breads, cereals, and sugar. Fiber is not digested. It provides the bulky part of chyme for elimination.
• *Fats*—provide energy. They provide flavor and help the body use certain vitamins. Sources include meats, lard, butter, shortening, oils, milk, cheese, egg yolks, and nuts. Unneeded dietary fat is stored as body fat (*adipose tissue*).
• *Vitamins*—are needed for certain body functions. The body stores vitamins A, D, E, and K. Vitamins C and the B complex vitamins are not stored. They must be ingested daily. The lack of a certain vitamin results in illness.
• *Minerals*—are needed for bone and tooth formation, nerve and muscle function, fluid balance, and other body processes. Foods containing calcium help prevent musculo-skeletal changes.
• *Water*—is needed for all body processes (Chapter 24).

FACTORS AFFECTING EATING AND NUTRITION

Factors affecting eating and nutrition begin in childhood and continue throughout life.

- *Culture.* Culture influences dietary practices, food choices, and food preparation. Frying, baking, smoking, or roasting food and eating raw food are some cultural practices. So is using sauces, herbs, and spices. See *Caring About Culture: Food Practices.*
- *Religion.* Selecting, preparing, and eating food often involve religion. A person may follow all, some, or none of the dietary practices of his or her faith. Respect the person's religious practices.
- *Finances.* People with limited incomes often buy cheaper carbohydrate foods. Their diets often lack protein and certain vitamins and minerals.
- *Appetite.* Appetite relates to the desire for food. *Loss of appetite* (*anorexia*) can occur. Causes include illness, drugs, anxiety, pain, and depression. Unpleasant sights, thoughts, and smells are other causes.
- *Personal choice.* Food likes and dislikes are influenced by foods served in the home. Usually food likes expand with age and social experiences.
- *Body reactions.* People should avoid foods that cause allergic reactions. Foods causing nausea, vomiting, diarrhea, indigestion, gas, or headaches are avoided.
- *Illness.* Appetite often decreases during illness and recovery from injuries. However, nutritional needs increase. The body must fight infection, heal tissue, and replace lost blood cells. Nutrients lost through vomiting and diarrhea need to be replaced.
- *Drugs.* Drugs can cause appetite loss, confusion, nausea, constipation, impaired taste, or changes in gastro-intestinal (GI) function. They can cause inflammation of the mouth, throat, esophagus, and stomach.
- *Chewing problems.* Mouth, teeth, and gum problems can affect chewing. Examples include oral pain, dry or sore mouth, gum disease (Chapter 18), dental problems, and dentures that fit poorly.
- *Swallowing problems.* Stroke; pain; confusion; dry mouth; and diseases of the mouth, throat, and esophagus can affect swallowing. See "The Dysphagia Diet" on p. 339.
- *Disability.* Disease or injury can affect the hands, wrists, and arms. Adaptive equipment (assistive devices) let the person eat independently.
- *Impaired cognitive function.* Cognitive changes may affect the ability to use eating utensils. And it may affect eating, chewing, and swallowing.
- *Age.* Many GI changes occur with aging.
  See *Focus on Older Persons: Factors Affecting Eating and Nutrition.*

CARING ABOUT CULTURE
Food Practices

Rice, corn, and beans are protein sources in *Mexico*. In the *Philippines,* rice is a main food. And fish, vegetables, and native fruits are preferred. A diet high in sugar and animal fat is common in *Poland.* In *China,* a meal of rice with meat, fish, and vegetables is common. High sodium content is from using soy sauce and dried and preserved foods.

(*NOTE: Each person is unique. A person may not follow all of the beliefs and practices of his or her culture. Follow the care plan.*)

Modified from D'Avanzo CE: *Pocket guide to cultural health assessment,* ed 4, St Louis, 2008, Mosby.

FOCUS ON OLDER PERSONS
Factors Affecting Eating and Nutrition

GI changes occur with aging.
- Taste and smell dull.
- Appetite decreases.
- Secretion of digestive juices decreases. Hard to digest, fried and fatty foods may cause indigestion.

Some people avoid the high-fiber foods needed for bowel elimination—apricots, celery, and fruits and vegetables with skins and seeds. High-fiber foods are hard to chew and can irritate the intestines.

Foods providing soft bulk are often ordered for persons with chewing problems or constipation. Whole-grain cereals and cooked fruits and vegetables are examples.

Calorie needs are lower. Energy and activity levels are lower. Foods that contain calcium help prevent musculo-skeletal changes. Protein is needed for tissue growth and repair. Because of cost, diets may lack high-protein foods.

OBRA DIETARY REQUIREMENTS

The *Omnibus Budget Reconciliation Act of 1987 (OBRA)* has requirements for food served in nursing centers.

- Each person's nutritional and dietary needs are met.
- The person's diet is well-balanced. It is nourishing and tastes good. Food is well-seasoned. It is not too salty or too sweet.
- Food is appetizing. It has an appealing aroma and is attractive.
- Hot food is served hot. Cold food is served cold.
- Food is served promptly. If not, hot food cools and cold food warms.
- Food is prepared to meet each person's needs. Some people need food cut, ground, or chopped. Others have special diets.
- Other foods are offered if the food served is refused. The substituted food must have a similar nutritional value to the first foods served.
- Each person receives at least 3 meals a day. A bedtime snack is offered.

The center provides needed adaptive equipment (assistive devices) and utensils (Fig. 23-2, p. 336). They promote independence. Make sure the person has needed equipment.

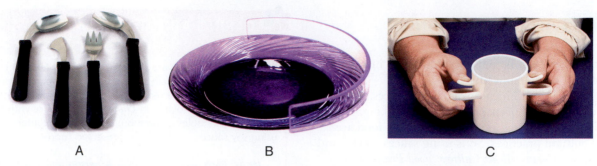

A B C

FIGURE 23-2 Adaptive equipment (assistive devices) for eating. **A,** Eating utensils have tapered and angled handles. The knife cuts with slicing and rocking motions. **B,** The plate guard helps keep food on the plate. **C,** The thumb grips on the cup help prevent spilling. (Images courtesy Elderstore, Alpharetta, Ga.)

SPECIAL DIETS

Doctors may order special diets (Table 23-2).
- For a nutritional deficiency or a disease
- For weight gain or loss
- To remove or decrease certain substances in the diet

Regular diet, *general diet*, and *house diet* mean no dietary limits or restrictions. The sodium-controlled diet is often ordered (p. 338). So is a diabetes meal plan (p. 338). Persons with swallowing problems may need a dysphagia diet (p. 339).

TABLE 23-2	Special Diets	
Diet	**Use**	**Foods Allowed/Restricted**
Clear liquid—foods liquid at room temperature and clear or able to see through; non-irritating; non–gas forming; leave a small amount of residue	After surgery; for acute illness, infection, nausea, and vomiting; and to prepare for GI exams	Water, tea, and coffee *(without milk or cream)*; carbonated drinks; gelatin; fruit juices *without pulp* (apple, grape, cranberry); fat-free broth; hard candy, sugar, and Popsicles; *may need to avoid liquids with red coloring*
Full liquid—foods liquid at room temperature	Advance from clear-liquid diet after surgery; for stomach irritation, fever, nausea, and vomiting; for persons unable to chew, swallow, or digest solid foods	Foods on the clear-liquid diet; custard; eggnog; strained soups; strained fruit and vegetable juices; milk and milk-shakes; cooked cereals; plain ice cream and sherbet; plain pudding; yogurt
Mechanical soft—semi-solid foods that are easily digested	Advance from full-liquid diet; chewing problems, GI disorders, and infections	All liquids; eggs *(not fried)*; broiled, baked, or roasted meat, fish, or poultry that is chopped or shredded; mild cheeses (American, Swiss, cheddar, cream, cottage); strained fruit juices; refined bread *(no crust)* and crackers; cooked cereal; cooked or pureed vegetables; cooked or canned fruit *without skin or seeds*; plain pudding; plain cakes and soft cookies *without fruit or nuts*
Fiber- and residue-restricted—foods that leave a small amount of residue in the colon	Diseases of the colon and diarrhea	Coffee, tea, milk, carbonated drinks, strained fruit and vegetable juices; refined bread and crackers; creamed and refined cereal; rice; cottage and cream cheese; eggs *(not fried)*; plain puddings and cakes; gelatin; custard; sherbet and ice cream; canned or cooked fruit *without skin or seeds*; potatoes *(not fried)*; strained cooked vegetables; plain pasta; *no raw fruits or vegetables*
High-fiber—foods that increase residue and fiber in the colon to stimulate peristalsis	Constipation and GI disorders	All fruits and vegetables; whole-wheat bread; whole-grain cereals; fried foods; whole-grain rice; milk, cream, butter, and cheese; meats

TABLE 23-2	Special Diets—cont'd	
Diet	**Use**	**Foods Allowed/Restricted**
Bland—foods that are non-irritating and low in roughage; foods served at moderate temperatures; no strong spices or condiments	Ulcers, gallbladder disorders, and some intestinal disorders; after abdominal surgery	Lean meats; white bread; creamed and refined cereals; cream or cottage cheese; gelatin; plain puddings, cakes, and cookies; eggs *(not fried);* butter and cream; canned fruits and vegetables *without skin and seeds;* strained fruit juices; potatoes *(not fried);* pastas and rice; strained or soft cooked carrots, peas, beets, spinach, squash, and asparagus tips; creamed soups from allowed vegetables; *no fried or spicy foods*
High-calorie—3000 to 4000 calories daily; includes 3 full meals and between-meal snacks	Weight gain and some thyroid problems	Dietary increases in all foods; large portions of regular diet with 3 between-meal snacks
Calorie-controlled—adequate nutrients while controlling calories to promote weight loss and reduce body fat	Weight loss	Foods low in fats and carbohydrates and lean meats; *avoid butter, cream, rice, gravies, salad oils, noodles, cakes, pastries, carbonated and alcoholic drinks, candy, potato chips, and similar foods*
High-iron—foods high in iron	Anemia; after blood loss; for women during the reproductive years	Liver and other organ meats; lean meats; egg yolks; shellfish; dried fruits; dried beans; green leafy vegetables; lima beans; peanut butter; enriched breads and cereals
Fat-controlled (low cholesterol)—foods low in fat and prepared without adding fat	Heart, gallbladder, and liver diseases; disorders of fat digestion; diseases of the pancreas	Skim milk (fat-free) or buttermilk; cottage cheese *(no other cheeses allowed);* gelatin; sherbet; fruit; lean meat, poultry, and fish (baked, broiled, or roasted); fat-free broth; soups made with skim milk (fat-free); margarine; rice, pasta, breads, and cereals; vegetables; potatoes
High-protein—aids and promotes tissue healing	Burns, high fever, infection, and some liver diseases	Meat, milk, eggs, cheese, fish, poultry; breads and cereals; green leafy vegetables
Sodium-controlled—a certain amount of sodium is allowed	Heart disease, fluid retention, liver diseases, and some kidney diseases	Fruits and vegetables and unsalted butter are allowed; *adding salt at the table is not allowed; highly salted foods and foods high in sodium are not allowed; the use of salt during cooking may be restricted*
Gluten-free—foods without the gluten protein	Celiac disease	Beans; seeds; nuts; eggs; meats, fish, and poultry *(without breading, batter, or marinade);* fruits and vegetables; most dairy foods; gluten-free grains and starches (arrowroot, corn, cornmeal, hominy, flax, millet, rice, soy, and tapioca); gluten-free flours (rice, soy, corn, potato, bean); *no foods containing wheat, barley, triticale, or rye*
Diabetes meal plan—the same amount of carbohydrates, protein, and fat are eaten at the same time each day	Diabetes	Determined by nutritional and energy requirements

The Sodium-Controlled Diet

According to the American Heart Association (AHA), the average amount of sodium in the daily diet is greater than 3400 mg (milligrams). For most adults, the AHA recommends limiting sodium intake to no more than 1500 mg a day. Doing so reduces the risk of high blood pressure, heart disease, and stroke (Chapter 33).

Heart, liver, and kidney diseases and certain drugs cause the body to retain extra sodium. Sodium causes the body to retain water. With too much sodium, water is retained. Tissues swell with water. There is excess fluid in the blood vessels. The heart works harder. With heart disease, the extra workload can cause serious problems or death.

Sodium control decreases the amount of sodium in the body. Less water is retained. Less water in the tissues and blood vessels reduces the heart's workload.

The doctor orders the amount of sodium allowed. Sodium-controlled diets involve:
- Omitting high-sodium foods (Box 23-2)
- Not adding salt to food at the table
- Limiting the amount of salt used in cooking
- Diet planning

Diabetes Meal Plan

Diabetes is a chronic illness in which the body cannot produce or use insulin properly (Chapter 33). The pancreas produces and secretes insulin. Insulin lets the body use sugar. Without enough insulin, sugar builds up in the bloodstream. It is not used by cells for energy. Diabetes is usually treated with insulin or other drugs, diet, and exercise.

A meal plan for healthy eating is developed. Consistency is key. It involves:
- Food preferences (likes, eating habits, meal times, culture, and life-style). Food amounts and preparation methods may be restricted.
- Calories needed. The same amount of carbohydrates, protein, and fat are eaten each day.
- Eating meals and snacks at regular times. The person eats at regular times to maintain a certain blood sugar level.

Serve meals and snacks on time. Always check what was eaten. Report what the person did and did not eat. A between-meal snack makes up for what was not eaten (p. 345). The nurse tells you what to provide. The amount of insulin given depends on daily food intake. Report changes in the person's eating habits.

BOX 23-2	High-Sodium Foods

Grains
- Baked goods—biscuits, muffins, cakes, cookies, pies, pastries, sweet rolls, donuts, and so on
- Breads and rolls
- Cereals—cold, instant hot
- Noodle mixes
- Pancakes
- Salted snack foods—pretzels, corn chips, popcorn, crackers, chips, and so on
- Stuffing mixes
- Waffles

Vegetables
- Canned vegetables
- Olives
- Pickles and other pickled vegetables
- Relish
- Sauerkraut
- Tomato sauce or paste
- Vegetable juices—tomato, V8, Bloody Mary mixes
- Vegetables with sauces, creams, or seasonings

Fruits
- None—fruits are not high in sodium

Dairy Group
- Buttermilk
- Cheese
- Commercial dips made with sour cream

Protein Foods
- Bacon and Canadian bacon
- Canned meats and fish—chicken, tuna, salmon, anchovies, sardines
- Caviar
- Chipped, dried, and corned beef and other meats
- Deli meats—turkey, ham, bologna, salami, pastrami, and so on

Protein Foods—cont'd
- Dried fish
- Ham
- Herring
- Hot dogs (frankfurters)
- Liverwurst
- Lox and smoked salmon
- Mackerel
- Pepperoni
- Salt pork
- Sausages
- Scrapple
- Shellfish—shrimp, crab, clams, oysters, scallops, lobster

Other
- Asian foods—Chinese, Japanese, East Indian, Thai, Vietnamese
- Baking soda and baking powder
- Catsup (ketchup)
- Cocoa mixes
- Commercially prepared dinners—frozen, canned, boxed, and so on
- Mayonnaise
- Mexican foods
- Mustard
- Pasta dishes—lasagna, manicotti, ravioli
- Peanut butter
- Pizzas
- Pot pies
- Salad dressings
- Salted nuts or seeds
- Sauces—soy, teriyaki, Worcestershire, steak, barbecue, pasta, chili, cocktail
- Seasoning salts—garlic, onion, celery, meat tenderizers, monosodium glutamate (MSG), and so on
- Soups—canned, packaged, instant, dried, bouillon

The Dysphagia Diet

Dysphagia means difficulty (dys) swallowing (phagia). See Box 23-3 for signs and symptoms.

- A *slow swallow* means the person has difficulty getting enough food and fluids for good nutrition and fluid balance.
- An *unsafe swallow* means that food enters the airway (aspiration). *Aspiration is breathing fluid, food, vomitus, or an object into the lungs* (p. 346).

Food thickness is changed for the person's needs (see Box 23-3). Safety and comfort are important when feeding a person with dysphagia. You must:

- Know the signs and symptoms of dysphagia (see Box 23-3).
- Feed the person according to the care plan.
- Follow aspiration precautions (Box 23-4) and the care plan.
- Report changes in how the person eats.
- Report signs and symptoms of aspiration at once: choking, coughing, or difficulty breathing during or after meals and abnormal breathing or respiratory sounds.

BOX 23-4   Aspiration Precautions

- Help the person with meals and snacks. Follow the care plan.
- Position the person upright as the nurse and care plan direct. The person remains upright for at least 1 hour after eating.
- Support the upper back, shoulders, and neck with a pillow.
- Follow the care plan for straw use. A straw may not be allowed.
- Observe for signs and symptoms of aspiration during meals and snacks.
- Check the person's mouth after eating for pocketing. Check inside the cheeks, under the tongue, and on the roof of the mouth. Remove any food.
- Provide mouth care after eating.
- Report and record your observations.

FOOD INTAKE

Food intake is measured in different ways. Follow agency policy for the method used.

- *Percentage of food eaten.* Intake ranges from 0 to 100 percent (%). Some agencies record the percent of the whole meal tray. Others record the percent of each food item eaten. See Figure 23-3.
- *Calorie counts.* Note what the person ate and how much. For example, a chicken breast, rice, beans, a roll, pudding, and 2 pats of butter were served. The person ate all the chicken, half the rice, and the roll. One pat of butter was used. The beans and pudding were not eaten. Note these on the flow sheet. A nurse or dietitian converts these portions into calories. See *Focus on Math: Food Intake*, p. 340.

BOX 23-3   Dysphagia

Signs and Symptoms

- Avoids food that needs chewing.
- Avoids food with certain textures and temperatures.
- Tires during a meal.
- Has food spill out of the mouth while eating.
- "Pockets" or "squirrels" food in the cheeks. This means that food remains or is hidden in the mouth.
- Eats slowly, especially solid foods.
- Complains that food will not go down or that the food is stuck.
- Coughs or chokes before, during, or after swallowing.
- Regurgitates food after eating (p. 346).
- Spits out food suddenly and almost violently.
- Has food come up through the nose.
- Has hoarseness—especially after eating.
- Makes gurgling sounds while talking or breathing after swallowing.
- Has a runny nose, sneezes, or has excessive drooling.
- Complains of frequent heartburn.
- Has a decreased appetite.

Dysphagia Diet

- *Thickened liquid*—No lumps. Pureed with milk, gravy, or broth to thickness of baby food. Thickener is added to some foods and fluids as needed. Does not mound on a plate. May be called *creamy* or a *sauce*. Stir before serving if the food settles.
- *Medium thick (nectar-like)*—The thickness of nectar or V8 juice (does not hold its shape). Stir right before serving.
- *Extra thick (honey-like)*—Thick like honey. Mounds a bit on a spoon. Can drink from a cup. Stir before serving.
- *Yogurt-like*—Thick like yogurt or pudding. Holds its shape. Served with a spoon.
- *Puree*—No lumps; mounds on a plate. May be thick like mashed potatoes.

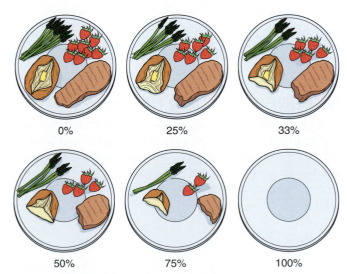

FIGURE 23-3 Percent of food eaten from the plate.

FOCUS ON MATH
Food Intake

To measure food intake, you need to understand percents. Percents measure parts of a whole (Fig. 23-4). The "whole" is written as 100%.

To measure food intake, compare the food left to that served. Depending on agency policy and the food type, *estimate* or *calculate* food intake. *To estimate*, record the approximate amount of food eaten. See Figure 23-3. *To calculate*:

1 Subtract the amount left from the amount served. (This is the amount the person ate.)
2 Divide the number from step 1 by the amount served (the number of pieces making up the whole).
3 Multiply the number from step 2 by 100 for a percent. (*Percent* means *out of 100*.)

For example, 8 apple slices were served; 2 remain on the tray.

$$8 \text{ slices} - 2 \text{ slices} = 6 \text{ slices}$$

The person ate 6 apple slices; 8 were served.

$$6 \text{ slices} \div 8 \text{ slices} = 0.75 \text{ of the slices served}$$

$$0.75 \times 100 = 75\%$$

75% of the apple slices were eaten.

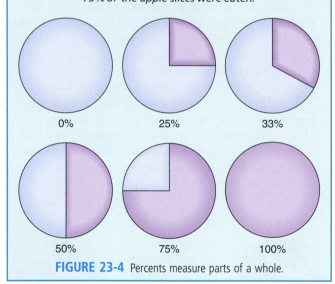

FIGURE 23-4 Percents measure parts of a whole.

MEETING NUTRITION NEEDS

Weakness, illness, and confusion can affect appetite and ability to eat. So can unpleasant odors, sights, and sounds. An uncomfortable position, oral hygiene needs, elimination needs, and pain also affect appetite.

See *Focus on Communication: Meeting Nutrition Needs.*

FOCUS ON COMMUNICATION
Meeting Nutrition Needs

The person may not eat everything served. You need to ask why and tell the nurse. You can say:
- "Please tell me why you didn't eat everything."
- "Was there something wrong with your food?"
- "Did your food taste okay?"
- "Was there something you didn't like?"
- "Was your food too hot or too cold?"
- "Would you like something else?"
- "Weren't you hungry?"

Preparing for Meals

Preparing patients and residents for meals promotes comfort. If they are ready to eat, you can serve meals faster. Foods stay at the correct temperature.

See *Delegation Guidelines: Preparing for Meals.*
See *Promoting Safety and Comfort: Preparing for Meals.*
See procedure: *Preparing the Person for a Meal.*

DELEGATION GUIDELINES
Preparing for Meals

To prepare a person for a meal, you need this information from the nurse and the care plan.
- How much help the person needs
- Where the person will eat—room or dining room
- What the person uses for elimination—toilet, commode, bedpan, urinal, or specimen pan
- What type of oral hygiene to give
- If the person wears dentures
- If the person wears eyeglasses or hearing aids
- How to position the person—in bed, a chair, or wheelchair
- How the person gets to the dining room—by self or with help
- If the person uses a wheelchair, walker, or cane
- When to report observations
- What patient or resident concerns to report at once

PROMOTING SAFETY AND COMFORT
Preparing for Meals

Safety
Before meals, the person needs to eliminate and have oral hygiene. Follow Standard Precautions and the Bloodborne Pathogen Standard (Chapter 13). Also follow them to clean equipment and the room.

Comfort
The meal setting must be free of unpleasant sights, sounds, and odors. If allowed, remove unpleasant equipment from the room.

Preparing the Person for a Meal

QUALITY OF LIFE

- Knock before entering the person's room.
- Address the person by name.
- Introduce yourself by name and title.

- Explain the procedure before starting and during the procedure.
- Protect the person's rights during the procedure.
- Handle the person gently during the procedure.

PRE-PROCEDURE

1 Follow *Delegation Guidelines: Preparing for Meals.* See *Promoting Safety and Comfort: Preparing for Meals.*
2 Practice hand hygiene.
3 Collect the following.
   - Equipment for oral hygiene (Chapter 18)
   - Bedpan and cover, urinal, commode, or specimen pan

- Toilet tissue
- Wash basin
- Soap
- Washcloth and towel
- Gloves

4 Provide for privacy.

PROCEDURE

5 Make sure eyeglasses and hearing aids are in place.
6 Assist with oral hygiene. Make sure dentures are in place. Wear gloves and practice hand hygiene after removing and discarding them.
7 Assist with elimination. Make sure the incontinent person is clean and dry. Wear gloves and practice hand hygiene after removing and discarding them.
8 Assist with hand-washing. Wear gloves and practice hand hygiene after removing and discarding them.
9 *If the person will sit in a chair:*
   a Position the person in a chair or wheelchair.
   b Remove items from the over-bed table. Clean the table.
   c Adjust the over-bed table in front of the person.

10 *For the person who eats in the dining room,* assist the person to the dining room.
11 *If the person will eat in bed:*
   a Raise the head of the bed to a comfortable position— Fowler's (45 to 60 degrees) or high-Fowler's (60 to 90 degrees). (Note: Some state competency tests require at least 45 degrees, others require 75 to 90 degrees.)
   b Remove items from the over-bed table. Clean the table.
   c Adjust the over-bed table in front of the person.

POST-PROCEDURE

12 Provide for comfort. (See the inside of the front cover.)
13 Place the call light and other needed items within reach.
14 Empty, clean, rinse, disinfect, and dry equipment. Use clean, dry paper towels for drying. Return equipment to its proper place. Wear gloves and practice hand hygiene after removing and discarding them.

15 Straighten the room. Eliminate unpleasant noise, odors, or equipment.
16 Unscreen the person.
17 Complete a safety check of the room. (See the inside of the front cover.)
18 Practice hand hygiene.

Dining Programs

The needs of nursing center residents vary. The following dining programs are common in nursing centers.

- *Social dining.* A table seats 4 to 6 residents (Fig. 23-5). Food is served as in a restaurant. Residents are oriented and can feed themselves.
- *Family dining.* Food is served in bowls and on platters. Residents serve and feed themselves as at home.
- *Low-stimulation dining.* Distractions are prevented. The health team decides where each person should sit.
- *Restaurant-style menus.* Food is selected from a menu to allow more food choices. The person is served as in a restaurant.
- *Open dining.* A buffet is open for several hours. Residents can eat any time while the buffet is open.

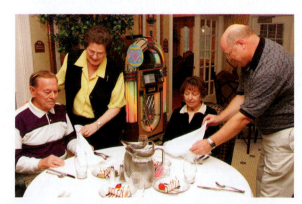

FIGURE 23-5 Residents eating in the dining room. Volunteers help as needed.

Serving Meals

Food is served in containers with covers that keep foods at the correct temperature. Hot food is kept hot. Cold food is kept cold. Uncover food just before the person eats. Uncovered food changes temperature quickly.

If food is not served within 15 minutes, re-check food temperatures. Follow agency policy. If not at the correct temperature, get fresh food. Temperature guides and food thermometers are in dining rooms and in nursing unit kitchens. Some agencies allow re-heating in microwave ovens.

See *Delegation Guidelines: Serving Meals.*
See *Promoting Safety and Comfort: Serving Meals.*
See procedure: *Serving Meal Trays.*

DELEGATION GUIDELINES
Serving Meals

To serve meal trays, you need this information from the nurse and the care plan.

- The person's food allergies (if any)
- What adaptive equipment (assistive devices) the person uses
- If the person needs help opening cartons, cutting food, buttering bread, and so on
- If the person's food intake (p. 339) and fluid intake (Chapter 24) are measured
- If calorie counts are done (p. 339)
- When to report observations
- What patient or resident concerns to report at once

PROMOTING SAFETY AND COMFORT
Serving Meals

Safety
Always check food temperature after re-heating. Food that is too hot can cause burns.

Comfort
Check the person's position when serving a meal. The position may have changed after the person was prepared to eat. Provide other comfort measures as needed. See the inside of the front cover.

Serving Meal Trays

QUALITY OF LIFE

- Knock before entering the person's room.
- Address the person by name.
- Introduce yourself by name and title.

- Explain the procedure before starting and during the procedure.
- Protect the person's rights during the procedure.
- Handle the person gently during the procedure.

PRE-PROCEDURE

1 Follow *Delegation Guidelines: Serving Meals.* See *Promoting Safety and Comfort: Serving Meals.*
2 Practice hand hygiene.

3 Prepare the person for the meal if not already done. See procedure: *Preparing the Person for a Meal,* p. 341.

PROCEDURE

4 Check items on the tray with the dietary card. Make sure the tray is complete and has adaptive equipment (assistive devices).
5 Identify the person. Check the ID (identification) bracelet against the dietary card. Use 2 identifiers (Chapter 10). Also call the person by name.
6 Place the tray within the person's reach. Adjust the over-bed table as needed.
7 Remove food covers. Open cartons, cut food into bite-sized pieces, butter bread, and so on as needed. Season food as the person prefers and the care plan allows.
8 Place the napkin, clothes protector, adaptive equipment (assistive devices), and eating utensils within reach. Help the person apply the clothes protector if needed.

9 Place the call light within reach.
10 Do the following when the person is done eating.
  a Measure and record fluid intake if ordered (Chapter 24).
  b Note the amount and type of foods eaten (p. 339).
  c Check for and remove any food in the mouth (pocketing). Wear gloves. Practice hand hygiene after removing and discarding them.
  d Remove the tray.
  e Clean spills. Change used linens and soiled clothing.
  f Help the person return to bed if needed.
  g Assist with oral hygiene and hand-washing. Wear gloves. Practice hand hygiene after removing and discarding the gloves.

POST-PROCEDURE

11 Provide for comfort. (See the inside of the front cover.)
12 Place the call light and other needed items within reach.
13 Raise or lower bed rails. Follow the care plan.
14 Complete a safety check of the room. (See the inside of the front cover.)

15 Follow agency policy for used linens.
16 Practice hand hygiene.
17 Report and record your observations.

Feeding the Person

Weakness, paralysis, casts, confusion, and other limits can make self-feeding impossible. These persons are fed.

Serve food and fluids in the order the person prefers. Offer fluids during the meal. Fluids help the person chew and swallow.

Use teaspoons to feed the person. They are less likely to cause injury than forks. The teaspoon should be only one-third (⅓) full. This portion is chewed and swallowed easily. Some people need smaller portions. Follow the care plan.

Persons who need to be fed are often angry, humiliated, and embarrassed. Some are depressed, resentful, or refuse to eat. Let them do what they can. Some can handle "finger foods" (bread, cookies, crackers). If strong enough, let them hold milk or juice cups (never hot drinks). Follow ordered activity limits. Provide support. Encourage them to try, even if food is spilled.

Visually impaired persons often recognize foods from their aromas. Describe what is on the tray and what you are offering. For persons who feed themselves, describe foods and fluids and their place on the tray. Use the numbers on a clock for the location of foods (Fig. 23-6).

Many people pray before eating. Allow time and privacy for prayer. This shows respect and caring.

Meals provide social contact with others. Engage the person in pleasant conversation. However, allow time to chew and swallow. Also, sit facing the person. Sitting is more relaxing. It shows that you have time for the person. By facing the person, you can see how well the person is eating. You can also see swallowing problems.

See *Focus on Older Persons: Feeding the Person.*
See *Focus on Surveys: Feeding the Person.*
See *Delegation Guidelines: Feeding the Person.*
See *Promoting Safety and Comfort: Feeding the Person,* p. 344.
See procedure: *Feeding the Person,* p. 344.

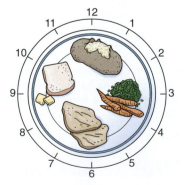

FIGURE 23-6 The numbers on a clock are used to help a visually impaired person locate food.

PROMOTING SAFETY AND COMFORT
Feeding the Person

Safety

Check food temperature. Very hot foods and fluids can burn the person.

Prevent aspiration. Check the person's mouth before offering more food or fluids. The person's mouth must be empty between bites and swallows.

Comfort

The person will eat better if not rushed. Sit to show that you have time. Standing communicates being in a hurry.

Wipe the person's hands, face, and mouth as needed during the meal. Use the napkin or a wet washcloth. Then dry the person with a towel.

Feeding the Person

QUALITY OF LIFE

- Knock before entering the person's room.
- Address the person by name.
- Introduce yourself by name and title.

- Explain the procedure before starting and during the procedure.
- Protect the person's rights during the procedure.
- Handle the person gently during the procedure.

PRE-PROCEDURE

1 Follow *Delegation Guidelines: Feeding the Person*, p. 343. See *Promoting Safety and Comfort: Feeding the Person.*
2 Practice hand hygiene.

3 Position the person in a comfortable position for eating—sitting in a chair or in Fowler's (45 to 60 degrees) or high-Fowler's (60 to 90 degrees). (NOTE: Some state competency tests require at least 45 degrees, others require 75 to 90 degrees.)
4 Get the tray. Place the tray on the over-bed table or dining table where the person can reach it.

PROCEDURE

5 Check items on the tray with the dietary card. Make sure the tray is complete.
6 Identify the person. Check the ID bracelet against the dietary card. Use 2 identifiers (Chapter 10). Also call the person by name.
7 Drape a napkin across the person's chest and underneath the chin. Or apply a clothes protector. Clean the person's hands with a hand wipe.
8 Tell the person what foods and fluids are on the tray.
9 Prepare food for eating. Cut food into bite-sized pieces. Season food as the person prefers and the care plan allows.
10 Place the chair where you can sit comfortably. Sit facing the person at eye level.
11 Serve foods in the order the person prefers. Identify foods as you serve them. Alternate between solid and liquid foods. Use a spoon for safety (Fig. 23-7). Allow enough time to chew and swallow. Do not rush the person. Also offer water, coffee, tea, or other fluids on the tray.
12 Check the person's mouth before offering more food or fluids. Make sure the mouth is empty between bites and swallows. Ask if the person is ready for the next bite or drink.

13 Use straws (if allowed) for liquids if the person cannot drink out of a glass or cup. Have 1 straw for each liquid. Provide short straws for weak persons. Follow the care plan for using straws.
14 Wipe the person's hands, face, and mouth as needed during the meal. Use the napkin or a hand wipe.
15 Follow the care plan if the person has dysphagia. (Some persons with dysphagia do not use straws.) Give thickened liquid with a spoon.
16 Talk with the person in a pleasant manner.
17 Encourage him or her to eat as much as possible.
18 Wipe the person's mouth with a napkin or a hand wipe. Discard the napkin or hand wipe.
19 Note how much and which foods were eaten (p. 339).
20 Measure and record fluid intake if ordered (Chapter 24).
21 Remove the tray.
22 Take the person to his or her room (if in a dining area).
23 Assist with oral hygiene and hand-washing. Provide for privacy. Wear gloves. Practice hand hygiene after removing and discarding gloves.

POST-PROCEDURE

24 Provide for comfort. (See the inside of the front cover.)
25 Place the call light and other needed items within reach.
26 Raise or lower bed rails. Follow the care plan.
27 Complete a safety check of the room. (See the inside of the front cover.)

28 Return the food tray to the food cart.
29 Practice hand hygiene.
30 Report and record your observations.

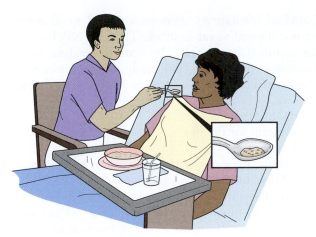

FIGURE 23-7 A spoon is used to feed the person. The spoon is one-third (⅓) full.

Between-Meal Snacks

Many special diets involve between-meal snacks. Snacks provide extra nutrients. Common snacks are crackers, milk, juice, a milk-shake, cake, wafers, a sandwich, gelatin, and custard.

Snacks are served upon arrival on the nursing unit. Provide needed utensils, a straw, and a napkin. Follow the same considerations and procedures for serving meals and feeding the person.

ASSISTING WITH SPECIAL NEEDS

Some persons cannot eat or drink because of chewing, swallowing, or other eating problems. Or food cannot pass from the mouth into the esophagus and into the stomach or small intestine. The doctor may order nutritional support to meet nutrition needs.

See *Delegation Guidelines: Assisting With Special Needs.*

DELEGATION GUIDELINES
Assisting With Special Needs

Your state and agency may not allow you to assist with some care measures or procedures involving nutritional support. Before assisting, make sure that:

- Your state allows you to perform the task.
- The task is in your job description.
- You have the necessary education and training.
- You know how to use the agency's equipment and supplies.
- You review the task in the agency's procedure manual.
- You review the task with the nurse.
- A nurse is available to answer questions and to supervise you.
- An RN (registered nurse) has identified and labeled all tubes, catheters, and needles.

Enteral Nutrition

Some persons require enteral nutrition. *Enteral nutrition is giving nutrients into the gastro-intestinal (GI) tract (enteral) through a feeding tube. Gavage is the process of giving a tube feeding* (Fig. 23-8).

These feeding tubes are common.

- *Naso-gastric (NG) tube.* A feeding tube is inserted through the nose *(naso)* into the stomach *(gastro)* (Fig. 23-9).
- *Gastrostomy tube.* A feeding tube is inserted through a surgically created opening *(stomy)* in the stomach *(gastro)* (Fig. 23-10).

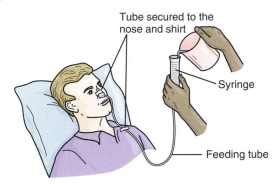

FIGURE 23-8 A tube feeding is given with a syringe.

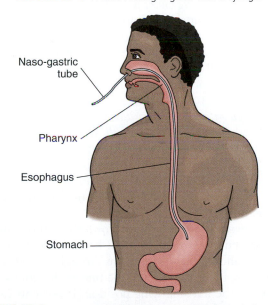

FIGURE 23-9 A naso-gastric (NG) tube is inserted through the nose and esophagus and into the stomach.

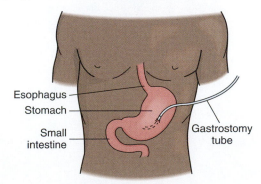

FIGURE 23-10 A gastrostomy tube.

Observations. Diarrhea, constipation, delayed stomach emptying, and aspiration are risks. Report the following at once.

- Nausea
- Discomfort during the feeding
- Vomiting
- Distended (enlarged and swollen) abdomen
- Coughing
- Complaints of indigestion or heartburn
- Redness, swelling, drainage, odor, or pain at the gastrostomy site
- Fever
- Signs and symptoms of respiratory distress (Chapter 30)
- Increased pulse rate
- Complaints of flatulence (Chapter 22)
- Diarrhea (Chapter 22)

Preventing Aspiration. Aspiration is a major risk from tube feedings. It can cause pneumonia and death. Aspiration can occur:

- *During insertion.* An NG tube can slip into the airway. An x-ray is taken after insertion to check tube placement.
- *From a tube moving out of place.* Coughing, sneezing, vomiting, suctioning, and poor positioning are common causes. A tube can move from the stomach or intestines into the esophagus and then into the airway. The RN (registered nurse) checks tube placement before a feeding. *You never check feeding tube placement.*
- *From regurgitation.* **Regurgitation** *is the backward flow of stomach contents into the mouth.* Delayed stomach emptying and over-feeding are common causes. To help prevent regurgitation and aspiration:
  - Position the person in Fowler's or semi-Fowler's position for the feeding. Follow the care plan and the nurse's directions.
  - Maintain Fowler's or semi-Fowler's position after the feeding. Do so for 1 to 2 hours or at all times. This allows formula to move through the GI tract. Follow the care plan and the nurse's directions.
  - Avoid the left side-lying position. It prevents the stomach from emptying into the small intestine.

Comfort Measures. Persons with feeding tubes usually are not allowed to eat or drink. They are NPO—nothing per mouth (Chapter 24). Dry mouth, dry lips, and sore throat cause discomfort. Hard candy or gum may be allowed. These measures are common every 2 hours while the person is awake.

- Oral hygiene
- Lubricant for the lips
- Mouth rinses

Feeding tubes can irritate and cause pressure on the nose. These measures are common.

- Clean the nose and nostrils every 4 to 8 hours.
- Secure the tube to the nose (Fig. 23-11). Use tape or a tube holder. Tube holders have foam cushions that prevent pressure on the nose. Re-taping is not needed. Re-taping irritates the nose.
- Secure the tube to the person's garment at the shoulder area (see Fig. 23-8). Do 1 of the following according to agency policy.
  - Loop a rubber band around the tube. Then pin the rubber band to the garment with a safety pin.
  - Tape the tube to the garment.

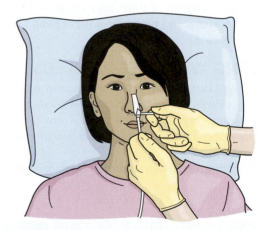

FIGURE 23-11 The feeding tube is secured to the nose.

FOCUS ON P R I D E

The Person, Family, and Yourself

Personal and Professional Responsibility

Many agencies serve food in new ways. For example:

- *24-hour catering*. Meals and snacks are served 24 hours a day. The person chooses when to eat. Food is ordered from the food service department. Food choices must be allowed on the person's ordered diet.
- *Mobile food carts*. Food service staff bring a food cart to the nursing unit. The person selects food and a tray is prepared.

With such systems, you have new responsibilities. You may serve food trays more often. Or you may read and fill out menus. Take pride in helping others meet their nutritional needs.

Rights and Respect

Cultural, social, religious, medical, and personal factors affect food choices throughout life. These do not change when in a hospital or nursing center. People often comment about food likes and dislikes. A person may say that the food is cold, bland, or tastes bad.

People have the right to express what they prefer. Do not get angry or upset. The person should not feel as if he or she is complaining or being picky. Learning the person's likes and dislikes can improve nutrition. It also shows interest and concern for the person.

Independence and Social Interaction

Meals provide a time for social contact. A friendly, social setting is important. Some nursing centers have areas for residents to dine with guests. They can enjoy holidays, birthdays, anniversaries, and other events. Food is provided by guests or the dietary department.

Families and friends may bring food from home. This helps meet love and belonging needs. The person usually enjoys home-made food. Tell the nurse when the person receives food. The food must not interfere with the person's diet.

Delegation and Teamwork

Some agencies deliver trays in meal carts. Trays are served in the order that they are slotted in the cart. The entire nursing team serves trays. The team works together to serve food promptly.

Ethics and Laws

Each person is different. For example, a person with an NG tube sits upright after a tube feeding. Lowering the head of the bed may cause aspiration. Or a person has a food allergy or special diet. You must know what the person can and cannot have.

You must protect the person from harm. If not, legal action can be taken. You can lose your ability to work as a nursing assistant. Know each person's needs and special care measures. If unsure, ask the nurse.

FOCUS ON PRIDE: *Application*

Meal time should be as pleasant as possible. How do sights, sounds, smells, and personal preferences affect meal time? How can you help make it pleasant?

Circle the BEST answer.

1 Nutrition is
   a Fats, proteins, carbohydrates, vitamins, and minerals
   b The processes involved in the ingestion, digestion, absorption, and use of food and fluids by the body
   c The MyPlate food guidance system
   d The balance between calories taken in and used by the body

2 MyPlate encourages
   a The same diet for everyone
   b Eating less
   c Increasing the amount of high-sodium foods
   d Eating more refined grains

3 What is the amount of grains needed daily for an adult woman?
   a 1 oz
   b 2 to 2½ oz
   c 3 oz
   d 5 to 6 oz

4 Which would meet an adult male's daily dairy needs?
   a 1 slice of bread, 1 cup of cheese, and ½ oz of nuts
   b 2 cups of milk and 1 cup of cooked rice
   c 1 cup of milk, 1 cup of yogurt, and 1½ oz of cheese
   d 2 tablespoons of peanut butter and 1 egg

5 Which food group contains the *most* cholesterol?
   a Grains
   b Vegetables
   c Fruit
   d Protein foods

6 These statements are about oils. Which is *true?*
   a The best oil choices come from fish, nuts, and vegetable oils.
   b Oils are low in calories.
   c Oils from plant sources contain cholesterol.
   d Oils are a food group.

7 Protein is needed for
   a Tissue growth and repair
   b Energy and the fiber for bowel elimination
   c Body heat and to protect organs from injury
   d Improving the taste of food

8 Which foods provide the *most* protein?
   a Butter and cream
   b Tomatoes and potatoes
   c Meats and fish
   d Corn and lettuce

9 The sodium-controlled diet involves
   a Omitting high-sodium foods
   b Adding salt to food at the table
   c Using 3000 mg of salt in cooking
   d A sodium-intake flow sheet

10 Diabetes meal planning involves
   a Changing the thickness of foods
   b Varying the amount of carbohydrates each day
   c Controlling sodium
   d Eating at regular times

11 Which does OBRA require?
   a 2 meals a day and a bedtime snack
   b Serving food promptly
   c Serving food at room temperature to avoid burns
   d A sodium-controlled diet

12 A resident eats half of the food on the meal tray. Food intake for this meal is
   a 25%
   b 33%
   c 50%
   d 75%

13 Persons with dysphagia
   a Use straws for all liquids
   b Have a regular diet
   c Are fed according to the care plan
   d Eat alone in their rooms

14 A person coughs and drools while eating. You should
   a Give the person a drink
   b Puree the person's food
   c Give mouth care and continue feeding
   d Tell the nurse

15 When feeding a person
   a Ask in what order the person likes foods served
   b Use a fork
   c Stand facing the person
   d Talk with your co-workers

16 Which position prevents regurgitation after a tube feeding?
   a Fowler's or semi-Fowler's position
   b The supine position
   c The left or right side-lying position
   d The prone position

17 A person with a feeding tube is NPO. Which should you question?
   a Provide oral hygiene.
   b Provide mouth rinses.
   c Give clear liquids.
   d Apply lubricant to the lips.

18 A person has an NG tube. To prevent nasal irritation
   a Clean the tube every 4 to 8 hours
   b Replace the tape on the nose every 4 hours
   c Remove the tube every 4 hours
   d Secure the tube to the person's gown

Answers to Chapter 23 questions are on p. 552.

FOCUS ON PRACTICE

Problem Solving

After receiving a breakfast tray, a resident says: "I didn't ask for eggs this morning." You check the dietary card and notice the tray is for another person. What will you do? Why is this a problem?

Fluid Needs

OBJECTIVES

- Define the key terms and key abbreviations in this chapter.
- Describe adult fluid requirements.
- Identify the causes and signs and symptoms of dehydration.
- Explain how to assist with special fluid orders.
- Explain the purpose of intake and output records.
- Identify what to count as fluid intake and output.

- Explain how to assist with fluid needs.
- Explain how to provide drinking water.
- Explain how to assist with IV therapy.
- Perform the procedures described in this chapter.
- Explain how to promote PRIDE in the person, the family, and yourself.

KEY TERMS

dehydration A decrease in the amount of water in body tissues
edema The swelling of body tissues with water
flow rate The number of drops per minute (gtt/min) or milliliters per hour (mL/hr)
graduate A measuring container for fluid

hydration Having an adequate amount of water in body tissues
intake The amount of fluid taken in; input
intravenous (IV) therapy Giving fluids through a needle or catheter inserted into a vein; IV and IV infusion
output The amount of fluid lost

KEY ABBREVIATIONS

gtt	Drops		mL	Milliliter
gtt/min	Drops per minute		mL/hr	Milliliters per hour
I&O	Intake and output		NPO	*Non per os;* nothing per mouth; nothing by mouth
IV	Intravenous		oz	Ounce

Water is needed to live. Water is ingested through fluids and foods. Water is lost through urine, feces, and vomit. It is also lost through the skin (perspiration) and the lungs (expiration).

Fluid balance is needed for health. Fluid balance involves these terms.

- *Hydration means having an adequate amount of water in body tissues.*
- *Intake (input) is the amount of fluid taken in.*
- *Output is the amount of fluid lost.*
- *Edema is the swelling of body tissues with water.*
- *Dehydration is a decrease in the amount of water in body tissues.*

Death can result from too much or too little water. To stay hydrated, intake must roughly equal output. Edema occurs when fluid intake exceeds fluid output. Edema is common in people with heart and kidney diseases.

Dehydration occurs when output exceeds intake. Common causes and signs and symptoms of dehydration are listed in Box 24-1, p. 350.

You will help meet fluid needs. Measuring intake and output and providing drinking water are examples.

NOTE: A task may require more than 1 pair of gloves. Change gloves as needed. Use careful judgment. Remember to practice hand hygiene after removing gloves.

NORMAL FLUID REQUIREMENTS

An adult needs 1500 mL (milliliters) of water daily to survive. About 2000 to 2500 mL are needed for normal fluid balance. Water requirements increase with hot weather, exercise, fever, illness, and excess fluid losses.

See *Focus on Older Persons: Normal Fluid Requirements,* p. 350.

BOX 24-1	Dehydration

Common Causes
- Bleeding
- Coma
- Dementia
- Diarrhea
- Drug therapy
- Fever
- Fluid intake: poor
- Fluid restriction
- Fluids: refusing
- Function problems: difficulty drinking, reaching fluids, communicating fluid needs
- Sweating: excess
- Urine production: increased
- Vomiting

Signs and Symptoms
- Blood pressure: low
- Confusion, delirium (Chapter 35)
- Dark yellow or amber colored urine
- Dizziness, feeling light-headed
- Dry, cool skin
- Dry mouth, coated tongue
- Fatigue
- Headache
- Irritability
- Muscle cramps
- *Oliguria* (Chapter 20)—scant amount of urine
- Orthostatic hypotension (Chapter 27)
- Poor *skin turgor*—when pinched and released, skin slowly returns to its normal position
- Pulse: fast
- Respirations: fast
- Shock (Chapter 36)
- Thirst
- Unconsciousness

FOCUS ON OLDER PERSONS

Normal Fluid Requirements

The amount of body water decreases with age. So does the thirst sensation. Older persons need water but may not feel thirsty. Offer water often.

Older persons are at risk for diseases affecting fluid balance. Dehydration and edema are risks. Some persons have special fluid orders.

SPECIAL FLUID ORDERS

The doctor may order the amount of fluid a person can have during 24 hours. This is done for fluid balance. Intake and output (I&O) records are kept. Common fluid orders are:

- *Encourage fluids.* The person drinks an increased amount of fluid. The order states the amount. Keep a variety of fluids within the person's reach. Offer fluids often to persons who cannot feed themselves.
- *Restrict fluids.* Fluids are limited to a certain amount. Offer fluids in small amounts and in small containers. Remove the water mug from the room or keep it out of sight. Frequent oral hygiene keeps the mouth moist.
- *Nothing per mouth.* The person cannot eat or drink anything. *NPO* stands for *non per os*— nothing (*non*) by (*per*) mouth (*os*). NPO is ordered before and after surgery, before some laboratory tests and diagnostic procedures, and to treat certain illnesses. An NPO sign is posted above the bed. The water mug is removed. Frequent oral hygiene is needed but the person must not swallow fluid. The person is NPO for 6 to 12 hours before surgery and before some laboratory tests and diagnostic procedures. Follow agency policy.
- *Thickened liquids.* Water and all fluids are thickened. The thickness depends on the person's ability to swallow (see Chapter 23). Thickener is added before serving fluids or thickened commercial fluids are used.

INTAKE AND OUTPUT

You will measure and record intake and output (I&O).
- *Intake.* All oral fluids are measured and recorded— water, milk, coffee, tea, juices, soups, and soft drinks. So are foods that melt at room temperature—ice cream, sherbet, custard, gelatin, and Popsicles. The nurse measures and records intravenous (IV) fluids (p. 355) and tube feedings (Chapter 23).
- *Output.* Urine, vomitus, diarrhea, and wound drainage amounts are measured and recorded.

Intake and output are measured in milliliters (mL). See Box 24-2 for amounts to know.

BOX 24-2	I&O Measures

1 cubic centimeter (cc) = 1 mL
1 teaspoon = 5 mL
1 tablespoon = 15 mL
1 oz = 30 mL
1 cup = 240 mL
1 pint = about 500 mL
1 quart = about 1000 mL
1 liter (L) = 1000 mL

Measuring Intake and Output

I&O records are used to plan and evaluate medical treatment (Fig. 24-1). They also are kept when the person has special fluid orders.

You must know the serving sizes of bowls, dishes, cups, pitchers, mugs, glasses, and other containers. This information may be on the I&O record. Or the serving size is on the container.

A measuring container for fluid is called a **graduate**. You use it to measure left-over fluids and urine, vomitus, and drainage from suction. Like a measuring cup, the graduate is marked in ounces (oz) and milliliters. Separate graduates are used for intake and for output. For an accurate measurement, place the device on a flat surface and read it at eye level (Fig. 24-2, p. 352).

When intake or output is measured, the amount is recorded in the correct column on the I&O record (see Fig. 24-1). Amounts are totaled at the end of the shift and 24-hour day. The totals are recorded in the person's chart.

The urinal, commode, bedpan, or specimen pan (Chapter 26) is used to void. Remind the person not to void in the toilet. Also remind the person to put toilet tissue into the wastebasket.

See *Focus on Math: Measuring Intake and Output*, p. 352.
See *Delegation Guidelines: Measuring Intake and Output*, p. 353.
See *Promoting Safety and Comfort: Measuring Intake and Output*, p. 353.
See procedure: *Measuring Intake and Output*, p. 353.

Text continued on p. 354.

FLUID INTAKE AND OUTPUT FLOW SHEET
DATE Oct 12

RECORD TOTALS IN PATIENT'S MEDICAL RECORD		DIET/FLUID ORDERS Regular	
Water glass	240 mL	Gelatin	120 mL
Juice glass	120 mL	Ice cream	90 mL
Milk carton	240 mL	Broth/strained soup	180 mL
Coffee cup	240 mL	Styrofoam cup	180 mL
Soft drink can	360 mL	Water mug	1000 mL
Tea glass	180 mL	Ice chips	½ amount of mL in cup

		INTAKE				OUTPUT		
	SHIFT	ORAL	TIME	IV	ENTERAL	TIME	SOURCE	AMOUNT
2300-0700	FLUIDS					2330	Void	225 mL
						0545	Void	325 mL
	MUG/OTHER	Water 200 mL						
	8-HOUR SUB-TOTAL				200 mL	**8-HOUR SUB-TOTAL**		550 mL
0700-1500	BREAKFAST	Coffee 240 mL				0750	Void	200 mL
		Milk 160 mL				0930	Void	225 mL
						1145	Void	250 mL
						1330	Void	200 mL
	SNACK	Juice 120 mL						
	LUNCH	Soft drink 240 mL						
		Ice cream 90 mL						
		Soup 90 mL						
	SNACK	Gelatin 120 mL						
	MUG/OTHER	Water 300 mL						
	8-HOUR SUB-TOTAL				1360 mL	**8-HOUR SUB-TOTAL**		875 mL
1500-2300	DINNER	Tea 180 mL				1505	Void	275 mL
		Soft drink 100 mL				1655	Void	150 mL
						2010	Void	150 mL
						2115	Vomitus	100 mL
	SNACK							
	MUG/OTHER	Water 325 mL						
	8-HOUR SUB-TOTAL		605 mL			**8-HOUR SUB-TOTAL**		675 mL
	24-HOUR TOTAL		2165 mL			**24-HOUR TOTAL**		2100 mL

FIGURE 24-1 A sample intake and output (I&O) record.

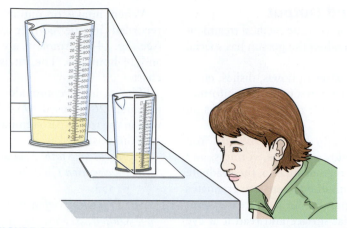

FIGURE 24-2 A graduate is on a flat surface. The amount is read at eye level.

FOCUS ON MATH
Measuring Intake and Output

To measure I&O, you must accurately read measurements. You may have to do some math.

Measuring Intake

To measure intake, subtract the amount left in each liquid served from the full serving amount. For total intake, add the intake amounts from each liquid together.

Intake is measured in mL (milliliters). Some containers show the serving amount in oz (ounces). You need to convert (change) the serving amount from oz to mL. One oz equals 30 mL (1 oz = 30 mL). To convert, multiply the number of oz by 30. For example:

A coffee cup holds 8 oz. Multiply 8 oz by 30 (the number of mL in each oz). The full serving amount is 240 mL.

$$8\ oz \times 30\ mL/oz = 240\ mL$$
(mL/oz is read as "milliliters per ounce")

You measure 90 mL left in the cup. Subtract 90 mL (amount left) from 240 mL (serving amount). The person drank 150 mL.

$$240\ mL\ (full\ serving) - 90\ mL\ (amount\ left) = 150\ mL\ intake$$

Measuring Output

Measuring containers are marked in oz and mL. Urinals and specimen pans used to measure output may not have all lines labeled. To calculate unlabeled measurements (Fig. 24-3):

1   Choose the labeled line above the fluid level and the labeled line below it.

400 mL and 300 mL

2   Subtract these 2 numbers. The result is called the *difference.*

400 mL − 300 mL = 100 mL

3   Count the number of spaces between the 2 labeled lines in step 1.

4 spaces

4   Divide the difference in step 2 by the number of spaces.

100 mL ÷ 4 spaces = 25 mL
Each line increases by 25 mL.

Totaling Intake and Output

Intake and output amounts are each totaled at the end of the shift and 24-hour day. See Figure 24-1. Add the amounts for intake and the amounts for output. For example:

- Total 24-hour intake amount: *A person had 125 mL during the first shift, 1100 mL during the second shift, and 600 mL during the third shift. The total 24-hour day intake amount is 1825 mL.*

$$125\ mL + 1100\ mL + 600\ mL = 1825\ mL$$

- Total shift output amount: *A person voided 3 times during your shift—200 mL, 250 mL, and 100 mL. The total output for your shift is 550 mL.*

$$200\ mL + 250\ mL + 100\ mL = 550\ mL$$

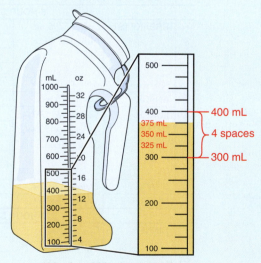

400 mL − 300 mL = 100 mL
100 mL ÷ 4 = 25 mL
Each line increases by 25 mL.

FIGURE 24-3 Calculating unlabeled measurements. Divide the difference between 2 labeled lines by the number of spaces between the 2 lines. For example, each line on the urinal increases by 25 mL. The measurements between 300 mL and 400 mL are 325 mL, 350 mL, and 375 mL.

DELEGATION GUIDELINES
Measuring Intake and Output

When measuring I&O, you need this information from the nurse and the care plan.

- If the person has a special fluid order (p. 350)
- When to report measurements—hourly or end-of-shift
- What the person uses for voiding—urinal, bedpan, commode, or specimen pan (Chapters 20 and 26)
- If the person has a catheter (Chapter 21)
- What patient or resident concerns to report at once

PROMOTING SAFETY AND COMFORT
Measuring Intake and Output

Safety
Urine, vomitus, feces, and wound drainage may contain microbes and blood. Microbes can grow in urinals, commodes, bedpans, specimen pans, kidney basins, and drainage systems. Follow Standard Precautions and the Bloodborne Pathogen Standard. Thoroughly clean the item with a disinfectant after it is used.

Remember to use separate graduates for intake and output.

Comfort
Promptly measure the contents of urinals, bedpans, commodes, specimen pans, and kidney basins. This helps prevent or reduce odors. Odors can disturb the person.

Measuring Intake and Output

QUALITY OF LIFE

- Knock before entering the person's room.
- Address the person by name.
- Introduce yourself by name and title.
- Explain the procedure before starting and during the procedure.
- Protect the person's rights during the procedure.
- Handle the person gently during the procedure.

PRE-PROCEDURE

1 Follow *Delegation Guidelines: Measuring Intake and Output.* See *Promoting Safety and Comfort: Measuring Intake and Output.*
2 Practice hand hygiene.

3 Collect the following.
- I&O record
- 2 graduates:
  - For intake
  - For output
- Gloves
- Paper towels

PROCEDURE

4 Put on gloves.
5 Measure intake.
  a Pour liquid remaining in the container into the graduate used to measure intake. Avoid spills and splashes on the outside of the graduate.
  b Place the graduate on a flat surface. Measure the amount at eye level (see Fig. 24-2).
  c Check the serving amount on the I&O record. Or check the serving size of each container.
  d Subtract the remaining amount from the full serving amount. Note the amount. (For example, a cup holds 240 mL. The amount in the graduate is 50 mL. 240 mL – 50 mL = 190 mL.)
  e Pour fluid in the graduate back into the container.
  f Repeat steps 5, a–e for each liquid.
  g Add the amounts from each liquid together.
  h Record the time and amount on the I&O record.

6 Measure output.
  a Pour the fluid into the graduate used to measure output. Avoid spills and splashes on the outside of the graduate.
  b Place the device on a paper towel on a flat surface. Measure the amount at eye level.
  c Dispose of fluid in the toilet. Avoid splashes.
7 Clean, rinse, disinfect, and dry the graduates. Dispose of rinse in the toilet and flush. Use clean, dry paper towels for drying. Return the graduates to their proper place.
8 Clean, rinse, disinfect, and dry the voiding receptacle or drainage container. Dispose of rinse in the toilet and flush. Use clean, dry paper towels for drying. Return the item to its proper place.
9 Remove and discard the gloves. Practice hand hygiene.
10 Record the output amount on the person's I&O record.

POST-PROCEDURE

11 Provide for comfort. (See the inside of the front cover.)
12 Place the call light and other needed items within reach.

13 Complete a safety check of the room. (See the inside of the front cover.)
14 Report and record your observations.

PROVIDING DRINKING WATER

You provide fresh drinking water each shift and when the water mug is empty (Fig. 24-4).

Some agencies do not use the following procedure. Each mug is filled as needed. You take the mug to an ice and water dispenser. Fill the mug with ice first. Then add water. Follow the agency's procedure for providing fresh drinking water.

See *Focus on Communication: Providing Drinking Water.*
See *Delegation Guidelines: Providing Drinking Water.*
See *Promoting Safety and Comfort: Providing Drinking Water.*
See procedure: *Providing Drinking Water.*

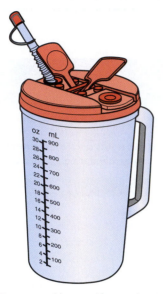

FIGURE 24-4 Water mug with straw. The mug is marked in milliliters (mL) and ounces (oz).

FOCUS ON COMMUNICATION

Providing Drinking Water

People vary about ice in their water. Ask what the person prefers. You can say:
- "Do you want ice in your water?"
- "How much ice do you want in your water?"
- "Do you like more ice or more water?"
  Also ask where to place the mug. Be sure the person can reach it.

DELEGATION GUIDELINES

Providing Drinking Water

To provide drinking water, you need this information from the nurse and the care plan.
- The person's fluid orders
- If the person can have ice
- If the person uses a straw

PROMOTING SAFETY AND COMFORT

Providing Drinking Water

Safety
Water mugs can spread microbes. To prevent the spread of microbes:
- Label the mug with the person's name and room and bed number.
- Do not touch the rim or inside of the mug or lid.
- Do not let the ice scoop touch the mug, lid, or straw.
- Place the ice scoop in the scoop holder or on a towel for the scoop. Do not place it in the ice container or dispenser.
- Keep the ice chest closed when not in use.
- Make sure the mug is clean. Also check for cracks and chips. Provide a new mug as needed.

Providing Drinking Water

QUALITY OF LIFE

- Knock before entering the person's room.
- Address the person by name.
- Introduce yourself by name and title.

- Explain the procedure before starting and during the procedure.
- Protect the person's rights during the procedure.
- Handle the person gently during the procedure.

PRE-PROCEDURE

1 Follow *Delegation Guidelines: Providing Drinking Water.* See *Promoting Safety and Comfort: Providing Drinking Water.*
2 Obtain a list of special fluid orders from the nurse. Or use your assignment sheet.
3 Practice hand hygiene.
4 Collect the following.
   - Cart
   - Ice chest filled with ice

- Cover for the ice chest
- Scoop
- Paper towels
- Water mugs
- Water pitcher filled with cold water (optional depending on agency procedure)
- Towel for the scoop
5 Cover the cart with paper towels. Arrange equipment on top of the paper towels.

Providing Drinking Water—cont'd

PROCEDURE

6 Take the cart to the person's room door. Do not take the cart into the room.

7 Check the person's fluid orders. Use the list from the nurse or your assignment sheet.

8 Identify the person. Check the identification (ID) bracelet against the fluid orders sheet or your assignment sheet. Use 2 identifiers (Chapter 10). Also call the person by name.

9 Take the mug from the over-bed table. Empty it into the bathroom sink.

10 Determine if a new mug is needed.

11 Use the scoop to fill the mug with ice (Fig. 24-5). Do not let the scoop touch the mug, lid, or straw.

12 Place the ice scoop on the towel.

13 Fill the mug with water. Get water from the room sink or bathroom sink or the water pitcher on the cart.

14 Place the mug on the over-bed table.

15 Make sure the mug is within the person's reach.

POST-PROCEDURE

16 Provide for comfort. (See the inside of the front cover.)

17 Place the call light and other needed items within reach.

18 Complete a safety check of the room. (See the inside of the front cover.)

19 Practice hand hygiene.

20 Repeats steps 6 through 19 for each person.

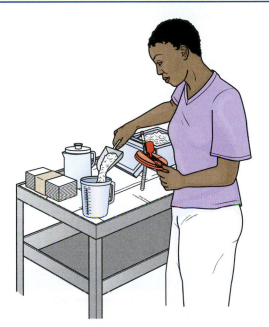

FIGURE 24-5 Providing drinking water.

IV THERAPY

Intravenous (IV) therapy (IV, IV infusion) is giving fluids through a needle or catheter inserted into a vein. See Figure 24-6 for the basic equipment used.

- The solution container is a plastic bag—*IV bag*.
- A *catheter* or *needle* is inserted into a vein (see Fig. 24-6).
- The *IV tube* or *infusion tubing* connects the IV bag to the catheter or needle.
  - Fluid drips from the bag into the *drip chamber*.
  - The *clamp* is used to regulate the flow rate.
- The IV bag hangs from an IV pole (IV standard) or ceiling hook.

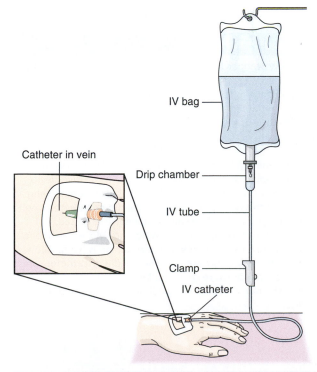

FIGURE 24-6 Equipment for IV therapy.

Flow Rate

The doctor orders the amount of fluid to give (*infuse*) and the amount of time to give it in. With this information, the RN (registered nurse) figures the flow rate. The *flow rate is the number of drops per minute (gtt/min) or milliliters per hour (mL/hr)*. The abbreviation *gtt* means *drops*. The Latin word *guttae* means *drops*.

The RN sets the clamp for the flow rate. An electronic pump is often used. The flow rate is displayed in mL/hr. An alarm sounds if something is wrong. Tell the nurse at once if you hear an alarm. *Never change the position of the clamp or adjust any controls on IV pumps.*

You can check the flow rate if a pump is not used. The RN tells you the number of drops per minute (gtt/min). To check the flow rate, count the number of drops in 1 minute (Fig. 24-7). Tell the RN at once if:

- No fluid is dripping.
- The rate is too fast.
- The rate is too slow.
- The bag is empty or close to being empty.
  See *Promoting Safety and Comfort: Flow Rate.*

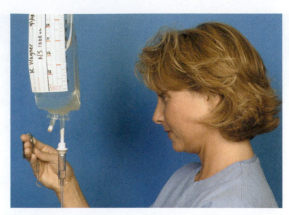

FIGURE 24-7 The flow rate is checked by counting the number of drops per minute.

Assisting With IV Therapy

You help meet the safety, hygiene, and activity needs of persons with IVs. Follow the safety measures in Box 24-3. Report any sign or symptom listed in Box 24-3 at once.

You never start or maintain IV therapy. Nor do you regulate the flow rate or change IV bags. You never give blood or IV drugs.

See *Focus on Communication: Assisting With IV Therapy.*

PROMOTING SAFETY AND COMFORT
Flow Rate

Safety

The person can suffer serious harm if the flow rate is too fast or too slow. The flow rate can change from:
- Position changes
- Kinked tubes
- Lying on the tube

Never change the position of the clamp or adjust any controls on infusion pumps. Tell the nurse at once about a problem with the flow rate.

BOX 24-3   IV Therapy

- Follow Standard Precautions and the Bloodborne Pathogen Standard.
- Do not move the needle or catheter. Correct position must be maintained. If the needle or catheter is moved, it may come out of the vein. Then fluid flows into tissues (*infiltration*). Or the flow stops.
- Follow the safety measures for restraints (Chapter 12). The nurse may splint or restrain the extremity to prevent movement. Or the nurse may apply a protective device. This helps prevent the needle or catheter from moving.
- Protect the IV bag, tubing, and needle or catheter when the person walks. Portable IV standards are used.
- Assist with turning and re-positioning. Move the IV bag to the side of the bed on which the person is lying. Allow enough slack in the tubing. The needle or catheter can move from pressure on the tube.
- Tell the nurse at once if bleeding occurs at the insertion site.

- Report signs and symptoms of IV therapy complications. Report the following at once.
  - Local—at the IV site
    - Bleeding
    - Blood backing up into the IV tube
    - Puffiness or swelling
    - Pale or reddened skin
    - Complaints of pain at or above the IV site
    - Hot or cold skin near the site
  - Systemic—involving the whole body
    - *Fever* (elevated body temperature)
    - Itching
    - Drop in blood pressure
    - Pulse rate greater than 100 beats per minute
    - Irregular pulse
    - *Cyanosis* (bluish color)
    - Confusion or changes in mental function
    - Loss of consciousness
    - Difficulty breathing or shortness of breath
    - Decreasing or no urine output
    - Chest pain
    - Nausea

FOCUS ON COMMUNICATION

Assisting With IV Therapy

Arm position is important during IV therapy. You may need to remind the person:

- To position the arm a certain way
- About position limits

    For example, IV tubing is kinked from a bent arm. The fluid flow stops. You can say: "Please keep your arm straight. The fluid will not flow through your IV when your arm is bent."

FOCUS ON P R I D E

The Person, Family, and Yourself

Personal and Professional Responsibility

Being attentive is a valuable quality for nursing assistants. When *attentive*, you are careful, alert, exact, and thorough. You meet the person's needs. You report problems at once.

These qualities are important when assisting with fluid needs. Special fluid orders and IV therapy maintain fluid balance. I&O measurements affect treatment decisions. Your observations, measurements, and care affect health and well-being. How you do your job matters.

Rights and Respect

Patients and residents may complain about orders and treatments. For example:

- A resident complains about thickened liquids.
- A patient who is NPO complains of thirst.
- A resident has an order to encourage fluids. The resident is tired of being reminded to drink.

Do not ignore complaints. They communicate needs. Listen and show respect. Do what you can to meet the need within the limits of the person's orders. Ask the nurse if you do not know how to help.

Independence and Social Interaction

IV therapy can affect independence. An IV in the arm can limit hand and arm movement. You may need to assist with hygiene, grooming, food and fluid, or activity needs. If the person can have oral fluids, make sure the water mug is within reach. Provide a variety of fluids as allowed. Assist only to the extent necessary. The person should do as much as safely possible.

Delegation and Teamwork

Before any task, you must know how to protect IVs. For example:

- A person with an IV needs a shower. The IV site must remain clean and dry. The nurse may have you apply a plastic bag, plastic wrap, or glove. Follow the nurse's instructions.
- A person receiving IV therapy needs to move from the bed to the chair. You must plan the move to avoid pulling on the IV site.

Ethics and Laws

When you hear an IV pump alarm, tell the nurse. Do so even if not assigned to the person. You do not adjust controls on IV pumps or clamps on IV tubing.

Know the limits of your role. If asked to do something outside those limits, politely refuse and explain why. Performing tasks outside the limits of your role can harm the person. Legal action can be taken. You can lose your ability to work as a nursing assistant.

FOCUS ON PRIDE: *Application*

A person restricted to 1000 mL in 24 hours complains of thirst. How can you meet the person's needs?

Circle the BEST answer.

1 For normal fluid balance, an adult requires
   a 500 to 1000 mL daily
   b 1500 mL daily
   c 2000 to 2500 mL daily
   d 5000 mL daily

2 A person is NPO. You should
   a Provide a variety of fluids
   b Remove the water mug from the room
   c Offer fluids in small amounts and in small containers
   d Remove oral hygiene equipment from the room

3 A person with diarrhea has scant, dark yellow urine. This is a sign of
   a Normal hydration
   b Edema
   c Infection
   d Dehydration

4 Which are counted as fluid intake?
   a Broths and ice cream
   b Sauces and melted cheese
   c Thick stews and mashed potatoes
   d Butter and syrup

5 A person drank all of an 8-oz carton of milk. How many mL of fluid would you chart on the I&O record?
   a 8 mL
   b 60 mL
   c 120 mL
   d 240 mL

6 A person was served 240 mL of coffee and 120 mL of juice. You measure 50 mL of coffee and 60 mL of juice left. What do you chart for intake on the I&O record?
   a 110 mL
   b 250 mL
   c 370 mL
   d 480 mL

7 When measuring intake and output
   a Convert measurements to ounces
   b Use the same graduate for intake and output
   c Place the graduate on a flat surface and read it at eye level
   d Gloves are not needed

8 During your shift a patient vomited twice—125 mL and 75 mL. The patient had diarrhea once—50 mL. You empty 500 mL from the urine drainage bag. What is the total shift output amount?
   a 200 mL
   b 250 mL
   c 500 mL
   d 750 mL

9 Before providing fresh drinking water, you need to know the person's
   a Intake
   b Fluid orders
   c Diet
   d Preferred beverages

10 Which prevents contamination when passing drinking water?
   a Labeling the mug with the person's name
   b Keeping the ice chest open when not in use
   c Leaving the ice scoop in the ice container
   d Touching the mug with the ice scoop

11 What is the *correct* way to check an IV flow rate?
   a Count the drops in 30 seconds. Multiply the number by 2.
   b Count the drops for 1 minute.
   c Check if the fluid is dripping.
   d Measure the amount of fluid.

12 The IV flow rate is
   a The number of gtt/hr
   b The amount of fluid given in 1 minute
   c The number of gtt/min or mL/hr
   d The amount of fluid in the IV bag

13 You note that the IV bag is almost empty. You should
   a Clamp the IV tubing
   b Tell the nurse
   c Remove the IV
   d Adjust the flow rate

14 You see bleeding from an IV site. You should
   a Tell the nurse
   b Move the needle or catheter
   c Remove the IV
   d Clamp the IV tubing

Answers to Chapter 24 questions are on p. 552.

FOCUS ON PRACTICE

Problem Solving

A resident with an order for thickened liquids was served coffee without thickener. What will you do? What is the purpose of thickened liquids?

Measurements

OBJECTIVES

- Define the key terms and key abbreviations in this chapter.
- Explain why vital signs are measured.
- List the factors affecting vital signs.
- Identify the normal ranges for each temperature site.
- Explain when to use each temperature site.
- Explain how to use thermometers.
- Identify the pulse sites.
- Describe a normal pulse and normal respirations.
- Describe the practices for measuring blood pressure.

- Describe the normal ranges for blood pressure.
- Describe the 4 types of pain.
- Explain why pain is personal.
- List the signs and symptoms of pain.
- Explain how to prepare the person for weight and height measurements.
- Perform the procedures described in this chapter.
- Explain how to promote PRIDE in the person, the family, and yourself.

KEY TERMS

blood pressure (BP) The amount of force exerted against the walls of an artery by the blood

body temperature The amount of heat in the body that is a balance between the amount of heat produced and the amount lost by the body

diastolic pressure The pressure in the arteries when the heart is at rest

discomfort See "pain"

fever Elevated body temperature

hypertension When the systolic pressure is 130 mm Hg or higher *(hyper)* or the diastolic pressure is 80 mm Hg or higher

hypotension When the systolic pressure is below *(hypo)* 90 mm Hg or the diastolic pressure is below 60 mm Hg

pain To ache, hurt, or be sore; discomfort

pulse The beat of the heart felt at an artery as a wave of blood passes through the artery

pulse rate The number of heartbeats or pulses in 1 minute

respiration Breathing air into *(inhalation)* and out of *(exhalation)* the lungs

stethoscope An instrument used to listen to the sounds produced by the heart, lungs, and other body organs

systolic pressure The pressure in the arteries when the heart contracts

thermometer A device used to measure *(meter)* temperature *(thermo)*

vital signs Temperature, pulse, respirations, and blood pressure; and pain in some agencies

KEY ABBREVIATIONS

BP	Blood pressure	ID	Identification
C	Centigrade	mm	Millimeter
F	Fahrenheit	mm Hg	Millimeters of mercury
Hg	Mercury	TPR	Temperature, pulse, and respirations

Measurements are used for the nursing process. They help the nurse plan for and evaluate care.

To assist with the nursing process, you will measure vital signs and weight and height. And you will collect information about the person's pain.

NOTE: A task may require more than 1 pair of gloves. Change gloves as needed. Use careful judgment. Remember to practice hand hygiene after removing gloves.

VITAL SIGNS

Vital signs reflect the function of 3 body processes—regulation of body temperature, breathing, and heart function. The *vital signs of body function are:*

- *Temperature*
- *Pulse*
- *Respirations*
- *Blood pressure*
- *Pain (in some agencies)*

Vital signs are often called TPR (temperature, pulse, and respirations) and BP (blood pressure). Some agencies include "pain" as a vital sign (p. 378 and Chapter 17). Also see "Pulse Oximetry" in Chapter 30.

A person's vital signs vary within certain limits. Box 25-1 lists the factors affecting vital signs.

Vital signs detect changes in normal body function. They show even minor changes in the person's condition. They tell about treatment response. They often signal life-threatening events.

You must accurately measure, record, and report vital signs. If unsure of your measurements, promptly ask the nurse to take them again. Unless otherwise ordered, take vital signs with the person at rest—lying or sitting. Report the following at once.

- Any vital sign changed from a prior measurement
- A vital sign above or below the normal range
  See *Focus on Communication: Vital Signs.*
  See *Focus on Older Persons: Vital Signs.*

BOX 25-1 Factors Affecting Vital Signs

- Activity
- Age
- Anger
- Anxiety
- Drugs
- Eating
- Exercise
- Fear
- Gender (male or female)
- Illness
- Noise
- Pain
- Sleep
- Smoking
- Stress
- Weather
- Weight

FOCUS ON COMMUNICATION

Vital Signs

Some persons like to know their vital signs. If agency policy allows, tell the person the measurements. With the person's consent, you can tell family members if they ask. This information is private and confidential. Roommates and visitors must not hear what you say. For greater privacy, write the measurements for the person.

A measurement may be abnormal. Or you are not able to feel a pulse or hear a blood pressure. Do not alarm the person. You can say:

- "I'm not sure I counted your pulse correctly. I'll have the nurse take it."
- "I'm not sure I heard your blood pressure correctly. I'll have the nurse take it again."
- "Your pulse is a little slow (or fast). I'll have the nurse check it."
- "Your temperature is higher than normal. I'll use another thermometer and have the nurse check you."

FOCUS ON OLDER PERSONS

Vital Signs

When measuring vital signs, the person with dementia may move, hit at you, or grab equipment. This is not safe for the person or you. Two staff members may be needed. One uses touch and a soothing voice to calm and distract the person. The other measures the vital signs.

Try the procedure when the person is calmer. Or take the respirations and pulse at one time. Then take the temperature and blood pressure later.

Approach the person calmly. Use a soothing voice. Explain what you will do. Do not rush. Follow the care plan. If you cannot measure vital signs, tell the nurse at once.

Body Temperature

Body temperature is the amount of heat in the body. It is a balance between the amount of heat produced and the amount lost by the body. Heat is produced as cells use food for energy. It is lost through the skin, breathing, urine, and feces. Body temperature is fairly stable. It is lower in the morning and higher in the afternoon and evening. See Box 25-1 for the factors affecting body temperature.

You use thermometers to measure temperature. A *thermometer is a device used to measure* (meter) *temperature* (thermo). Thermometers have Fahrenheit (F) or centigrade (C) scales. Use the degrees symbol (°) to record temperatures.

Temperature Sites. Temperature sites are the mouth, rectum, axilla (underarm), tympanic membrane (ear), and temporal artery (forehead) (Box 25-2). Each site has a normal range (Table 25-1). *Fever means an elevated body temperature.* Always report temperatures above or below the normal range.

See *Focus on Communication: Temperature Sites.*

See *Focus on Older Persons: Temperature Sites.*

See *Promoting Safety and Comfort: Temperature Sites.*

TABLE 25-1	Normal Body Temperatures	
Site	**Baseline**	**Normal Range**
Oral	98.6°F (37.0°C)	97.6°F to 99.6°F (36.5°C to 37.5°C)
Rectal	99.6°F (37.5°C)	98.6°F to 100.6°F (37.0°C to 38.1°C)
Axillary	97.6°F (36.5°C)	96.6°F to 98.6°F (35.9°C to 37.0°C)
Tympanic membrane	98.6°F (37.0°C)	98.6°F (37.0°C)
Temporal artery	99.6°F (37.5°C)	99.6°F (37.5°C)

BOX 25-2   Temperature Sites

Oral Site

Oral temperatures are *not* taken if the person:
- Is under 4 or 5 years of age.
- Is unconscious.
- Has had surgery or an injury to the face, neck, nose, or mouth.
- Is receiving oxygen.
- Breathes through the mouth.
- Has a naso-gastric tube.
- Is delirious, restless, confused, or disoriented.
- Is paralyzed on 1 side of the body.
- Has a sore mouth.
- Has a convulsive (seizure) disorder.

Rectal Site

The rectal site is used for infants and children under 3 years old. Rectal temperatures are taken when the oral site cannot be used. Rectal temperatures are *not* taken if the person:
- Has diarrhea.
- Has a rectal disorder or injury.
- Has heart disease.
- Had rectal surgery.
- Is confused or agitated.

Tympanic Membrane Site

The site has fewer microbes than the mouth or rectum. The risk of spreading infection is reduced. This site is *not* used if the person has:
- An ear disorder
- Ear drainage

Temporal Artery Site

Body temperature is measured at the temporal artery in the forehead. The site is non-invasive.

Axillary Site

The axillary site is less reliable than the other sites. It is used when the other sites cannot be used.

FOCUS ON COMMUNICATION

Temperature Sites

Taking a rectal temperature can be embarrassing and uncomfortable. Be professional. Explain what you will do and why you must use the rectal site. For example:

Mr. Presney, I need to take a rectal temperature because you have a sore mouth. This electronic thermometer stays in place until it beeps. It takes a few seconds. Please tell me if you feel pain.

A glass thermometer (p. 365) remains in the rectum for at least 2 minutes. To promote comfort, talk the person through the procedure. You can say: "I'm almost done. There's about 1 minute left. Are you doing okay?"

FOCUS ON OLDER PERSONS

Temperature Sites

Older persons have lower body temperatures than younger persons. An oral temperature of 98.6°F may signal fever in an older person.

Tympanic membrane and temporal artery sites are used for persons who are confused and resist care. Oral and rectal sites are unsafe. The person may move, resist care, or bite down on the thermometer. This can injure the mouth, teeth, or rectum.

PROMOTING SAFETY AND COMFORT

Temperature Sites

Safety

Rectal temperatures are dangerous for persons with heart disease. The thermometer can stimulate the vagus nerve and slow the heart rate to dangerous levels.

Taking Temperatures. The nurse and care plan indicate:
• When to take the person's temperature
• What site to use
• What thermometer to use

    See *Delegation Guidelines: Taking Temperatures.*
    See *Promoting Safety and Comfort: Taking Temperatures.*

DELEGATION GUIDELINES

Taking Temperatures

Before taking temperatures, you need this information from the nurse and the care plan.
• What site to use for each person—oral, rectal, axillary, tympanic membrane, or temporal artery
• What thermometer to use for each person
• How long to leave a glass thermometer in place (p. 365)
• When to take temperatures
• Which persons are at risk for a fever
• What observations to report and record
• When to report observations
• What patient or resident concerns to report at once:
   • A temperature changed from a past measurement
   • A temperature above or below the normal range

PROMOTING SAFETY AND COMFORT

Taking Temperatures

Safety

The mouth, rectum, axilla, and ear have many microbes and may contain blood. Therefore each person has his or her own digital or glass thermometer. This prevents the spread of microbes and infection. Follow Standard Precautions and the Bloodborne Pathogen Standard when taking temperatures.

    With rectal temperatures, your gloved hands may have contact with feces. If so, remove gloves and practice hand hygiene. Then note the temperature on your note pad or assignment sheet. Put on clean gloves to complete the procedure.

Comfort

Do not leave a thermometer in place longer than needed. This affects comfort. For example, an oral glass thermometer is left in place for 2 to 3 minutes. Do not leave it in place longer than that.

Electronic Thermometers.
Electronic thermometers show the temperature on the front of the device. Battery operated, they are kept in chargers when not in use.

• *Standard electronic thermometers*—measure temperature at the oral, rectal, and axillary sites in a few seconds. The blue probe is used for oral and axillary temperatures. The red probe is used for rectal temperatures. A disposable cover (sheath) protects the probe and prevents the spread of infection. See Figure 25-1, *A.*

• *Tympanic membrane thermometers*—measure temperature at the tympanic membrane in the ear in 1 to 3 seconds (Fig. 25-1, *B*). They are comfortable and not invasive. To use one, gently insert the covered probe into the ear.

• *Temporal artery thermometers*—measure temperature at the temporal artery in the forehead in 3 to 4 seconds (Fig. 25-1, *C*). The temperature of the blood in the temporal artery is the same as the temperature of the blood coming from the heart. To use one:

  1 Use the side of the head that is exposed. Do not use the side covered by hair, a dressing, a hat, or other covering. Do not use the side that was on a pillow.
  2 Place a disposable cap or cover on the thermometer.
  3 Place the device in the center of the forehead.
  4 Press the scan button.
  5 Slide the device across the forehead and across the temporal artery (see Fig. 25-1, *C*).
  6 Release the scan button.
  7 Read the temperature display.

• *Digital thermometers*—measure temperature at the oral, rectal, and axillary sites. Depending on the type, the temperature is measured in 6 to 60 seconds. See Figure 25-1, *D.*

There are many types of electronic thermometers. Follow the manufacturer's instructions. The procedure that follows is used as a guide.

    See procedure: *Taking a Temperature With an Electronic Thermometer.*

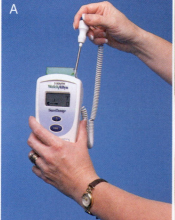
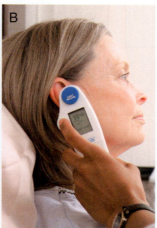
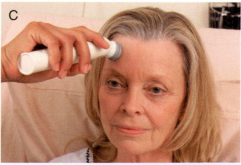
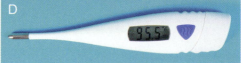

FIGURE 25-1 Electronic thermometers. **A,** Standard electronic thermometer. **B,** Tympanic membrane thermometer. **C,** Temporal artery thermometer. **D,** Digital thermometer.

Taking a Temperature With an Electronic Thermometer

QUALITY OF LIFE

- Knock before entering the person's room.
- Address the person by name.
- Introduce yourself by name and title.

- Explain the procedure before starting and during the procedure.
- Protect the person's rights during the procedure.
- Handle the person gently during the procedure.

PRE-PROCEDURE

1 Follow *Delegation Guidelines: Taking Temperatures*. See *Promoting Safety and Comfort: Taking Temperatures*.
2 For an oral temperature, ask the person not to eat, drink, smoke, or chew gum for at least 15 to 20 minutes before the measurement or as required by agency policy.
3 Practice hand hygiene.
4 Collect the following.
  - Thermometer—electronic or tympanic membrane
  - Probe (blue—oral or axillary temperature; red—rectal temperature)
  - Probe covers
  - Toilet tissue (rectal temperature)
  - Water-soluble lubricant (rectal temperature)
  - Gloves
  - Towel (axillary temperature)

5 Plug the probe into the thermometer if using a standard electronic thermometer.
6 Practice hand hygiene.
7 Identify the person. Check the identification (ID) bracelet against the assignment sheet. Use 2 identifiers (Chapter 10). Also call the person by name.

PROCEDURE

8 Provide for privacy. Position the person for an oral, rectal, axillary, or tympanic membrane temperature. The Sims' position is used for a rectal temperature.
9 Put on gloves if contact with blood, body fluids, secretions, or excretions is likely.
10 Insert the probe into a probe cover.
11 *For an oral temperature:*
  a Have the person open the mouth and raise the tongue.
  b Place the covered probe at the base of the tongue and to 1 side (Fig. 25-2, p. 364).
  c Have the person lower the tongue and close the mouth.
12 *For a rectal temperature:*
  a Place some lubricant on toilet tissue.
  b Lubricate the end of the covered probe.
  c Expose the anal area.
  d Raise the upper buttock (Fig. 25-3, p. 364).
  e Insert the probe ½ inch into the rectum.
  f Hold the probe in place.
13 *For an axillary temperature:*
  a Help the person remove an arm from the gown. Do not expose the person.
  b Dry the axilla with the towel.
  c Place the covered probe in the center of the axilla (Fig. 25-4, p. 364).
  d Place the person's arm over the chest.
  e Hold the probe in place.

14 *For a tympanic membrane temperature:*
  a Have the person turn his or her head so the ear is in front of you.
  b Pull up and back on the adult's ear to straighten the ear canal (Fig. 25-5, p. 364).
  c Insert the covered probe gently.
15 Start the thermometer.
16 Hold the probe in place until you hear a tone or see a flashing or steady light.
17 Read the temperature on the display.
18 Remove the probe. Press the eject button to discard the cover.
19 Note the person's name, temperature, and temperature site on your note pad or assignment sheet.
20 Return the probe to the holder.
21 Help the person put the gown back on (axillary temperature). For a rectal temperature:
  a Wipe the anal area with toilet tissue to remove lubricant.
  b Cover the person.
  c Dispose of used toilet tissue.
  d Remove and discard the gloves. Practice hand hygiene.

POST-PROCEDURE

22 Provide for comfort. (See the inside of the front cover.)
23 Place the call light and other needed items within reach.
24 Unscreen the person.
25 Complete a safety check of the room. (See the inside of the front cover.)

26 Return the thermometer to the charging unit.
27 Practice hand hygiene.
28 Report and record the temperature. Note the temperature site. Report an abnormal temperature at once.

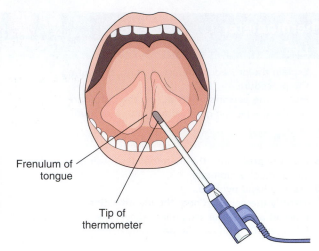

Frenulum of tongue

Tip of thermometer

FIGURE 25-2 The thermometer is placed at the base of the tongue and to 1 side.

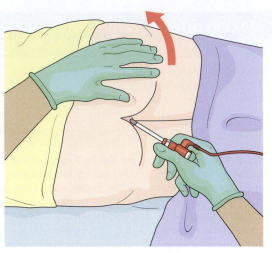

FIGURE 25-3 The rectal temperature is taken with the person in Sims' position. The buttock is raised to expose the anus.

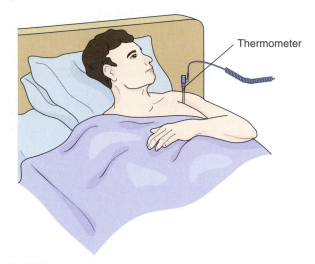

Thermometer

FIGURE 25-4 The thermometer is in the center of the axilla and the person's arm is over the chest.

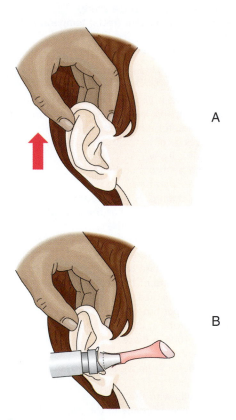

A

B

FIGURE 25-5 Tympanic membrane thermometer. **A,** The adult's ear is pulled up and back. **B,** The probe is inserted into the ear canal.

Glass Thermometers. Glass thermometers have a hollow glass tube and a bulb tip (Fig. 25-6). The device is filled with a substance that expands and rises in the tube when heated. When cooled, the substance contracts and moves down the tube.

Long- or slender-tip thermometers are used for oral and axillary temperatures. So are those with stubby and pear-shaped tips. Rectal thermometers have stubby tips. See Figure 25-6.

Glass thermometers are color-coded.

- Blue—oral and axillary thermometers
- Red—rectal thermometers

Glass thermometers are re-usable. However, the following are problems.

- They take a long time to register—3 to 10 minutes depending on the site.
- They break easily. Broken rectal thermometers can injure the rectum and colon.
- The person may bite down and break an oral thermometer. Cuts in the mouth are risks. If the thermometer contains mercury, swallowed mercury can cause mercury poisoning.

See Box 25-3 for how to use and read glass thermometers.

See *Focus on Math: Glass Thermometers,* p. 366.

See *Promoting Safety and Comfort: Glass Thermometers,* p. 367.

See procedure: *Taking a Temperature With a Glass Thermometer,* p. 367.

Text continued on p. 368.

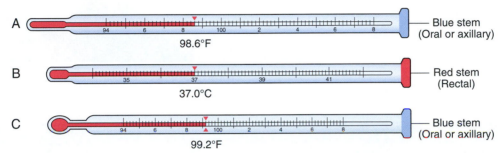

FIGURE 25-6 Glass thermometers. **A,** Fahrenheit thermometer with a long or slender tip. The temperature measurement is 98.6°F. **B,** Centigrade thermometer with a stubby tip. The temperature measurement is 37.0°C. **C,** Fahrenheit thermometer with a pear-shaped tip. The temperature measurement is 99.2°F.

BOX 25-3   Glass Thermometers

Using a Glass Thermometer

- Follow Standard Precautions and the Bloodborne Pathogen Standard.
- Use the person's thermometer.
- Use a rectal thermometer only for rectal temperatures.
- Rinse the thermometer under cold, running water if it was soaking in a disinfectant. Dry it from the stem to the bulb end with tissues.
- Check the thermometer for breaks, cracks, and chips. Discard it following agency policy if it is broken, cracked, or chipped.
- Shake down the thermometer to move the substance down in the tube. Hold it at the stem and stand away from walls, tables, or other hard surfaces. Flex and snap your wrist until the substance is below 94°F or 34°C. See Figure 25-7, p. 366.
- Insert the thermometer into a plastic cover (Fig. 25-8, p. 366). Remove the cover to read the device. Discard the cover after use.
- Clean and store the thermometer following agency policy. Wipe it with tissues first to remove mucus, feces, or sweat. Do not use hot water. It causes the substance to expand so much that the thermometer could break. After cleaning, rinse the thermometer under cold, running water. Then store it in a container with a disinfectant solution.

Taking Temperatures

- The oral site:
  - The glass thermometer remains in place 2 to 3 minutes or as required by agency policy.

Taking Temperatures—cont'd

- The rectal site:
  - Provide for privacy. The buttocks and anus are exposed. This can embarrass the person.
  - Lubricate the bulb end of the rectal thermometer for easy insertion and to prevent injury.
  - Hold the device in place so it is not lost into the rectum or broken.
  - Leave the thermometer in the rectum for 2 minutes or as required by agency policy.
- The axillary site:
  - Make sure the axilla (underarm) is dry. Do not use the site right after bathing.
  - Leave the thermometer in place for 5 to 10 minutes or as required by agency policy.

Reading a Glass Thermometer

- Hold it at the stem (Fig. 25-9, p. 366). Bring it to eye level.
- Turn it until you can see the numbers and the long and short lines.
- Turn it back and forth slowly until you can see the silver or red line.
- Read from the tip toward the stem.
- Read the nearest degree (long line) to the left of the silver or red line.
- Read the nearest tenth of a degree (short line)—an even number on a Fahrenheit thermometer.

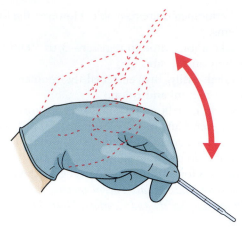

FIGURE 25-7 The wrist is snapped to shake down the thermometer.

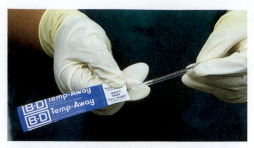

FIGURE 25-8 The thermometer is inserted into a plastic cover.

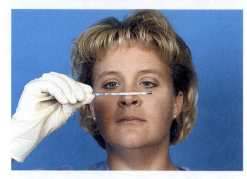

FIGURE 25-9 The thermometer is held at the stem. It is read at eye level.

FOCUS ON MATH
Glass Thermometers

To read a thermometer, you must understand whole numbers and decimals. Whole numbers are 0, 1, 2, 3, and so on. They are to the *left* of the decimal point. The numbers to the *right* of the decimal point (decimal place values) are part of a whole number. Each whole number has 10 parts—the decimal place values. Decimal place values are read as "tenths"—1-tenth, 2-tenths, 3-tenths, and so on. Thermometers are read to 1 number past the decimal point (the "tenths" place). See Figure 25-10.

To read a glass thermometer (Fig. 25-11):

1 Read the nearest long line to the left of the silver or red line.
   • Fahrenheit—each long line is 1 degree from 94°F to 108°F.
   • Centigrade—each long line is 1 degree from 34°C to 42°C.
2 Read the nearest tenth of a degree (short line).
   • Fahrenheit—each short line is 0.2 (2-tenths) of a degree (2-tenths, 4-tenths, 6-tenths, and 8-tenths).
   • Centigrade—each short line is 0.1 (1-tenth) of a degree (1-tenth, 2-tenths, 3-tenths, and so on to 9-tenths).

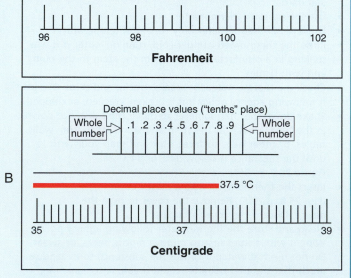

FIGURE 25-11 Reading thermometers. **A,** Fahrenheit thermometer. Every other long line is marked in even degrees (ending in 0, 2, 4, 6, or 8). Each long line increases by 1 degree. Each short line increases by 0.2 (2-tenths) of a degree. **B,** Centigrade thermometer. Each long line increases by 1 degree. Each short line increases by 0.1 (1-tenth) of a degree.

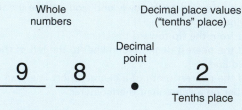

FIGURE 25-10 Values used to read thermometers.

PROMOTING SAFETY AND COMFORT
Glass Thermometers

Safety

Mercury-glass thermometers are not common today. Safer chemicals have replaced mercury. However, do not assume that a glass thermometer has a mercury-free mixture. If a thermometer breaks, tell the nurse at once.

Mercury is a hazardous substance. Do not touch the substance. Do not let the person do so. Follow agency procedures for handling hazardous materials. See Chapter 10.

Taking a Temperature With a Glass Thermometer

QUALITY OF LIFE

- Knock before entering the person's room.
- Address the person by name.
- Introduce yourself by name and title.

- Explain the procedure before starting and during the procedure.
- Protect the person's rights during the procedure.
- Handle the person gently during the procedure.

PRE-PROCEDURE

1 Follow *Delegation Guidelines: Taking Temperatures*, p. 362. See *Promoting Safety and Comfort:*
   a *Taking Temperatures*, p. 362
   b *Glass Thermometers*
2 For an oral temperature, ask the person not to eat, drink, smoke, or chew gum for at least 15 to 20 minutes before the measurement or as required by agency policy.
3 Practice hand hygiene.
4 Collect the following.
   - Oral or rectal thermometer and holder
   - Tissues
   - Plastic covers if used
   - Gloves
   - Toilet tissue (rectal temperature)
   - Water-soluble lubricant (rectal temperature)
   - Towel (axillary temperature)

5 Practice hand hygiene.
6 Identify the person. Check the ID bracelet against the assignment sheet. Use 2 identifiers (Chapter 10). Also call the person by name.
7 Provide for privacy.

PROCEDURE

8 Put on the gloves.
9 Rinse the thermometer under cold running water if it was soaking in a disinfectant. Dry it with tissues.
10 Check for breaks, cracks, or chips.
11 Shake down the thermometer below the lowest number. Hold the device by the stem. See Figure 25-7.
12 Insert it into a plastic cover if used (see Fig. 25-8).
13 *For an oral temperature:*
   a Have the person moisten his or her lips.
   b Place the bulb end of the thermometer under the tongue and to 1 side (see Fig. 25-2).
   c Have the person close the lips around the thermometer to hold it in place.
   d Ask the person not to talk or bite down on the thermometer.
   e Leave it in place for 2 to 3 minutes or as required by agency policy.

14 *For a rectal temperature:*
   a Position the person in the Sims' position.
   b Put a small amount of lubricant on a tissue.
   c Lubricate the bulb end of the thermometer.
   d Fold back top linens to expose the anal area.
   e Raise the upper buttock to expose the anus (see Fig. 25-3).
   f Insert the thermometer 1 inch into the rectum. Do not force the thermometer.
   g Hold the thermometer in place for 2 minutes or as required by agency policy. Continue to hold it while it is in the rectum.

Continued

Taking a Temperature With a Glass Thermometer—cont'd

PROCEDURE—cont'd

15 *For an axillary temperature:*
  a Help the person remove an arm from the gown. Do not expose the person.
  b Dry the axilla with the towel.
  c Place the bulb end of the thermometer in the center of the axilla.
  d Have the person place the arm over the chest to hold the thermometer in place (see Fig. 25-4). Hold it and the arm in place if he or she cannot help.
  e Leave the thermometer in place for 5 to 10 minutes or as required by agency policy.
16 Remove the thermometer.
17 *For an oral or axillary temperature:*
  a Use a tissue to remove the plastic cover.
  b Wipe the thermometer with a tissue if no cover was used. Wipe from the stem to the bulb end.
  c Discard the tissue and cover (if used).
  d Read the thermometer.
  e Help the person put the gown back on (axillary temperature).

18 *For a rectal temperature:*
  a Use toilet tissue to remove the plastic cover.
  b Wipe the thermometer with toilet tissue if no cover was used. Wipe from the stem to the bulb end.
  c Place used toilet tissue on several thicknesses of clean toilet tissue. Discard the cover (if used).
  d Read the thermometer.
  e Place the thermometer on clean toilet tissue.
  f Wipe the anal area with toilet tissue to remove lubricant and any feces. Set the used toilet tissue on several thicknesses of clean toilet tissue.
  g Cover the person.
  h Dispose of toilet tissue in the toilet.
  i Remove and discard the gloves. Practice hand hygiene.
19 Note the person's name, temperature, and temperature site on your note pad or assignment sheet.
20 Shake down the thermometer.
21 Clean the thermometer following agency policy. (Wear gloves.) Return it to the holder.
22 Remove and discard the gloves. Practice hand hygiene.

POST-PROCEDURE

23 Provide for comfort. (See the inside of the front cover.)
24 Place the call light and other needed items within reach.
25 Unscreen the person.
26 Complete a safety check of the room. (See the inside of the front cover.)
27 Practice hand hygiene.
28 Report and record the temperature. Note the temperature site. Report an abnormal temperature at once.

Pulse

The **pulse** *is the beat of the heart felt at an artery as a wave of blood passes through the artery.* A pulse occurs when the heart beats.

The temporal, carotid, brachial, radial, femoral, popliteal, posterior tibial, and dorsalis pedis (pedal) pulses are on each side of the body (Fig. 25-12). The radial pulse is used most often. It is easy to reach and find. The person is not exposed.

The apical pulse is over the heart. The apex (apical) of the heart is at the tip of the heart (p. 370). This pulse is taken with a stethoscope.

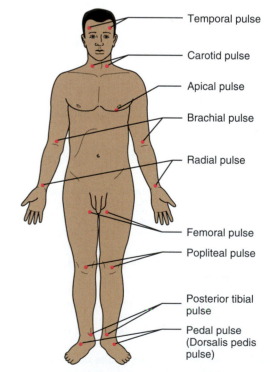

FIGURE 25-12 The pulse sites.

Temporal pulse
Carotid pulse
Apical pulse
Brachial pulse
Radial pulse
Femoral pulse
Popliteal pulse
Posterior tibial pulse
Pedal pulse (Dorsalis pedis pulse)

Using a Stethoscope. A *stethoscope* *is an instrument used to listen to the sounds produced by the heart, lungs, and other body organs* (Fig. 25-13). You use it for apical pulses and blood pressures. See Box 25-4 for how to use a stethoscope.

See *Focus on Communication: Using a Stethoscope.*
See *Promoting Safety and Comfort: Using a Stethoscope.*

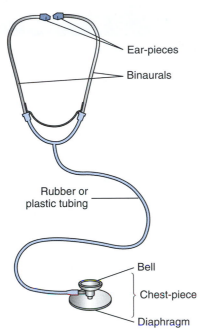

FIGURE 25-13 Parts of a stethoscope.

- Ear-pieces
- Binaurals
- Rubber or plastic tubing
- Bell
- Chest-piece
- Diaphragm

BOX 25-4   Using a Stethoscope

- Wipe the ear-pieces and chest-piece with antiseptic wipes before and after use.
- Place the ear-piece tips in your ears. The bend of the tips points forward. Ear-pieces should fit snugly to block out noises. They should not cause ear pain or discomfort.
- Tap the diaphragm gently. You should hear the tapping. If not, turn the chest-piece at the tubing. Gently tap the diaphragm again. Proceed if you hear the tapping sound. Check with the nurse if you do not hear the tapping.
- Place the diaphragm over the pulse site. Hold it in place as in Figure 25-14.
- Prevent noise. Do not let anything touch the tubing. Ask the person to be silent. Make sure the room is quiet.

Pulse Rate. The *pulse rate is the number of heartbeats or pulses in 1 minute.* Pulse rate is affected by the factors in Box 25-1. Some drugs increase the pulse rate. Other drugs slow the pulse.

The adult pulse rate is between 60 and 100 beats per minute. A rate of less than 60 or more than 100 is abnormal. Report abnormal pulses at once.

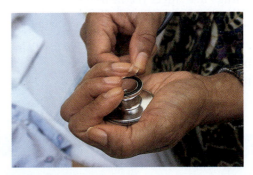

FIGURE 25-15 The diaphragm of the stethoscope is warmed in the palm of the hand.

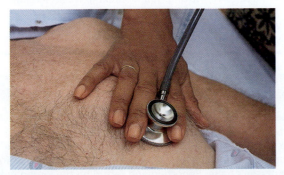

FIGURE 25-14 The stethoscope is held in place with the fingertips of the index and middle fingers.

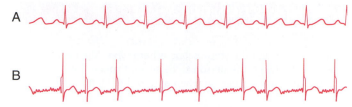

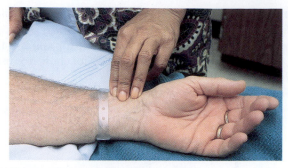

FIGURE 25-16 **A,** The electrocardiogram shows a regular pulse. The beats occur at regular intervals. **B,** These beats are at irregular intervals.

FIGURE 25-17 The 3 middle fingers are used to take the radial pulse.

Pulse Rhythm and Force. The pulse *rhythm* should be in a regular pattern. The same interval occurs between beats. An irregular pulse is when the beats are not evenly spaced or beats are skipped (Fig. 25-16).

Force relates to pulse strength. A forceful pulse is easy to feel. It is described as *strong*, *full*, or *bounding*. Hard-to-feel pulses are described as *weak*, *thready*, or *feeble*.

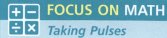 **Taking Pulses.** You will take radial and apical pulses. You must count, report, and record accurately.

The radial pulse is used for routine vital signs. Place the first 2 or 3 fingertips against the radial artery. The radial artery is on the thumb side of the wrist (Fig. 25-17). Follow agency policy for how long to count. The following is common.

- Regular pulses—count the pulse for 30 seconds. Multiply by 2 for the number of pulses in 1 minute.
- Irregular pulses—count the pulse for 1 minute.

The apical pulse is located 2 to 3 inches left of the sternum (Fig. 25-18). Use a stethoscope and count the pulse for 1 minute. The heartbeat normally sounds like a *lub-dub*. Count each *lub-dub* as 1 beat. Do not count the *lub* as 1 beat and the *dub* as another.

Apical pulses are taken on persons who:
- Have heart disease.
- Have irregular heart rhythms.
- Take drugs that affect the heart.
  See *Focus on Math: Taking Pulses.*
  See *Delegation Guidelines: Taking Pulses.*
  See *Promoting Safety and Comfort: Taking Pulses.*
  See procedure: *Taking a Radial Pulse.*
  See procedure: *Taking an Apical Pulse.*

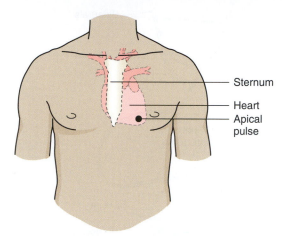

FIGURE 25-18 The apical pulse is located 2 to 3 inches to the left of the sternum (breastbone).

DELEGATION GUIDELINES
Taking Pulses

Before taking a pulse, you need this information from the nurse and the care plan.
- What pulse to take for each person—radial or apical
- When to take the pulse
- What other vital signs to measure
- How long to count the pulse—30 seconds or 1 minute
- If the nurse has concerns about certain patients or residents
- What observations to report and record:
  - The pulse site
  - The pulse rate—report a pulse rate less than 60 (*bradycardia*) or more than 100 (*tachycardia*) beats per minute at once
  - If the pulse is regular or irregular
  - Pulse force—strong, full, bounding, weak, thready, or feeble
- When to report the pulse rate
- What patient or resident concerns to report at once

FOCUS ON MATH
Taking Pulses

Pulse rate is measured in beats per minute. When you measure a regular pulse for 30 seconds, multiply the number by 2. This gives the number of beats per minute (60 seconds). For example, you count 36 beats in 30 seconds. For the number of beats per minute, multiply 36 by 2.

36 beats × 2 = 72 beats
The pulse is 72 beats per minute.

PROMOTING SAFETY AND COMFORT
Taking Pulses

Safety
Use your first 2 or 3 fingertips to take a pulse. Do not use your thumb. You could mistake the pulse in your thumb for the person's pulse. Reporting and recording the wrong pulse rate can harm the person.

Taking a Radial Pulse

QUALITY OF LIFE

- Knock before entering the person's room.
- Address the person by name.
- Introduce yourself by name and title.

- Explain the procedure before starting and during the procedure.
- Protect the person's rights during the procedure.
- Handle the person gently during the procedure.

PRE-PROCEDURE

1 Follow *Delegation Guidelines: Taking Pulses.* See *Promoting Safety and Comfort: Taking Pulses.*
2 Practice hand hygiene.

3 Identify the person. Check the ID bracelet against the assignment sheet. Use 2 identifiers (Chapter 10). Also call the person by name.
4 Provide for privacy.

PROCEDURE

5 Have the person sit or lie down.
6 Locate the radial pulse on the thumb side of the person's wrist. Use your first 2 or 3 middle fingertips (see Fig. 25-17).
7 Note if the pulse is strong or weak and regular or irregular.
8 Count the pulse for 30 seconds. Multiply the number of beats by 2 for the number of pulses in 60 seconds (1 minute). This is the pulse rate. For example:
- You count 45 beats in 30 seconds.
- Multiply 45 beats by 2.
- 45 beats × 2 = 90 beats per minute.

9 Count the pulse for 1 minute if:
  a Directed by the nurse and the care plan.
  b Required by agency policy.
  c The pulse was irregular.
  d Required for your state competency test.
10 Note the following on your note pad or assignment sheet.
  a The person's name
  b Pulse rate
  c Pulse strength
  d If the pulse was regular or irregular

POST-PROCEDURE

11 Provide for comfort. (See the inside of the front cover.)
12 Place the call light and other needed items within reach.
13 Unscreen the person.
14 Complete a safety check of the room. (See the inside of the front cover.)

15 Practice hand hygiene.
16 Report and record the pulse rate and your observations. Report an abnormal pulse at once.

Taking an Apical Pulse

QUALITY OF LIFE

- Knock before entering the person's room.
- Address the person by name.
- Introduce yourself by name and title.

- Explain the procedure before starting and during the procedure.
- Protect the person's rights during the procedure.
- Handle the person gently during the procedure.

PRE-PROCEDURE

1 Follow *Delegation Guidelines: Taking Pulses.* See *Promoting Safety and Comfort: Using a Stethoscope,* p. 369.
2 Practice hand hygiene.
3 Collect a stethoscope and antiseptic wipes.
4 Practice hand hygiene.

5 Identify the person. Check the ID bracelet against the assignment sheet. Use 2 identifiers (Chapter 10). Also call the person by name.
6 Provide for privacy.

PROCEDURE

7 Clean the stethoscope ear-pieces and chest-piece with the wipes.
8 Have the person sit or lie down.
9 Expose the upper part of the left chest. Expose a woman's breasts only to the extent necessary.
10 Warm the diaphragm in your palm.
11 Place the stethoscope ear-pieces in your ears.
12 Find the apical pulse. Place the diaphragm 2 to 3 inches to the left of the breastbone (see Fig. 25-18).

13 Count the pulse for 1 minute. (Count each lub-dub as 1 beat.) Note if it was regular or irregular.
14 Cover the person. Remove the stethoscope ear-pieces.
15 Note the person's name and pulse rate on your note pad or assignment sheet. Note if the pulse was regular or irregular.

Continued

Taking an Apical Pulse—cont'd

POST-PROCEDURE

16 Provide for comfort. (See the inside of the front cover.)
17 Place the call light and other needed items within reach.
18 Unscreen the person.
19 Complete a safety check of the room. (See the inside of the front cover.)
20 Clean the stethoscope ear-pieces and chest-piece with the wipes.

21 Return the stethoscope to its proper place.
22 Practice hand hygiene.
23 Report and record your observations. Record the pulse rate with *Ap* for apical. Report an abnormal pulse at once.

Respirations

Respiration means breathing air into (inhalation) *and out of* (exhalation) *the lungs.* Each respiration involves 1 inhalation and 1 exhalation. The chest rises during inhalation. It falls during exhalation.

The healthy adult has 12 to 20 respirations per minute. See Box 25-1 for the factors affecting vital signs. Heart and respiratory diseases often increase the respiratory rate.

Respirations are normally quiet, effortless, and regular. Both sides of the chest rise and fall equally. See Chapter 30 for abnormal respiratory patterns.

People tend to change their breathing patterns when they know their respirations are being counted. Therefore do not tell the person that you are counting them. Count respirations right after taking a pulse. Keep your fingers or stethoscope over the pulse site. The person assumes you are taking the pulse.

To count respirations, watch the chest rise and fall. Count chest rises for 30 seconds. Multiply the number by 2 for the number of respirations in 1 minute. If you note an abnormal pattern, count respirations for 1 minute.

See *Focus on Math: Respirations.*
See *Delegation Guidelines: Respirations.*
See procedure: *Counting Respirations.*

FOCUS ON MATH
Respirations

Respirations are measured in breaths per minute. When you count regular respirations for 30 seconds, multiply the number by 2. This gives the number of respirations per minute (60 seconds). For example, you count 8 breaths in 30 seconds. For the number of breaths per minute, multiply 8 by 2.

$$8 \text{ breaths} \times 2 = 16 \text{ breaths}$$
The respiratory rate is 16 breaths per minute.

DELEGATION GUIDELINES
Respirations

Before counting respirations, you need this information from the nurse and the care plan.
- How long to count respirations for each person—30 seconds or 1 minute
- When to count respirations
- If the nurse has concerns about certain patients or residents
- What other vital signs to measure
- What observations to report and record:
  - The respiratory rate
  - Equality and depth of respirations
  - If the respirations were regular or irregular
  - If the person has pain or difficulty breathing
  - Any respiratory noises
  - An abnormal respiratory pattern (Chapter 30)
- When to report observations
- What patient or resident concerns to report at once

Counting Respirations

PROCEDURE

1 Follow *Delegation Guidelines: Respirations.*
2 Keep your fingers or stethoscope over the pulse site.
3 Do not tell the person you are counting respirations.
4 Count chest rises. Each rise and fall of the chest is 1 respiration.
5 Note the following.
 • If respirations are regular
 • If both sides of the chest rise equally
 • The depth of respirations
 • If the person has any pain or difficulty breathing
 • An abnormal respiratory pattern

6 Count respirations for 30 seconds. Multiply the number by 2 for the number of respirations in 60 seconds (1 minute). This is the respiratory rate. For example:
 • You count 9 breaths in 30 seconds.
 • Multiply 9 breaths by 2.
 • 9 breaths × 2 = 18 breaths per minute.
7 Count respirations for 1 minute if:
 a Directed by the nurse and the care plan.
 b Required by agency policy.
 c They are abnormal or irregular.
 d Required for your state competency test.
8 Note the person's name, respiratory rate, and other observations on your note pad or assignment sheet.

POST-PROCEDURE

9 Provide for comfort. (See the inside of the front cover.)
10 Place the call light and other needed items within reach.
11 Unscreen the person.
12 Complete a safety check of the room. (See the inside of the front cover.)

13 Practice hand hygiene.
14 Report and record the respiratory rate and your observations. Report abnormal respirations at once.

Blood Pressure

Blood pressure (BP) is the amount of force exerted against the walls of an artery by the blood. Systole is the period of heart muscle contraction. The heart is pumping blood. *Diastole* is the period of heart muscle relaxation. The heart is at rest.

You measure systolic and diastolic pressures. The *systolic pressure is the pressure in the arteries when the heart contracts.* It is the higher pressure. The *diastolic pressure is the pressure in the arteries when the heart is at rest.* It is the lower pressure.

BP is measured in millimeters (mm) of mercury (Hg). The systolic pressure is recorded over the diastolic pressure. A systolic pressure of 120 mm Hg (millimeters of mercury) and a diastolic pressure of 80 mm Hg are written as 120/80 mm Hg. This is read as "120 over 80 millimeters of mercury."

Normal and Abnormal Blood Pressures. BP can change from minute to minute. Therefore BP has normal ranges.
• *Systolic pressure*—90 mm Hg or higher but lower than 120 mm Hg
• *Diastolic pressure*—60 mm Hg or higher but lower than 80 mm Hg
Treatment is indicated for:
• *Hypertension—The systolic pressure is 130 mm Hg or higher (hyper) or the diastolic pressure is 80 mm Hg or higher.* Report any systolic measurement at or above 120 mm Hg. Also report a diastolic pressure at or above 80 mm Hg.
• *Hypotension—The systolic pressure is below (hypo) 90 mm Hg or the diastolic pressure is below 60 mm Hg.* Report a systolic pressure below 90 mm Hg. Also report a diastolic pressure below 60 mm Hg.
See *Focus on Communication: Normal and Abnormal Blood Pressures.*

FOCUS ON COMMUNICATION

Normal and Abnormal Blood Pressures

If agency policy allows, tell the person the BP if he or she wants to know. If the BP is high or low, the person may worry and say: "That is higher (lower) than normal for me." Be calm and professional. You can say: "Yes, it was a little high (low). I will tell your nurse." Report abnormal blood pressures to the nurse.

You must report some concerns at once. For example, a BP is 82/58 and the person is dizzy. You help the person lie down and press the call light to report your concern. After identifying yourself, you say: "Please have the nurse come to room 216 right away." When the nurse arrives, you say: "I measured the BP at 82/58 with the complaint of dizziness. How can I help?"

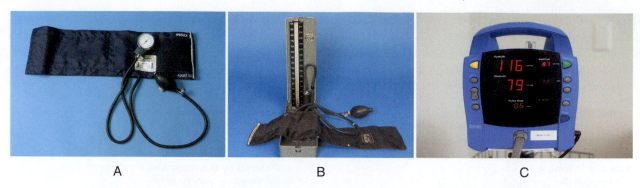

FIGURE 25-19 Blood pressure equipment. **A,** Aneroid manometer and cuff. **B,** Mercury manometer and cuff. **C,** Electronic manometer.

Blood Pressure Equipment. A *sphygmomanometer* has a cuff and a measuring device for measuring blood pressure. *Sphygmo* means *pulse*. A device for measuring pressure is called a *manometer*.

- The *aneroid type* has a round dial and a needle that points to the numbers (Fig. 25-19, *A*).
- The *mercury type* has a column of mercury within a calibrated tube (Fig. 25-19, *B*).
- The *electronic type* shows the systolic and diastolic pressures and the pulse rate (Fig. 25-19, *C*).

You wrap the blood pressure cuff around the upper arm. Tubing connects the cuff to the manometer. When inflated, the cuff causes pressure over the brachial artery. BP is measured as the cuff deflates.

- *Aneroid and mercury types.* A tube connects the cuff to a small, hand-held bulb. See Figure 25-20. Hold the bulb with the air-release valve up. To inflate the cuff, turn the air-release valve on the bulb clockwise to close the valve. Squeeze the bulb. To deflate the cuff, turn the valve counter-clockwise. Using a stethoscope, listen and measure BP as the cuff deflates. Blood flowing through the arteries produces sounds.
- *Electronic type.* No stethoscope is needed. A button is pressed to inflate the cuff. The cuff deflates automatically. The BP is displayed. Follow the manufacturer's instructions.

See *Promoting Safety and Comfort: Blood Pressure Equipment.*

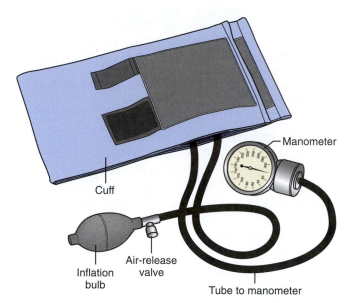

FIGURE 25-20 Parts of an aneroid sphygmomanometer.

PROMOTING SAFETY AND COMFORT
Blood Pressure Equipment

Safety

Mercury is a hazardous substance. Mercury manometers are being phased out of health care. Some agencies may still use them. Handle mercury manometers carefully. If one breaks, call for the nurse at once. Do not touch the mercury. Do not let the person touch it. The agency follows special procedures for handling hazardous substances. See Chapter 10.

Comfort

Inflate the cuff only to the extent necessary. (See procedure: *Measuring Blood Pressure*, p. 376.) The inflated cuff causes discomfort. The higher the inflation, the greater the discomfort.

■ **Measuring Blood Pressure.** You measure blood pressure in the brachial artery. Box 25-5 lists the guidelines for measuring blood pressure.

See *Focus on Math: Measuring Blood Pressure.*

See *Delegation Guidelines: Measuring Blood Pressure,* p. 376.

See procedure: *Measuring Blood Pressure,* p. 376.

Text continued on p. 378.

BOX 25-5	Measuring Blood Pressure—Guidelines

- Do not take BP on an arm:
  - With an IV (intravenous) infusion
  - With an arm cast
  - With a dialysis access site
  - On the side of breast surgery
  - That is injured
- Ask the nurse if unsure of which arm to use.
- Let the person rest for 10 to 20 minutes before measuring BP.
- Measure BP with the person sitting or lying. Sometimes BP is measured in the standing position.
- Apply the cuff to the bare upper arm. Clothing can affect the measurement.
- Make sure the cuff is snug. A loose cuff causes a wrong reading.
- Use a larger cuff if the person is obese or has a large arm. Use a small cuff for a very small arm. Ask the nurse what size to use. Also check the care plan.

- Make sure the room is quiet. Talking, TV, music, and sounds from the hallway can affect hearing through a stethoscope.
- Have the manometer where you can clearly see it.
- Place the diaphragm of the stethoscope firmly over the brachial artery. The entire diaphragm has contact with the skin.
- Measure the systolic and diastolic pressures.
  - Expect the first sound at the point where you last felt the radial or brachial pulse. (See procedure: *Measuring Blood Pressure,* p. 376.) The first sound is the systolic pressure.
  - The point where the sound disappears (the last sound heard) is the diastolic pressure.
- Take the BP again if you are not sure of accuracy. Wait 30 to 60 seconds to repeat the measurement. Ask the nurse to take the BP if you are unsure of the measurement.
- Tell the nurse at once if you cannot hear the blood pressure.

⊞ FOCUS ON MATH
Measuring Blood Pressure

Manometers are marked with long and short lines (Fig. 25-21).

- Long lines mark 10 mm Hg values.
- Short lines mark 2 mm Hg values.

Read the manometer as the cuff deflates. The needle or mercury column is dropping.

- If the needle or mercury column is at a long line, note this value. Long line values end in 0. For example: 70, 80, 90, 100, 110, 120, and so on.
- If the needle or mercury column is between 2 long lines:
  - Note the value of the long line below the needle or mercury column.
  - Note the short line. Count up from the long line below by even numbers. Short line values end with 2, 4, 6, or 8. See Figure 25-21.

For example, the needle is at the 3rd short line between 90 and 100. Count up by even numbers from 90. Line 1 is 92. Line 2 is 94. Line 3 is 96. The value is 96.

If needed, round up to the nearest 2 mm Hg. When you *round up* you choose the higher value. For example, the needle is between 82 and 80. Report and record the value as 82 mm Hg.

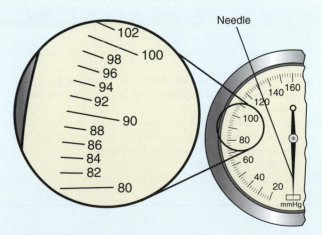

FIGURE 25-21 Reading the manometer. Long lines mark 10 mm Hg values. Short lines mark 2 mm Hg values.

DELEGATION GUIDELINES
Measuring Blood Pressure

Before measuring BP, you need this information from the nurse and the care plan.
- When to measure BP
- What sphygmomanometer to use (p. 374)
- What arm to use
- The person's normal blood pressure range
- If the nurse has concerns about certain patients or residents
- If the person needs to be lying down, sitting, or standing
- What size cuff to use—regular, child-sized, extra-large
- What observations to report and record
- When to report the BP measurement
- What patient or resident concerns to report at once

Measuring Blood Pressure

QUALITY OF LIFE

- Knock before entering the person's room.
- Address the person by name.
- Introduce yourself by name and title.

- Explain the procedure before starting and during the procedure.
- Protect the person's rights during the procedure.
- Handle the person gently during the procedure.

PRE-PROCEDURE

1 Follow *Delegation Guidelines: Measuring Blood Pressure.*
  See *Promoting Safety and Comfort:*
  a *Using a Stethoscope*, p. 369
  b *Blood Pressure Equipment*, p. 374
2 Practice hand hygiene.
3 Collect the following.
  - Sphygmomanometer
  - Stethoscope
  - Antiseptic wipes

4 Practice hand hygiene.
5 Identify the person. Check the ID bracelet against the assignment sheet. Use 2 identifiers (Chapter 10). Also call the person by name.
6 Provide for privacy.

PROCEDURE

7 Have the person sit or lie down.
8 Position the person's arm level with the heart. The palm is up.
9 Wipe the stethoscope ear-pieces and chest-piece with the wipes. Warm the diaphragm in your palm. Discard the wipes.
10 Stand no more than 3 feet away from the manometer. The mercury type is vertical, on a flat surface, and at eye level. The aneroid type is directly in front of you.
11 Expose the upper arm.
12 Squeeze the cuff to expel any air. Close the valve on the bulb.

13 Find the brachial artery at the inner aspect of the elbow. (The brachial artery is on the little finger side of the arm.) Use your fingertips.
14 Locate the arrow on the cuff (Fig. 25-22, *A*). Align the arrow with the brachial artery (Fig. 25-22, *B*). Wrap the cuff around the upper arm at least 1 inch above the elbow. It is even and snug.
15 Place the stethoscope ear-pieces in your ears. Place the diaphragm over the brachial artery (Fig. 25-22, *C*). Do not place it under the cuff.
16 Find the radial pulse. This step is for Methods 1 and 2.

Continued

Measuring Blood Pressure—cont'd

PROCEDURE—cont'd

17 *Method 1:*
   a Inflate the cuff until you cannot feel the pulse. Note this point.
   b Inflate the cuff 30 mm Hg beyond where you last felt the pulse.
18 *Method 2:*
   a Inflate the cuff until you cannot feel the pulse. Note this point.
   b Inflate the cuff 30 mm Hg beyond where you last felt the pulse.
   c Deflate the cuff slowly. Note the point when you feel the pulse.
   d Wait 30 seconds.
   e Inflate the cuff again, 30 mm Hg beyond where you felt the pulse return.
19 *Method 3:*
   a Inflate the cuff 160 mm Hg to 180 mm Hg.
   b Deflate the cuff if you hear a blood pressure sound. Re-inflate the cuff to 200 mm Hg.

20 Deflate the cuff at an even rate of 2 to 4 millimeters per second. Turn the valve counter-clockwise to deflate the cuff.
21 Note the point where you hear the first sound (Fig. 25-23, A). This is the systolic reading. It is near the point where the pulse disappeared (Method 1) or returned (Method 2).
22 Continue to deflate the cuff completely. Note the point where the sound disappears (the last sound heard). This is the diastolic reading (Fig. 25-23, B).
23 Deflate the cuff completely. Remove the cuff. Remove the stethoscope ear-pieces.
24 Note the person's name and blood pressure on your note pad or assignment sheet.
25 Return the cuff to the case or wall holder.

POST-PROCEDURE

26 Provide for comfort. (See the inside of the front cover.)
27 Place the call light and other needed items within reach.
28 Unscreen the person.
29 Complete a safety check of the room. (See the inside of the front cover.)

30 Clean the stethoscope ear-pieces and chest-piece with the wipes. Discard the wipes.
31 Return the equipment to its proper place.
32 Practice hand hygiene.
33 Report and record the BP. Note which arm was used. Report an abnormal BP at once.

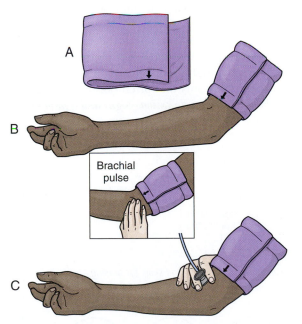

FIGURE 25-22 Measuring blood pressure. **A,** The arrow is used for correct cuff alignment. **B,** The cuff is placed so the arrow is aligned with the brachial artery. **C,** The diaphragm of the stethoscope is over the brachial artery.

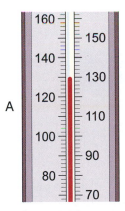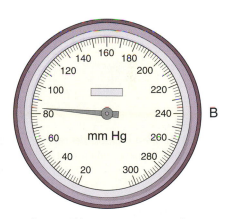

FIGURE 25-23 Manometer readings. **A,** This mercury manometer is at 130 mm Hg for a systolic pressure. **B,** This aneroid manometer is at 84 mm Hg for a diastolic pressure.

PAIN

Pain or discomfort means to ache, hurt, or be sore. Often called the fifth vital sign, pain signals tissue damage. Pain often causes the person to seek health care.

Types of Pain

There are different types of pain.

- *Acute pain* is felt suddenly from injury, disease, trauma, or surgery. There is tissue damage. Acute pain lasts a short time and lessens with healing.
- *Chronic pain (persistent pain)* continues for a long time (months or years) or occurs off and on. There is no longer tissue damage. Chronic pain remains long after healing. Arthritis is a common cause.
- *Radiating pain* is felt at the site of tissue damage and in nearby areas. Pain from a heart attack is often felt in the left chest, left jaw, left shoulder, and left arm. Gallbladder disease can cause pain in the right upper abdomen, the back, and the right shoulder (Fig. 25-24).
- *Phantom pain* is felt in a body part that is no longer there. For example, a person with an amputated leg still senses leg pain.

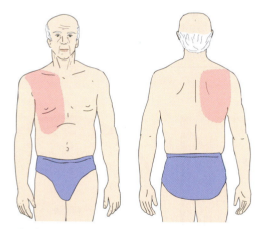

FIGURE 25-24 Gallbladder pain may radiate to the right upper abdomen, the back, and the right shoulder.

Signs and Symptoms

You cannot see, hear, feel, or smell the person's pain. Rely on what the person tells you. Promptly report information you collect about pain. Write down what the person says. Use the person's exact words to report and record. The nurse needs the following information.

- *Location.* Where is the pain? Ask the person to point to the area. Pain can radiate. Ask the person if the pain is anywhere else and to point to those areas.
- *Onset and duration.* When did the pain start? How long has it lasted?
- *Intensity.* Does the person complain of mild, moderate, or severe pain? Ask the person to rate the pain on a scale of 0 to 10, with 10 as the most severe (Fig. 25-25). Or use the *Wong-Baker FACES® Pain Rating Scale* (Fig. 25-26). Tell the person that each face shows how a person feels. Read the description for each face. Then ask the person to choose the face best describing how he or she feels.
- *Description.* Ask the person to describe the pain. *Ache, dull,* and *sharp* are examples.
- *Factors causing pain.* These are called *precipitating factors.* To *precipitate* means *to cause.* Such factors include moving or turning in bed, coughing or deep breathing, and exercise. Ask what the person was doing before the pain started and when it started.
- *Factors affecting pain.* Ask what makes the pain better. Also ask what makes it worse.
- *Vital signs.* Measure pulse, respirations, and blood pressure. Increases in these vital signs often occur with acute pain. Vital signs may be normal with chronic pain.
- *Other signs and symptoms.* Does the person have other symptoms—dizziness, nausea, vomiting, weakness, numbness or tingling, or others? Box 25-6 lists the signs and symptoms that often occur with pain. See *Focus on Communication: Signs and Symptoms.*

PAIN: Ask patient to rate pain on scale of 0-10	
No pain	Worst pain imaginable
0 1 2 3 4 5 6 7 8 9 10	

FIGURE 25-25 Pain rating scale. (From deWit SC, O'Neill P: *Fundamental concepts and skills for nursing,* ed 4, St Louis, 2014, Saunders.)

FIGURE 25-26 Wong-Baker FACES® Pain Rating Scale. (From Hockenberry MJ and others: *Wong's nursing care of infants and children,* ed 10, St Louis, 2015, Mosby.)

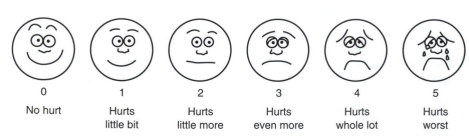

0	1	2	3	4	5
No hurt	Hurts little bit	Hurts little more	Hurts even more	Hurts whole lot	Hurts worst

BOX 25-6	Pain—Signs and Symptoms

Body Responses
- Appetite: changes in
- Dizziness
- Nausea; vomiting
- Numbness; tingling
- Skin: pale (*pallor*)
- Sleep: difficulty with
- Sweating (*diaphoresis*)
- Vital signs (pulse, respirations, and blood pressure): increased
- Weakness
- Weight loss

Behaviors
- Clenching the jaw
- Crying
- Frowning
- Gait: changes in; limping
- Gasping
- Grimacing
- Groaning; grunting; moaning
- Holding the affected body part (splinting; guarding)
- Irritability
- Mood: changes in; depressed
- Pacing
- Positioning: maintaining 1 position; refusing to move; frequent position changes
- Pulling away when touched
- Quietness
- Resisting care
- Restlessness
- Rubbing a body part or area
- Screaming
- Speech: slow or rapid; loud or quiet
- Whimpering

WEIGHT AND HEIGHT

Weight and height are measured on admission to the agency. Then the person is weighed daily, weekly, or monthly. Doing so measures weight gain or loss.

Standing scales are common. Chair, wheelchair, bed, and lift scales are used for persons who cannot stand. Follow the manufacturer's instructions and agency procedures.

To measure weight and height, follow these guidelines.
- The person wears only a patient gown or pajamas. Clothes add weight. Footwear adds to the weight and height measurements.
- The person voids before being weighed. A full bladder adds weight.
- A dry incontinence product is worn. A wet product adds weight.
- Weigh the person at the same time of day. Before breakfast is best. Food and fluids add weight.
- Use the same scale for daily, weekly, and monthly weights. Scales weigh differently.
- Balance the scale at zero (0) before weighing the person. For balance scales, move the weights to zero. A digital scale should read at zero.

See *Focus on Communication: Weight and Height.*
See *Focus on Math: Weight and Height,* p. 380.
See *Delegation Guidelines: Weight and Height,* p. 381.
See *Promoting Safety and Comfort: Weight and Height,* p. 381.
See procedure: *Measuring Weight and Height,* p. 381.

FOCUS ON COMMUNICATION

Signs and Symptoms

A person may say "hurt" or "discomfort" instead of "pain." Use words that the person uses.

Some persons have trouble rating pain intensity on a 0 to 10 scale. Instead, ask if the pain is mild, moderate, or severe.

FOCUS ON COMMUNICATION

Weight and Height

Some agencies use pounds (lb) for weight. Others use kilograms (kg) (2.2 lb = 1 kg). For height, some agencies use feet and inches. Others only use inches.

Ask the nurse what measurements to use. Follow agency policy for reporting and recording height and weight.

FOCUS ON MATH
Weight and Height

Weight—Reading the Scale

Standing scales (balance scales) have 2 bars with measurements (Fig. 25-27).

- The lower bar is divided into 50 lb values.
- The upper bar has long and short lines.
  - Long lines are 1 lb values.
  - Short lines are ¼, ½, and ¾ lb values.

The lower and upper bar values are added for the weight. For example, the lower bar is at 150 lb and the upper bar is at 22½ lb. The person's weight is 172½ lb.

$$150 \text{ lb} + 22\frac{1}{2} \text{ lb} = 172\frac{1}{2} \text{ lb}$$

Height—Reading the Height Rod

The height rod has 2 sections—upper and lower. Raise or lower the upper section to adjust to the person's height. If the person is taller than the lower section, read the height at the movable part of the height rod.

The rod is marked with 1 inch (in) and ¼ inch values (¼, ½, and ¾). Read height to the nearest ¼ inch. The numbers on the lower section increase moving up the rod. The numbers on the upper section increase moving down the rod. See Figure 25-28.

Height—Converting Inches Into Feet and Inches

There are 12 inches (in) in 1 foot (ft) (1 ft = 12 in). To convert inches into feet and inches, divide the number of inches by 12. If it does not divide evenly by 12, the number left over is the number of inches.

For example: Convert 64 inches into feet and inches.

```
                    5 Number of feet
12 Inches per foot | 64 Inches
                   −60
                     4 Number of inches
          64 inches = 5 ft 4 in
```

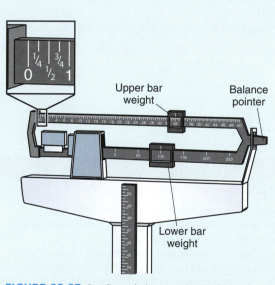

FIGURE 25-27 Reading a balance scale. On this scale the lower bar weight is at 100 lb. The upper bar weight is at 34 lb. The weight is 134 lb (100 lb + 34 lb = 134 lb).

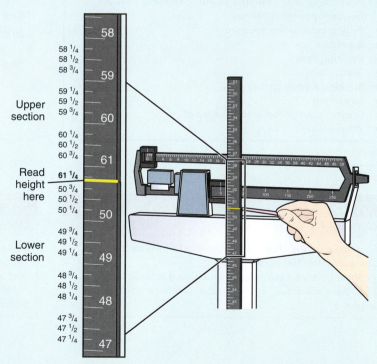

FIGURE 25-28 Height is read at the movable part of the height rod. (NOTE: The movable part of the height rod is marked with a yellow line.) This height rod measures 61¼ inches (5 feet 1¼ inches).

DELEGATION GUIDELINES
Weight and Height

To measure weight and height, you need this information from the nurse and the care plan.
- When to measure weight and height
- What scale to use
- When to report the measurements
- What patient or resident concerns to report at once

PROMOTING SAFETY AND COMFORT
Weight and Height

Safety

Follow the manufacturer's instructions for chair, wheelchair, bed, or lift scales. Also follow the agency's procedures. Practice safety measures to prevent falls.

Comfort

The person wears only a patient gown or pajamas for the weight measurement. Prevent chilling and drafts (Chapter 17).

 Measuring Weight and Height

QUALITY OF LIFE

- Knock before entering the person's room.
- Address the person by name.
- Introduce yourself by name and title.
- Explain the procedure before starting and during the procedure.
- Protect the person's rights during the procedure.
- Handle the person gently during the procedure.

PRE-PROCEDURE

1 Follow *Delegation Guidelines: Weight and Height.* See *Promoting Safety and Comfort: Weight and Height.*
2 Have the person void.
3 Practice hand hygiene.
4 Bring the scale and paper towels (for a standing scale) to the person's room.
5 Practice hand hygiene.
6 Identify the person. Check the ID bracelet against the assignment sheet. Use 2 identifiers (Chapter 10). Also call the person by name.
7 Provide for privacy.

PROCEDURE

8 Place the paper towels on the scale platform.
9 Raise the height rod.
10 Move the weights to zero (0). The pointer is in the middle.
11 Have the person remove the robe and footwear. Assist as needed. (NOTE: For some state competency tests, shoes are worn.)
12 Help the person stand in the center of the scale. Arms are at the sides. The person does not hold on to anyone or anything. See Figure 25-29, p. 382.
13 Move the lower and upper weights until the balance pointer is in the middle (see Fig. 25-27).
14 Note the weight on your note pad or assignment sheet.
15 Ask the person to stand very straight.
16 Lower the height rod until it rests on the person's head (Fig. 25-30, p. 382).
17 Read the height at the movable part of the height rod. Record the height in inches (or in feet and inches) to the nearest ¼ inch. See Figure 25-28.
18 Note the height on your note pad or assignment sheet.
19 Raise the height rod. Help the person step off the scale.
20 Help the person put on a robe and non-skid footwear if he or she will be up. Or help the person back to bed.
21 Lower the height rod. Adjust the weights to zero (0) if this is your agency's policy.

POST-PROCEDURE

22 Provide for comfort. (See the inside of the front cover.)
23 Place the call light and other needed items within reach.
24 Raise or lower bed rails. Follow the care plan.
25 Unscreen the person.
26 Complete a safety check of the room. (See the inside of the front cover.)
27 Discard the paper towels.
28 Return the scale to its proper place.
29 Practice hand hygiene.
30 Report and record the measurements.

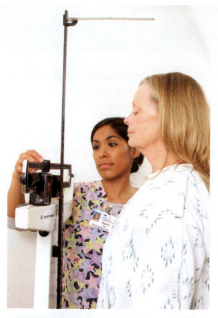

FIGURE 25-29 The person is weighed.

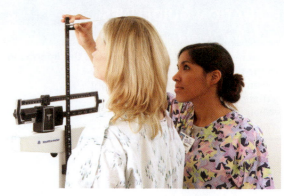

FIGURE 25-30 The height rod rests on the person's head.

FOCUS ON P R I D E

The Person, Family, and Yourself

Personal and Professional Responsibility

Measurements are an important part of your role. All measurements affect the person's health and well-being—vital signs, pain rating, and weight and height.

For vital signs, you must know the normal ranges. For an adult:

- Oral temperature—98.6 °F (37.0 °C). See Table 25-1 for normal temperatures at other sites.
- Pulse—60 to 100 beats per minute.
- Respirations—12 to 20 breaths per minute.
- Blood pressure—90/60 mm Hg or higher but lower than 120/80 mm Hg.

Learning to measure vital signs takes practice. Do not be upset if you struggle at first. Plan when and what you will practice. Use class time wisely. Tell your instructor if you need more practice. Never be ashamed to ask for more practice time. Practice builds confidence.

Rights and Respect

The nurse may ask you to re-take a measurement. You may need to use different equipment or change the person's position. For example, you need to weigh a person with a different scale. Or you need to use a different blood pressure cuff. Follow the nurse's directions.

The nurse may re-check the measurements. Do not be offended. Show respect. Avoid negative thoughts or statements about the nurse or yourself. It does not mean the nurse does not trust you or that you have done something wrong. The nurse checks the measurements for safe care.

Independence and Social Interaction

Personal choice promotes independence. The person may prefer a certain arm for pulses and blood pressures. If safe to do so, use the arm the esperson prefers. Unless directed otherwise, let the person choose to sit or lie when vital signs are measured.

Delegation and Teamwork

You may care for persons needing Transmission-Based Precautions (Chapter 13). You must prevent the spread of infection from equipment. Some agencies have isolation carts or kits with equipment. A stethoscope, blood pressure cuff, and thermometer are common. The equipment is left in the person's room. Do not use your own stethoscope or bring other equipment into the room. For example, do not bring a scale into the room. If equipment must be brought in, clean it after use. Special cleansers may be needed. Follow agency policy to protect others from infection.

Ethics and Laws

You may question the person's pain. For example, a patient rates a headache as a 9 on the 0 to 10 pain rating scale. The patient is working on a crossword puzzle. For a headache that severe, you rest. You question a pain rating of 9. You do not tell the nurse.

The patient's pain was severe. The crossword puzzle was a distraction. The pain was not relieved because it was not reported.

Pain is personal. It is handled in different ways. Ignoring pain is wrong. Reporting a different pain rating is wrong. Avoid making judgments about the person's pain. Accurate reporting is needed for proper pain management.

FOCUS ON PRIDE: Application

Plan to practice measurements at school and at home. Practice on classmates, family, and friends. Who will you practice with? What will you practice most at school? What can you practice at home?

REVIEW QUESTIONS

Circle the BEST answer.

1 Which should you report at once?
   a An oral temperature of 98.4°F
   b A rectal temperature of 101.6°F
   c An axillary temperature of 97.6°F
   d An oral temperature of 99.0°F

2 A rectal temperature is taken when the person
   a Is unconscious
   b Has heart disease
   c Is confused
   d Has diarrhea

3 To use an electronic thermometer
   a Shake down the thermometer before each use
   b Leave the thermometer in place for 2 minutes
   c Cover the probe with a probe cover
   d Use the blue probe for a rectal temperature

4 Which is usually used to take an adult's pulse?
   a The radial pulse
   b The apical pulse
   c The carotid pulse
   d The brachial pulse

5 For an adult, which pulse do you report at once?
   a A regular pulse at 64 beats per minute
   b A strong pulse at 78 beats per minute
   c A regular pulse at 90 beats per minute
   d An irregular pulse at 124 beats per minute

6 You count a regular pulse for 30 seconds. Which is *true*?
   a Divide the number of beats by 2 for the pulse rate.
   b If you count 44 beats, record a pulse rate of 44.
   c If you count 44 beats, record a pulse rate of 88.
   d Ask the nurse to check a regular pulse.

7 Which statement about measuring respirations is *true*?
   a Count the rise and fall of the chest as 2 respirations.
   b Count an abnormal pattern for 30 seconds.
   c A rate of 14 is abnormal for an adult.
   d Respirations are normally quiet.

8 Respirations are usually counted
   a After taking the temperature
   b Before taking the pulse
   c After taking the pulse
   d After taking the blood pressure

9 Which adult blood pressure is normal?
   a 88/54 mm Hg
   b 140/90 mm Hg
   c 112/78 mm Hg
   d 100/58 mm Hg

10 When measuring BP
   a Apply the cuff to the bare upper arm
   b Use the arm with an IV infusion
   c Make sure the cuff is loose
   d Place the stethoscope under the cuff

11 The systolic blood pressure is the point
   a Where the pulse is no longer felt
   b 30 mm Hg above where the pulse was felt
   c Where the first sound is heard
   d Where the last sound is heard

12 When taking a BP, you hear the last sound at the 1st short line above 70. You record the
   a Systolic pressure as 70
   b Diastolic pressure as 71
   c Systolic pressure as 72
   d Diastolic pressure as 72

13 You are not sure you heard a BP correctly. You should
   a Record what you think you heard
   b Measure the BP again after 60 seconds
   c Repeat the BP using the bell part of the stethoscope
   d Ask another nursing assistant to take the BP

14 A person has pain in the left chest, the left jaw, and the left shoulder and arm. This is
   a Gallbladder pain
   b Chronic pain
   c Radiating pain
   d Phantom pain

15 A person is restless and complains of pain. You should
   a Rate the intensity based on the person's behavior
   b Give a pain-relief drug and tell the nurse
   c Tell the nurse only if you think the person has pain
   d Report the person's exact words

16 You are about to measure weight with a standing scale. Which should you correct before weighing the person?
   a The person is wearing footwear.
   b The scale is balanced at zero (0).
   c There is a paper towel on the scale platform.
   d The person is in the center of the scale with arms at the sides.

17 When measuring height with a standing scale
   a Balance the height rod at zero (0)
   b Be sure footwear is worn
   c Read the height at the movable part of the rod
   d Record height to the nearest inch

18 What is 68 inches in feet and inches?
   a 4 ft 0 in
   b 5 ft 6 in
   c 5 ft 8 in
   d 6 ft 8 in

Answers to Chapter 25 questions are on p. 552.

FOCUS ON PRACTICE

Problem Solving

A person's pulse is 110. The respiratory rate is 24. The oral temperature is 100.8°F. You think you heard the BP at 86/52. You are unsure of the measurement. What will you do? Are any of the vital signs abnormal? What must you do?

OBJECTIVES

- Define the key terms and key abbreviations in this chapter.
- Explain why specimens are collected.
- Explain the rules for collecting specimens.
- Describe 3 types of urine specimens.
- Describe 5 urine tests.
- Explain how to use reagent strips.
- Describe how to collect a stool specimen.
- Describe how to collect a sputum specimen.
- Perform the procedures described in this chapter.
- Explain how to promote PRIDE in the person, the family, and yourself.

KEY TERMS

acetone See "ketone"
glucosuria Sugar (glucose) in the urine (uria)
hematuria Blood (hemat) in the urine (uria)
hemoptysis Bloody (hemo) sputum (ptysis means to spit)
ketone A substance appearing in urine from the rapid breakdown of fat for energy; acetone, ketone body

ketone body See "ketone"
sputum Mucus from the respiratory system that is expectorated (expelled) through the mouth

KEY ABBREVIATIONS

BM Bowel movement
ID Identification
I&O Intake and output

mL Milliliter
oz Ounce
U/A Urinalysis

Specimens (*samples*) are collected and tested to prevent, detect, and treat disease. Some specimens are tested at the bedside. Most are tested in the laboratory. All laboratory specimens require requisition slips with identifying information and the test ordered. The specimen container is labeled following agency policy. To collect specimens, follow the rules in Box 26-1.

See *Promoting Safety and Comfort: Collecting Specimens.*

| | | |

BOX 26-1   Collecting Specimens

- Follow the rules for medical asepsis.
- Follow Standard Precautions and the Bloodborne Pathogen Standard.
- Use a clean container for each specimen.
- Use the correct container.
- Do not touch the inside of the container or the inside of the lid.
- Identify the person. Check the ID (identification) bracelet against the laboratory requisition slip or assignment sheet. Compare all information. Ask the person to state his or her first and last name and birthdate.
- Label the container in the person's presence. Provide clear, accurate information.
- Collect the specimen at the correct time.
- Ask a female if she is having a menstrual period. Tell the nurse. Menstruating may cause blood to be in the urine specimen.
- Ask the person not to have a bowel movement (BM) when collecting a urine specimen. Urine specimens must not contain stools.
- Ask the person to void before collecting a stool specimen. Stool specimens must not contain urine.
- Have the person put toilet tissue in the toilet or wastebasket. Urine and stool specimens must not contain tissue.
- Secure the lid on the specimen container tightly.
- Place the specimen container in a labeled *BIOHAZARD* plastic bag. Do not let the container touch the outside of the bag. Seal the bag.
- Take the specimen and requisition slip to the laboratory or storage area.

PROMOTING SAFETY AND COMFORT
Collecting Specimens

Safety

Correct identification is important when collecting and testing specimens. To identify the person, check the ID bracelet against all information on the requisition slip. Agency policy may require asking the person to identify himself or herself by both of the following.
- Stating or spelling his or her first and last name
- Stating his or her birthdate

Blood, body fluids, secretions, and excretions may contain microbes and blood. This includes urine, stool, and sputum specimens. Follow Standard Precautions and the Bloodborne Pathogen Standard when collecting, testing, and handling specimens.

NOTE: A task may require more than 1 pair of gloves. Change gloves as needed. Use careful judgment. Remember to practice hand hygiene after removing gloves.

URINE SPECIMENS

Urine specimens are collected for urine tests. Follow the rules in Box 26-1.

See *Delegation Guidelines: Urine Specimens.*
See *Promoting Safety and Comfort: Urine Specimens.*

The Random Urine Specimen

The random urine specimen is used for a routine urinalysis (U/A). No special measures are needed. It is collected any time in a 24-hour period. Many people collect the specimen themselves. Weak and very ill persons need help.

See procedure: *Collecting a Random Urine Specimen, p. 386.*

DELEGATION GUIDELINES
Urine Specimens

To collect a urine specimen, you need this information from the nurse and the care plan.
- Voiding device—bedpan, urinal, commode, or toilet with specimen pan
- The type of specimen needed
- What time to collect the specimen
- What special measures are needed
- If you need to test the specimen (p. 389)
- If measuring intake and output (I&O) is ordered (Chapter 24)
- What observations to report and record:
  - Problems obtaining the specimen
  - Color, clarity, and odor of urine
  - Blood in the urine
  - Particles in the urine
  - Complaints of pain, burning, urgency, difficulty voiding, or other problems
  - The time the specimen was collected
- When to report observations
- What patient or resident concerns to report at once

PROMOTING SAFETY AND COMFORT
Urine Specimens

Comfort

Clear specimen containers show urine. This may embarrass some people. Cloudy urine specimen containers are common.

Collecting a Random Urine Specimen

QUALITY OF LIFE

- Knock before entering the person's room.
- Address the person by name.
- Introduce yourself by name and title.

- Explain the procedure before starting and during the procedure.
- Protect the person's rights during the procedure.
- Handle the person gently during the procedure.

PRE-PROCEDURE

1 Follow *Delegation Guidelines: Urine Specimens*, p. 385. See *Promoting Safety and Comfort:*
   a *Collecting Specimens*, p. 385
   b *Urine Specimens*, p. 385
2 Practice hand hygiene.
3 Collect the following before going to the person's room.
   - Laboratory requisition slip
   - Specimen container and lid
   - Voiding device (clean, un-used)—bedpan and cover, urinal, or specimen pan (Fig. 26-1)
   - Specimen label
   - Plastic bag
   - *BIOHAZARD* label (if needed)
   - Gloves

4 Arrange your work area.
5 Practice hand hygiene.
6 Identify the person. Check the ID bracelet against the requisition slip. Compare all information. Also call the person by name. Ask the person to state his or her first and last name and birthdate.
7 Label the container in the person's presence.
8 Put on gloves
9 Collect a commode (if needed) and a graduate to measure output.
10 Provide for privacy.

PROCEDURE

11 Place the specimen pan on the toilet or commode container (see Fig. 26-1).
12 Have the person urinate into the voiding device. Remind him or her to put toilet tissue into the wastebasket or toilet. Toilet tissue is not put in the bedpan or specimen pan.
13 Take the voiding device or commode container to the bathroom.
14 Pour about 120 mL (milliliters) (4 oz [ounces]) into the specimen container.
15 Place the lid on the specimen container tightly. Put the container in the plastic bag. Do not let the container touch the outside of the bag. Apply a *BIOHAZARD* label.

16 Measure urine if I&O are ordered. Include the specimen amount.
17 Empty, rinse, clean, disinfect, and dry equipment. Use clean, dry paper towels for drying. Return equipment to its proper place.
18 Remove and discard the gloves. Practice hand hygiene. Put on clean gloves.
19 Assist with hand-washing.
20 Remove and discard the gloves. Practice hand hygiene.

POST-PROCEDURE

21 Provide for comfort. (See the inside of the front cover.)
22 Place the call light and other needed items within reach.
23 Raise or lower bed rails. Follow the care plan.
24 Unscreen the person.
25 Complete a safety check of the room. (See the inside of the front cover.)

26 Practice hand hygiene.
27 Take the specimen and requisition slip to the laboratory or storage area. Wear gloves if that is agency policy.
28 Remove and discard the gloves. Practice hand hygiene.
29 Report and record your observations.

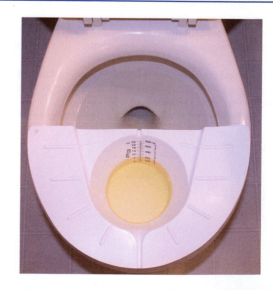

FIGURE 26-1 The specimen pan is at the front of the toilet on the toilet rim for a urine specimen. (NOTE: The toilet seat is lowered over the specimen pan for voiding.)

The Midstream Specimen

The midstream specimen is also called a *clean-voided specimen* or *clean-catch specimen*. The perineal area is cleaned first to reduce the number of microbes in the urethral area. The person starts to void into a device. Then the person stops the urine stream and a sterile specimen container is positioned. The person voids into the container until the specimen is obtained.

Stopping and starting the urine stream is hard for many people. You may need to position and hold the specimen container after the person starts to void (Fig. 26-2).

See *Focus on Communication: The Midstream Specimen.*
See procedure: *Collecting a Midstream Specimen.*

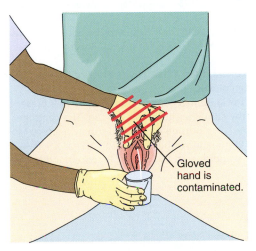

Gloved hand is contaminated.

FIGURE 26-2 The labia are separated to collect a midstream specimen.

FOCUS ON COMMUNICATION

The Midstream Specimen

Some persons can collect the midstream specimen without help. To explain the procedure, use words the person understands. Show the supplies and how to use them. Also, ask if the person has questions. For example:

> Ms. Jacobs, I need a midstream urine specimen. This means I need urine from the middle of your urine stream. First, wipe well with this towelette (show the towelette) from the front to back. The specimen goes in this cup (show the specimen cup). Please do not touch the inside of the cup. Start urinating and then stop. Position the cup to catch urine and start urinating again. If you cannot stop the stream, position the cup during the middle of the stream. I need at least this much urine if possible (point to the 30 mL measure on the cup). Remove the cup when it is about that full. Finish urinating. Secure the lid on top of the cup. Please do not touch the inside of the lid. I will take the specimen when you are done.

Then ask if the person has questions. Make sure the person understands what to do. You can say: "Please tell me what you will do so I know that you understand."

Collecting a Midstream Specimen

QUALITY OF LIFE

- Knock before entering the person's room.
- Address the person by name.
- Introduce yourself by name and title.

- Explain the procedure before starting and during the procedure.
- Protect the person's rights during the procedure.
- Handle the person gently during the procedure.

PRE-PROCEDURE

1 Follow *Delegation Guidelines: Urine Specimens, p. 385.* See *Promoting Safety and Comfort:*
   a *Collecting Specimens*, p. 385
   b *Urine Specimens*, p. 385
2 Practice hand hygiene.
3 Collect the following before going to the person's room.
   - Laboratory requisition slip
   - Midstream specimen kit—specimen container, label, towelettes, sterile gloves
   - Plastic bag
   - Sterile gloves (if not part of the specimen kit and required by agency policy)
   - Disposable gloves
   - *BIOHAZARD* label (if needed)

4 Arrange your work area.
5 Practice hand hygiene.
6 Identify the person. Check the ID bracelet against the requisition slip. Compare all information. Also call the person by name. Ask the person to state his or her first and last name and birthdate.
7 Put on gloves.
8 Collect the following.
   - Voiding device—bedpan and cover, urinal, commode, or specimen pan if needed
   - Supplies for perineal care (Chapter 18)
   - Graduate to measure output
   - Paper towels
9 Provide for privacy.

Continued

Collecting a Midstream Specimen—cont'd

PROCEDURE

10 Provide perineal care (Chapter 18). (Wear gloves for this step. Practice hand hygiene after removing and discarding them.)
11 Open the sterile kit.
12 Put on the gloves. Apply sterile gloves if required by agency policy.
13 Open the packet of towelettes.
14 Open the sterile specimen container. Do not touch the inside of the container or lid. Set the lid down with the inside up.
15 *For a female*—clean the perineal area with towelettes.
   a Spread the labia with your thumb and index finger. Use your non-dominant hand. (This hand is now contaminated. It must not touch anything sterile.)
   b Clean down the urethral area from front to back (top to bottom). Use a clean towelette for each stroke.
   c Keep the labia separated to collect the specimen (steps 17 through 20).
16 *For a male*—clean the penis with towelettes.
   a Hold the penis with your non-dominant hand. (This hand is now contaminated. It must not touch anything sterile.)
   b Clean the penis starting at the meatus. (Retract the foreskin if the male is uncircumcised.) Clean in a circular motion. Start at the center and work outward.
   c Hold the penis (and keep the foreskin retracted in the uncircumcised male) until the specimen is collected (steps 17 through 20).

17 Have the person void into a device.
18 Pass the specimen container into the urine stream. Keep the labia separated (see Fig. 26-2).
19 Collect about 30 to 60 mL (1 to 2 oz) of urine.
20 Remove the specimen container before the person stops voiding. Release the foreskin of the uncircumcised male.
21 Release the labia or penis. Let the person finish voiding into the device.
22 Put the lid on the specimen container. Touch only the outside of the container and lid. Wipe the outside of the container. Set the container on a paper towel.
23 Provide toilet tissue when the person is done voiding.
24 Take the voiding device to the bathroom.
25 Measure urine if I&O are ordered. Include the specimen amount.
26 Empty, rinse, clean, disinfect, and dry equipment. Use clean, dry paper towels for drying. Return equipment to its proper place.
27 Remove and discard the gloves. Practice hand hygiene. Put on clean gloves.
28 Label the specimen container in the person's presence. Place the container in the plastic bag. The container must not touch the outside of the bag. Apply a *BIOHAZARD* label.
29 Assist with hand-washing.
30 Remove and discard the gloves. Practice hand hygiene.

POST-PROCEDURE

31 Provide for comfort. (See the inside of the front cover.)
32 Place the call light and other needed items within reach.
33 Raise or lower the bed rails. Follow the care plan.
34 Unscreen the person.
35 Complete a safety check of the room. (See the inside of the front cover.)

36 Practice hand hygiene.
37 Take the specimen and requisition slip to the laboratory or storage area. Wear gloves if that is agency policy.
38 Remove and discard the gloves. Practice hand hygiene.
39 Report and record your observations.

The 24-Hour Urine Specimen

All urine voided during 24 hours is collected for a 24-hour urine specimen. To prevent microbe growth, the urine is chilled on ice or refrigerated. A preservative may be added to the collection container.

The person voids to start the test with an empty bladder. Discard this voiding. Save *all voidings* for the next 24 hours. The person and staff must clearly understand the procedure and the test period. This test is re-started if:

- A voiding was not saved.
- Toilet tissue was discarded into the specimen.
- The specimen contains stools.

Testing Urine

The doctor orders the type and frequency of urine tests. Random urine specimens are needed. The nurse may have you do these simple tests.

- *Testing for pH*—Urine pH measures if urine is acidic or alkaline. Changes in normal pH (4.6 to 8.0) occur from illness, food, and drugs.
- *Testing for blood*—Injury and disease can cause hematuria. ***Hematuria** means blood* (hemat) *in the urine* (uria). Sometimes blood is seen in the urine. At other times it is unseen *(occult).*
- *Testing for glucose and ketones*—In diabetes, the pancreas does not secrete enough insulin (Chapter 33). The body needs insulin to use sugar for energy. If not used, sugar builds up in the blood. Some sugar appears in the urine. ***Glucosuria** means sugar* (glucose) *in the urine* (uria). Diabetes may cause ketones in the urine. ***Ketones (ketone bodies, acetone) are substances appearing in urine from the rapid breakdown of fat for energy.*** The body uses fat for energy if it cannot use sugar. Tests for glucose and ketones are usually done 4 times a day—30 minutes before meals and at bedtime. Test results are used for drug and diet decisions.
- *Testing for infection*—The presence of certain white blood cells can signal a urinary tract infection.
- *Testing for protein*—Protein in the urine can signal kidney and other diseases.

■ Using Reagent Strips. Reagent strips (test strips) have sections that change color when reacting with urine. To use a reagent (test) strip:

- Do not touch the test area on the strip.
- Dip the strip into urine.
- Compare the strip with the color chart on the bottle (Fig. 26-3).
  See *Delegation Guidelines: Testing Urine.*
  See *Promoting Safety and Comfort: Testing Urine.*
  See procedure: *Testing Urine With Reagent Strips,*
  p. 390.

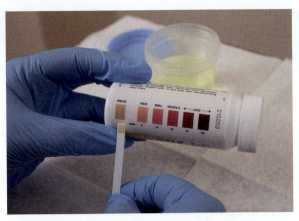

FIGURE 26-3 Reagent (test) strip for sugar and ketones.

DELEGATION GUIDELINES
Testing Urine

When testing urine is delegated to you, you need this information from the nurse and the care plan.

- What test is needed
- What equipment to use
- When to test urine
- Instructions for the test ordered
- If the nurse will observe test results
- What observations to report and record:
  - The time you collected and tested the specimen
  - Test results
  - Problems obtaining the specimen
  - Color, clarity, and odor of urine
  - Blood in the urine
  - Particles in the urine
  - Complaints of pain, burning, urgency, difficulty voiding, or other problems
- When to report test results and observations
- What patient or resident concerns to report at once

PROMOTING SAFETY AND COMFORT
Testing Urine

Safety
Accuracy is important. Promptly report results. Ordered drugs may depend on the results.
    When using reagent (test) strips:

- Check the color of the strips. Do not use discolored strips.
- Check the expiration date on the bottle. Do not use the strips if the date has passed.
- Follow the manufacturer's instructions for an accurate result. Test results are used for diagnosis and treatment. A wrong result can cause serious harm.

Testing Urine With Reagent Strips

QUALITY OF LIFE

- Knock before entering the person's room.
- Address the person by name.
- Introduce yourself by name and title.

- Explain the procedure before starting and during the procedure.
- Protect the person's rights during the procedure.
- Handle the person gently during the procedure.

PRE-PROCEDURE

1 Follow *Delegation Guidelines: Testing Urine*, p. 389. See *Promoting Safety and Comfort:*
   a *Collecting Specimens*, p. 385
   b *Testing Urine*, p. 389
2 Practice hand hygiene.
3 Collect gloves and the reagent (test) strips ordered.
4 Practice hand hygiene.

5 Identify the person. Check the ID bracelet against the assignment sheet. Use 2 identifiers (Chapter 10). Also call the person by name. Ask the person to state his or her first and last name and birthdate.
6 Put on gloves.
7 Collect equipment for the urine specimen. (See procedure: *Collecting a Random Urine Specimen*, p. 386.)
8 Provide for privacy.

PROCEDURE

9 Collect the urine specimen. (See procedure: *Collecting a Random Urine Specimen*, p. 386.)
10 Remove a strip from the bottle. Put the cap tightly on the bottle at once.
11 Dip the strip test area into the urine.
12 Remove the strip after the correct amount of time. See the manufacturer's instructions.
13 Tap the strip gently against the urine container. This removes excess urine.

14 Wait the required amount of time. See the manufacturer's instructions.
15 Compare the strip with the color chart on the bottle (see Fig. 26-3). Read the results.
16 Discard disposable items and the specimen.
17 Empty, rinse, clean, disinfect, and dry equipment. Use clean, dry paper towels for drying. Return equipment to its proper place.
18 Remove and discard the gloves. Practice hand hygiene.

POST-PROCEDURE

19 Provide for comfort. (See the inside of the front cover.)
20 Place the call light and other needed items within reach.
21 Raise or lower bed rails. Follow the care plan.
22 Unscreen the person.

23 Complete a safety check of the room. (See the inside of the front cover.)
24 Practice hand hygiene.
25 Report and record the test results and other observations.

STOOL SPECIMENS

Stools are studied for fat, microbes, worms, blood, and other abnormal contents. Urine must not contaminate the stool specimen. The person uses 1 device for voiding and another for a BM.

Some tests require a warm stool. The specimen is taken at once to the laboratory or storage area. Follow the rules in Box 26-1.

See *Focus on Communication: Stool Specimens.*
See *Delegation Guidelines: Stool Specimens.*
See *Promoting Safety and Comfort: Stool Specimens.*
See procedure: *Collecting a Stool Specimen.*

FOCUS ON COMMUNICATION

Stool Specimens

Before you begin, explain what the person needs to do and what you will do. Show the equipment and supplies and how to use them. For example:

I need to collect a specimen from a bowel movement. I'm going to place the specimen pan (show specimen pan) at the back of the toilet. Urinate into the toilet (urinal). Your bowel movement collects in the specimen pan. Please put toilet tissue in the toilet, not in the specimen pan. After your bowel movement, put your call light on right away. I'll collect the specimen in this container (show the specimen container).

Then ask if the person has questions. If you do not know the answer, tell the nurse.

Make sure the person understands what to do. You can say: "Please tell me what you will do so I know that you understand."

DELEGATION GUIDELINES

Stool Specimens

Before collecting a stool specimen, you need this information from the nurse.
- What time to collect the specimen
- What equipment and special measures are needed
- If the nurse wants to observe the stool
- What observations to report and record:
  - The time you collected the specimen
  - Problems obtaining the specimen
  - Color, amount, consistency, and odor of stools
  - Complaints of pain or discomfort
- When to report observations
- What patient or resident concerns to report at once

PROMOTING SAFETY AND COMFORT
Stool Specimens

Comfort
Stools normally have an odor. A person may be embarrassed that you need a specimen. Complete the task quickly and carefully. Act in a professional manner.

Collecting a Stool Specimen

QUALITY OF LIFE

- Knock before entering the person's room.
- Address the person by name.
- Introduce yourself by name and title.

- Explain the procedure before starting and during the procedure.
- Protect the person's rights during the procedure.
- Handle the person gently during the procedure.

PRE-PROCEDURE

1 Follow *Delegation Guidelines: Stool Specimens.* See *Promoting Safety and Comfort:*
   a *Collecting Specimens,* p. 385
   b *Stool Specimens*
2 Practice hand hygiene.
3 Collect the following before going to the person's room.
   - Laboratory requisition slip
   - Specimen pan for the toilet
   - Stool specimen container and lid
   - Specimen label
   - Tongue blades
   - Disposable bag
   - Plastic bag
   - *BIOHAZARD* label (if needed)
   - Gloves

4 Arrange collected items in the person's bathroom.
5 Practice hand hygiene.
6 Identify the person. Check the ID bracelet against the requisition slip. Compare all information. Also call the person by name. Ask the person to state his or her first and last name and birthdate.
7 Label the specimen container in the person's presence.
8 Put on gloves.
9 Collect the following.
   - Device for voiding—bedpan and cover, urinal, commode, or specimen pan
   - Toilet tissue
10 Provide for privacy.

PROCEDURE

11 Have the person void. Provide the voiding device if not using the bathroom. Empty, rinse, clean, disinfect, and dry the device. Use clean, dry paper towels for drying. Return it to its proper place.
12 Put the specimen pan on the toilet for bathroom use. Place it at the back of the toilet (Fig. 26-4, p. 392). Or provide the bedpan or commode.
13 Ask the person not to put toilet tissue into the bedpan, commode, or specimen pan. Provide a bag for toilet tissue.
14 Place the call light and toilet tissue within reach. Raise or lower bed rails. Follow the care plan.
15 Remove and discard the gloves. Practice hand hygiene. Leave the room if the person can be left alone.
16 Return when the person signals. Or check on the person every 5 minutes. Knock before entering.
17 Practice hand hygiene. Put on clean gloves.
18 Lower the bed rail near you if up. Remove the bedpan (if used). Or assist the person off the toilet or commode (if used). Provide perineal care if needed.
19 Note the color, amount, consistency, and odor of stools.

20 Collect the specimen.
   a Use a tongue blade to take about 2 tablespoons of stool to the specimen container (Fig. 26-5, p. 392). Take the sample from:
      1 The middle of a formed stool
      2 Areas of pus, mucus, or blood and watery areas
      3 The middle and both ends of a hard stool
   b Put the lid on the specimen container.
   c Place the container in the plastic bag. Do not let the container touch the outside of the bag. Apply a *BIOHAZARD* label according to agency policy.
   d Wrap the tongue blade in toilet tissue. Discard it in the disposable bag.
21 Remove and discard the gloves. Practice hand hygiene. Put on clean gloves.
22 Empty, rinse, clean, disinfect, and dry equipment. Use clean, dry paper towels for drying. Return equipment to its proper place.
23 Remove and discard the gloves. Practice hand hygiene. Put on clean gloves.
24 Assist with hand-washing.
25 Remove and discard the gloves. Practice hand hygiene.

POST-PROCEDURE

26 Provide for comfort. (See the inside of the front cover.)
27 Place the call light and other needed items within reach.
28 Raise or lower bed rails. Follow the care plan.
29 Unscreen the person.
30 Complete a safety check of the room. (See the inside of the front cover.)

31 Deliver the specimen and requisition slip to the laboratory or storage area. Follow agency policy. Wear gloves if that is agency policy.
32 Remove and discard the gloves. Practice hand hygiene.
33 Report and record your observations.

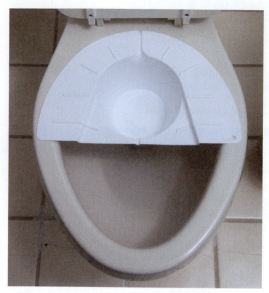

FIGURE 26-4 The specimen pan is placed at the back of the toilet for a stool specimen. (NOTE: The toilet seat is lowered over the specimen pan for the BM.)

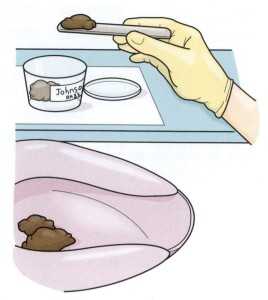

FIGURE 26-5 A tongue blade is used to transfer a small amount of stool from the bedpan to the specimen container.

SPUTUM SPECIMENS

Respiratory disorders cause the lungs, bronchi, and trachea to secrete mucus. *Mucus from the respiratory system is called* **sputum** *when expectorated (expelled) through the mouth.* Sputum specimens are studied for blood, microbes, and abnormal cells.

Sputum is coughed up from the bronchi and trachea. This is often painful and hard to do. Collecting a specimen is easier in the morning. Secretions collect in the trachea and bronchi during sleep. They are coughed up on awakening.

Follow the rules in Box 26-1. Also have the person rinse the mouth with water. Rinsing decreases saliva and removes food particles. Mouthwash is not used. It destroys some of the microbes in the mouth.

See *Delegation Guidelines: Sputum Specimens.*
See *Promoting Safety and Comfort: Sputum Specimens.*
See procedure: *Collecting a Sputum Specimen.*

Collecting a Sputum Specimen

QUALITY OF LIFE

- Knock before entering the person's room.
- Address the person by name.
- Introduce yourself by name and title.

- Explain the procedure before starting and during the procedure.
- Protect the person's rights during the procedure.
- Handle the person gently during the procedure.

PRE-PROCEDURE

1 Follow *Delegation Guidelines: Sputum Specimens.* See *Promoting Safety and Comfort:*
  a *Collecting Specimens,* p. 385
  b *Sputum Specimens*
2 Practice hand hygiene.
3 Collect the following before going to the person's room.
  - Laboratory requisition slip
  - Sputum specimen container and lid
  - Specimen label
  - Plastic bag
  - *BIOHAZARD* label (if needed)

4 Arrange collected items in the person's bathroom.
5 Practice hand hygiene.
6 Identify the person. Check the ID bracelet against the requisition slip. Compare all information. Also call the person by name. Ask the person to state his or her first and last name and birthdate.
7 Label the specimen container in the person's presence.
8 Collect gloves and tissues.
9 Provide for privacy. If able, the person uses the bathroom for the procedure.

PROCEDURE

10 Put on gloves.
11 Have the person rinse the mouth with clear water.
12 Have the person hold the container. Only the outside is touched.
13 Have the person cover the mouth and nose with tissues when coughing. Follow agency policy for used tissues.
14 Have the person take 2 or 3 breaths and cough up the sputum.
15 Have the person expectorate (spit) directly into the container (Fig. 26-6). Sputum must not touch the outside of the container.

16 Collect 1 to 2 teaspoons of sputum unless told to collect more.
17 Put the lid on the container.
18 Place the container in the plastic bag. Do not let the container touch the outside of the bag. Apply a *BIOHAZARD* label according to agency policy.
19 Remove and discard the gloves. Practice hand hygiene. Put on clean gloves.
20 Assist with hand-washing.
21 Remove and discard the gloves. Practice hand hygiene.

POST-PROCEDURE

22 Provide for comfort. (See the inside of the front cover.)
23 Place the call light and other needed items within reach.
24 Raise or lower bed rails. Follow the care plan.
25 Unscreen the person.
26 Complete a safety check of the room. (See the inside of the front cover.)

27 Practice hand hygiene.
28 Deliver the specimen and the requisition slip to the laboratory or storage area. Follow agency policy. Wear gloves if that is agency policy.
29 Remove and discard the gloves. Practice hand hygiene.
30 Report and record your observations.

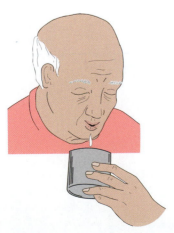

FIGURE 26-6 The person expectorates into the center of the specimen container.

BLOOD GLUCOSE TESTING

Blood glucose testing is used for persons with diabetes. The skin is punctured and a drop of blood is collected and tested (Fig. 26-7). Results are used to regulate drugs and diet.

If your state and agency allow you to perform blood glucose testing, make sure that:

- You have the necessary training.
- You know how to use the agency's equipment.
- You review the procedure with a nurse.
- The nurse is available to answer questions and to supervise you.

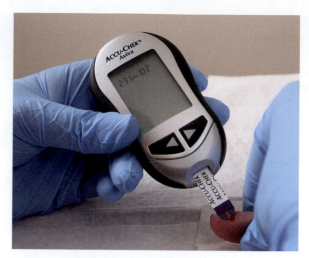

FIGURE 26-7 A blood glucose test.

FOCUS ON **P R I D E**

The Person, Family, and Yourself

Personal and Professional Responsibility

You must collect specimens on the right person. Otherwise, one or both persons could be harmed. Before collecting a specimen, carefully identify the person. Compare all information on the requisition slip and ID bracelet, not just the person's name. Also ask the person to state his or her first and last name and state his or her birthdate.

In some agencies, collection information is written on the specimen container. Collection date and time and the collector's name or initials are examples. Follow agency policy to label specimens. Take pride in properly collecting and labeling specimens.

Rights and Respect

Specimen collection can be embarrassing. To respect the right to privacy:

- Politely ask visitors to leave the room.
- Close doors, privacy curtains, and window coverings.
- Leave the room if it is safe to do so. If you cannot leave, tell the person why.

Independence and Social Interaction

Some persons can collect their own specimens. Doing so promotes independence and reduces embarrassment.

Explain the procedure and show the person the container. Ask the person where to place the container. When ready to collect the specimen, the person knows where to find the container.

Delegation and Teamwork

Before taking a specimen to the laboratory, tell the nurse and your co-workers. Ask if other staff need specimens delivered. Doing so saves staff time. This also prevents having too many staff members off the unit at the same time. Return from the laboratory promptly.

Ethics and Laws

If you did not collect a specimen correctly, do not send it to the laboratory. Tell the nurse. Then collect the specimen at the next opportunity. Test results must be accurate for correct diagnosis and treatment. Take pride in honestly reporting mistakes.

FOCUS ON PRIDE: *Application*

What mistakes could occur in specimen collection? What can you do to prevent such mistakes? Explain why failing to report a mistake can be harmful.

REVIEW QUESTIONS

Circle the BEST answer.

1 Which specimen was collected *correctly*?
   a A stool specimen that contains urine
   b A urine specimen that contains toilet tissue
   c A sputum specimen with a label and requisition slip
   d A urine specimen with a loose lid

2 A random urine specimen is collected
   a After sleep
   b Before meals
   c After meals
   d Any time

3 Perineal care is given before collecting a
   a Random specimen
   b Midstream specimen
   c 24-hour specimen
   d Stool specimen

4 To collect a midstream specimen on a female
   a Spread the labia to expose the urethral area
   b Clean the urethral area from back to front
   c Collect urine at the start of the urine stream
   d Collect about 10 mL of urine

5 Urine is tested for glucose
   a To measure the pH
   b To check for blood
   c To check for sugar
   d To check for ketones

6 A warm stool specimen is needed. After collecting the specimen
   a Put it in an oven
   b Put it in a paper bag
   c Cover it with a towel
   d Take it to the laboratory or storage area

7 The best time to collect a sputum specimen is
   a On awakening
   b After meals
   c At bedtime
   d After oral hygiene

8 A sputum specimen is needed. Have the person
   a Use mouthwash
   b Rinse the mouth with clear water
   c Brush the teeth
   d Remove dentures

Answers to Chapter 26 questions are on p. 552.

FOCUS ON PRACTICE

Problem Solving

A midstream urine specimen is ordered. You give the patient the specimen cup and pack of towelettes and ask: "Do you know what to do?" The patient says: "Yes, I've done this before." You tell the patient to leave the specimen in the bathroom and signal for you when done.

You return and notice the towelettes are unopened. What do you do? Should you send the specimen to the laboratory? How could this have been prevented?

Exercise and Activity Needs

OBJECTIVES

- Define the key terms and key abbreviations in this chapter.
- Describe bedrest.
- Explain how to prevent the complications from bedrest.
- Describe the devices that support and maintain body alignment.
- Describe range-of-motion exercises.
- Describe 4 walking aids.
- Perform the procedures described in this chapter.
- Explain how to promote PRIDE in the person, the family, and yourself.

KEY TERMS

abduction Moving a body part away from the mid-line of the body
adduction Moving a body part toward the mid-line of the body
ambulation The act of walking
atrophy The decrease in size or wasting away of tissue
contracture The lack of joint mobility caused by abnormal shortening of a muscle
dorsiflexion Bending the toes and foot up at the ankle
extension Straightening a body part
external rotation Turning the joint outward
flexion Bending a body part
footdrop The foot falls down at the ankle; permanent plantar flexion
hyperextension Excessive straightening of a body part
internal rotation Turning the joint inward

opposition Touching an opposite finger with the thumb
orthostatic hypotension Abnormally low (hypo) blood pressure when the person suddenly stands up (ortho and static); postural hypotension
orthotic device A device used to support a muscle, promote a certain motion, or correct a deformity; ortho means to straighten
plantar flexion The foot (plantar) is bent (flexion); bending the foot down at the ankle
postural hypotension See "orthostatic hypotension"
pronation Turning the joint downward
range of motion (ROM) The movement of a joint to the extent possible without causing pain
rotation Turning the joint
supination Turning the joint upward

KEY ABBREVIATIONS

ADL	Activities of daily living		PROM	Passive range of motion
ID	Identification		ROM	Range of motion

Illness, surgery, injury, pain, and aging cause weakness and some activity limits. Inactivity, whether mild or severe, affects every body system and mental well-being.

You help promote exercise and activity in all persons to the extent possible. The care plan and your assignment sheet include the person's activity level and needed exercises.

See *Focus on Older Persons: Exercise and Activity Needs.*

FOCUS ON OLDER PERSONS

Exercise and Activity Needs

Persons with dementia may resist exercise and activity. They do not understand what is happening and may fear harm. They may become agitated and combative. Some cry out for help. Do not force the person to exercise or take part in activities. Stay calm and ask the nurse for help. Follow the care plan.

BEDREST

The doctor orders bedrest to treat a health problem. Or it is a nursing measure if the person's condition changes. Bedrest is ordered to:

- Reduce physical activity.
- Reduce pain.
- Encourage rest.
- Regain strength.
- Promote healing.
  These types of bedrest are common.
- *Strict bedrest.* Everything is done for the person. All activities of daily living (ADL) are done in bed.
- *Bedrest.* The person performs some ADL. Self-feeding, oral hygiene, bathing, shaving, and hair care are often allowed.
- *Bedrest with commode privileges.* The commode is used at the bedside for elimination.
- *Bedrest with bathroom privileges (bedrest with BRP).* The bathroom is used for elimination.

The care plan and your assignment sheet state the activities allowed. Always ask the nurse what bedrest means for each person. Ask the nurse if you have questions about a person's activity limits.

Complications From Bedrest

Bedrest and lack of exercise and activity can cause serious complications. Pressure injuries, constipation, and fecal impaction can result. Urinary tract infections and renal calculi (kidney stones) can occur. So can blood clots (thrombi) and pneumonia (inflammation and infection of the lung).

The musculo-skeletal system is affected too. For normal movement, you must help prevent the following.

- A ***contracture*** *is the lack of joint mobility caused by abnormal shortening of a muscle.* The contracted muscle is fixed into position, is deformed, and cannot stretch (Fig. 27-1). Common sites are the fingers, wrists, elbows, toes, ankles, knees, and hips. They can also occur in the neck and spine. The site is deformed and stiff.
- ***Atrophy*** *is the decrease in size or the wasting away of tissue.* Tissues shrink in size. *Muscle atrophy* is a decrease in size or a wasting away of muscle (Fig. 27-2).

Orthostatic hypotension *is abnormally low (hypo) blood pressure when the person suddenly stands up (ortho and static).* When a person moves from a lying to sitting to standing position, the blood pressure drops. The person is dizzy, weak, and has spots before the eyes. *Orthostatic hypotension also is called* **postural hypotension.** *(Postural relates to posture or standing.)* Slowly changing positions is key. Have the person sit or lie down if orthostatic hypotension occurs.

Good nursing care prevents complications from bedrest. Good alignment, range-of-motion exercises (p. 399), and frequent position changes are important measures. These are part of the care plan.

See *Focus on Communication: Complications of Bedrest.*

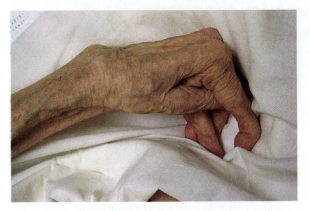

FIGURE 27-1 A contracture.

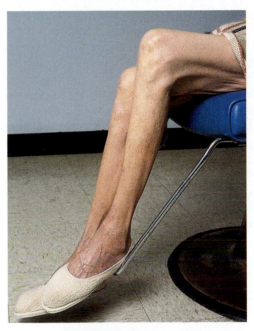

FIGURE 27-2 Muscle atrophy.

FOCUS ON COMMUNICATION

Complications of Bedrest

Orthostatic hypotension can occur when moving from lying to sitting or standing. To check for orthostatic hypotension, ask these questions.

- "Do you feel weak?"
- "Do you feel dizzy?"
- "Do you see spots before your eyes?"
- "Do you feel like fainting?"

Positioning

Body alignment and positioning were discussed in Chapter 14. Supportive devices are often used to support and maintain a certain position.

- *Foot-board*—prevents plantar flexion that can lead to footdrop. In ***plantar flexion***, *the foot* (plantar) *is bent* (flexion). ***Footdrop*** *is when the foot falls down at the ankle (permanent plantar flexion).* The foot-board is placed so the soles of the feet are flush against it (Fig. 27-3). Foot-boards also serve as bed cradles by keeping top linens off the feet and toes.
- *Trochanter roll*—prevents the hips and legs from turning outward (external rotation) (Fig. 27-4). A bath blanket is folded to the desired length and rolled up. The loose end is under the person from the hip to the knee. The roll is tucked alongside the body.
- *Hip abduction wedge*—keeps the hips abducted (apart) (Fig. 27-5). The wedge is placed between the person's legs. The device is common after hip replacement surgery.
- *Splints*—keep the elbows, wrists, thumbs, fingers, ankles, or knees in normal position. They are usually secured in place with Velcro (Fig. 27-6).
- *Hand roll or hand grip*—prevents contractures of the thumb, fingers, and wrist (Fig. 27-7). Foam rubber sponges, rubber balls, and finger cushions (Fig. 27-8) also are used.
- *Bed cradle*—keeps the weight of top linens off the feet and toes (Fig. 27-9). Heavy top linens can cause footdrop and pressure injuries.

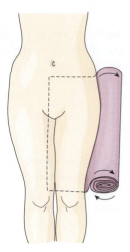

FIGURE 27-4 A trochanter roll is made from a bath blanket. It extends from the hip to the knee.

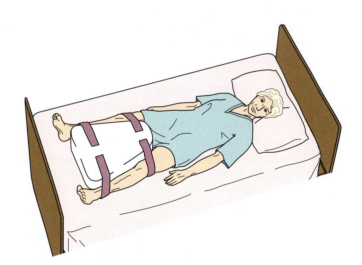

FIGURE 27-5 Hip abduction wedge.

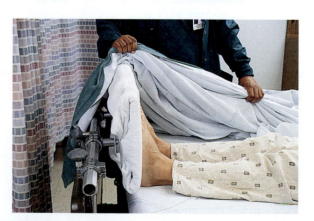

FIGURE 27-3 A foot-board. Feet are flush with the board to keep them in normal alignment.

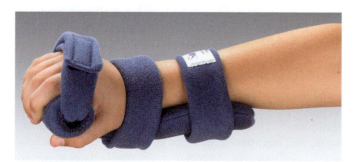

FIGURE 27-6 A splint. (Courtesy Ongoing Care Solutions, Inc., Pinellas Park, Florida.)

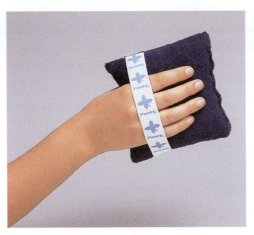

FIGURE 27-7 Hand grip. (Image courtesy Posey Company, Arcadia, Calif.)

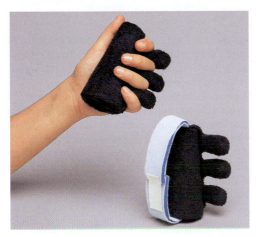

FIGURE 27-8 Finger cushion. (Image courtesy Posey Company, Arcadia, Calif.)

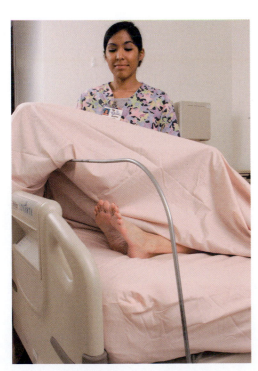

FIGURE 27-9 A bed cradle.

Exercise

Exercise helps prevent contractures, muscle atrophy, and other complications from bedrest. Some exercise occurs with ADL. Other exercises are needed for muscles and joints. (See "Range-of-Motion Exercises" and "Ambulation," p. 404.)

RANGE-OF-MOTION EXERCISES

*The movement of a joint to the extent possible without causing pain is the **range of motion (ROM)** of the joint.* Range-of-motion exercises involve moving the joints through their complete range of motion (Box 27-1). They are usually done at least 2 times a day.

* *Active* ROM exercises—are done by the person.
* *Passive* ROM (PROM) exercises—you move the joints through their range of motion.
* *Active-assistive* ROM exercises—the person does the exercises with some help.

See *Focus on Communication: Range-of-Motion Exercises,* p. 400.

See *Focus on Surveys: Range-of-Motion Exercises,* p. 400.

See *Delegation Guidelines: Range-of-Motion Exercises,* p. 400.

See *Promoting Safety and Comfort: Range-of-Motion Exercises,* p. 400.

See procedure: *Performing Range-of-Motion Exercises,* p. 401.

Text continued on p. 404.

BOX 27-1	Range-of-Motion Exercises

Joint Movements
* *Abduction*—moving a body part away from the mid-line of the body
* *Adduction*—moving a body part toward the mid-line of the body
* *Opposition*—touching an opposite finger with the thumb
* *Flexion*—bending a body part
* *Extension*—straightening a body part
* *Hyperextension*—excessive straightening of a body part
* *Dorsiflexion*—bending the toes and foot up at the ankle
* *Plantar flexion*—bending the foot down at the ankle
* *Rotation*—turning the joint
* *Internal rotation*—turning the joint inward
* *External rotation*—turning the joint outward
* *Pronation*—turning the joint downward
* *Supination*—turning the joint upward

Safety Measures
* Cover the person with a bath blanket for warmth and privacy.
* Exercise only the joints the nurse tells you to exercise.
* Expose only the body parts being exercised.
* Use good body mechanics.
* Support the part being exercised.
* Move the joint slowly, smoothly, and gently.
* Do not force a joint beyond its present range of motion.
* Do not force a joint to the point of pain.
* Ask the person if he or she has pain or discomfort.

FOCUS ON COMMUNICATION

Range-of-Motion Exercises

Do not force a joint beyond its present range of motion or to the point of pain. Ask if the person:
- Feels that the joint cannot move any farther.
- Feels pain or discomfort in the joint.
- Needs to stop or rest.

The person may not be able to tell you about discomfort or limited joint movement. Observe for signs of pain (Chapter 25). Restlessness and grimacing are examples. Stop if you suspect pain or meet resistance. Tell the nurse.

FOCUS ON SURVEYS

Range-of-Motion Exercises

The person's care plan must focus on his or her ROM. The goal may be 1 of the following.
- Increase range of motion.
- Prevent loss or further decreases in range of motion.

During a survey, surveyors may observe you performing ROM activities.

DELEGATION GUIDELINES

Range-of-Motion Exercises

When delegated ROM exercises, you need this information from the nurse and the care plan.
- If ROM exercises are active, passive, or active-assistive
- Which joints to exercise
- What ROM exercises to do—abduction, adduction, flexion, extension, and so on (see Box 27-1)
- When to do the exercises
- How many times to repeat each exercise
- What observations to report and record:
  - The time the exercises were performed
  - The joints exercised and the exercises performed
  - The number of times the exercises were performed on each joint
  - Complaints of pain or signs of stiffness or spasm; specify the joint or body part involved
  - The degree to which the person took part in the exercises
  - When to report observations
- What patient or resident concerns to report at once

PROMOTING SAFETY AND COMFORT

Range-of-Motion Exercises

Safety

ROM exercises can cause injury if not done correctly. Muscle strain, joint injury, and pain are possible. Practice the measures in Box 27-1. Remind the person to tell you about any pain during the procedure.

ROM exercises to the neck can cause serious injury if not done correctly. Some agencies give nursing assistants special training before doing such exercises. Other agencies do not let nursing assistants do them. Know your agency's policy. Perform ROM exercises to the neck only if allowed by your agency, if you received needed training, and if the nurse instructs you to do so. In some agencies, only physical therapists do neck exercises.

Comfort

To promote physical comfort during ROM exercises, see Box 27-1. Provide privacy to promote mental comfort.

Performing Range-of-Motion Exercises

QUALITY OF LIFE

- Knock before entering the person's room.
- Address the person by name.
- Introduce yourself by name and title.

- Explain the procedure before starting and during the procedure.
- Protect the person's rights during the procedure.
- Handle the person gently during the procedure.

PRE-PROCEDURE

1 Follow *Delegation Guidelines: Range-of-Motion Exercises.* See *Promoting Safety and Comfort: Range-of-Motion Exercises.*
2 Practice hand hygiene.
3 Identify the person. Check the ID (identification) bracelet against the assignment sheet. Use 2 identifiers (Chapter 10). Also call the person by name.

4 Obtain a bath blanket.
5 Provide for privacy.
6 Raise the bed for body mechanics. Bed rails are up if used.

PROCEDURE

7 Lower the bed rail near you if up.
8 Position the person supine.
9 Cover the person with the bath blanket. Fan-fold top linens to the foot of the bed.
10 Exercise the neck *if allowed by your agency and if the nurse instructs you to do so* (Fig. 27-10, p. 402).
   a Place your hands over the ears to support the head. Support the jaw with your fingers.
   b Flexion—bring the head forward. The chin touches the chest.
   c Extension—straighten the head.
   d Hyperextension—bring the head backward until the chin points up.
   e Rotation—turn the head from side to side.
   f Lateral flexion—move the head to the right and to the left.
   g Repeat flexion, extension, hyperextension, rotation, and lateral flexion 5 times—or the number of times stated on the care plan.
11 Exercise the shoulder (Fig. 27-11, p. 402).
   a Grasp the wrist with 1 hand. Grasp the elbow with the other hand.
   b Flexion—raise the arm straight in front and over the head.
   c Extension—bring the arm down to the side.
   d Hyperextension—move the arm behind the body. (Do this if the person is in a straight-backed chair or is standing.)
   e Abduction—move the straight arm away from the side of the body.
   f Adduction—move the straight arm to the side of the body.
   g Internal rotation—bend the elbow. Place it at the same level as the shoulder. Move the forearm and hand so the fingers point down.
   h External rotation—move the forearm and hand so the fingers point up.
   i Repeat flexion, extension, hyperextension, abduction, adduction, and internal and external rotation 5 times—or the number of times stated on the care plan.

12 Exercise the elbow (Fig. 27-12, p. 403).
   a Grasp the wrist with 1 hand. Grasp the elbow with your other hand.
   b Flexion—bend the arm so the same-side shoulder is touched.
   c Extension—straighten the arm.
   d Repeat flexion and extension 5 times—or the number of times stated on the care plan.
13 Exercise the forearm (Fig. 27-13, p. 403).
   a Continue to support the wrist and elbow.
   b Pronation—turn the hand so the palm is down.
   c Supination—turn the hand so the palm is up.
   d Repeat pronation and supination 5 times—or the number of times stated on the care plan.
14 Exercise the wrist (Fig. 27-14, p. 403).
   a Hold the wrist with both of your hands.
   b Flexion—bend the hand down.
   c Extension—straighten the hand.
   d Hyperextension—bend the hand back.
   e Radial flexion (deviation)—turn the hand toward the thumb.
   f Ulnar flexion (deviation)—turn the hand toward the little finger.
   g Repeat flexion, extension, hyperextension, radial flexion (deviation), and ulnar flexion (deviation) 5 times—or the number of times stated on the care plan.
15 Exercise the thumb (Fig. 27-15, p. 403).
   a Hold the person's hand with 1 hand. Hold the thumb with your other hand.
   b Abduction—move the thumb out from the inner part of the index finger.
   c Adduction—move the thumb back next to the index finger.
   d Opposition—touch each fingertip with the thumb.
   e Flexion—bend the thumb into the hand.
   f Extension—move the thumb out to the side of the fingers.
   g Repeat abduction, adduction, opposition, flexion, and extension 5 times—or the number of times stated on the care plan.

Continued

Performing Range-of-Motion Exercises—cont'd

PROCEDURE—cont'd

16 Exercise the fingers (Fig. 27-16).
  a Abduction—spread the fingers and thumb apart.
  b Adduction—bring the fingers and thumb together.
  c Flexion—make a fist.
  d Extension—straighten the fingers so the fingers, hand, and arm are straight.
  e Repeat abduction, adduction, flexion, and extension 5 times—or the number of times stated on the care plan.

17 Exercise the hip (Fig. 27-17).
  a Support the leg. Place 1 hand under the knee. Place your other hand under the ankle.
  b Flexion—raise the leg.
  c Extension—straighten the leg.
  d Hyperextension—move the leg behind the body. (Do this if the person is standing.)
  e Abduction—move the leg away from the body.
  f Adduction—move the leg toward the other leg.
  g Internal rotation—turn the leg inward.
  h External rotation—turn the leg outward.
  i Repeat flexion, extension, hyperextension, abduction, adduction, and internal and external rotation 5 times— or the number of times stated on the care plan.

18 Exercise the knee (Fig. 27-18).
  a Support the knee. Place 1 hand under the knee. Place your other hand under the ankle.
  b Flexion—bend the knee.
  c Extension—straighten the knee.
  d Repeat flexion and extension 5 times—or the number of times stated on the care plan.

19 Exercise the ankle (Fig. 27-19).
  a Support the foot and ankle. Place 1 hand under the foot. Place your other hand under the ankle.
  b Dorsiflexion—pull the foot upward. Push down on the heel at the same time.
  c Plantar flexion—turn the foot down. Or point the toes.
  d Repeat dorsiflexion and plantar flexion 5 times—or the number of times stated on the care plan.

20 Exercise the foot (Fig. 27-20).
  a Continue to support the foot and ankle.
  b Pronation—turn the outside of the foot up and the inside down.
  c Supination—turn the inside of the foot up and the outside down.
  d Repeat pronation and supination 5 times—or the number of times stated on the care plan.

21 Exercise the toes (Fig. 27-21).
  a Flexion—curl the toes.
  b Extension—straighten the toes.
  c Abduction—spread the toes.
  d Adduction—put the toes together.
  e Repeat flexion, extension, abduction, and adduction 5 times—or the number of times stated on the care plan.

22 Cover the leg. Raise the bed rail if used.

23 Go to the other side. Lower the bed rail near you if up.

24 Repeat steps 11 through 21. Cover the leg when done.

POST-PROCEDURE

25 Provide for comfort. (See the inside of the front cover.)

26 Cover the person with the top linens. Remove the bath blanket.

27 Place the call light and other needed items within reach.

28 Lower the bed to a safe and comfortable level. Follow the care plan.

29 Raise or lower bed rails. Follow the care plan.

30 Fold and return the bath blanket to its proper place. Or follow agency policy for used linens.

31 Unscreen the person.

32 Complete a safety check of the room. (See the inside of the front cover.)

33 Practice hand hygiene.

34 Report and record your observations.

Flexion   Extension   Hyperextension   Rotation   Lateral flexion

FIGURE 27-10 Range-of-motion exercises for the neck.

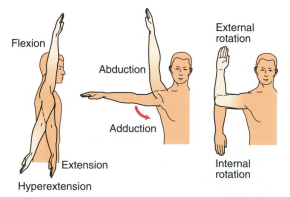

Flexion

Abduction

External rotation

Adduction

Extension

Hyperextension

Internal rotation

FIGURE 27-11 Range-of-motion exercises for the shoulder.

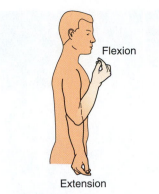

Flexion

Extension

FIGURE 27-12 Range-of-motion exercises for the elbow.

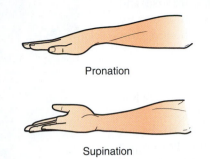

Pronation

Supination

FIGURE 27-13 Range-of-motion exercises for the forearm.

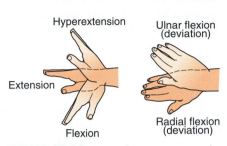

Hyperextension

Ulnar flexion (deviation)

Extension

Flexion

Radial flexion (deviation)

FIGURE 27-14 Range-of-motion exercises for the wrist.

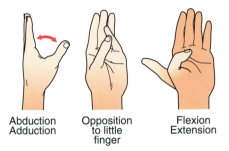

Abduction
Adduction

Opposition to little finger

Flexion
Extension

FIGURE 27-15 Range-of-motion exercises for the thumb.

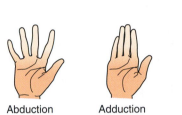

Abduction

Adduction

Flexion

Extension

FIGURE 27-16 Range-of-motion exercises for the fingers.

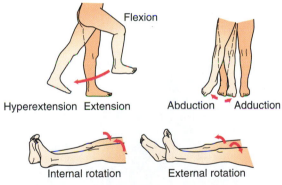

Flexion

Hyperextension Extension

Abduction Adduction

Internal rotation

External rotation

FIGURE 27-17 Range-of-motion exercises for the hip.

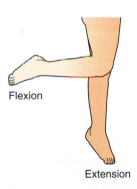

Flexion

Extension

FIGURE 27-18 Range-of-motion exercises for the knee.

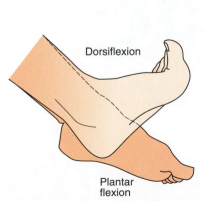

Dorsiflexion

Plantar flexion

FIGURE 27-19 Range-of-motion exercises for the ankle.

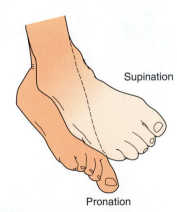

Supination

Pronation

FIGURE 27-20 Range-of-motion exercises for the foot.

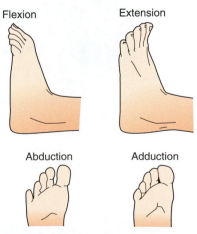

Flexion

Extension

Abduction

Adduction

FIGURE 27-21 Range-of-motion exercises for the toes.

AMBULATION

Ambulation is the act of walking. Some people are weak and unsteady and need help walking. Walkers and canes are common for safety. Sometimes crutches and orthotic devices are needed (p. 408).

Canes

Canes are used for weakness on 1 side of the body. They help provide balance and support (Fig. 27-22).

A cane is held on the *strong side* of the body. (If the left leg is weak, the cane is held in the right hand.) For proper cane position, the cane is held to the side and in front of the *strong foot*.

- Side—the cane tip is about 6 to 10 inches to the side of the strong foot.
- Front—the cane tip is about 6 to 10 inches in front of the strong foot.

The grip is level with the hip on the strong side. The person walks as follows.

- *Step 1:* The cane (on the strong side) is moved forward 6 to 10 inches (Fig. 27-23, *A*).
- *Step 2:* The weak leg (opposite the cane) is moved forward even with the cane (Fig. 27-23, *B*).
- *Step 3:* The strong leg is moved forward and ahead of the cane and the weak leg (Fig. 27-23, *C*).

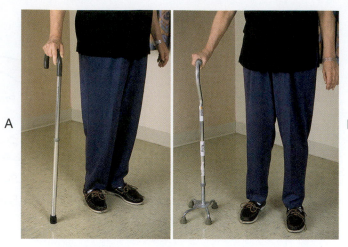

FIGURE 27-22 **A,** Single-tip cane. **B,** Four-point cane.

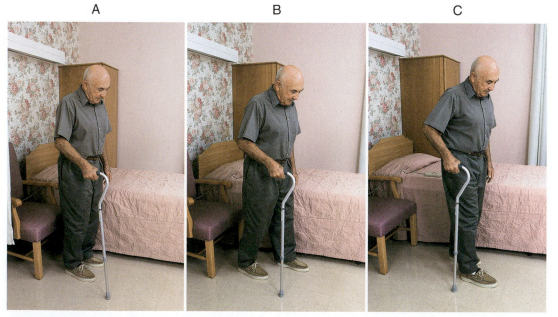

FIGURE 27-23 Walking with a cane. **A,** The cane (on the strong side) is moved forward about 6 to 10 inches. **B,** The leg opposite the cane (weak leg) is brought forward even with the cane. **C,** The leg on the cane side (strong side) is moved ahead of the cane and the weak leg.

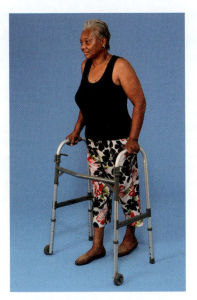

FIGURE 27-24 Wheeled walker.

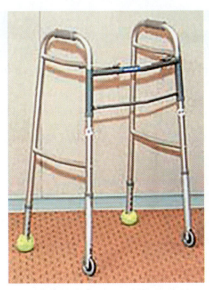

FIGURE 27-25 Walker tennis balls on the rear legs of a walker. (From Fairchild SL, Kuchler R, Washington RD: *Pierson and Fairchild's principles & techniques of patient care*, ed 6, St Louis, 2018, Elsevier.)

Walkers

A walker gives more support than a cane. Wheeled walkers have wheels on the front legs and rubber tips on the back legs (Fig. 27-24). Rubber tips on the back legs prevent the walker from moving while the person is standing. To walk, the person pushes the walker about 6 to 8 inches in front of the feet.

Baskets, pouches, and trays attach to the walker for needed items. This allows more independence. The hands are free to grip the walker.

See *Promoting Safety and Comfort: Walkers.*

Helping the Person Walk

After bedrest, activity increases slowly and in steps. First the person sits on the side of the bed (dangles). Sitting in a chair follows. Next the person walks in the room and then in the hallway.

Follow the care plan when helping a person walk. Use a gait (transfer) belt if the person is weak or unsteady. The person also uses wall hand rails or a cane or walker. Always check for orthostatic hypotension (p. 397).

See *Focus on Communication: Helping the Person Walk.*
See *Delegation Guidelines: Helping the Person Walk,* p. 406.
See *Promoting Safety and Comfort: Helping the Person Walk,* p. 406.
See procedure: *Helping the Person Walk,* p. 406.

See procedure: *Helping the Person Walk,* p. 406.

PROMOTING SAFETY AND COMFORT

Walkers

Safety

Wheels are usually on the outside of the walker (see Fig. 27-24). With wheels on the outside, the walker may be too wide for some doorways. Moving the wheels to the inside of the walker reduces the width. The person can go through narrower doorways.

Walker tennis balls are common. Placed on the rear legs, they allow the walker to slide more easily on carpets and other surfaces (Fig. 27-25).

Walkers vary in design. Some have a braking action when weight is applied to the back legs. Some walkers have seats. The person sits to rest. Never push the walker when the person is seated.

FOCUS ON COMMUNICATION

Helping the Person Walk

Before ambulating, explain the activity. This promotes comfort and reduces fear. Explain:

- How far to walk
- What assistive (adaptive) devices are used
- That you will use a gait belt
- How you will assist
- What the person is to report to you
- How you will help if the person begins to fall
  For example, you can say:

I am going to help you walk from your bed to the doorway and back. This belt helps support you while you walk. I will be at your side holding the belt at all times. Tell me right away if you feel unsteady, dizzy, weak, or faint. Also tell me if you feel any pain or discomfort. If you begin to fall, I will use the belt to pull you close to me and gently lower you to the floor. Do you have any questions?

Helping the Person Walk

QUALITY OF LIFE

- Knock before entering the person's room.
- Address the person by name.
- Introduce yourself by name and title.
- Explain the procedure before starting and during the procedure.
- Protect the person's rights during the procedure.
- Handle the person gently during the procedure.

PRE-PROCEDURE

1 Follow *Delegation Guidelines: Helping the Person Walk.* See *Promoting Safety and Comfort: Helping the Person Walk.*
2 Practice hand hygiene.
3 Collect the following.
- Robe and non-skid footwear
- Paper or towel to protect bottom linens
- Gait (transfer) belt
- Walker or cane (if needed)

4 Identify the person. Check the ID bracelet against the assignment sheet. Use 2 identifiers (Chapter 10). Also call the person by name.
5 Provide for privacy.

PROCEDURE

6 Lower the bed to a safe and comfortable level. Follow the care plan. Lock (brake) the bed wheels. Lower the bed rail if up.
7 Fan-fold top linens to the foot of the bed.
8 Place the paper or towel under the person's feet to protect bottom linens. Put the shoes on and fasten.
9 Help the person sit on the side of the bed. (See procedure: *Sitting on the Side of the Bed [Dangling]* in Chapter 15.)
10 Make sure the person's feet are flat on the floor.
11 Help the person put on the robe.
12 Apply the gait belt at the waist over clothing. (See procedure: *Using a Transfer/Gait Belt* in Chapter 11.)
13 Position the walker (if used) in front of the person. Or have the person hold the cane (if used) on the strong side.
14 Help the person stand. (See procedure: *Transferring the Person to a Chair or Wheelchair* in Chapter 16.) Grasp the gait belt at each side.

15 Stand at the weak side while the person gains balance. Hold the belt at the side and back.
16 Encourage the person to stand erect with the head up and the back straight.
17 *Positioning a walker or cane:*
   a Walker—the walker is 6 to 8 inches in front of the person.
   b Cane—the cane is held on the strong side.
     1 The cane tip is 6 to 10 inches to the side of the strong foot.
     2 The cane tip is 6 to 10 inches in front of the strong foot.
18 Help the person walk. Walk to the side and slightly behind the person on the person's weak side. Provide support with the gait belt (Fig. 27-26). Have the person use the hand rail on his or her strong side (unless using a walker or cane).

Helping the Person Walk—cont'd

PROCEDURE—cont'd

19 *If using a walker or cane:*
   a Walker—with both hands, the person pushes the walker 6 to 8 inches in front of the feet.
   b Cane:
   1 The cane (on the strong side) is moved forward 6 to 10 inches (see Fig. 27-23, *A*).
   2 The weak leg (opposite the cane) is moved forward even with the cane (see Fig. 27-23, *B*).
   3 The strong leg is moved forward and ahead of the cane and the weak leg (see Fig. 27-23, *C*).
20 Encourage the person to walk normally. The heel strikes the floor first. Discourage shuffling, sliding, or walking on tip-toes.

21 Walk the required distance if the person tolerates the activity. Do not rush the person.
22 Help the person return to bed. Remove the gait belt. (See procedure: *Transferring the Person From a Chair or Wheelchair to Bed* in Chapter 16.)
23 Lower the head of the bed. Help the person to the center of the bed.
24 Remove the shoes. Remove the paper or towel over the bottom sheet. Discard the paper or follow agency policy for used linens.

POST-PROCEDURE

25 Provide for comfort. (See the inside of the front cover.)
26 Place the call light and other needed items within reach.
27 Raise or lower bed rails. Follow the care plan.
28 Return the robe and shoes to their proper place.
29 Unscreen the person.

30 Complete a safety check of the room. (See the inside of the front cover.)
31 Practice hand hygiene.
32 Report and record your observations.

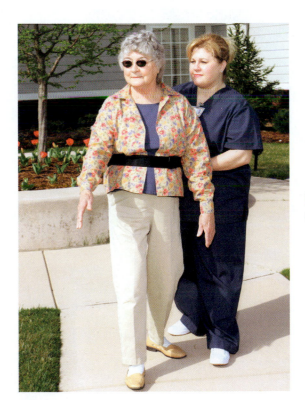

FIGURE 27-26 Assisting with ambulation. The nursing assistant walks at the person's side and slightly behind her. A gait belt is used for safety.

Other Walking Aids

Injury, surgery, and deformity are some reasons for crutches or orthotic devices. The need may be temporary or permanent.

Crutches. Crutches are used when the person cannot use 1 leg or when 1 or both legs need to gain strength. Some persons with permanent leg weakness can use crutches.

Falls are a risk. Follow these safety measures.
- Check the crutch tips. They must not be worn down, torn, or wet. Replace worn or torn crutch tips. Dry wet tips with a towel or paper towels.
- Check crutches for flaws. Check wooden crutches for cracks and metal crutches for bends.
- Tighten all bolts.
- Have the person wear street shoes. They must be flat and have non-skid soles.
- Make sure clothes fit well. Loose clothes may get caught between the crutches and underarms. Loose clothes and long skirts can hang forward and block the person's view of the feet and crutch tips.
- Practice safety rules to prevent falls (Chapter 11).
- Keep crutches within the person's reach. Put them by the person's chair or against a wall.

Orthotic Devices. An *orthotic device is used to support a muscle, promote a certain motion, or correct a deformity.* (*Ortho means to straighten.*) Paralysis and muscle weakness are common reasons for orthotic devices.
- *Braces.* Braces support weak body parts. They also prevent or correct deformities or prevent joint movement. A brace is applied over the ankle, knee, or back (Fig. 27-27).
- *Ankle-foot orthosis (AFO).* An AFO is worn with a shoe (Fig. 27-28). The AFO is secured with a Velcro strap. This type of brace is common after a stroke.

Keep skin and bony points under orthotic devices clean and dry. This prevents skin breakdown. Report redness or signs of skin breakdown at once. Also report complaints of pain or discomfort. The care plan tells you when to apply and remove a brace or AFO.

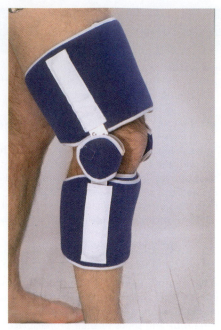

FIGURE 27-27 Knee brace. (Courtesy AliMed, Inc., Dedham, Massachusetts.)

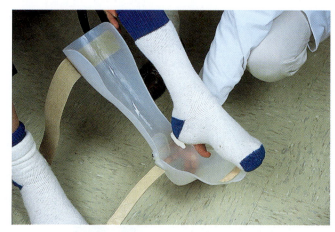

FIGURE 27-28 Ankle-foot orthosis (AFO).

FOCUS ON **P R I D E**
The Person, Family, and Yourself

Personal and Professional Responsibility

Exercise and activity promote normal function of all body systems. The more active a person is now, the more likely he or she will remain active in the future.

To promote activity, exercise, and well-being, you can:

- Encourage the person to be as active as possible.
- Resist the urge to do things that the person can safely do alone or with some help.
- Focus on the person's abilities.
- Tell the person when he or she is doing well or making progress.
- Tell the person you are proud of what he or she did or tried to do.

Rights and Respect

Garments must provide privacy during exercise and activity. When ambulating, the person's gown must not be open in the back. During ROM exercises, cover the person with a bath blanket. Expose only the body part being exercised. Protect the right to privacy. Privacy promotes dignity and mental comfort.

Independence and Social Interaction

Nursing center activity programs promote physical and mental well-being. Joints and muscles are exercised. Circulation is stimulated. Social interaction is mentally stimulating.

Bingo, movies, dances, exercise groups, shopping and museum trips, concerts, and guest speakers are common. Residents may share ideas or tell you about favorite pastimes. Share these with the health team. They are given to the resident group that plans activities.

Encourage residents to be involved. Listen to the person's interests. Suggest options that the person may like. Allow personal choice to promote independence and well-being. Do not force the person to take part in activities that are not of interest.

Delegation and Teamwork

The person's care plan and your assignment sheet tell you the person's activity limits and allowed activities. Ask the nurse what bedrest means for each person. Ask the nurse if you have questions about activity limits. Take pride in providing safe care by following the person's activity level.

Ethics and Laws

You can lose your ability to work as a nursing assistant for handling persons in ways that cause harm. Work carefully. Move patients and residents in a way that shows you care for their comfort, safety, and well-being.

FOCUS ON PRIDE: *Application*

Emotional responses to activity limits vary. What emotional changes might you expect? How can you encourage independence and self-worth in persons needing help with exercise and activity?

Circle **T** *if the statement is TRUE or* **F** *if it is FALSE.*

1   **T F**   You must know the person's activity level.

2   **T F**   A hip abduction wedge keeps the legs together.

3   **T F**   A person is dizzy when walking. Help the person to sit.

4   **T F**   A walker and a cane give the same support.

5   **T F**   When using a cane, the feet move first.

6   **T F**   When using a wheeled walker, the walker is pushed 6 to 8 inches in front of the person's feet.

7   **T F**   An orthotic device is used to support a muscle or promote a certain motion.

8   **T F**   A person has a brace. Bony areas need protection from skin breakdown.

9   **T F**   Bedrest prevents pressure injuries and blood clots.

10 **T F**   An abduction wedge helps prevent plantar flexion.

Circle the BEST answer.

11 Which prevents the hip from turning outward?
   a   A cane
   b   A foot-board
   c   A trochanter roll
   d   A leg brace

12 A contracture is
   a   The loss of muscle strength from inactivity
   b   A decrease in the size of a muscle
   c   A blood clot in the muscle
   d   The lack of joint mobility from shortening of a muscle

13 Active ROM exercises are performed by
   a   The person
   b   The physical therapist
   c   You
   d   The person with the help of another

14 When performing ROM exercises, which may cause injury?
   a   Supporting the part being exercised
   b   Moving the joint slowly, smoothly, and gently
   c   Forcing the joint through its full range of motion
   d   Exercising only the joints indicated by the nurse

15 Flexion involves
   a   Bending the body part
   b   Straightening the body part
   c   Moving the body part toward the body
   d   Moving the body part away from the body

16 Turning the joint downward is called
   a   Dorsiflexion
   b   Rotation
   c   Supination
   d   Pronation

17 When ambulating a person
   a   A gait belt is used if the person is weak or unsteady
   b   The person can shuffle or slide when walking after bedrest
   c   Encourage the person to walk quickly
   d   You walk on the person's strong side

18 A cane is held
   a   At waist level
   b   On the strong side
   c   On the weak side
   d   On either side

Answers to Chapter 27 questions are on p. 552.

FOCUS ON PRACTICE

Problem Solving

You are ambulating a resident in the hallway with a walker and gait belt. The resident says: "I feel dizzy." A chair is not nearby. A wheelchair is at the nurses' station at the end of the hallway. What will you do?

Wound Care

OBJECTIVES

- Define the key terms and key abbreviations in this chapter.
- Describe skin tears, circulatory ulcers, and diabetic foot ulcers and the persons at risk.
- Explain how to help prevent skin tears, circulatory ulcers, and diabetic foot ulcers.
- Describe what to observe about wounds.
- Explain how to secure dressings.

- Explain the rules for applying dressings.
- Explain the purpose, effects, and complications of heat and cold applications.
- Describe the rules for applying heat and cold.
- Perform the procedures described in this chapter.
- Explain how to promote PRIDE in the person, the family, and yourself.

KEY TERMS

constrict To narrow
dilate To expand or open wider
skin tear A break or rip in the outer layers of the skin; the epidermis (top skin layer) separates from the underlying tissues

ulcer A shallow or deep crater-like sore of the skin or mucous membrane
wound A break in the skin or mucous membrane

KEY ABBREVIATIONS

AE	Anti-embolism; anti-embolic
C	Centigrade
F	Fahrenheit

ID	Identification
PPE	Personal protective equipment

A **wound** *is a break in the skin or mucous membrane.* Wounds commonly result from:

- Surgery
- *Trauma*—an accident or violent act that injures the skin, mucous membranes, bones, and organs
- Unrelieved pressure or friction (Chapter 29)
- Decreased blood flow through arteries or veins
- Nerve damage

Wounds are portals of entry for microbes. Infection is a major threat. Wound care includes preventing infection and further injury to the wound and nearby tissues.

See *Delegation Guidelines: Wound Care.*
See *Promoting Safety and Comfort: Wound Care,* p. 412.

DELEGATION GUIDELINES
Wound Care

Your state and agency may not allow you to perform the procedures in this chapter. Before performing a procedure, make sure that:

- Your state allows you to perform the procedure.
- The procedure is in your job description.
- You have the necessary education and training.
- You review the procedure with a nurse.
- A nurse is available to answer questions and to supervise you.

PROMOTING SAFETY AND COMFORT
Wound Care

Safety

Wound care may involve contact with blood, body fluids, secretions, or excretions. Follow Standard Precautions and the Bloodborne Pathogen Standard. Wear personal protective equipment (PPE) as needed. Gloves, gowns, masks, and eye protection are necessary when blood splashes and splatters are likely.

> NOTE: A task may require more than 1 pair of gloves. Change gloves as needed. Use careful judgment. Remember to practice hand hygiene after removing gloves.

SKIN TEARS

A **skin tear** *is a break or rip in the outer layers of the skin* (Fig. 28-1). *The epidermis (top skin layer) separates from the underlying tissues* (Chapter 8). The hands, arms, and lower legs are common sites for skin tears. Skin tears are caused by:

- Friction, shearing (Chapter 15), pulling, or pressure on the skin.
- Falls or bumping a hard surface. Beds, bed rails, chairs, wheelchair parts, walkers, and tables are dangers.
- Holding an arm or leg too tight.
- Removing tape or adhesives.
- Bathing, dressing, and other tasks.
- Pulling buttons and zippers across fragile skin.
- Jewelry—yours or the person's. Rings, watches, and bracelets are examples.
- Long or jagged fingernails (yours or the person's) and long or jagged toenails.

Skin tears are painful. They are portals of entry for microbes. Infection is a risk. Tell the nurse at once if you cause or find a skin tear. To prevent skin tears, follow the care plan and the measures in Box 28-1.

See *Focus on Older Persons: Skin Tears.*

BOX 28-1   Preventing Skin Tears

- Follow the care plan and safety rules to:
  - Move, turn, position, or transfer the person.
    - Prevent shearing and friction.
    - Use an assist device to move and turn the person in bed.
    - Use pillows to support arms and legs.
  - Pad bed rails and wheelchair arms, footplates, and leg supports.
  - Bathe the person.
  - Keep the skin moisturized and apply lotion.
  - Offer fluids.
- Keep your fingernails short and smoothly filed.
- Keep the person's fingernails short and smoothly filed. Report long, tough, or jagged toenails.
- Do not wear rings with large or raised stones. Do not wear bracelets.
- Be patient and calm when the person is confused, agitated, or resists care.
- Dress and undress the person carefully. The person wears soft clothes with long sleeves and long pants.
- Apply arm or leg protectors as ordered.
- Provide good lighting so the person can see. The person must avoid bumping into furniture, walls, and equipment.
- Provide a safe area for wandering (Chapter 35).
- Remove tape carefully (p. 418). To remove tape, gently pull the tape ends toward the wound.
- Do not apply adhesive tape (p. 418).

FOCUS ON OLDER PERSONS
Skin Tears

Very thin and fragile skin is common in older persons. Slight pressure can cause a skin tear. Persons who are confused may resist care. They often move quickly and without warning. Or they pull away during care. Some try to hit or kick. These sudden movements can cause skin tears.

Never force care on a person. Chapter 35 describes how to care for persons who are confused and resist care. Always follow the care plan.

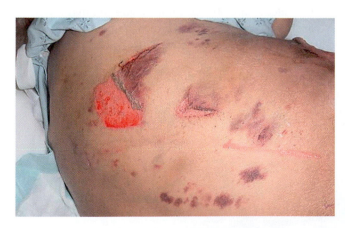

FIGURE 28-1 Skin tear. (Used with permission from Rosemary Kohr, RN, PhD, ACNP (cert), www.lhsc.on.ca/wound, Rosemary.Kohr@Lhasa.on.ca.)

CIRCULATORY ULCERS

An **ulcer** *is a shallow or deep crater-like sore of the skin or mucous membrane.* *Circulatory ulcers (vascular ulcers)* are open sores on the lower legs or feet. They are caused by decreased blood flow through the arteries or veins. These wounds are painful and hard to heal. Infection and gangrene can develop. *Gangrene* is a condition in which there is death of tissue.

Circulatory ulcers include:

- *Venous ulcers (stasis ulcers)* are open sores on the lower legs or feet caused by poor venous blood flow (Fig. 28-2). *Stasis* means *stopped or slowed fluid flow.* The heels and inner part of the ankles are common sites. They can occur from skin injury. Scratching and trauma are examples. Venous ulcers are painful. Infection is a risk. Healing is slow.
- *Arterial ulcers* are open wounds on the lower legs or feet caused by poor arterial blood flow. They are found between the toes, on top of the toes, and on the outer side of the ankle (Fig. 28-3).
- *Diabetic foot ulcers* are open wounds on the foot caused by complications from diabetes. Diabetes (Chapter 33) can affect the nerves and blood vessels. With nerve damage, the person can lose sensation in a foot or leg. The person may not feel pain, heat, or cold. When blood vessels are affected, blood flow decreases. Tissues and cells do not get needed oxygen and nutrients. Sores heal poorly. Infection and tissue death (gangrene) are risks. Sometimes the affected part must be amputated.

Prevention and Treatment

Check the person's feet and legs daily. Report any sign of a problem at once. You must help prevent skin breakdown on the legs and feet. Follow the care plan to prevent and treat circulatory ulcers (Box 28-2). Diabetes foot care can prevent foot problems that cause diabetic foot ulcers (Box 28-3, p. 414). The doctor orders drugs and treatments as needed.

Persons at risk need professional foot care. *You do not cut the toenails of persons with diseases affecting circulation.*

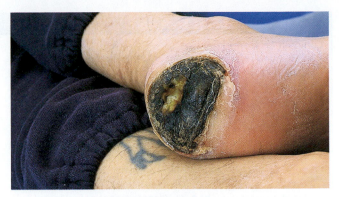

FIGURE 28-2 Venous ulcer.

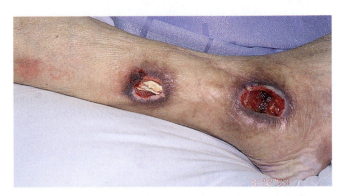

FIGURE 28-3 Arterial ulcer. (From Black JM, Hawks JH: *Medical-surgical nursing: clinical management for positive outcomes,* ed 8, St Louis, 2009, Saunders.)

BOX 28-2	Preventing Circulatory Ulcers

- Remind the person not to sit with the legs crossed.
- Re-position the person according to the care plan—at least every 2 hours.
- Do not use elastic or rubber band–type garters to hold socks or hose in place.
- Do not dress the person in tight clothes.
- Provide good skin care daily and as needed. Keep the feet clean and dry. Clean and dry between the toes.
- Do not scrub or rub the skin during bathing and drying.
- Keep linens clean, dry, and wrinkle-free.
- Avoid injury to the legs and feet.
- Make sure shoes fit well.
- Keep pressure off the heels and other bony areas. Use pillows or other devices as directed.
- Check the person's legs and feet. Report skin breaks or changes in skin color.
- Do not massage over pressure points (Chapter 29). *Never rub or massage reddened areas.*
- Use protective devices as directed.
- Follow the care plan for walking and exercises.

BOX 28-3   Diabetes Foot Care

Common Problems

- *Corns and calluses* (Fig. 28-4, *A*). These are thick layers of skin caused by too much rubbing or pressure on the same spot.
- *Blisters* (Fig. 28-4, *B*). These form when shoes rub on the same spot.
- *Ingrown toenails* (Fig. 28-4, *C*). An edge of a toenail grows into the skin.
- *Bunions* (Fig. 28-4, *D*). A bunion is a bump on the outside edge of the big toe. The big toe slants toward the small toes.
- *Plantar warts* (Fig. 28-4, *E*). *Plantar* means *sole*. Plantar warts occur on the soles (bottoms) of the feet.
- *Hammer toes* (Fig. 28-4, *F*). One or more toes are flexed.
- *Dry and cracked skin* (Fig. 28-4, *G*). The dry skin can crack, causing portals of entry for microbes. Infection can occur.
- *Athlete's foot* (Fig. 28-4, *H*). This is a fungus causing itching, burning, redness, and cracked skin between the toes and on the soles of the feet.
- *Fungal infection of the toenails* (Figure 28-4, *I*). The toenails become thick and hard to cut. They may be yellow, brown, or black.

Care Measures

- Check the feet daily for:
  - Cuts
  - Sores
  - Blisters
  - Redness
  - Calluses
  - Infected toenails
  - Pus
  - Warm skin

Care Measures—cont'd

- Wash the feet daily in warm water with mild soap.
  - Do not use hot water.
  - Test the water temperature with your elbow or use a water thermometer. Because burns are a risk, water temperature should be 90°F to 95°F (Fahrenheit).
  - Do not soak the feet in water. The skin could dry out.
  - Dry the feet well, especially between the toes.
- Apply talcum powder or cornstarch between the toes. This keeps the skin between the toes dry.
- Apply a thin layer of lotion, cream, or petroleum jelly on the tops and bottoms of the feet (not between the toes). Do so after washing and drying to keep the skin soft and smooth.
- Have the person wear closed-toed shoes and clean socks, stockings, or nylons. This prevents blisters and sores.
  - Socks, stockings, and nylons do not have holes or seams.
  - Lightly padded socks are best.
  - Tight socks or knee-high stockings are avoided.
  - Athletic and walking shoes are best. They have laces, Velcro, or buckles for easy adjustment.
  - Open-toed shoes, sandals, flip-flops, pointy shoes, and high-heels are not worn.
  - Vinyl and plastic shoes are not worn. They do not stretch and do not allow air movement inside the shoes.
- Check shoes for sharp edges or objects in the shoes. Make sure the lining is smooth.
- Do not allow the person to walk barefoot.
- Provide socks at night for cold feet.
- Promote blood flow to the feet. Have the person:
  - Elevate the feet when sitting.
  - Wiggle the toes for 5 minutes 2 or 3 times a day.
  - Move the ankles up and down and in and out.
  - Avoid crossing the legs.
- Do not trim or cut toenails or cut corns or calluses or try to smooth them. Professional foot care is needed.

Modified from National Institute of Diabetes and Digestive and Kidney Diseases: *Prevent diabetes problems: keep your feet healthy,* NIH Publication No. 14-4282, Bethesda, Md, February 2014, U.S. Department of Health and Human Services.

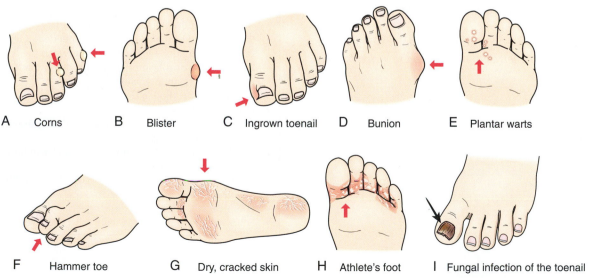

| A Corns | B Blister | C Ingrown toenail | D Bunion | E Plantar warts |

| F Hammer toe | G Dry, cracked skin | H Athlete's foot | I Fungal infection of the toenail |

FIGURE 28-4 Foot problems common with diabetes. (Redrawn from National Institute of Diabetes and Digestive and Kidney Diseases: *Prevent diabetes problems: keep your feet healthy,* NIH Publication No. 14-4282, Bethesda, Md, February 2014, U.S. Department of Health and Human Services.)

Elastic Stockings. Elastic stockings put pressure on the veins. This promotes venous blood return to the heart. The stockings help prevent blood clots *(thrombi)* in leg veins. A blood clot is called a *thrombus*.

If blood flow is sluggish, blood clots may form. They can form in the deep leg veins in the lower leg or thigh (Fig. 28-5, *A*). A blood clot *(thrombus)* can break loose and travel through the bloodstream. It then becomes an *embolus*—a blood clot that travels through the vascular system until it lodges in a blood vessel (Fig. 28-5, *B*). An embolus from a vein lodges in the lungs *(pulmonary embolism)* and can cause severe respiratory problems and death. Report chest pain or shortness of breath at once.

Persons at risk for thrombi include those who:
- Have heart and circulatory disorders.
- Are on bedrest.
- Have had surgery.
- Are older.
- Are pregnant.

Elastic stockings also are called AE stockings (AE means *anti-embolism* or *anti-embolic*). They also are called TED hose (TED means *thrombo-embolic disease*).

The person usually has 2 pairs of stockings. Wash 1 pair while the other pair is worn. Wash them by hand with a mild soap. Hang them to dry.

See *Delegation Guidelines: Elastic Stockings.*
See *Promoting Safety and Comfort: Elastic Stockings.*
See procedure: *Applying Elastic Stockings,* p. 416.

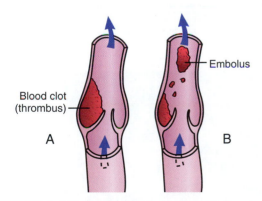

FIGURE 28-5 A, A blood clot is attached to the wall of a vein. The *arrows* show the direction of blood flow. **B,** Part of the thrombus breaks off and becomes an embolus. The embolus travels through the vascular system until it lodges in a distant vessel.

DELEGATION GUIDELINES
Elastic Stockings

To apply elastic stockings, you need this information from the nurse and the care plan.
- What size to use—small, medium, large, or extra-large
- What length to use—thigh-high or knee-high
- When to remove them and for how long—usually every 8 hours for 30 minutes
- What observations to report and record:
  - The size and length of stockings applied
  - When you applied the stockings
  - Skin color and temperature
  - Leg and foot swelling
  - Skin tears, wounds, or signs of skin breakdown
  - Complaints of pain, tingling, or numbness
  - When you removed the stockings and for how long
  - When you re-applied the stockings
  - When you washed the stockings
- When to report observations
- What patient or resident concerns to report at once

PROMOTING SAFETY AND COMFORT
Elastic Stockings

Safety
Apply the stocking so the toe opening is over the top of the toes or under the toes. Follow the manufacturer's instructions. Use the opening to check circulation, skin color, and skin temperature in the toes.

Stockings must not have twists, creases, or wrinkles. Twists can affect circulation. So can stockings that roll up, bunch up, or have the toe opening wrapped around the toes. Creases and wrinkles can cause skin breakdown.

Loose stockings do not exert pressure on the veins. Stockings that are too tight can affect circulation. Tell the nurse if the stockings are too loose or too tight.

Comfort
Apply stockings before the person gets out of bed. Otherwise the legs can swell from sitting or standing. Stockings are hard to put on swollen legs. The person is in bed while they are off. This prevents the legs from swelling.

Gently handle and move the person's foot and leg. Do not force the joints (toes, foot, ankle, knee, and hip) beyond their range of motion or to the point of pain.

Applying Elastic Stockings

QUALITY OF LIFE

- Knock before entering the person's room.
- Address the person by name.
- Introduce yourself by name and title.

- Explain the procedure before starting and during the procedure.
- Protect the person's rights during the procedure.
- Handle the person gently during the procedure.

PRE-PROCEDURE

1 Follow *Delegation Guidelines: Elastic Stockings,* p. 415. See *Promoting Safety and Comfort: Elastic Stockings,* p. 415.
2 Practice hand hygiene.
3 Obtain elastic stockings in the correct size and length. Note the location of the toe opening.

4 Identify the person. Check the ID (identification) bracelet against the assignment sheet. Use 2 identifiers (Chapter 10). Also call the person by name.
5 Provide for privacy.
6 Raise the bed for body mechanics. Bed rails are up if used.

PROCEDURE

7 Lower the bed rail.
8 Position the person supine.
9 Expose 1 leg. Fan-fold top linens to the foot of the bed or toward the other leg.
10 Gather or turn the stocking inside out down to the heel.
11 Slip the foot of the stocking over the toes, foot, and heel (Fig. 28-6, *A*). Properly position the heel pocket on the heel. The toe opening is over or under the toes. Follow the manufacturer's instructions.

12 Grasp the stocking top. Roll or pull the stocking up the leg. It turns right side out as it is rolled or pulled up.
13 Adjust the stocking as needed. Make sure the stocking does not cause pressure on the toes.
14 Remove twists, creases, or wrinkles. Make sure the stocking is even, snug, smooth, and wrinkle-free (Fig. 28-6, *B*).
15 Cover the leg. Repeat steps 9 through 14 for the other leg.
16 Cover the person.

POST-PROCEDURE

17 Provide for comfort. (See the inside of the front cover.)
18 Place the call light and other needed items within reach.
19 Lower the bed to a safe and comfortable level. Follow the care plan.
20 Raise or lower bed rails. Follow the care plan.

21 Unscreen the person.
22 Complete a safety check of the room. (See the inside of the front cover.)
23 Practice hand hygiene.
24 Report and record your observations.

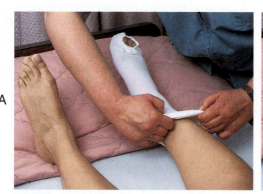 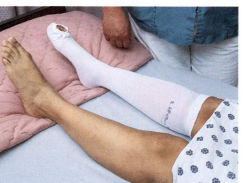

FIGURE 28-6 Applying elastic stockings. **A,** The stocking is slipped over the toes, foot, and heel. **B,** The stocking turns right side out as it is pulled up over the leg. The heel is positioned in the heel pocket of the stocking.

Elastic Bandages. Elastic bandages have the same purposes as elastic stockings. They also provide support and reduce swelling from injuries. Another use is to hold dressings in place. They are applied to arms and legs. To apply bandages:

- Start at the lower (*distal*) part of the extremity. Work upward to the top (*proximal*) part.
- Expose the fingers or toes if possible. This allows circulation checks.
- Check the color and temperature of the extremity every hour.
- Re-apply a loose or wrinkled bandage.
- Replace a moist or soiled bandage.
  See *Focus on Communication: Elastic Bandages.*
  See *Delegation Guidelines: Elastic Bandages.*
  See *Promoting Safety and Comfort: Elastic Bandages.*
  See procedure: *Applying an Elastic Bandage.*

DELEGATION GUIDELINES
Elastic Bandages

To apply elastic bandages, you need this information from the nurse and the care plan.

- Where to apply the bandage
- What width and length to use
- When to remove the bandage and for how long—usually every 8 hours for 30 minutes
- What observations to report and record:
  - The width and length applied
  - When you applied the bandage
  - Skin color and temperature
  - Swelling of the part
  - Skin tears, wounds, or signs of skin breakdown
  - Complaints of pain, itching, tingling, or numbness
  - A wet or soiled bandage
  - When you removed the bandage and for how long
  - When you re-applied the bandage
- When to report observations
- What patient or resident concerns to report at once

FOCUS ON COMMUNICATION
Elastic Bandages

Elastic bandages should promote comfort. To check for comfort, ask:

- "Does the bandage feel too tight?"
- "Do you feel pain, itching, or numbness?" If yes: "What do you feel?" "Where do you feel it?"

PROMOTING SAFETY AND COMFORT
Elastic Bandages

Safety

Elastic bandages must be firm and snug but not tight. A tight bandage can affect circulation.

Bandages are secured with clips, tape, or Velcro. Metal or plastic clips can injure the skin if they are loose, fall off, or cause pressure. Use clips only if the nurse tells you to. Check the clips often for correct placement.

Some agencies do not allow you to apply elastic bandages. Know your agency's policy.

Comfort

A tight bandage can cause pain and discomfort. If the person complains of pain, tingling, or numbness, remove the bandage. Tell the nurse at once.

Applying an Elastic Bandage

QUALITY OF LIFE

- Knock before entering the person's room.
- Address the person by name.
- Introduce yourself by name and title.
- Explain the procedure before starting and during the procedure.
- Protect the person's rights during the procedure.
- Handle the person gently during the procedure.

PRE-PROCEDURE

1 Follow *Delegation Guidelines: Elastic Bandages.* See *Promoting Safety and Comfort: Elastic Bandages.*
2 Practice hand hygiene.
3 Collect the following.
   - Elastic bandage as directed by the nurse
   - Tape or clips (unless the bandage has Velcro)
4 Identify the person. Check the ID bracelet against the assignment sheet. Use 2 identifiers (Chapter 10). Also call the person by name.
5 Provide for privacy.
6 Raise the bed for body mechanics. Bed rails are up if used.

Continued

Applying an Elastic Bandage—cont'd

PROCEDURE

7　Lower the bed rail near you if up.

8　Help the person to a comfortable position in good alignment. Expose the part to bandage.

9　Make sure the area is clean and dry.

10　Hold the bandage with the roll up. The loose end is on the bottom (Fig. 28-7, A).

11　Apply the bandage to the lower (distal) and smallest part of the wrist, foot, ankle, or knee (Fig. 28-7, B).

12　Make 2 circular turns around the part.

13　Make over-lapping spiral turns in an upward (proximal) direction. Each turn over-laps ½ to ¾ of the previous turn (Fig. 28-7, C). Each over-lap is equal.

14　Apply the bandage smoothly with firm, even pressure. It is not tight.

15　End the bandage with 2 circular turns.

16　Secure the bandage in place with Velcro, tape, or clips. Clips are not under the body part.

17　Check the fingers or toes for coldness or cyanosis (bluish color). Ask about pain, itching, numbness, or tingling. Remove the bandage if any are noted. Report your observations.

POST-PROCEDURE

18　Provide for comfort. (See the inside of the front cover.)

19　Place the call light and other needed items within reach.

20　Lower the bed to a safe and comfortable level. Follow the care plan.

21　Raise or lower bed rails. Follow the care plan.

22　Unscreen the person.

23　Complete a safety check of the room. (See the inside of the front cover.)

24　Practice hand hygiene.

25　Report and record your observations.

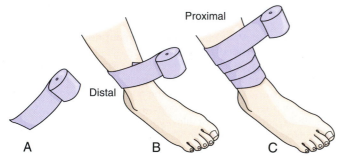

FIGURE 28-7 Applying an elastic bandage. **A,** The bandage roll is up. The loose end is at the bottom. **B,** The bandage is applied to the lower (distal) and smallest part with 2 circular turns. **C,** The bandage is applied with spiral turns in an upward (proximal) direction.

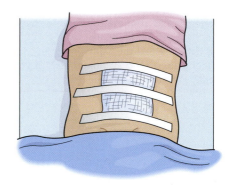

FIGURE 28-8 Tape is applied at the top, middle, and bottom of the dressing. The tape extends beyond both sides of the dressing.

DRESSINGS

Wound dressings have many functions. They:

- Protect wounds from injury and microbes.
- Absorb drainage.
- Remove dead tissue.
- Promote comfort.
- Cover unsightly wounds.
- Provide a moist environment for wound healing.
- Apply pressure (pressure dressings) to help control bleeding.

Securing Dressings

Dressings must be secured over wounds. Microbes can enter the wound and drainage can escape if the dressing is dislodged. Tape and Montgomery ties secure dressings. Binders (p. 421) hold dressings in place.

Tape. Adhesive, paper, plastic, cloth, and elastic tapes are common. Adhesive tape sticks well. However, problems with adhesive include:

- It is hard to remove from the skin.
- It can irritate the skin.
- Skin tears or abrasions can occur when tape is removed.
- Many people are allergic to adhesive tape.

Paper, plastic, and cloth tapes usually do not cause allergic reactions. Elastic tape allows movement of the body part.

Tape comes in ½, ¾, 1, 2, and 3 inch widths. Tape is applied to the top, middle, and bottom of the dressing. The tape extends beyond each side of the dressing (Fig. 28-8). *Do not apply tape to circle the entire body part. If swelling occurs, circulation to the part is impaired.*

See *Focus on Communication: Tape.*

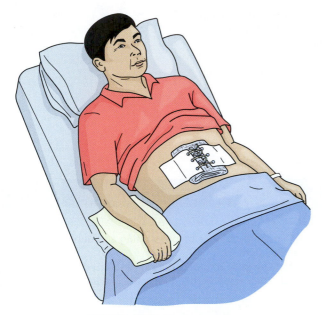

FIGURE 28-9 Montgomery ties.

BOX 28-4 Applying Dressings

- Let pain-relief drugs take effect, usually 30 minutes. The dressing change can cause discomfort. The nurse gives the drug and tells you how long to wait.
- Meet fluid and elimination needs before you begin.
- Collect equipment and supplies before you begin.
- Do not bend or reach over your work area.
- Control your nonverbal communication. Wound odors, appearance, and drainage may be unpleasant. Do not communicate your thoughts or reaction to the person.
- Remove soiled dressings so the person cannot see the soiled side. The drainage and its color may upset the person.
- Do not force the person to look at the wound. A wound can affect body image and self-esteem. The nurse helps the person deal with the wound.
- Remove tape by gently pulling the tape ends toward the wound.
- Remove dressings gently. They may stick to the wound, drain, or surrounding skin. If the dressing sticks, the nurse may have you wet the dressing with a saline solution. A wet dressing is easier to remove.
- Touch only the outer edges of old and new dressings.
- Report and record your observations. See *Delegation Guidelines: Applying Dressings.*

Montgomery Ties. Montgomery ties (Fig. 28-9) are used for large dressings and frequent dressing changes. A Montgomery tie has a tape strip and cloth tie. With the dressing in place, the tape strips are placed on both sides of the dressing. Then the cloth ties are secured over the dressing.

A wound may need 2 or 3 Montgomery ties on each side. The ties are undone for the dressing change. The tape strips stay in place. They are removed if soiled. Montgomery ties protect the skin from frequent tape application and removal.

Applying Dressings

Some agencies let you apply simple, dry, non-sterile dressings to simple wounds. Follow the rules in Box 28-4.

See *Delegation Guidelines: Applying Dressings.*
See *Promoting Safety and Comfort: Applying Dressings,* p. 420.
See procedure: *Applying a Dry, Non-Sterile Dressing,* p. 420.

DELEGATION GUIDELINES

Applying Dressings

When applying a dressing is delegated to you, you need this information from the nurse.
- When to change the dressing
- When a pain-relief drug will take effect
- What to do if the dressing sticks to the wound
- How to clean the wound
- What dressings to use
- How to secure the dressing—tape or Montgomery ties
- What kind of tape to use—adhesive, paper, plastic, cloth, or elastic
- What size tape to use—½, ¾, 1, 2, or 3 inch width
- What observations to report and record:
  - What you used to dress the wound and secure the dressing
  - A red or swollen wound
  - An area around the wound that is warm to touch
  - If wound edges are closed or separated
  - A wound that has broken open
  - Drainage appearance—clear, bloody, or watery and blood-tinged; thick and green, yellow, or brown
  - The amount of drainage
  - Wound or drainage odor
  - Intactness and color of surrounding tissues
  - Possible dressing contamination—urine; feces; other body fluids, secretions, or excretions; dislodged dressing
  - Pain
  - Fever
- When to report observations
- What patient or resident concerns to report at once

PROMOTING SAFETY AND COMFORT
Applying Dressings

Safety

Tape removal can cause skin tears in persons with thin, fragile skin. Use extreme care to remove tape. Do not apply tape to irritated, injured, or non-intact skin. Tape can further damage the skin.

Comfort

Wounds and dressing changes can cause discomfort or pain. Allow time for a pain-relief drug to take effect before a dressing change. Gently apply and remove tape and dressings.

The person may not report discomfort from a dressing. You should ask:

- "Is the dressing comfortable?"
- "Does the tape cause pain or itching?"

Applying a Dry, Non-Sterile Dressing

QUALITY OF LIFE

- Knock before entering the person's room.
- Address the person by name.
- Introduce yourself by name and title.
- Explain the procedure before starting and during the procedure.
- Protect the person's rights during the procedure.
- Handle the person gently during the procedure.

PRE-PROCEDURE

1 Follow *Delegation Guidelines:*
  a *Wound Care,* p. 411
  b *Applying Dressings,* p. 419
  See *Promoting Safety and Comfort:*
  a *Wound Care,* p. 412
  b *Applying Dressings*
2 Practice hand hygiene.
3 Collect the following.
- Gloves
- PPE (personal protective equipment) as needed
- Tape or Montgomery ties
- Dressings as directed by the nurse
- 4 × 4 gauze
- Saline solution as directed by the nurse

- Cleaning solution as directed by the nurse
- Adhesive remover
- Dressing set with scissors and forceps
- Plastic bag
- Bath blanket
4 Practice hand hygiene.
5 Identify the person. Check the ID bracelet against the assignment sheet. Use 2 identifiers (Chapter 10). Also call the person by name.
6 Provide for privacy.
7 Arrange your work area. You should not have to reach over or turn your back on your work area.
8 Raise the bed for body mechanics. Bed rails are up if used.

PROCEDURE

9 Lower the bed rail near you if up.
10 Help the person to a comfortable position.
11 Cover the person with a bath blanket. Fan-fold top linens to the foot of the bed.
12 Expose the affected body part.
13 Make a cuff on the plastic bag. Place the bag within reach.
14 Practice hand hygiene.
15 Put on needed PPE. Put on gloves.

16 Remove tape or undo Montgomery ties.
  a *Tape:* hold the skin down. Gently pull the tape ends toward the wound.
  b *Montgomery ties:* undo the ties. Fold the ties away from the wound.
17 Remove any adhesive from the skin. Pick up a gauze square with the forceps. Wet a 4 × 4 gauze dressing with adhesive remover. Clean away from the wound.
18 Remove gauze dressings. Start with the top dressing and remove each layer. Keep the soiled side away from the person's sight. Put dressings in the plastic bag. They must not touch the outside of the bag.

Applying a Dry, Non-Sterile Dressing—cont'd

PROCEDURE—cont'd

19 Remove the dressing over the wound very gently. It may stick to the wound or drain site. Moisten the dressing with saline if it sticks to the wound. Discard the dressing as in step 18.
20 Observe the wound, drain site, and wound drainage.
21 Remove the gloves and put them in the bag. Practice hand hygiene.
22 Open the new dressings.
23 Put on clean gloves.
24 Clean the wound with saline as directed by the nurse. See Figure 28-10.
25 Apply dressings as directed by the nurse.
26 Secure the dressings. Use tape or Montgomery ties.
27 Remove the gloves. Put them in the bag.
28 Remove and discard PPE.
29 Practice hand hygiene.
30 Cover the person. Remove the bath blanket.

POST-PROCEDURE

31 Provide for comfort. (See the inside of the front cover.)
32 Place the call light and other needed items within reach.
33 Lower the bed to a safe and comfortable level. Follow the care plan.
34 Raise or lower bed rails. Follow the care plan.
35 Return equipment and supplies to their proper place. Leave extra dressings and tape in the room.
36 Discard used supplies in the bag. Tie the bag closed. Discard the bag following agency policy. (Wear gloves for this step.)
37 Clean your work area. Follow the Bloodborne Pathogen Standard.
38 Unscreen the person.
39 Complete a safety check of the room. (See the inside of the front cover.)
40 Remove and discard the gloves. Practice hand hygiene.
41 Report and record your observations.

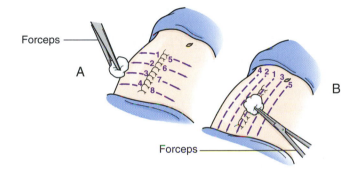

FIGURE 28-10 Cleaning a wound. **A,** Start at the wound and stroke out to the surrounding skin. Use new gauze for each stroke. **B,** Clean the wound from the top to the bottom. Start at the wound. Then clean the surrounding areas. Use new gauze for each stroke. (From Potter PA, Perry AG, Stockert PA, Hall AM: *Fundamentals of nursing,* ed 9, St Louis, 2017, Elsevier.)

BINDERS AND COMPRESSION GARMENTS

Binders are wide bands of elastic fabric. They support wounds and hold dressings in place. They also prevent or reduce swelling, promote comfort, and prevent injury. These binders are common.
- *Abdominal binder*—provides abdominal support and holds dressings in place (Fig. 28-11). The top part is at the waist. The lower part is over the hips. Binders are secured in place with Velcro or with hook and loop closures.
- *Breast binder*—supports the breasts after surgery (Fig. 28-12, p. 422). It is secured in place with Velcro or padded zippers.

Compression garments are made of a tight, stretchy fabric (Fig. 28-13, p. 422). Common after plastic surgery, they help:
- Reduce swelling.
- Prevent fluid buildup at the surgical site.
- Hold the skin against the body.
- Achieve the desired shape.

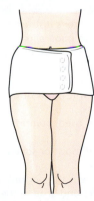

FIGURE 28-11 Abdominal binder. The top part is at the waist. The lower part is over the hips.

Box 28-5 (p. 422) lists the rules for applying binders and compression garments.
See *Focus on Communication: Binders and Compression Garments*, p. 422.
See *Promoting Safety and Comfort: Binders and Compression Garments*, p. 422.

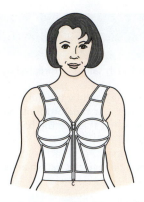

FIGURE 28-12 Breast binder.

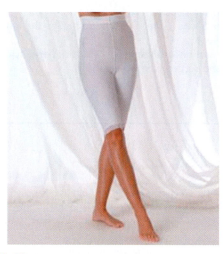

FIGURE 28-13 Compression garment. (Courtesy Rainey Compression Essentials, Atlanta, Ga.)

HEAT AND COLD APPLICATIONS

Heat and cold applications:
- Promote healing.
- Promote comfort.
- Reduce tissue swelling.

See *Focus on Older Persons: Heat and Cold Applications.*

BOX 28-5   Binders and Compression Garments

- Follow the manufacturer's instructions.
- Position the person in good alignment.
- Apply the device for firm, even pressure over the area.
- Apply the device so it is snug. It must not interfere with breathing or circulation.
- Re-apply the device if it is out of position or causes discomfort.
- Secure safety pins, if used, pointing away from the wound.
- Change the device if moist or soiled. This prevents the growth of microbes.
- Tell the nurse at once if the person's breathing changes.
- Check the skin under and around the device. Tell the nurse at once if there is redness, irritation, or other signs of a skin problem.

Heat Applications

Heat applications can be applied to almost any body part. They are used for musculo-skeletal injuries or problems (sprains, arthritis). Heat:

- Relieves pain.
- Relaxes muscles.
- Promotes healing.
- Reduces tissue swelling.
- Decreases joint stiffness.

When heat is applied to the skin, blood vessels in the area dilate. *Dilate means to expand or open wider* (Fig. 28-14). Blood flow increases. Tissues have more oxygen and nutrients for healing. Excess fluid is removed from the area faster. The skin is red and warm.

Complications.
High temperatures can cause burns. Report pain, excess redness, and blisters at once. Also observe for pale skin. When heat is applied too long, blood vessels *constrict (narrow)* (see Fig. 28-14). Blood flow decreases. Tissues receive less blood. Tissue damage occurs and the skin is pale.

Metal implants pose risks. Metal conducts heat. Deep tissues can be burned. Pacemakers (cardiac devices) and some joint replacements are made of metal. Do not apply heat to an implant area.

Heat is not applied to a pregnant woman's abdomen. The heat can affect fetal growth.

Moist and Dry Heat Applications.
With a *moist heat application*, water has contact with the skin. Water conducts heat. Moist heat has greater and faster effects than dry heat. Heat penetrates deeper with a moist application. To prevent injury, moist heat applications have lower (cooler) temperatures than dry heat applications. Moist heat applications (Fig. 28-15) include:

- *Hot compress.* A *compress* is a soft pad applied over a body area. It is usually made of cloth.
- *Hot soak.* A body part is put into water.
- *Sitz bath.* The perineal and rectal areas are immersed in warm or hot water. (*Sitz* means *seat* in German.)
- *Hot pack.* A *pack* involves wrapping a body part with a wet or dry application.

With *dry heat applications*, water does not have contact with the skin. A dry heat application stays at the desired temperature longer. Dry heat does not penetrate as deep as moist heat. Because water is not used, dry heat needs higher (hotter) temperatures for the desired effect. Therefore burns are still a risk.

Some *hot packs* and warming therapy pads are dry heat applications. The *aquathermia pad* (Aqua-K, K-Pad) is a common therapy pad (Fig. 28-16, p. 424). Tubes inside the pad are filled with distilled water. Heated water flows to the pad through a hose. Another hose returns water to the electric heating unit. Reheated water flows back into the pad.

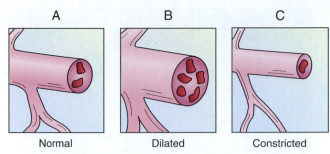

Normal · Dilated · Constricted

FIGURE 28-14 A, A blood vessel under normal conditions. **B,** Dilated blood vessel. **C,** Constricted blood vessel.

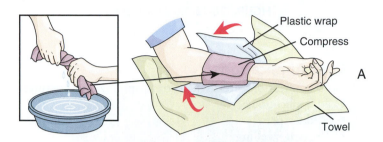

Plastic wrap
Compress
Towel
A

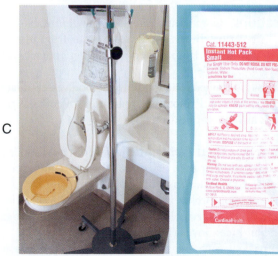

B

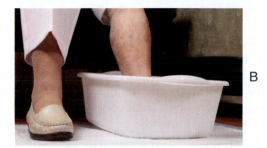

C

D

Cat. 11443-512
Instant Hot Pack
Small

FIGURE 28-15 Moist heat applications. **A,** Compress. **B,** Hot soak. **C,** Disposable sitz bath. **D,** Hot pack. (NOTE: Compresses can be hot or cold. And some hot packs can also be used as cold packs.)

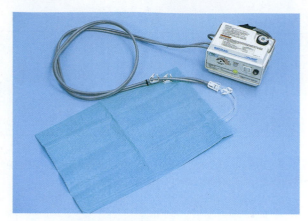

FIGURE 28-16 The aquathermia pad.

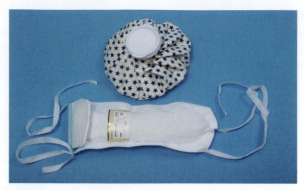

FIGURE 28-17 Ice bags.

Cold Applications

Cold applications are used to treat sprains and fractures. Cold applications:

- Reduce pain.
- Prevent swelling.
- Decrease circulation and bleeding.
- Cool the body when fever is present.

Cold has the opposite effect of heat. When cold is applied to the skin, blood vessels constrict (see Fig. 28-14). Blood flow decreases. Tissues receive less oxygen and nutrients.

Cold is useful right after an injury. Decreased blood flow reduces bleeding. Less fluid collects in the tissues. Cold numbs the skin. This helps reduce or relieve pain in the part.

Complications. Complications include pain, burns, blisters, and poor circulation. Burns and blisters occur from intense cold. They also occur from dry cold in direct contact with the skin.

When cold is applied for a long time, blood vessels dilate. Blood flow increases. Prolonged application of cold has the same effect as heat applications.

Moist and Dry Cold Applications. Moist cold applications penetrate deeper than dry ones. Therefore moist cold applications are warmer than dry cold applications.

The cold compress is a moist cold application (see Fig. 28-15, A). Dry cold applications include ice bags, ice collars, and ice gloves (Fig. 28-17).

Cold packs can be moist or dry applications (see Fig. 28-15, D). Commercial cold packs are single-use (disposable) or re-usable. To activate the cold, you will strike, knead, or squeeze the pack. Keep re-usable cold packs in the freezer. Clean them after use.

Applying Heat and Cold

Protect the person from injury during heat and cold applications. Follow the rules in Box 28-6. See Table 28-1 for heat and cold temperature ranges.

See *Focus on Communication: Applying Heat and Cold.*

See *Delegation Guidelines: Applying Heat and Cold.*

See *Promoting Safety and Comfort: Applying Heat and Cold.*

See procedure: *Applying Heat and Cold Applications,* p. 426.

BOX 28-6	Applying Heat and Cold

- Know how to use the equipment. Follow the manufacturer's instructions for commercial devices.
- Measure the temperature of moist applications. Follow agency policy or use a water thermometer.
- Follow agency policies for safe temperature ranges. See Table 28-1.
- Do not apply *very hot* (above 106°F or 41.1°C) applications. Tissue damage can occur. A nurse applies *very hot* applications.
- Ask the nurse what temperature to use.
  - Heat—cooler temperatures for persons at risk.
  - Cold—warmer temperatures for persons at risk.
- Have the nurse show you the application site.
- Cover dry heat or cold applications before applying them. Use a flannel cover, towel, or other cover as directed.
- Provide for privacy. Properly screen and drape the person. Expose only the body part involved.
- Maintain comfort and body alignment during the procedure.
- Observe the skin every 5 minutes during the procedure. See *Delegation Guidelines: Applying Heat and Cold.*
- Do not let the person change the temperature of the application.
- Know how long to leave the application in place. Heat and cold are applied no longer than 15 to 20 minutes.
- Follow the rules for electrical safety when using electrical appliances for heat. See Chapter 10.
- Place the call light within the person's reach.
- Complete a safety check before leaving the room. (See the inside of the front cover.)

TABLE 28-1	Heat and Cold Temperature Ranges	
Temperature	Fahrenheit (F) Range	Centigrade (C) Range
Hot	99°F to 106°F	37°C to 41°C
Warm	93°F to 98°F	34°C to 37°C
Tepid	80°F to 92°F	26°C to 34°C
Cool	65°F to 79°F	18°C to 26°C
Cold	50°F to 64°F	10°C to 18°C

Modified from Perry AG, Potter PA, Ostendorf WR: Nursing interventions & clinical skills, ed 6, St Louis, 2016, Mosby.

FOCUS ON COMMUNICATION

Applying Heat and Cold

The person may not report pain or discomfort. The person may not know what symptoms to report. For heat and cold applications, you need to ask:
- "Does the application feel too hot or too cold?"
- "Do you feel any pain, numbness, or burning?"
- "Do you feel weak, faint, or drowsy?" If yes: "Tell me how you feel."

DELEGATION GUIDELINES

Applying Heat and Cold

To apply heat or cold, you need this information from the nurse and the care plan.
- What application to apply
- How to cover the application
- What temperature to use (see Table 28-1)
- The application site
- How long to leave the application in place
- What observations to report and record:
  - Complaints of pain or discomfort, numbness, or burning
  - Excess redness
  - Blisters
  - Pale, white, or gray skin
  - Cyanosis—bluish (cyano) color
  - Shivering
  - Rapid pulse, weakness, faintness, and drowsiness (sitz bath)
  - Time, site, and length of application
- When to report observations
- What patient or resident concerns to report at once

PROMOTING SAFETY AND COMFORT

Applying Heat and Cold

Safety

Keep the call light within reach and check the person every 5 minutes. Also follow these safety measures.
- *Sitz bath.* Blood flow increases to the perineum and rectum. Therefore less blood flows to other areas. Observe for signs of weakness, fainting, or fatigue. Also protect the person from injury. Prevent chills and burns.
- *Commercial hot and cold packs.* Read warning labels and follow the manufacturer's instructions.
- *Aquathermia pad:*
  - Follow electrical safety measures (Chapter 10).
  - Check the device for damage or flaws.
  - Follow the manufacturer's instructions.
  - Place the heating unit on an even, uncluttered surface. This prevents it from being knocked over or knocked off the surface.
  - Check the hoses for kinks or bubbles. Water must flow freely.
  - Place the pad in a flannel cover. The flannel absorbs perspiration at the application site. (Some agencies use towels or pillowcases.)
  - Secure the pad in place with ties, tape, or rolled gauze. Do not use pins. They can puncture the pad and cause leaks.
  - Do not place the pad under a body part. This prevents the escape of heat. Burns can result if heat cannot escape.
  - Give the temperature setting key to the nurse. This prevents anyone from changing the temperature. The temperature is usually set at 105°F (40.5°C) with a key.

Some persons have medicated patches or ointments applied to the skin. Do not apply heat over such areas.

Comfort

Cold applications can cause chills and shivering. Provide for warmth. Use bath blankets or other blankets as needed.

Applying Heat and Cold Applications

QUALITY OF LIFE

- Knock before entering the person's room.
- Address the person by name.
- Introduce yourself by name and title.

- Explain the procedure before starting and during the procedure.
- Protect the person's rights during the procedure.
- Handle the person gently during the procedure.

PRE-PROCEDURE

1 Follow *Delegation Guidelines:*
   a *Wound Care*, p. 411
   b *Applying Heat and Cold*, p. 425
   See *Promoting Safety and Comfort: Applying Heat and Cold*, p. 425.
2 Practice hand hygiene.
3 Collect equipment.
   - *For a hot compress:*
     - Basin
     - Water thermometer
     - Small towel, washcloth, or gauze squares
     - Plastic wrap or aquathermia pad
     - Ties, tape, or rolled gauze
     - Bath towel
     - Waterproof under-pad
   - *For a hot soak:*
     - Water basin or arm or foot bath
     - Water thermometer
     - Waterproof under-pad
     - Bath blanket
     - Towel
   - *For a sitz bath:*
     - Disposable sitz bath
     - Water thermometer
     - 2 bath blankets, bath towels, and a clean gown

   - *For an aquathermia pad:*
     - Aquathermia pad and heating unit
     - Distilled water
     - Flannel cover or other cover as directed
     - Ties, tape, or rolled gauze
   - *For a hot or cold pack:*
     - Commercial pack
     - Pack cover
     - Ties, tape, or rolled gauze (if needed)
     - Waterproof under-pad
   - *For an ice bag, ice collar, or ice glove:*
     - Ice bag, collar, or glove
     - Crushed ice
     - Flannel cover or other cover as directed
     - Paper towels
   - *For a cold compress:*
     - Large basin with ice
     - Small basin with cold water
     - Gauze squares, washcloths, or small towels
     - Waterproof under-pad
4 Identify the person. Check the ID bracelet against the assignment sheet. Use 2 identifiers (Chapter 10). Also call the person by name.

PROCEDURE

5 Provide for privacy.
6 Position the person for the procedure.
7 Place the waterproof under-pad (if needed) under the body part.
8 *For a hot compress* (see Fig. 28-15, A):
   a Fill the basin ½ to ⅔ full with hot water as directed. Measure water temperature.
   b Place the compress in the water and wring out.
   c Apply the compress over the area. Note the time.
   d Cover the compress as directed. Do 1 of the following.
     1 Apply plastic wrap and then a bath towel. Secure the towel in place with ties, tape, or rolled gauze.
     2 Apply an aquathermia pad.
9 *For a hot soak* (see Fig. 28-15, B):
   a Fill the container ½ full with hot water. Measure water temperature.
   b Place the part into the water. Pad the edge of the container with a towel (optional). Note the time.
   c Cover the person with a bath blanket for warmth.

10 *For a sitz bath* (see Fig. 28-15, C):
   a Place the disposable sitz bath on the toilet seat.
   b Fill the sitz bath ⅔ full with water. Measure water temperature.
   c Secure the gown above the waist.
   d Help the person sit on the sitz bath. Note the time.
   e Provide for warmth. Place a bath blanket around the shoulders. Place the other over the legs.
   f Stay with the person if he or she is weak or unsteady.
11 *For an aquathermia pad* (see Fig. 28-16):
   a Fill the heating unit to the fill line with distilled water.
   b Remove the bubbles. Place the pad and tubing below the heating unit. Tilt the heating unit from side to side.
   c Set the temperature as the nurse directs (usually 105°F [40.5°C]). Remove the key.
   d Place the pad in the cover.
   e Plug in the unit. Let water warm to the desired temperature.
   f Set the heating unit on the bedside stand. Keep the pad and connecting hoses level with the unit.
   g Apply the pad to the part. Note the time.
   h Secure the pad in place with ties, tape, or rolled gauze.

Applying Heat and Cold Applications—cont'd

PROCEDURE—cont'd

12 *For a hot or cold pack* (see Fig. 28-15, *D*):
  a Squeeze, knead, or strike the pack as directed by the manufacturer.
  b Place the pack in the cover.
  c Apply the pack. Note the time.
  d Secure the pack in place with ties, tape, or rolled gauze. Some packs are secured with Velcro straps.

13 *For an ice bag, collar, or glove* (see Fig. 28-17):
  a Fill the device with water. Put in the stopper. Turn the device upside down to check for leaks.
  b Empty the device.
  c Fill the device ½ to ⅔ full with crushed ice or ice chips.
  d Remove excess air. Bend, twist, or squeeze the device. Or press it against a firm surface.
  e Place the cap or stopper on securely.
  f Dry the device with paper towels.
  g Place the device in the cover.
  h Apply the device. Note the time.
  i Secure the device with ties, tape, or rolled gauze.

14 *For a cold compress* (see Fig. 28-15, *A*):
  a Place the small basin with cold water into the large basin with ice.
  b Place the compresses into the cold water.
  c Wring out a compress.
  d Apply the compress to the part. Note the time.

15 Place the call light and other needed items within reach. Unscreen the person if appropriate.

16 Raise or lower bed rails. Follow the care plan.

17 Do the following every 5 minutes.
  a Check the person for signs and symptoms of complications (see *Delegation Guidelines: Applying Heat and Cold*, p. 425). Remove the application if any occur. Tell the nurse at once.
  b Check the application for cooling (hot application) or warming (cold application).

18 Remove the application after 15 to 20 minutes.

POST-PROCEDURE

19 Provide for comfort. (See the inside of the front cover.)
20 Place the call light and other needed items within reach.
21 Raise or lower bed rails. Follow the care plan.
22 Unscreen the person.
23 Clean, rinse, dry (with clean, dry paper towels), and return re-usable items to their proper place. Follow agency policy for used linens. Wear gloves.
24 Complete a safety check of the room. (See the inside of the front cover.)
25 Remove and discard the gloves. Practice hand hygiene.
26 Report and record your observations.

FOCUS ON **P R I D E**

The Person, Family, and Yourself

Personal and Professional Responsibility
You are responsible for the tasks you perform. Never perform a task you are not comfortable doing. The person may be harmed. Do not be afraid, embarrassed, or ashamed to ask the nurse about your concerns. Take pride in acting responsibly.

Rights and Respect
A person may ask about a wound care measure. Avoid answers like: "It's to help you get better" or "The doctor (nurse) says you need it." The person has the right to be informed. Be kind, caring, and patient when the person asks questions. Tell the person that you will ask the nurse to explain reasons for care. Wait until the person's questions are answered before performing the care measure.

Independence and Social Interaction
Remember to explain procedures to patients and residents. They can plan if they know what will happen. For example, a person wants to make a phone call before a hot compress. Or a person may want a procedure done by a certain time—before visitors arrive or before an activity. You promote independence when you involve the person in planning.

Delegation and Teamwork
Wound care can be painful and tiring. To promote comfort and rest:
- Plan care with the nurse. Ask when drugs for pain will be given and when they will take effect. Allow rest periods before and after care that is tiring.
- Be prepared. Gather supplies. Leaving to get supplies causes delays. Care and procedures take longer than planned.
- Work with the nurse as instructed. You may need to position the person or raise a body part while the nurse changes a dressing. Teamwork reduces the amount of energy the person must use.

Ethics and Laws
Agency practices vary for charging supplies. The person's name and the type and amount of items used are recorded. Ethical practice involves honestly following agency rules. Not charging supplies correctly costs the nursing unit and agency money. Taking supplies home is unethical. This is stealing. Take pride in following agency rules and being an honest and reliable member of the nursing team.

FOCUS ON PRIDE: *Application*

Providing comfort is an important part of every task. What special considerations are needed for wound care? How will you know if you have met the person's comfort needs?

REVIEW QUESTIONS

Circle the BEST answer.

1 Which can cause skin tears?
   a Keeping your nails trimmed and smooth
   b Dressing the person in soft clothing
   c Wearing rings
   d Padding wheelchair footplates

2 A person has a circulatory ulcer. Which measure should you question?
   a Do not cut or trim toenails.
   b Hold socks in place with elastic garters.
   c Apply elastic stockings.
   d Re-position the person every hour.

3 A person has diabetes. When providing foot care
   a Dry well between the toes
   b Apply lotion between the toes
   c Trim the toenails
   d Use hot water

4 Elastic stockings
   a Hold dressings in place
   b Reduce swelling after injury
   c Prevent pressure injuries
   d Prevent blood clots

5 Elastic stockings are applied
   a When the person is standing
   b Before the person gets out of bed
   c After breakfast
   d For 30 minutes and then removed

6 The purpose of an elastic bandage is to
   a Prevent infection
   b Absorb drainage
   c Provide moisture for wound healing
   d Reduce swelling

7 When applying an elastic bandage
   a Position the part in good alignment
   b Cover the fingers or toes if possible
   c Apply it from the large to small part of the extremity
   d Apply it from the upper to lower part of the extremity

8 Dressings
   a Protect the wound from injury
   b Prevent drainage
   c Provide a dry environment for healing
   d Support the wound and reduce swelling

9 To secure a dressing, apply tape
   a Around the entire part
   b Along the sides of the dressing
   c To the top, middle, and bottom of the dressing
   d As the person prefers

10 To remove tape
   a Pull it away from the wound
   b Pull it toward the wound
   c Use forceps
   d Use a saline solution

11 An abdominal binder is used to
   a Prevent blood clots
   b Prevent wound infection
   c Provide support and hold dressings in place
   d Decrease swelling and circulation

12 The *greatest* threat from heat applications is
   a Infection
   b Burns
   c Chilling
   d Skin tears

13 A nurse asks you to apply a hot pack. Which should you question?
   a Check that the pack's temperature is at least 110°F (43.3°C).
   b Place the pack in a cover.
   c Secure the pack in place with ties.
   d Check the person for complications every 5 minutes.

14 When using an aquathermia pad
   a Do not cover the pad
   b Place the pad under the person
   c Check for kinks in the hoses
   d Secure the pad in place with pins

15 Which signals a complication of a cold application?
   a Cool skin
   b Cyanosis
   c Decreased swelling
   d Fever

16 Moist cold compresses are left in place no longer than
   a 20 minutes
   b 30 minutes
   c 45 minutes
   d 60 minutes

Answers to Chapter 28 questions are on p. 552.

FOCUS ON PRACTICE

Problem Solving

An older resident has thin, fragile skin. You notice a new skin tear on the person's arm. What do you do? How can you prevent skin tears?

Pressure Injuries

OBJECTIVES

- Define the key terms and key abbreviations in this chapter.
- Describe the causes and risk factors for pressure injuries.
- Identify the persons at risk for pressure injuries.
- Describe the stages of pressure injuries.
- Identify the sites for pressure injuries.

- Explain how to prevent pressure injuries.
- Identify the complications from pressure injuries.
- Explain how to promote PRIDE in the person, the family, and yourself.

KEY TERMS

bony prominence An area where the bone sticks out or projects from the flat surface of the body; pressure point
eschar Thick, leathery dead tissue that may be loose or adhered to the skin; it is often black or brown
intact skin Normal skin and skin layers without damage or breaks
pressure injury Localized damage to the skin and underlying soft tissue; the injury is usually over a bony prominence or related to a medical or other device and results from pressure or pressure in combination with shear

pressure point See "bony prominence"
shear When layers of the skin rub against each other; when the skin remains in place and underlying tissues move and stretch, tearing underlying capillaries and blood vessels and causing tissue damage
slough Dead tissue that is shed from the skin; it is usually light colored, soft, and moist; may be stringy at times

KEY ABBREVIATIONS

CMS	Centers for Medicare & Medicaid Services	**NPUAP**	National Pressure Ulcer Advisory Panel

Formerly called *pressure ulcers*, the National Pressure Ulcer Advisory Panel (NPUAP) defines *pressure injury* (Fig. 29-1) *as:*
- *Localized damage to the skin and underlying soft tissue.*
- *The injury is usually over a bony prominence or related to a medical or other device.*
- *The injury results from pressure or pressure in combination with shear.*

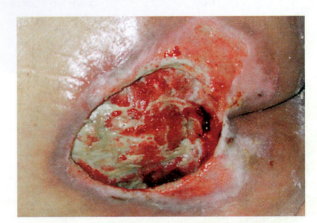

FIGURE 29-1 A pressure injury. (From Ostomy Wound Management, *Proceedings from the November National V.A.C.®* 51[2A, supp]: 7S, Feb 2005, HMP Communications. Used with permission.)

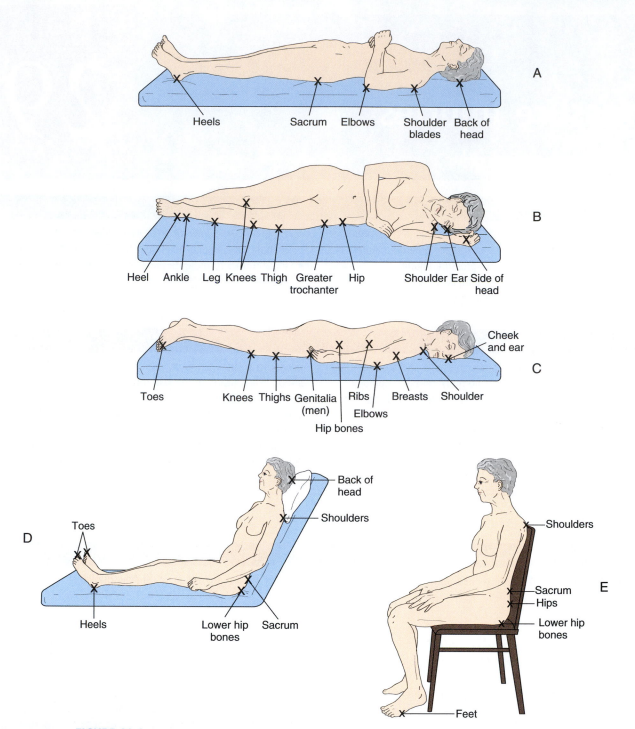

FIGURE 29-2 Bony prominences (pressure points). **A,** The supine position. **B,** The lateral position. **C,** The prone position. **D,** Fowler's position. **E,** Sitting position.

A **bony prominence (pressure point)** *is an area where the bone sticks out or projects from the flat surface of the body.* The backs of the hands, shoulder blades, elbows, hips, spine, sacrum, knees, ankles, heels, and toes are bony prominences (Fig. 29-2).

Pressure injuries result from intense or prolonged pressure and shear. **Shear** *is when layers of the skin rub against each other. Or shear is when the skin remains in place and underlying tissues move and stretch, tearing underlying capillaries and blood vessels. Tissue damage occurs.*

Possibly painful, a pressure injury may involve intact skin or an open ulcer.

- **Intact skin** *is normal skin and skin layers without damage or breaks* (Fig. 29-3).
- An *ulcer* is a shallow or deep crater-like sore of the skin or mucous membrane (see Fig. 29-1).

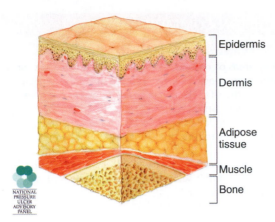

FIGURE 29-3 Intact skin. (From National Pressure Ulcer Advisory Panel.)

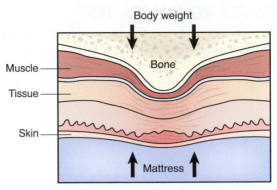

FIGURE 29-4 Tissue under pressure. The skin is squeezed between 2 hard surfaces—the bone and the mattress. (Redrawn from Agency for Healthcare Research and Quality: *Understanding your body: what are pressure ulcers?* Rockville, Md, November 2007, U.S. Department of Health and Human Services.)

RISK FACTORS

Pressure and shearing are the major causes of pressure injuries. Unrelieved pressure squeezes tiny blood vessels. For example, pressure occurs when the skin over a bony area is squeezed between hard surfaces (Fig. 29-4). The bone is 1 hard surface. The other is usually the mattress or chair. Squeezing or pressure prevents blood flow to the skin and underlying tissues. Oxygen and nutrients cannot get to the cells. Skin and tissues die.

Shear occurs when the person slides down in the bed or chair. Blood vessels and tissues are damaged. Blood flow to the area is reduced.

See Box 29-1 for pressure injury risk factors.

PERSONS AT RISK

Persons at risk for pressure injuries are those who:
- Are *bedfast* (confined to bed) or *chairfast* (confined to a chair).
- Need some or total help moving.
- Are agitated, have muscle spasms, or have involuntary muscle movements.
- Are incontinent of urine or feces.
- Are exposed to moisture—urine, feces, wound drainage, sweat, or saliva.
- Have poor nutrition or poor fluid balance.
- Have limited awareness.
- Have problems sensing pain or pressure.
- Have circulatory problems.
- Are obese, have weight loss, or are very thin.
- Have medical devices.
- Have a healed pressure injury.
  See *Focus on Older Persons: Persons at Risk.*

BOX 29-1   Pressure Injury Risk Factors

- Age-related skin changes
- Breaks in the skin
- Dry skin
- Fragile and weak capillaries
- General thinning of the skin
- Loss of the fatty layer under the skin
- Decreased sensation to touch, heat, and cold
- Decreased mobility
- Sitting in a chair or lying in bed most or all of the day
- Chronic diseases (diabetes, high blood pressure)
- Diseases that decrease circulation; poor circulation to an area
- Poor nutrition
- Poor hydration
- Incontinence: urinary, fecal
- Moisture in dark body areas: skin folds, under breasts, perineal area
- Pressure on bony parts
- Poor fingernail and toenail care
- Friction (rubbing of 1 surface against another) and shearing
- *Edema* (the swelling of body tissues with water)

FOCUS ON OLDER PERSONS

Persons at Risk

Older persons have thin, fragile skin that is easily injured. Some have chronic diseases affecting mobility, nutrition, circulation, and awareness.

PRESSURE INJURY STAGES

Pressure injuries range from reddened intact skin to tissue loss with bone exposure. See Box 29-2 for pressure injury stages.

See *Focus on Communication: Pressure Injury Stages.*

Text continued on p. 436.

FOCUS ON COMMUNICATION

Pressure Injury Stages

Report areas of redness, skin color changes, blisters, or skin or tissue loss. Describe what you see as best as you can. Tell the nurse the site. The nurse needs to assess the area. For example, you can say:

- "I saw a reddened area on Mr. Drake's left heel. It was about the size of a quarter. The skin looked intact. Please look at it."
- "I noticed a red area with a blister on Ms. Walsh's left buttock. I didn't see any drainage. Please look at it. I'll help you turn her."

BOX 29-2 | Pressure Injury Stages

Stage 1 Pressure Injury: Non-blanchable erythema of intact skin. *To blanch* means *to become white.* When pressure is applied to the skin, blood is pressed away. This causes the skin to become white or pale. When pressure is relieved, the skin returns to its normal color. *Erythema* means *red or redness. Non-blanchable erythema* means that *the reddened skin does not become white or pale when pressure is applied and removed* (Fig. 29-5). With Stage 1 Pressure Injury, intact skin has a reddened area that is non-blanchable. See Figures 29-6 and 29-7.

Stage 2 Pressure Injury: Partial-thickness skin loss with exposed dermis. The wound is pink or red and moist. It may involve a broken or intact blister. Fat and deeper tissues are not visible. See Figures 29-8 and 29-9.

Stage 3 Pressure Injury: Full-thickness skin loss. The skin is gone. Fat can be seen in the ulcer. Slough and/or eschar may be present. See Figures 29-10 and 29-11, p. 434.

- *Slough* is dead tissue that is shed from the skin. It is usually light colored, soft, and moist. It may be stringy at times.
- *Eschar* is thick, leathery dead tissue that may be loose or adhered to the skin. It is often black or brown.

Stage 4 Pressure Injury: Full-thickness skin and tissue loss. The skin is gone. Muscle, tendon, ligament, cartilage, or bone is exposed. Slough and/or eschar may be seen. See Figures 29-12 and 29-13, p. 434.

Unstageable Pressure Injury: Obscured full-thickness skin and tissue loss. *Obscure* means *not plain or clear.* There is skin and tissue loss. The extent of tissue damage cannot be seen because of slough or eschar. When slough or eschar is removed, the injury can be seen. See Figures 29-14, p. 434 and 29-15, p. 435.

Deep Tissue Pressure Injury: Persistent non-blanchable deep red, maroon, or purple discoloration. Intact or non-intact skin is deep red, maroon, or purple and remains non-blanchable. The wound is dark or is a blood-filled blister. See Figures 29-16 and 29-17, p. 435.

Modified from National Pressure Ulcer Advisory Panel: *NPUAP pressure injury stages,* April 2016.

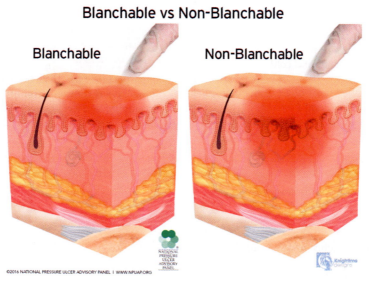

Blanchable vs Non-Blanchable

Blanchable   Non-Blanchable

©2016 NATIONAL PRESSURE ULCER ADVISORY PANEL | WWW.NPUAP.ORG

FIGURE 29-5 Blanchable and non-blanchable skin. (Used with permission of the National Pressure Ulcer Advisory Panel, January 2017.)

Stage 1 Pressure Injury - Lightly Pigmented

Stage 1 Pressure Injury – Darkly Pigmented

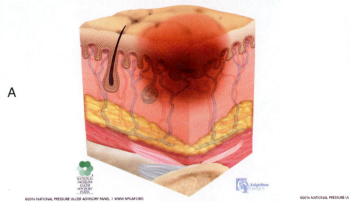

A

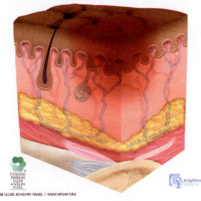

B

FIGURE 29-6 Stage 1 Pressure Injury: Non-blanchable erythema of intact skin. **A,** Light skin. **B,** Dark skin. (Used with permission of the National Pressure Ulcer Advisory Panel, January 2017.)

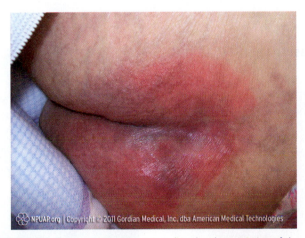

FIGURE 29-7 Stage 1 Pressure Injury. (Used with permission of the National Pressure Ulcer Advisory Panel, January 2017.)

Stage 2 Pressure Injury

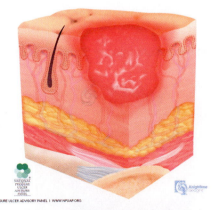

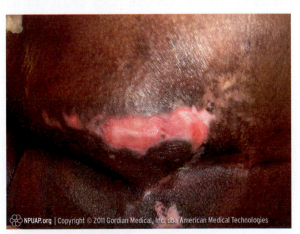

FIGURE 29-8 Stage 2 Pressure Injury: Partial-thickness skin loss with exposed dermis. (Used with permission of the National Pressure Ulcer Advisory Panel, January 2017.)

FIGURE 29-9 Stage 2 Pressure Injury. (Used with permission of the National Pressure Ulcer Advisory Panel, January 2017.)

Stage 3 Pressure Injury

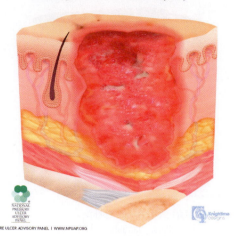

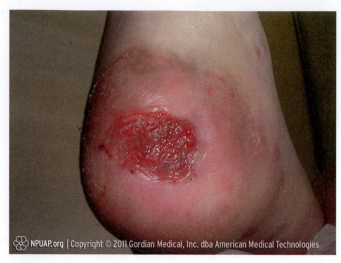

FIGURE 29-10 Stage 3 Pressure Injury: Full-thickness skin loss. (Used with permission of the National Pressure Ulcer Advisory Panel, January 2017.)

FIGURE 29-11 Stage 3 Pressure Injury. (Used with permission of the National Pressure Ulcer Advisory Panel, January 2017.)

Stage 4 Pressure Injury

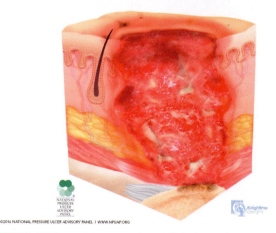

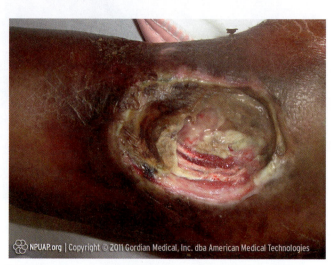

FIGURE 29-12 Stage 4 Pressure Injury: Full-thickness skin and tissue loss. (Used with permission of the National Pressure Ulcer Advisory Panel, January 2017.)

FIGURE 29-13 Stage 4 Pressure Injury. (Used with permission of the National Pressure Ulcer Advisory Panel, January 2017.)

Unstageable Pressure Injury – Dark Eschar   Unstageable Pressure Injury – Slough and Eschar

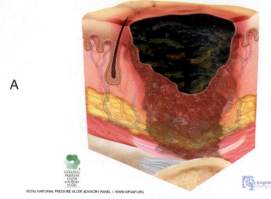

A

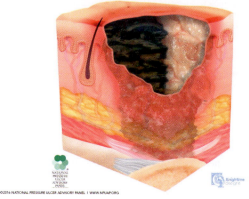

B

FIGURE 29-14 Unstageable Pressure Injury: Obscured full-thickness skin and tissue loss. **A,** Dark eschar. **B,** Slough and eschar. (Used with permission of the National Pressure Ulcer Advisory Panel, January 2017.)

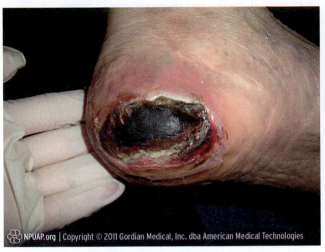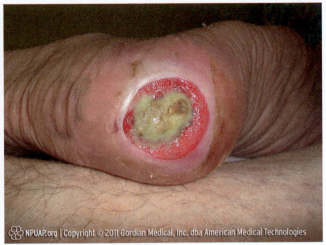

FIGURE 29-15 **A,** Unstageable Pressure Injury with eschar. **B,** Unstageable Pressure Injury with slough. (Used with permission of the National Pressure Ulcer Advisory Panel, January 2017.)

Deep Tissue Pressure Injury

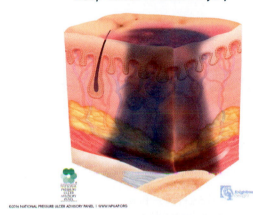

FIGURE 29-16 Deep Tissue Pressure Injury: Persistent non-blanchable deep red, maroon, or purple discoloration. (Used with permission of the National Pressure Ulcer Advisory Panel, January 2017.)

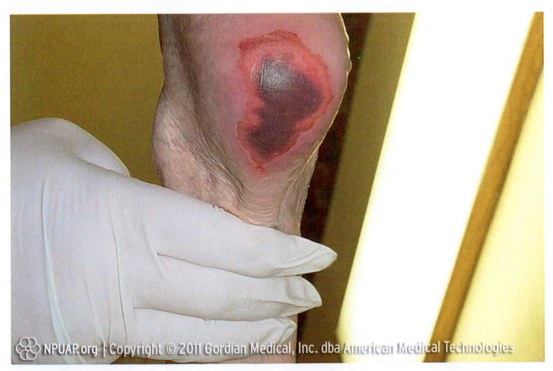

FIGURE 29-17 Deep Tissue Pressure Injury. (Used with permission of the National Pressure Ulcer Advisory Panel, January 2017.)

SITES

Pressure injuries usually occur over bony prominences (pressure points). These areas bear the body's weight in certain positions (see Fig. 29-2). Pressure from body weight can reduce the blood supply to the skin. According to the Centers for Medicare & Medicaid Services (CMS), the sacrum is the most common site for a pressure injury. However, pressure injuries on the heels often occur.

Medical device-related pressure injuries can develop at sites where devices are used for diagnostic or treatment purposes. For example, eyeglasses can cause pressure on the ears. Oxygen tubing (Chapter 30) places pressure on the nose, face, and ears. Pressure can occur on an ear from the mattress when in a side-lying position. Tubes, casts, braces, and other devices can cause pressure on hands, arms, legs, and feet. Pressure can occur on the buttocks from bedpans.

Mucosal membrane pressure injuries are found in mucous membranes where a medical device is used. A urinary catheter can cause pressure on the meatus. A feeding tube can cause pressure in the nose.

Pressure injuries can occur where skin has contact with skin. Common sites are between abdominal folds, the legs, the buttocks, the thighs, and under the breasts.

PREVENTION AND TREATMENT

Preventing pressure injuries is much easier than trying to heal them. Good nursing care, cleanliness, and skin care are essential. Pressure injury prevention involves:
- Identifying persons at risk. The nurse assesses the person's risk factors and skin condition.
- Prevention measures for those at risk. Managing moisture, good nutrition and fluid balance, and relieving pressure are key measures. Box 29-3 lists common measures used to prevent skin damage and pressure injuries. Always follow the care plan.

Some agencies use symbols or colored stickers as pressure injury alerts. Placed on the person's door or medical record, the alerts remind the staff that the person is at risk.

See *Focus on Surveys: Prevention and Treatment*, p. 438.

BOX 29-3	Preventing Pressure Injuries

Moving and Positioning
- Follow the person's re-positioning schedule (Fig. 29-18). Re-position bedfast persons at least every 1 to 2 hours. Re-position chairfast persons at least every hour. Some persons are re-positioned every 15 minutes.
- Remind persons in chairs to shift positions every 15 minutes.
- Position the person according to the care plan. Use pillows for support as directed. The 30-degree lateral position is recommended (Fig. 29-19).
- Do not position the person:
  - On a pressure injury
  - On a reddened area
  - On tubes or other medical devices
- Do not leave a person on a bedpan longer than needed.
- Do not let the person sit on donut-shaped cushions.
- Prevent shearing during moving and transfer procedures. Do not drag the person. Use assist devices as directed. See Chapters 15 and 16.

Moving and Positioning—cont'd
- Prevent shearing. Do not raise the head of the bed more than 30 degrees. Follow the care plan for:
  - When to raise the head of the bed
  - How far to raise the head of the bed
  - How long (in minutes) to raise the head of the bed
- Use pillows, foam wedges, or other devices to prevent bony areas from contact with bony areas. The ankles, knees, hips, and sacrum are examples.
- Keep the heels and ankles off the bed. Use pillows or other devices as directed. Place the pillows or devices under the lower legs from mid-calf to the ankles.
- Use protective devices as directed (p. 438).
- Support the feet properly. Use a footstool if the person's feet do not touch the floor when sitting in a chair. The body slides forward when the feet do not touch the floor. For the person in a wheelchair, position the feet on the footrests.

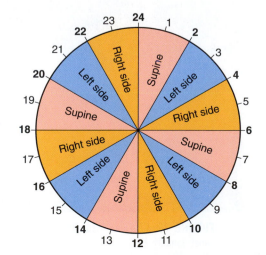

FIGURE 29-18 Turn clock. The clock shows the times to turn the person and to what position.

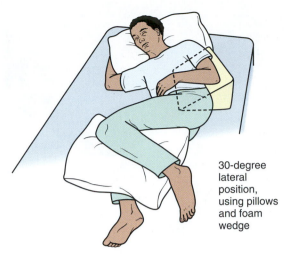

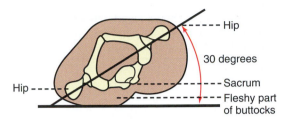

30-degree lateral position, using pillows and foam wedge

Hip

30 degrees

Hip

Sacrum

Fleshy part of buttocks

FIGURE 29-19 The 30-degree lateral position. Pillows are under the head, shoulder, and leg. This position inclines (lifts up) the hip to avoid pressure on the hip. The person does not lie on the hip as in the side-lying position.

BOX 29-3	Preventing Pressure Injuries—cont'd

Skin Care

- Inspect the skin every time you give care. This includes during or after transfers, re-positioning, bathing, and elimination procedures. Report any concern at once.
- Follow the person's bathing schedule. Some persons do not need a bath or shower every day.
- Do not use hot water to bathe or clean the skin. Hot water can irritate the skin.
- Use a cleansing agent as directed. Soap can dry and irritate the skin.
- Provide good skin care.
  - The skin is clean and dry after bathing.
  - The skin is free of moisture from a bath or shower, urine, feces, perspiration, wound drainage, and other secretions.
  - Skin under the breasts and in the groin area is clean and dry.
- Follow measures to prevent incontinence.
- Prevent skin exposure to moisture. Check persons who are incontinent of urine or feces often. Provide good skin care and change linens and garments at the time of soiling. Use incontinence products as directed.
- Apply an ointment or moisture barrier if the person is incontinent of urine or feces. Follow the care plan.
- Check persons often who perspire heavily or have wound drainage. Change linens and garments as needed. Provide good skin care.
- Apply moisturizer to dry areas—hands, elbows, hips, ankles, heels, and so on. The nurse tells you what to use and what areas need attention.
- Give a back massage when re-positioning the person. Do not massage bony areas.
- Do not massage over pressure points. *Never rub or massage reddened areas.*

Skin Care—cont'd

- Keep linens clean, dry, and wrinkle-free.
- Make sure the bed or chair is free of objects. Crumbs, pins, pencils, pens, and coins are examples.
- Do not irritate the skin. Avoid scrubbing or vigorous rubbing when bathing or drying the person.
- Use pillows and blankets to prevent skin from being in contact with skin. They also reduce moisture and friction.
- Make sure clothes do not increase the risk for pressure injuries.
  - Avoid seams, buttons, or zippers that press against the skin.
  - Avoid tight clothes.
  - Keep clothes from bunching up or wrinkling.
- Make sure socks and shoes are in good repair. Socks should not have holes, wrinkles, or creases. Make sure there is nothing in the shoes before the person puts them on.
- Do not apply heat or cold (Chapter 28) directly on a pressure injury.
- See Chapter 28 for care measures to prevent diabetic foot ulcers.

Medical Devices

- Check the skin under a medical device for edema and signs of skin breakdown or a pressure injury.
- Protect the skin under the device as directed by the nurse.
- Do not position the person on top of a medical device.
- Tell the nurse if the device is too loose or too tight.

Protective Devices

The doctor orders wound care products, drugs, treatments, dressings, and equipment to promote healing. Support surfaces relieve or reduce pressure. Such surfaces include foam, air, alternating air, gel, or water mattresses.

Protective devices are often used to prevent and treat skin breakdown and pressure injuries. These devices are common.

- *Bed cradle.* A bed cradle is a metal frame placed on the bed and over the person (Chapter 27). Top linens are brought over the cradle to prevent pressure on the legs, feet, and toes.
- *Heel and elbow protectors.* These devices are made of foam padding, pressure-relieving gel, sheepskin, and other cushioning materials. They fit the shape of heels and elbows (Fig. 29-20).
- *Heel and foot elevators.* These raise the heels and feet off the bed (Fig. 29-21). They prevent pressure. Some also prevent footdrop (Chapter 27).
- *Gel- or fluid-filled pads and cushions.* These devices have a pressure-relieving gel or fluid (Fig. 29-22). They are used for chairs and wheelchairs to prevent pressure. The outer case is vinyl. The device may be placed in a fabric cover to protect the skin.
- *Special beds.* Some beds have air flowing through the mattresses (Fig. 29-23). Body weight is distributed evenly. There is little pressure on body parts. Some beds allow re-positioning without moving the person. The person is turned to the prone or supine position or the bed is tilted various degrees. Alignment does not change. Pressure points change as the position changes. Some beds constantly rotate from side to side. They are useful for persons with spinal cord injuries.
- *Other equipment.* Pillows, trochanter rolls, foot-boards, and other positioning devices are used (Chapter 27). They maintain good alignment.

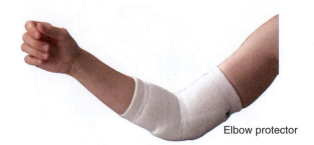

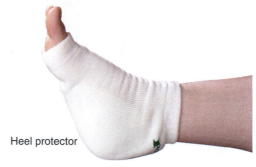

FIGURE 29-20 Elbow and heel protectors. (Images courtesy Posey Company, Arcadia, Calif.)

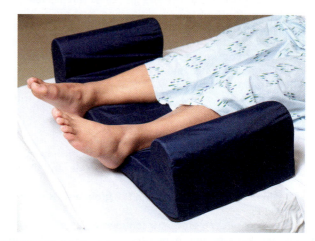

FIGURE 29-21 Heel elevator. (Image courtesy Posey Company, Arcadia, Calif.)

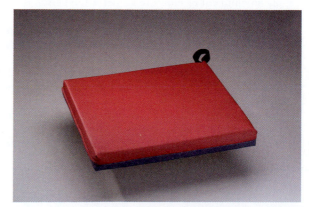

FIGURE 29-22 Two-color foam cushion. The colors remind the staff to re-position the person. (Image courtesy Posey Company, Arcadia, Calif.)

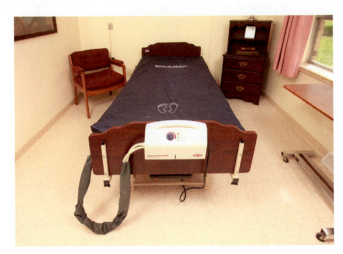

FIGURE 29-23 Air flotation bed.

COMPLICATIONS

Infection is the most common complication. According to the CMS, all Stage 2, 3, and 4 pressure injuries are colonized with bacteria. *Colonized* refers to the presence of bacteria on the wound surface or in wound tissue. The person does not have signs and symptoms of an infection. A wound is *infected* when bacteria invade the tissues around or in the pressure injury. The person has signs and symptoms of infection (Chapter 13). Pain and delayed healing may signal an infection.

Osteomyelitis is a risk if the pressure injury is over a bony prominence. The risk is great if the wound is not healing. *Osteomyelitis* means inflammation (*itis*) of the bone (*osteo*) and bone marrow (*myel*). Pain is severe. Treatment includes bedrest and antibiotics. Careful and gentle positioning is needed. Surgery may be done to remove dead bone and tissue.

Pressure injuries can cause pain. Pain management is important. Pain may affect movement and activity. Immobility is a risk factor for pressure injuries. And it may delay healing of an existing pressure injury.

FOCUS ON PRIDE
The Person, Family, and Yourself

Personal and Professional Responsibility

You have an important role in preventing and treating pressure injuries. Positioning, applying protective devices, and skin care may be delegated to you. Your care must promote quality of life, health, and safety. Your attitude and quality of work affect the person. If you take your role seriously and believe you have a positive impact, the person benefits. If you are careless and lack concern for the person's well-being, harm can result.

You are an important part of the nursing team. Take pride in your role. Work to the best of your ability.

Rights and Respect

You have the right and responsibility to speak for patients and residents. This is called being an *advocate*. You may be the first to notice a pressure injury. Telling the nurse can prevent further harm and result in prompt actions that promote healing. Take pride in being a voice for your patients and residents.

Independence and Social Interaction

A pressure injury is a serious matter. Infection, pain, amputation, and longer hospital or nursing center stays are complications. Healing can take a long time. As time passes, family and friends may not visit as often. Or the person may feel like a burden to others. Loneliness and depression can occur.

Physical needs are great. Do not neglect mental and social needs. Be kind. Show compassion. Take time to listen. Give care in a way that improves quality of life.

Delegation and Teamwork

Always report and record the completion of delegated tasks. Be accurate and honest. Never report or record something you did not do. Also, do not report or record before completing a task.

For example, a nursing assistant did not report placing a resident on the bedpan at 2250 (10:50 PM). The next shift began at 2300 (11:00 PM). At 0700 (7:00 AM), the resident was still on the bedpan. A pressure injury had developed. At risk for pressure injuries, the resident was to be re-positioned every 2 hours. The chart showed re-positioning had been done every 2 hours from 2300 (11:00 PM) to 0700 (7:00 AM).

Poor communication, false recording, and negligence will cause harm. You must be thorough, honest, and careful when completing, reporting, and recording delegated tasks.

Ethics and Laws

Agencies must have a plan to predict, prevent, and treat pressure injuries early. Many agencies use a form or screening tool to identify persons at risk. Assessments are done on admission and regularly. The agency must take action to address risks.

Know your agency's policies and procedures for identifying those at risk for pressure injuries. Follow the measures in Box 29-3 and the care plan to do your part to prevent pressure injuries.

FOCUS ON PRIDE: *Application*

Describe the physical, mental, and social effects a pressure injury can have. How can you help meet the person's needs?

REVIEW QUESTIONS

*Circle **T** if the statement is TRUE or **F** if it is FALSE.*

1 **T F** Unrelieved pressure squeezes tiny blood vessels. Tissues do not receive needed oxygen and nutrients.

2 **T F** Persons who are bedfast or chairfast are at risk for pressure injuries.

3 **T F** Pressure injuries can develop on the ears.

4 **T F** Pressure injuries can develop where medical devices are on the skin.

5 **T F** To prevent pressure injuries, the head of the bed is raised higher than 30 degrees.

6 **T F** You should inspect the person's skin every time you provide care.

7 **T F** A person is at risk for pressure injuries. A bath is needed every day.

8 **T F** You are giving a back massage. You should massage bony areas.

Circle the BEST answer.

9 A pressure injury is
  a An open wound
  b A localized injury to the skin and underlying tissue
  c A bony prominence
  d Dead tissue

10 A person is in Fowler's position. This places pressure on
  a The knees and ankles
  b The ribs and breasts
  c The cheek and ear
  d The sacrum and heels

11 Which contributes to the development of pressure injuries?
  a Shear
  b Slough
  c Eschar
  d Skin blanching

12 Which is a risk factor for pressure injuries?
  a Balanced diet
  b Intact skin
  c Incontinence
  d Increased circulation

13 In a light-skinned person, a Stage 1 Pressure Injury has
  a A blister
  b A reddened area
  c Drainage
  d Gangrene

14 A care plan includes the following. Which should you question?
  a Re-position the person every 2 hours.
  b Scrub the skin during bathing.
  c Apply lotion to dry areas.
  d Keep linens clean, dry, and wrinkle-free.

15 You should position the person
  a On an existing pressure injury
  b On a reddened area
  c On tubes or other medical devices
  d Using assist devices

16 What is the preferred position for preventing pressure injuries?
  a 30-degree lateral position
  b Semi-Fowler's position
  c Prone position
  d Supine position

17 Which keeps the heels and ankles off the bed?
  a Bed cradles
  b Pillows
  c Air flotation bed
  d Trochanter rolls

18 A person in a chair should shift position every
  a 15 minutes
  b 30 minutes
  c Hour
  d 2 hours

19 To prevent skin damage from moisture
  a Avoid using lotion on dry areas
  b Check incontinent persons every 4 hours
  c Dry under the breasts and in the groin area well
  d Change linens once daily for persons who perspire heavily

20 You see a reddened area on the person's skin. What should you do?
  a Rub the area.
  b Apply a moisturizer.
  c Apply a moisture barrier.
  d Tell the nurse.

21 Which can be delegated to you?
  a Assess pressure injury risk factors.
  b Diagnose pressure injury stages.
  c Perform pressure injury prevention measures.
  d Decide how to treat pressure injuries.

22 A pressure injury is colonized. This means that
  a The wound is infected
  b Bacteria are present
  c The person has osteomyelitis
  d The person has a gauze dressing

Answers to Chapter 29 questions are on p. 552.

FOCUS ON PRACTICE

Problem Solving

A resident at risk for pressure injuries complains when awakened for care. You and a co-worker enter the room for re-positioning. The person is asleep. What will you do? What is the risk of waiting to re-position? How can you provide safe, quality care that avoids causing frustration?

Oxygen Needs

OBJECTIVES

- Define the key terms and key abbreviations in this chapter.
- Describe hypoxia and abnormal respirations.
- Explain the measures that promote oxygenation.
- Describe the devices used to give oxygen.
- Explain how to safely assist with oxygen therapy.
- Perform the procedures described in this chapter.
- Explain how to promote PRIDE in the person, the family, and yourself.

KEY TERMS

apnea The lack or absence (a) of breathing (pnea)
bradypnea Slow (brady) breathing (pnea); respirations are fewer than 12 per minute
Cheyne-Stokes respirations Respirations gradually increase in rate and depth and then become shallow and slow; breathing may stop (apnea) for 10 to 20 seconds
cyanosis Bluish color (cyano) to the skin, lips, mucous membranes, and nail beds
dyspnea Difficult, labored, or painful (dys) breathing (pnea)
hyperventilation Breathing (ventilation) is rapid (hyper) and deeper than normal
hypoventilation Breathing (ventilation) is slow (hypo), shallow, and sometimes irregular

hypoxia Cells do not have enough (hypo) oxygen (oxia)
Kussmaul respirations Very deep and rapid respirations
orthopnea Breathing (pnea) deeply and comfortably only when sitting (ortho)
orthopneic position Sitting up (ortho) and leaning over a table to breathe (pneic)
oxygen concentration The amount (percent) of hemoglobin containing oxygen
pulse oximetry Measures (metry) the oxygen (oxi) concentration in arterial blood
tachypnea Rapid (tachy) breathing (pnea); respirations are more than 20 per minute

KEY ABBREVIATIONS

CO_2	Carbon dioxide	O_2	Oxygen
ID	Identification	SpO_2	Saturation of peripheral oxygen (oxygen concentration)
L/min	Liters per minute		

Oxygen (O_2) is a gas. It has no taste, odor, or color. It is a basic need required for life. Death occurs within minutes if breathing stops. Brain damage and serious illness can occur without enough oxygen. Illness, surgery, and injuries affect the amount of oxygen in the body.

NOTE: A task may require more than 1 pair of gloves. Change gloves as needed. Use careful judgment. Remember to practice hand hygiene after removing gloves.

ALTERED RESPIRATORY FUNCTION

Hypoxia means that cells do not have enough (hypo) *oxygen* (oxia). Cells cannot function properly. Anything affecting respiratory function can cause hypoxia. The brain is very sensitive to inadequate O_2. Restlessness, dizziness, and disorientation are early signs. Report the signs and symptoms in Box 30-1 (p. 442) at once.

Hypoxia threatens life. All organs need O_2 to function. Oxygen is given (p. 447). The cause of hypoxia is treated.

BOX 30-1	Altered Respiratory Function

- Hypoxia: signs and symptoms of
  - Restlessness
  - Dizziness
  - Disorientation and confusion
  - Behavior and personality changes
  - Concentrating and following directions: problems with
  - Anxiety and apprehension
  - Fatigue
  - Agitation
  - Pulse rate: increased
  - Respirations: increased rate and depth
  - Sitting position—upright, leaning forward, hunched over a table
  - *Cyanosis—bluish color (cyano) to the skin, lips, mucous membranes, and nail beds*
  - Dyspnea
- Breathing pattern: abnormal
- Shortness of breath or complaints of being "winded" or "short-winded"
- Cough (note type, frequency, and time of day)
  - Dry and hacking
  - Harsh and barking
  - Productive (produces sputum) or non-productive
- Sputum (mucus from the respiratory system)
  - Color—clear, white, yellow, green, brown, or red
  - Odor—none or foul odor
  - Consistency—thick, watery, or frothy (with bubbles or foam)
  - *Hemoptysis—bloody (hemo) sputum (ptysis means to spit);* note if the sputum is bright red, dark red, blood-tinged, or streaked with blood
- Respirations—noisy, wheezing, wet-sounding, crowing sounds
- Chest pain (note location)
  - Constant or comes and goes
  - Person's description—stabbing, knife-like, aching
  - What makes it worse—movement, coughing, yawning, sneezing, sighing, deep breathing, position
- Vital signs: changes in

Abnormal Respirations

Adults normally breathe 12 to 20 times per minute. Normal respirations are quiet, effortless, and regular. Both sides of the chest rise and fall equally. These breathing patterns are abnormal (Fig. 30-1).

- *Tachypnea—rapid* (tachy) *breathing* (pnea). *Respirations are more than 20 per minute.*
- *Bradypnea—slow* (brady) *breathing* (pnea). *Respirations are fewer than 12 per minute.*
- *Apnea—the lack or absence* (a) *of breathing* (pnea).
- *Hypoventilation—breathing* (ventilation) *is slow* (hypo), *shallow, and sometimes irregular.*
- *Hyperventilation—breathing* (ventilation) *is rapid* (hyper) *and deeper than normal.*
- *Dyspnea—difficult, labored, or painful* (dys) *breathing* (pnea).
- *Cheyne-Stokes respirations—respirations gradually increase in rate and depth and then become shallow and slow. Breathing may stop* (apnea) *for 10 to 20 seconds.*
- *Orthopnea—breathing* (pnea) *deeply and comfortably only when sitting* (ortho).
- *Kussmaul respirations—very deep and rapid respirations.*

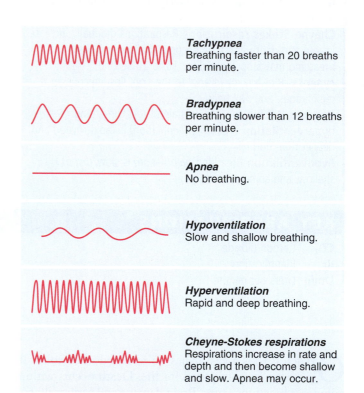

Tachypnea
Breathing faster than 20 breaths per minute.

Bradypnea
Breathing slower than 12 breaths per minute.

Apnea
No breathing.

Hypoventilation
Slow and shallow breathing.

Hyperventilation
Rapid and deep breathing.

Cheyne-Stokes respirations
Respirations increase in rate and depth and then become shallow and slow. Apnea may occur.

Kussmaul respirations
Very deep and rapid breathing.

FIGURE 30-1 Some abnormal breathing patterns.

RESPIRATORY TESTS

The doctor may order a chest x-ray to detect lung changes. Sometimes other complex tests are ordered. You may be involved in pulse oximetry and sputum specimens (Chapter 26). Assist with other tests as directed by the nurse.

Pulse Oximetry

Pulse oximetry measures (metry) *the oxygen* (oxi) *concentration in arterial blood. Oxygen concentration is the amount (percent) of hemoglobin containing O_2.* An agency may use 1 of these terms.

- *Pulse oximetry* or *pulse ox*
- *O_2 saturation* or *O_2 sat*
- *SpO_2* (saturation of peripheral oxygen)

The normal oxygen concentration range is 95% to 100%. For example, if 97% of all hemoglobin (100%) carries O_2, tissues get enough oxygen. If only 90% contains O_2, tissues do not get enough oxygen.

A sensor attaches to a finger, toe, earlobe, nose, or forehead (Fig. 30-2). A good sensor site is needed. Avoid swollen sites and sites with skin breaks. If there is poor blood flow to fingers or toes, use the earlobe, nose, or forehead site.

Bright light, nail polish, fake nails, and movements affect measurements.

- Place a towel over the sensor to block bright lights.
- Remove nail polish or use another site.
- Do not use finger sites with fake nails.
- Use the earlobe if there is shivering, seizure, or tremor movements.
- Do not measure blood pressure on the side of a finger site. Blood pressure cuffs affect blood flow.

Oxygen concentration is often measured with vital signs. The pulse rate may be shown on the pulse oximeter along with the oxygen concentration. Report and record measurements according to agency policy.

See *Delegation Guidelines: Pulse Oximetry.*
See *Promoting Safety and Comfort: Pulse Oximetry.*
See procedure: *Using a Pulse Oximeter*, p. 444.

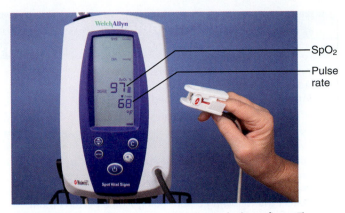

FIGURE 30-2 A pulse oximetry sensor is attached to a finger. The device displays the O_2 concentration and pulse.

DELEGATION GUIDELINES
Pulse Oximetry

To assist with pulse oximetry, you need this information from the nurse and the care plan.

- What site to use
- How to use the equipment
- What sensor to use
- What type of tape to use (if needed)
- The person's normal SpO_2 range
- Alarm limits for SpO_2 and pulse rate (if set)
- When to do the measurement
- What pulse site to use: apical or radial
- How often to check the site for continuous monitoring (usually every 2 hours)
- What observations to report and record:
  - The date and time
  - The SpO_2 and display pulse rate (see Fig. 30-2)
  - Apical or radial pulse rate
  - What the person was doing at the time
  - Oxygen flow rate (p. 448) and the device used (p. 448)
  - Reason for the measurement: routine, continuous monitoring, or condition change
- When to report observations
- What patient or resident concerns to report at once:
  - An SpO_2 below the alarm limit (usually 95%)
  - A pulse rate above or below the alarm limit
  - The signs and symptoms listed in Box 30-1

PROMOTING SAFETY AND COMFORT
Pulse Oximetry

Safety
The person's condition can change quickly. Pulse oximetry does not lessen the need for good observation. Observe for signs and symptoms of hypoxia and altered respiratory system function (see Box 30-1).

Comfort
A clip-on sensor feels like a clothespin. It should not hurt or cause discomfort. Ask the person to tell you at once if it causes pain, discomfort, or too much pressure. Change the sensor site as directed by the nurse.

Using a Pulse Oximeter

QUALITY OF LIFE

- Knock before entering the person's room.
- Address the person by name.
- Introduce yourself by name and title.

- Explain the procedure before starting and during the procedure.
- Protect the person's rights during the procedure.
- Handle the person gently during the procedure.

PRE-PROCEDURE

1 Follow *Delegation Guidelines: Pulse Oximetry*, p. 443. See *Promoting Safety and Comfort: Pulse Oximetry*, p. 443.
2 Practice hand hygiene.
3 Collect the following before going to the person's room.
   - Oximeter
   - Tape (if needed)
   - Towel

4 Arrange your work area.
5 Practice hand hygiene.
6 Identify the person. Check the identification (ID) bracelet against your assignment sheet. Use 2 identifiers (Chapter 10). Also call the person by name.
7 Provide for privacy.

PROCEDURE

8 Provide for comfort.
9 Dry the site with a towel.
10 Clip or tape the sensor to the site.
11 Turn on the oximeter.
12 *For continuous monitoring:*
   a Set the high and low alarm limits for SpO$_2$ and pulse rate.
   b Turn on audio and visual alarms.

13 Check the apical or radial pulse with the pulse on the display. The pulse rates should be about the same. Note both pulses on your assignment sheet.
14 Read the SpO$_2$ on the display. Note the value on the flow sheet and your assignment sheet.
15 Leave the sensor in place for continuous monitoring. Otherwise, turn off the device and remove the sensor.

POST-PROCEDURE

16 Provide for comfort. (See the inside of the front cover.)
17 Place the call light and other needed items within reach.
18 Unscreen the person.
19 Complete a safety check of the room. (See the inside of the front cover.)

20 Return the device to its proper place (unless monitoring is continuous).
21 Practice hand hygiene.
22 Report and record the SpO$_2$, the pulse rates, and your other observations.

MEETING OXYGEN NEEDS

Air must move deep into the lungs to alveoli where O$_2$ and CO$_2$ (carbon dioxide) are exchanged. Disease, injury, and surgery can prevent air from reaching the alveoli. Pain, immobility, and some drugs interfere with deep breathing and coughing. Therefore secretions collect in the airway and lungs. Microbes can grow in the secretions. Infection is a threat.

See *Focus on Communication: Meeting Oxygen Needs.*

FOCUS ON COMMUNICATION

Meeting Oxygen Needs

The questions you ask the person assist the nurse with the nursing process. For example:
- "Do you need more pillows?"
- "Do you want the head of your bed raised more?"
- "How often are you coughing?"
- "Are you coughing anything up?"
- "Are you coughing up mucus? Please use a tissue to cough up mucus, then put on your call light. The nurse will observe the mucus."

Positioning

Breathing is usually easier in the semi-Fowler's and Fowler's positions. Persons with difficulty breathing often prefer the *orthopneic position—sitting up* (ortho) *and leaning over a table to breathe* (pneic). Place a pillow on the table to increase comfort (Fig. 30-3).

If the person must lie flat for a procedure, raise the head of the bed as soon as possible. Raise it at once if the person has difficulty breathing.

Position changes are needed at least every 2 hours. Follow the care plan.

FIGURE 30-3 The person is in the orthopneic position. A pillow is on the over-bed table for comfort.

Deep Breathing and Coughing

Deep breathing moves air into most parts of the lungs. Coughing removes mucus. Deep-breathing and coughing exercises promote oxygenation. They are done after surgery or injury and during bedrest. The exercises are painful after surgery or injury. Breaking an incision open while coughing is a fear.

Deep breathing and coughing are usually done every 1 to 2 hours while awake.

See *Focus on Communication: Deep Breathing and Coughing.*

See *Delegation Guidelines: Deep Breathing and Coughing.*

See *Promoting Safety and Comfort: Deep Breathing and Coughing.*

See procedure: *Assisting With Deep-Breathing and Coughing Exercises.*

DELEGATION GUIDELINES

Deep Breathing and Coughing

When delegated deep-breathing and coughing exercises, you need this information from the nurse and the care plan.

- When to do them and how often
- How many deep breaths and coughs are needed
- What observations to report and record:
  - The number of deep breaths and coughs
  - How the person tolerated the procedure
- When to report observations
- What patient or resident concerns to report at once

PROMOTING SAFETY AND COMFORT

Deep Breathing and Coughing

Safety

Respiratory hygiene and cough etiquette are needed for a productive cough (Chapter 13). The person needs to:

- Cover the nose and mouth to cough or sneeze.
- Use tissues to contain respiratory secretions.
- Dispose of tissues in the nearest waste container after use.
- Wash the hands after coughing, sneezing, or contact with respiratory secretions.

While the person is covering the nose and mouth, you need to splint a chest or abdominal incision with your hands or a pillow. See step 8-b in procedure: *Assisting With Deep-Breathing and Coughing Exercises.* Wear gloves to splint the incision.

FOCUS ON COMMUNICATION

Deep Breathing and Coughing

To encourage cough etiquette (Chapter 13), you can say:

Please cover your nose and mouth with tissues when coughing. I'll put these tissues where you can reach them. Here is a waste container to dispose of your tissues. Where would you like it? Also, please wash your hands after coughing. Let me know if you need help.

Assisting With Deep-Breathing and Coughing Exercises

QUALITY OF LIFE

- Knock before entering the person's room.
- Address the person by name.
- Introduce yourself by name and title.

- Explain the procedure before starting and during the procedure.
- Protect the person's rights during the procedure.
- Handle the person gently during the procedure.

PRE-PROCEDURE

1 Follow *Delegation Guidelines: Deep Breathing and Coughing.* See *Promoting Safety and Comfort: Deep Breathing and Coughing.*
2 Practice hand hygiene.

3 Identify the person. Check the ID bracelet against the assignment sheet. Use 2 identifiers (Chapter 10). Also call the person by name.
4 Provide for privacy.

PROCEDURE

5 Lower the bed rail if up.
6 Help the person to a comfortable sitting position.
  - Sitting on the side of the bed
  - Semi-Fowler's
  - Fowler's
7 Have the person deep breathe.
  a Have the person place the hands over the rib cage (Fig. 30-4, p. 446).
  b Have the person breathe as deeply as possible. Remind the person to inhale through the nose.
  c Ask the person to hold the breath for 2 to 3 seconds.
  d Ask the person to exhale slowly through pursed lips (Fig. 30-5, p. 446). Ask the person to exhale until the ribs move as far down as possible.
  e Repeat this step 4 more times.

8 Ask the person to cough.
  a *If the person does not have a productive cough:* Have the person place both hands over the chest or abdominal incision. One hand is on top of the other (Fig. 30-6, A, p. 446). Or the person holds a pillow or folded towel over the chest or abdominal incision (Fig. 30-6, B, p. 446).
  b *If the person has a productive cough:*
    1 Have the person practice cough etiquette.
    2 Splint the chest or abdominal incision with your hands or a pillow. Wear gloves.
  c Have the person take in a deep breath as in step 7.
  d Ask the person to cough strongly 2 times with the mouth open.

Continued

Assisting With Deep-Breathing and Coughing Exercises—cont'd

POST-PROCEDURE

9 Provide for comfort. (See the inside of the front cover.)
10 Place the call light and other needed items within reach.
11 Raise or lower bed rails. Follow the care plan.
12 Unscreen the person.

13 Complete a safety check of the room. (See the inside of the front cover.)
14 Practice hand hygiene.
15 Report and record your observations.

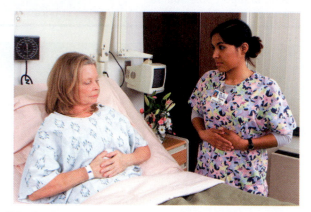

FIGURE 30-4 The hands are over the rib cage for deep breathing.

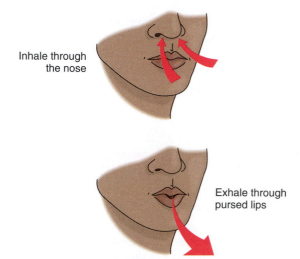

Inhale through the nose

Exhale through pursed lips

FIGURE 30-5 The person inhales through the nose and exhales through pursed lips during the deep-breathing exercise.

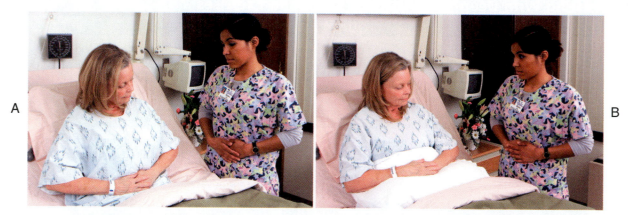

A

B

FIGURE 30-6 The incision is supported for the coughing exercise. **A,** The hands are over the incision. **B,** A pillow is held over the incision.

ASSISTING WITH OXYGEN THERAPY

Disease, injury, and surgery often interfere with breathing. The doctor orders oxygen therapy when the amount of O_2 in the blood is less than normal (*hypoxemia*).

Oxygen is treated as a drug. The doctor orders when to give O_2, the amount, and the device to use. Oxygen is needed constantly or for symptom relief—chest pain or shortness of breath. Persons with respiratory diseases may have enough oxygen at rest. With mild exercise or activity, they become short of breath. Oxygen helps relieve shortness of breath.

You do not give oxygen. The nurse and respiratory therapist start and maintain oxygen therapy. You help provide safe care.

Oxygen Sources

Oxygen is supplied as follows.

- *Wall outlet.* O_2 is piped into each person's unit (Fig. 30-7).
- *Oxygen tank.* The tank is placed at the bedside. Small tanks are used for emergencies and transfers. They also are used by persons who walk or use wheelchairs (Fig. 30-8). A gauge tells how much O_2 is left (Fig. 30-9).
- *Oxygen concentrator.* The machine removes oxygen from the air (Fig. 30-10). A power source is needed. A small oxygen tank is needed for power failures and mobility.
- *Liquid oxygen system.* A portable unit is filled from a stationary unit. Depending on unit size and the flow rate (p. 448), the portable unit has enough O_2 for about 8 to 20 hours of use. A dial shows the amount of O_2 in the unit. The portable unit is shown in Figure 30-11, p. 448.

See *Promoting Safety and Comfort: Oxygen Sources,* p. 448.

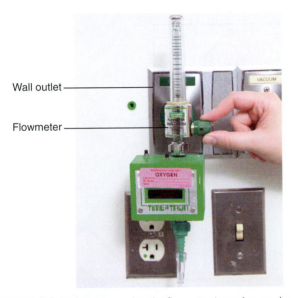

FIGURE 30-7 Wall oxygen outlet. The flowmeter is used to set the oxygen flow rate.

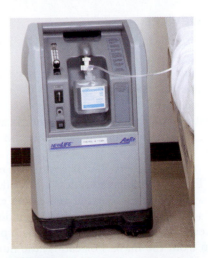

FIGURE 30-8 A portable oxygen tank is used when walking.

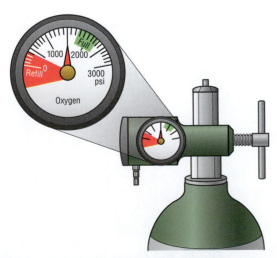

FIGURE 30-9 The gauge shows the amount of oxygen in the tank.

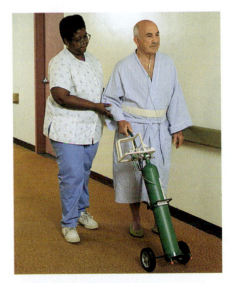

FIGURE 30-10 Oxygen concentrator.

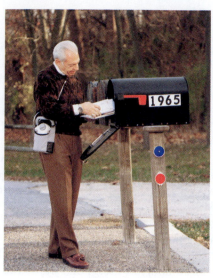

FIGURE 30-11 A portable liquid oxygen unit allows the person to be mobile. (Image used by permission from Nellcor Puritan Bennett LLC, Boulder, Colo; part of Covidien.)

PROMOTING SAFETY AND COMFORT

Oxygen Sources

Safety

Liquid oxygen is very cold. If touched, it can freeze the skin. Tampering with equipment is unsafe and could damage the equipment. Follow agency procedures and the manufacturer's instructions for liquid oxygen.

Many activities increase the need for O_2. These include moving in bed, transfer procedures, and walking. Do not remove the person's O_2. If needed, ask the nurse for longer tubing. Or ask the nurse to change to a portable oxygen tank.

Oxygen tanks and liquid oxygen systems contain a certain amount of O_2. When the O_2 level is low, a new tank is needed or the liquid oxygen system is refilled. Check the O_2 level often. Report a low O_2 level at once.

Oxygen Devices

The doctor orders the device for giving O_2. These devices are common.

- *Nasal cannula* (Fig. 30-12). The prongs are inserted into the nostrils. A band goes behind the ears and under the chin to keep the device in place. A cannula allows eating and drinking. Tight prongs can irritate the nose. Pressure on the ears and cheekbones is possible.
- *Simple face mask* (Fig. 30-13). It covers the nose and mouth. The mask has small holes in the sides. CO_2 escapes when exhaling. Talking and eating are hard to do with a mask. Moisture can build up under the mask. Keep the face clean and dry to help prevent irritation from the mask. For eating, the nurse changes the oxygen mask to a cannula.

Oxygen Flow Rates

The *flow rate* is the amount of oxygen given. It is measured in liters per minute (L/min). The doctor orders 1 to 15 liters of O_2 per minute. The nurse or respiratory therapist sets the flow rate with a flowmeter (see Fig. 30-7).

The nurse and care plan tell you the person's flow rate. Always check the flow rate. Tell the nurse at once if it is too high or too low. A nurse or respiratory therapist will adjust the flow rate. Some states and agencies let nursing assistants adjust O_2 flow rates. Know your agency's policy.

Oxygen Safety

You assist the nurse with oxygen therapy. *You do not give oxygen. You do not adjust the flow rate unless allowed by your state and agency.* However, you must give safe care. Follow the rules in Box 30-2. Also follow the rules for fire and the use of oxygen (Chapter 10).

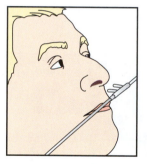

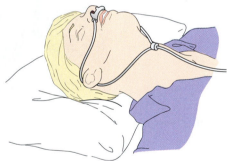

FIGURE 30-12 Nasal cannula. NOTE: The prong openings face downward.

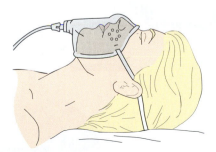

FIGURE 30-13 Simple face mask.

BOX 30-2   Oxygen Safety

- Do not remove the oxygen device.
- Make sure the device is secure but not tight.
- Check for irritation from the device:
  - Behind the ears
  - Under the nose (cannula)
  - Around the face (mask)
  - On the cheekbones
- Keep the face clean and dry when a mask is used.
- Do not shut off the O_2 flow. *However, turn off the O_2 flow if there is a fire. Remove the oxygen device.*
- Do not adjust the flow rate unless allowed by your state and agency.
- Tell the nurse at once if the:
  - Flow rate is too high or too low.
  - Humidifier is not bubbling (Fig. 30-14). Humidified (moist) oxygen prevents drying of the airway's mucous membranes. Bubbling means that moisture is being produced.
- Maintain an adequate water level in the humidifier.
- Secure tubing in place. Tape, clamp, or pin it to the person's garment following agency policy. Do not puncture the tubing.
- Make sure there are no kinks in the tubing.
- Make sure the person does not lie on any part of the tubing.
- Make sure the oxygen tank is secure in its holder.
- Report at once signs and symptoms of altered respiratory function or abnormal breathing patterns. See p. 442.
- Follow the care plan for oral hygiene.
- Make sure the oxygen device is clean and free of mucus.
- See "Fire and Oxygen" in Chapter 10.

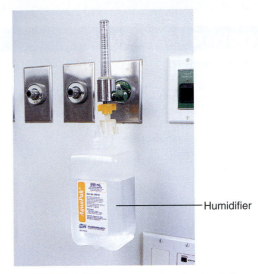
— Humidifier

FIGURE 30-14 Oxygen set-up with a humidifier.

FOCUS ON P R I D E

The Person, Family, and Yourself

Personal and Professional Responsibility

You are responsible for reporting the person's complaints. A person may say: "I can't breathe" or "I'm not getting enough air." Yet you see the person breathing. Do not dismiss the complaint. Tell the nurse at once. You cannot feel what the person does. Trust what the person tells you.

Rights and Respect

People have the right to a safe setting. For safety, smoking is not allowed where oxygen is used and stored. NO SMOKING signs are common in rooms and hallways. You may need to remind the person or visitors not to smoke. Be polite and respectful. Show the person where smoking is allowed.

Independence and Social Interaction

Needing long-term oxygen therapy changes a person's life. Work, daily activities, and hobbies can be a challenge. The person may feel alone and depressed. Social support from family and friends is important.

Portable oxygen sources increase independence. Small oxygen tanks and portable liquid oxygen units are examples. Such devices allow freedom and promote quality of life.

Delegation and Teamwork

Oxygen is treated as a drug. You assist with oxygen therapy. You do not give oxygen. You do not adjust the flow rate unless allowed by your state and agency and instructed to do so by the nurse.

If asked to give oxygen or adjust a flow rate, politely refuse. Refusing to perform a task is your right and duty when the task is beyond the legal limits of your role. Do not ignore the request. Tell the nurse that you can assist. Gathering supplies is an example. Or ask if you can help with a different task.

Ethics and Laws

Performing tasks that you are not trained to do can cause harm. You can lose your job and your ability to work as a nursing assistant. Take pride in following the limits of your role and providing safe care.

FOCUS ON PRIDE: *Application*

What are the limits to your role when assisting with oxygen therapy? Why are such limits important? Explain the value of your role. How do you help the nurse and patient or resident?

Circle the BEST answer.

1 Hypoxia is
   a Not enough oxygen in the blood
   b The amount of hemoglobin that contains oxygen
   c Not enough oxygen in the cells
   d The lack of carbon dioxide

2 An early sign of hypoxia is
   a Cyanosis
   b Increased pulse
   c Restlessness
   d Dyspnea

3 A person breathes deeply and comfortably only while sitting. This is called
   a Apnea
   b Orthopnea
   c Bradypnea
   d Kussmaul respirations

4 Tachypnea means that respirations are
   a Slow
   b Rapid
   c Absent
   d Difficult or painful

5 Which should you report to the nurse at once?
   a A respiratory rate of 18 per minute
   b An SpO_2 of 97%
   c Bubbling in a humidifier
   d Dyspnea

6 A person's SpO_2 is 98%. Which is *true?*
   a The pulse oximeter is wrong.
   b The pulse is 98 beats per minute.
   c The measurement is within normal range.
   d The person has hypoxia.

7 A person has fake nails. Which is a good pulse oximetry sensor site?
   a The wrist
   b A finger
   c The upper arm
   d An earlobe

8 You are assisting with deep breathing and coughing. You need to explain the procedure again if the person
   a Inhales through pursed lips
   b Sits in a comfortable position
   c Inhales deeply through the nose
   d Holds a pillow over an incision

9 A person has a productive cough. You remind the person to
   a Use a face mask
   b Cover the nose and mouth when coughing
   c Cough and deep breathe twice daily
   d Inhale through the mouth

10 Liquid oxygen can freeze the skin.
   a True
   b False

11 Oxygen flow rate is measured in
   a mm Hg
   b mL/hr
   c L/min
   d SpO_2

12 When assisting with oxygen therapy, you can
   a Turn the oxygen on and off
   b Start the oxygen
   c Decide what device to use
   d Keep connecting tubing secure and free of kinks

13 A person complains of pressure on the ears from nasal cannula tubing. You should
   a Check for irritation and tell the nurse
   b Change the cannula to a mask
   c Remove the device
   d Explain that the pressure is normal

14 A person is receiving O_2. Which should you question?
   a Provide oral hygiene.
   b Use a portable tank for walking.
   c Adjust the flow rate if it is too high or too low.
   d Secure tubing in place.

Answers to Chapter 30 questions are on p. 552.

FOCUS ON PRACTICE

Problem Solving

You are a student training in the clinical setting. A nursing assistant asks you to change a person's O_2 flow rate. Nursing assistants in your state are not allowed to adjust O_2 flow rates. How will you respond? What will you do if the nursing assistant adjusts the flow rate?

Rehabilitation Needs

OBJECTIVES

- Define the key terms and key abbreviations in this chapter.
- Describe how rehabilitation involves the whole person.
- Identify the complications to prevent.
- Identify the common reactions to rehabilitation.

- Explain your role in rehabilitation.
- List the common rehabilitation programs and services.
- Explain how to promote PRIDE in the person, the family, and yourself.

KEY TERMS

activities of daily living (ADL) The activities usually done during a normal day in a person's life
disability Any lost, absent, or impaired physical or mental function
prosthesis An artificial replacement for a missing body part
rehabilitation The process of restoring the person to his or her highest possible level of physical, psychological, social, and economic function

restorative aide A nursing assistant with special training in restorative nursing and rehabilitation skills
restorative nursing care Care that helps persons regain health, strength, and independence

KEY ABBREVIATIONS

ADL   Activities of daily living

ROM   Range of motion

Disease, injury, and surgery can affect body function. Often more than 1 function is lost.

A *disability* is any lost, absent, or impaired physical or mental function.

- An *acute problem* has a short course with complete recovery. A fracture (broken bone) is an example.
- A *chronic problem* has a long course. The problem is controlled—not cured—with treatment. Arthritis and paralysis are chronic health problems.

Disabilities can affect eating, bathing, dressing, walking, and work ability. The degree of disability affects how much function is possible. The person may depend totally or in part on others for basic needs.

Rehabilitation is the process of restoring the person to his or her highest possible level of physical, psychological, social, and economic function. The goals are to:

- Prevent or reduce the degree of disability.
- Improve abilities for the highest level of independence. Self-care or returning to work may be a goal. If improved function is not possible, the goal is to prevent further loss of function for the best possible quality of life.
- Help the person adjust to the disability.

Some persons return home after rehabilitation. The process may continue in home or community settings. See *Focus on Older Persons: Rehabilitation Needs, p. 452.*

RESTORATIVE NURSING

Some persons cannot perform daily functions. *Restorative nursing care is care that helps persons regain health, strength, and independence.* With progressive illnesses, disabilities increase. Restorative nursing:
- Helps maintain the highest level of function.
- Prevents unnecessary decline in function.
  Restorative nursing measures promote:
- Self-care
- Elimination
- Positioning
- Mobility
- Communication
- Cognitive function

Many persons need restorative nursing and rehabilitation. In many agencies, they mean the same thing. Both focus on the whole person.

Restorative Aides

A *restorative aide is a nursing assistant with special training in restorative nursing and rehabilitation skills.* These aides assist the nursing and health teams as needed. Required training varies among states. If there are no state requirements, the agency provides needed training.

THE WHOLE PERSON

A health problem affects the whole person with physical, psychological, and social effects. So does a disability. Adjustments are physical, psychological, social, and economic. Abilities—what the person can do—are stressed. Complications may cause further disability.

See *Focus on Older Persons: The Whole Person.*

Physical Aspects

Rehabilitation starts when the person first seeks health care. Complications are prevented from bedrest, a long illness, surgery, or injury. Bowel and bladder problems are prevented. So are contractures and pressure injuries. Good alignment, turning and re-positioning, range-of-motion (ROM) exercises, and supportive devices are needed (Chapters 14, 15, 16, and 27). Good skin care also prevents pressure injuries (Chapters 18 and 29).

Elimination. Some persons need bladder training (Chapter 20). The method depends on the person's problems, abilities, and needs. Some need bowel training (Chapter 22). Bowel control and regular elimination are goals. Fecal impaction, constipation, and fecal incontinence are prevented.

Self-Care. Self-care is a major goal. *Activities of daily living (ADL) are the activities usually done during a normal day in a person's life.* ADL include bathing, oral hygiene, dressing, eating, elimination, and moving about. The health team evaluates the person's ADL abilities and the need for self-help devices.

Sometimes the hands, wrists, and arms are affected. Adaptive (assistive) devices are often changed, made, or bought for the person's needs.
- Eating devices include glass holders, plate guards, and silverware with curved handles or cuffs (Chapter 23). Some devices attach to splints (Fig. 31-1).
- Electric toothbrushes have back-and-forth brushing motions for oral hygiene.
- Adaptive (assistive) devices for hygiene promote independence.

Adaptive (assistive) devices are useful for cooking, dressing, writing, phone calls, and other tasks. Some are shown in Figure 31-2. Also see Chapters 18 and 19.

See *Focus on Surveys: Self-Care.*

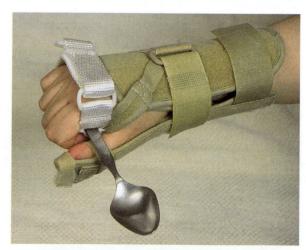

FIGURE 31-1 Eating device attached to a splint.

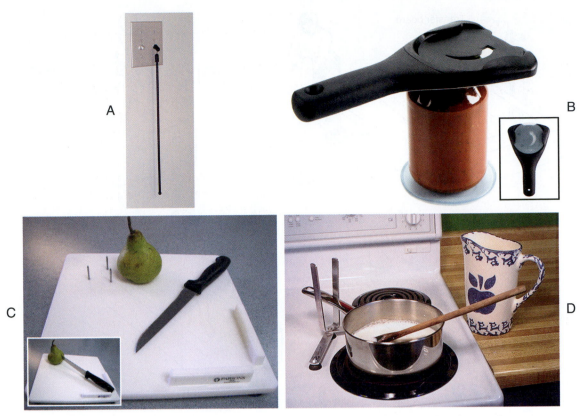

FIGURE 31-2 A, Light switch extender. **B,** Jar opener. **C,** Cutting board. **D,** Pot stabilizer. (A, C, and D, Courtesy Parsons ADL, Inc. Tottenham, Ontario. B, Courtesy OXO International, Inc., New York, NY.)

Nutrition. Difficulty swallowing (*dysphagia*) may occur after a stroke. The person may need a dysphagia diet (Chapter 23). If possible, the person learns exercises to improve swallowing. Persons who cannot swallow need enteral nutrition (Chapter 23).

Mobility. The person may need crutches or a walker, cane, or brace (Chapter 27). Physical and occupational therapies are common for musculo-skeletal and nervous system problems. Some people need wheelchairs. If possible, they learn wheelchair transfers. Such transfers include to and from the bed, toilet, bathtub, sofa, and chair and in and out of vehicles (Fig. 31-3, p. 454).

A ***prosthesis*** *is an artificial replacement for a missing body part.* The person learns how to use the artificial arm or leg (Chapter 33). The goal is for the device to be like the missing body part in function and appearance.

Communication

Aphasia (Chapter 32) may occur from a stroke. *Aphasia* is the total or partial loss (*a*) of the ability to use or understand language (*phasia*). It results from damage to parts of the brain responsible for language and speech. Speech therapy and communication devices are helpful (Chapter 7).

See *Focus on Communication: Communication,* p. 454.

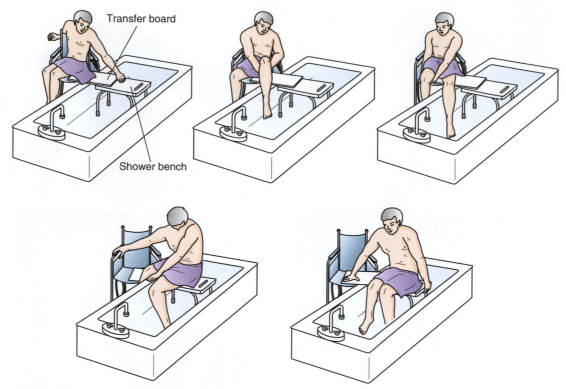

FIGURE 31-3 A wheelchair to tub transfer. A transfer board (sliding board) and shower bench are used.

FOCUS ON COMMUNICATION

Communication

Speaking presents problems for some persons. Persons with speech disorders may need other communication methods. Pictures, reading, writing, facial expressions, and gestures are examples. All health team members and the family use the same method with the person. Changing methods can cause confusion and delay progress.

Psychological and Social Aspects

A disability can affect function and appearance. Self-esteem and relationships may suffer. Feelings of being unwhole, useless, unattractive, unclean, or undesirable are common. Some deny the disability, expecting therapy to correct the problem. Some persons are depressed, angry, and hostile.

A good attitude is important. The person must be motivated and accept limits. The focus is on abilities and strengths. Progress may be slow. Learning a new task is a reminder of the disability.

Remind persons of their progress. Give support, reassurance, and encouragement. Psychological and social needs are part of the care plan. Spiritual support helps some persons.

See *Focus on Communication: Psychological and Social Aspects.*

FOCUS ON COMMUNICATION

Psychological and Social Aspects

Emotional needs are great during rehabilitation. Good communication and support provide encouragement.
- Listen to the person.
- Show concern, not pity.
- Focus on what the person can do. Point out even slight progress.
- Be polite but firm. Do not let the person control you.
- Do not shout at or insult the person. Such behaviors are abuse and mistreatment.
- Do not argue with the person.
- Tell the nurse about problems. The person may need other support measures.

THE REHABILITATION TEAM

Rehabilitation is a team effort. The person is the key team member. The person, family, doctor, and nursing and health teams set goals and plan care. The focus is to regain function and independence.

The team meets often to discuss the person's progress. The rehabilitation plan is changed as needed. The person and family attend the meetings when possible. Families provide support and encouragement. Often they help with home care.

Your Role

You help promote the person's independence. Preventing decline in function also is a goal. The many procedures, care measures, and rules in this book apply. Safety, communication, legal, and ethical aspects apply. So do the measures in Box 31-1.

See *Focus on Communication: Your Role.*

FOCUS ON COMMUNICATION

Your Role

You may need to guide and direct the person during care. Listen to how the nurse or therapist guides and directs the person. Use those words. Hearing the same thing helps the person learn and remember what to do.

REHABILITATION PROGRAMS

Common rehabilitation programs include:

- *Cardiac rehabilitation*—for heart disorders
- *Brain injury rehabilitation*—for nervous system disorders including traumatic brain injury
- *Spinal cord rehabilitation*—for spinal cord injuries
- *Stroke rehabilitation*—after a stroke
- *Respiratory rehabilitation*—for respiratory system disorders such as chronic obstructive pulmonary disease, after lung surgery, and for respiratory complications from other health problems
- *Orthopedic rehabilitation*—for fractures, joint replacement surgery, and other musculo-skeletal problems
- *Amputee rehabilitation*—for amputation of a limb
- *Hearing, speech, and vision rehabilitation*—for persons who are deaf, have speech problems, are blind, or have severe vision problems
- *Drug and alcohol treatment*—for persons addicted to drugs or alcohol
- *Behavioral health treatment*—for those with mental health problems
- *Rehabilitation for complex medical and surgical conditions*—wound care, diabetes, and burns are examples

After hospital care, the person may transfer to a nursing center or rehabilitation agency. Home care agencies and adult day-care centers also provide rehabilitation services.

QUALITY OF LIFE

Successful rehabilitation improves quality of life. A hopeful and winning outlook is needed. The more the person can do alone, the better his or her quality of life. To promote quality of life:

- Protect the right to privacy.
- Encourage personal choice.
- Protect the right to be free from abuse and mistreatment.
- Learn to deal with your anger and frustration.
- Encourage activities.
- Provide a safe setting.
- Show patience, understanding, and sensitivity.

BOX 31-1 Assisting With Rehabilitation Needs

Physical Needs

- Follow the care plan and the nurse's instructions.
- Follow the person's daily routine.
- Provide for safety.
- Report early signs and symptoms of complications. They include pressure injuries, contractures, and bowel and bladder problems.
- Keep the person in good alignment.
- Turn and re-position the person as directed.
- Use safe transfer methods.
- Practice measures to prevent pressure injuries.
- Perform ROM exercises as instructed.
- Remember that muscles will atrophy if not used. And contractures can develop.
- Know how to use and apply assistive (adaptive) devices.
- Provide and apply needed assistive (adaptive) devices.

Psychological and Social Needs

- Protect the person's rights. Privacy and personal choice are very important.
- Encourage performing ADL to the extent possible.
- Allow time to complete tasks. Do not rush the person.
- Give praise for even a little progress.
- Provide emotional support and reassurance.
- Try to understand and appreciate the person's situation, feelings, and concerns.
- Do not pity the person or give sympathy.
- Provide for spiritual needs.
- Practice the methods developed by the rehabilitation team. You will better assist the person.
- Practice the task that the person must do. This helps you guide and direct the person.
- Stress what the person can do. Focus on abilities and strengths, not on disabilities and weaknesses.
- Have a hopeful outlook.

FOCUS ON P R I D E

The Person, Family, and Yourself

Personal and Professional Responsibility

Often nursing assistants are promoted to restorative aide positions. Professional behaviors are highly valued for promotions. Patience, kindness, and good communication skills are needed. Staff with a positive attitude, good work ethics, and excellent job performance are considered first.

Becoming a restorative aide allows you to advance as a nursing assistant. Seek out learning opportunities and practice positive work habits. Take pride in continuing to learn, improve, and grow as a nursing assistant.

Rights and Respect

Rehabilitation is challenging for the person, the family, and the nursing staff. No matter how difficult the situation, the person's rights are always protected. See Chapter 2.

Simple things are often hard. You, other staff, or the family may become upset and short-tempered. Protect the person from abuse and mistreatment. No one can shout at, scream at, yell at, or call the person names. They cannot hit or strike the person. Unkind remarks are not allowed. Report signs of abuse or mistreatment.

The setting must be safe and meet the person's needs. Needed changes are made. For example, the over-bed table, bedside stand, call light, and other needed items are moved to the person's strong (unaffected) side. If unable to use the call light, another communication aid is used. The rehabilitation team suggests needed changes to the person and family.

Independence and Social Interaction

Quality of life improves the more the person can do for himself or herself. To promote independence:

- Stress the person's abilities and strengths.
- Let the person choose activities of interest.
- Remain patient. Avoid rushing the person.
- Resist the urge to do things for the person that he or she can do.
- Offer encouragement and support. The person may worry about how others view the disability. A caring and positive attitude can help motivate them.
- Have the person use assistive (adaptive) devices as needed.
- Encourage personal choice. Personal choice allows control.

Delegation and Teamwork

Disability affects the whole person. Frustration is common. Many persons are angry and discouraged. Such feelings can be hard to control. Outbursts may occur.

You must learn to deal with your frustration. The person does not choose loss of function. If the process upsets you, think how the person must feel. You must:

- Show patience, understanding, sensitivity, and respect.
- Be calm and act in a professional manner.
- Control your words and actions.

The nurse can suggest ways to help you control or express your feelings. You may need to assist with other persons for a while. Take pride in being a part of a strong, supportive team.

Ethics and Laws

The person may not want to practice rehabilitation procedures or methods. He or she may want you to give care instead. To make progress, the person needs to follow the rehabilitation plan. Do not let the person control you. Report any problems to the nurse.

FOCUS ON PRIDE: *Application*

Explain how a disability affects the whole person. Write a brief scenario describing a person with a disability. Discuss the impact on the whole person and family.

Circle T if the statement is TRUE and F if it is FALSE.

1 **T F** You should give praise for even slight progress.
2 **T F** Only chronic health problems require rehabilitation.
3 **T F** A person is not allowed food until exercises are done. This is abuse and mistreatment.
4 **T F** Personal preferences are considered in the rehabilitation plan.
5 **T F** Rehabilitation for older persons is usually faster-paced than for younger persons.
6 **T F** You need to stress what the person can do.
7 **T F** You should know how to use and apply assistive (adaptive) devices.
8 **T F** You need to convey hopefulness to the person.

Circle the BEST answer.

9 Rehabilitation focuses on
   a What the person cannot do
   b Self-care
   c The whole person
   d Mobility and communication

10 Rehabilitation involves preventing
   a Angry feelings
   b Contractures and pressure injuries
   c The use of assistive (adaptive) devices
   d Nursing center care

11 A person has weakness on the right side. ADL are
   a Done by the person to the extent possible
   b Done by you
   c Delayed until the right side can be used
   d Supervised by a therapist

12 To provide emotional support during rehabilitation
   a Remind the person of his or her limits
   b Give sympathy and show pity
   c Talk about your feelings
   d Listen and give praise

13 During therapy, a person wants music played. You should
   a Explain that music is not allowed
   b Choose some music
   c Ask the person to choose some music
   d Ask a therapist to choose some music

14 A person's right side is weak. You move the call light to the left side. You promote quality of life by
   a Encouraging self-care
   b Allowing personal choice
   c Providing for safety
   d Taking part in activities

Answers to Chapter 31 questions are on p. 552.

FOCUS ON PRACTICE

Problem Solving

A person's care plan includes long-handled devices for dressing and bathing. During the bath, you provide a long-handled sponge. The person says: "I don't feel like using that today. Will you wash my feet for me?" What will you say and do? How will your response affect the person's progress?

OBJECTIVES

- Define the key terms and key abbreviations in this chapter.
- Describe the common ear, speech, and eye disorders.
- Describe how to communicate with persons who have hearing loss.
- Explain the purpose of a hearing aid.
- Describe how to care for hearing aids.
- Explain how to communicate with persons who have speech disorders.

- Explain how to assist persons who are visually impaired or blind.
- Perform the procedure described in this chapter.
- Explain how to promote PRIDE in the person, the family, and yourself.

KEY TERMS

aphasia The total or partial loss *(a)* of the ability to use or understand language *(phasia)*

blindness The absence of sight

braille A touch reading and writing system that uses raised dots for each letter of the alphabet; the first 10 letters also represent the numbers 0 through 9

deafness Hearing loss in which it is impossible for the person to understand speech through hearing alone

hearing loss Not being able to hear the range of sounds associated with normal hearing

low vision Vision loss that cannot be corrected with eyeglasses, contact lenses, drugs, or surgery; vision loss interferes with every-day activities

tinnitus A ringing, roaring, hissing, or buzzing sound in the ears or head

vertigo Dizziness

KEY ABBREVIATIONS

AMD	Age-related macular degeneration	**ASL**	American Sign Language

Hearing, speech, and vision are important for self-care, work, most activities, and safety and security needs. For example, you see dark clouds and hear tornado warning sirens. You know to seek shelter. With speech, you alert others.

Hearing, speech, and vision disorders occur in all age-groups. Common causes are birth defects, injuries, infections, diseases, and aging. See Chapter 8 as you study this chapter.

HEARING DISORDERS

The ear functions in hearing and balance. Hearing is needed for clear speech, responding to others, safety, and awareness of surroundings.

Meniere's Disease

Meniere's disease involves the inner ear. Symptoms include:

- *Vertigo—dizziness*
- *Tinnitus—a ringing, roaring, hissing, or buzzing sound in the ears or head*
- Hearing loss
- Feeling of fullness or pressure in the ear
  Fluid buildup in the inner ear causes swelling and pressure in the inner ear. Symptoms are sudden.

An attack usually involves vertigo, tinnitus, and hearing loss. Vertigo causes whirling and spinning sensations. The dizziness causes severe nausea and vomiting. An episode can last 20 minutes or 2 to 24 hours.

Drugs and a low-salt diet decrease fluid in the inner ear. Smoking, caffeine, and alcohol are avoided. Safety is needed during vertigo.

- Have the person lie down.
- Prevent falls. Assist with walking and use bed rails according to the care plan.
- Have the person keep the head still. The person avoids turning the head. To talk to the person, stand directly in front of him or her.
- Avoid sudden movements. The person moves slowly.
- Prevent bright or glaring lights.

Hearing Loss

Hearing loss is not being able to hear the range of sounds associated with normal hearing. Losses are mild to deafness. *Deafness is hearing loss in which it is impossible for the person to understand speech through hearing alone.*

Common in older persons, causes include damage to the outer, middle, or inner ear or to the acoustic nerve. See Box 32-1 for some signs and symptoms of hearing loss.

Hearing is needed for clear speech. Pronouncing words and voice volume depend on hearing yourself. Hearing loss may result in slurred speech or pronouncing words wrong. Some people have monotone speech or drop word endings. It may be hard to understand the person. Do not assume or pretend that you understand. Serious problems can result. See "Speech Disorders" on p. 461.

Communication. Persons with hearing loss may wear hearing aids or lip-read (speech-read). They watch facial expressions, gestures, and body language. Some people learn American Sign Language (ASL) (Fig. 32-1). ASL uses signs made with the hands and other movements such as facial expressions, gestures, and postures.

Some people have *hearing dogs.* The dog alerts the person to sounds. Phones, doorbells, smoke alarms, alarm clocks, babies' cries, sirens, and on-coming cars are examples.

See Box 32-2 (p. 460) for measures to promote hearing. See *Focus on Communication: Communication.*

FOCUS ON COMMUNICATION

Communication

The National Association of the Deaf (NAD) uses the terms *deaf* and *hard of hearing* to describe persons with hearing loss. Do not use the terms *deaf and dumb, deaf-mute,* or *hearing-impaired.* Such terms offend persons who are hard of hearing.

BOX 32-1	Hearing Loss—Signs and Symptoms

- Problems:
  - Hearing on the phone
  - Hearing with background noise or in noisy areas
  - Following conversations when 2 or more people are speaking
  - Understanding women and children
- Straining to understand a conversation
- Hearing voices as mumbled or slurred
- Misunderstanding what others say
- Answering questions or responding inappropriately
- Asking others to repeat themselves
- Speaking too loudly
- Leaning forward to hear
- Turning and cupping the better ear toward the speaker
- Turning up the TV, radio, music, or other sound sources so loud that others complain

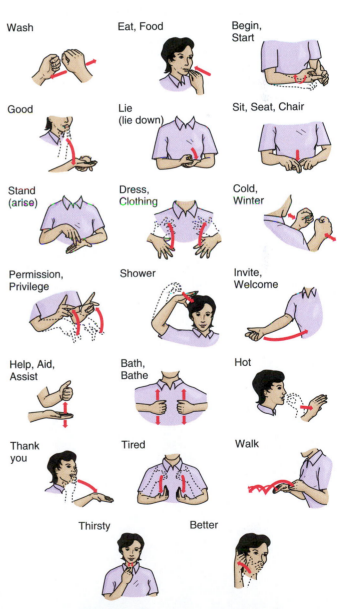

FIGURE 32-1 American Sign Language examples.

BOX 32-2	Measures to Promote Hearing

The Setting

- Reduce or eliminate background noises. Turn off radios, music players, TVs, air conditioners, fans, and so on.
- Provide a quiet place to talk. Avoid areas with loud sound.
- Have the person sit where able to hear best.

The Person

- Have the person wear his or her hearing aid. It must be turned on and working.
- Have the person wear needed eyeglasses or contact lenses. The person needs to see your face to lip-read (speech-read).

You

- Gain attention. Alert the person to your presence. Raise an arm or hand or lightly touch the person's hand, arm, or shoulder. Do not startle or approach the person from behind.
- Position yourself at the person's level. Sit if the person is sitting. Stand if the person is standing.
- Face the person when speaking. Do not turn or walk away while you are talking. Do not talk from the doorway or another room.
- Have light shine on your face. Shadows and glares affect the ability to see your face clearly.
- Maintain eye contact with the person.
- Speak clearly, distinctly, and at a normal rate. Do not talk too fast or too slow.
- Speak in a normal tone of voice. Do not shout or mumble.
- State the person's name before starting a conversation. This gains the person's attention and focus.

You—cont'd

- Adjust the pitch of your voice as needed. Ask if the person can hear you better.
  - If no hearing aid, lower the pitch. Higher-pitched voices are harder to hear than lower-pitched voices.
  - If a hearing aid is worn, raise the pitch slightly.
- Do not cover your mouth, smoke, eat, or chew gum while talking. Mouth movements are affected.
- Keep your hands away from your face. The person needs to see your face clearly.
- Stand or sit on the side of the better ear.
- State the topic of conversation first.
- Say when you are changing the subject. State the new topic.
- Use short sentences and simple words.
- Pause between sentences. Ensure understanding before speaking again.
- Use gestures and facial expressions as useful clues.
- Write out important names, words, numbers, addresses, appointments, and so on.
- Re-phrase if the person does not seem to understand. Do not repeat the same words again and again.
- Keep conversations and discussions short. This avoids tiring the person.
- Be alert to messages sent by your facial expressions, gestures, and body language.
- Be alert to the person's nonverbal communication. For example, watch for puzzled looks and expressions of anger, frustration, excitement, fatigue, and so on.

Hearing Aids. *Hearing aids* fit inside or behind the ear (Fig. 32-2). They make sounds louder. They do not correct, restore, or cure hearing problems. The person hears better because the device makes sounds louder. Background noise and speech are louder. The measures in Box 32-2 apply.

Hearing aids are costly. See Box 32-3 for hearing aid care measures.

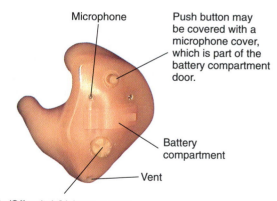

Microphone

Push button may be covered with a microphone cover, which is part of the battery compartment door.

Battery compartment

Vent

On/Off switch/Volume control

FIGURE 32-2 A hearing aid. (Courtesy Siemens Hearing Instruments, Inc., Piscataway, NJ.)

BOX 32-3   Hearing Aids—Care Measures

- Hold and handle hearing aids gently. This includes when removing, inserting, or cleaning the device and when inserting batteries.
- Do the following if a hearing aid does not seem to work properly.
  - Check if the hearing aid is *on*. The device has an *on* and *off* switch.
  - Check the battery position.
  - Insert a new battery if needed. Use the correct battery size.
  - Clean the hearing aid. Follow the manufacturer's instructions.
- Hold the hearing aid over a soft cloth or soft surface to change the battery or to clean the device.
- Do not expose the hearing aid to heat or extreme cold.
- Have the person remove the hearing aid before using a hair dryer, hair spray, spray perfumes, shaving lotions, or powders.
- Protect the hearing aid from water. The person does not wear a hearing aid during a bath or shower.
- Clean the hearing aid according to the manufacturer's instructions.
- Check meal trays and bed linens for hearing aids. The person may have removed the hearing aid and set it aside.
- Remove and turn off the hearing aid at bedtime. This saves battery life. Remove the battery if the person prefers.
- Place the hearing aid in its storage case when not worn. Place the storage case in the top drawer of the bedside stand.

BOX 32-4   Communicating With Speech-Impaired Persons

The Person
- Have the person repeat or re-phrase statements as needed.
- Repeat what the person has said. Ask if you understood correctly.
- Have the person write down key words or the message.
- Have the person point, gesture, or draw key words.

You
- Follow the care plan. A consistent approach is needed.
- Provide a calm, quiet setting. Turn off the TV, radio, music, and other distractions.
- Include the person in conversations.
- Listen and give the person your full attention.
- Use short, simple sentences.
- Repeat as needed.
- Write down key words as needed.
- Speak in a normal tone. Do not treat or talk to an adult in a babyish or child-like way.
- Ask questions to which you know the answers. This helps you learn how the person speaks.
- Allow the person plenty of time to talk.
- Determine the topic being discussed. This helps you understand main points. Watch lip movements.
- Watch facial expressions, gestures, and body language. They give clues about what is being said.
- Do not correct the person's speech.

SPEECH DISORDERS

Speech disorders affect oral communication. Hearing loss and brain injury are common causes. These problems are common.
- *Aphasia.* See "Aphasia" below.
- *Apraxia of speech.* Apraxia means not (*a*) to act, do, or perform (*praxia*). The person with *apraxia of speech* cannot use speech muscles for understandable speech. The person understands and knows what to say. However, the person cannot make the words.
- *Dysarthria.* Dysarthria means difficult or poor (*dys*) speech (*arthria*). Mouth and face muscles are affected. Slurred, soft, slow, or hoarse speech can occur.

To communicate with the speech-impaired person, practice the measures in Box 32-4.

Aphasia

Aphasia is the total or partial loss (a) *of the ability to use or understand language* (phasia). Parts of the brain responsible for language are damaged. Stroke, head injury, brain infections, dementia, and cancer are common causes.

Expressive aphasia (motor aphasia, Broca's aphasia) relates to difficulty expressing or sending out thoughts through speech or writing. The person knows what to say but has problems speaking, spelling, counting, gesturing, or writing. The person may:
- Omit small words such as "is," "and," "of," and "the."
- Speak in 1-word or short sentences. "Walk dog" can mean "I will take the dog for walk" or "You take the dog for a walk."
- Put words in the wrong order. The person may say "room bath" for "bathroom."
- Think one thing but say another. The person may want food but asks for a book.
- Call people the wrong names.
- Make up words.
- Produce sounds and no words.
- Cry or swear for no reason.

Receptive aphasia (Wernicke's aphasia) is difficulty understanding language. The person has trouble understanding what is said or written. Words do not make sense. What the person says has no meaning. People and common objects are not recognized. The person may not know how to use every-day items—fork, toilet, cup, TV, phone, or other items.

Some people have both expressive and receptive aphasia. *Global aphasia (mixed aphasia)* involves difficulty expressing or sending out thoughts and difficulty understanding language. The person has problems speaking and understanding language.

EYE DISORDERS

Vision problems range from mild loss to complete blindness. *Blindness is the absence of sight.* Vision loss is sudden or gradual. One or both eyes are affected.

Cataracts

A cataract is clouding of the lens. The normal lens is clear. *Cataract* comes from the Greek word for *waterfall*. Trying to see is like looking through a waterfall. Cataracts can occur in 1 or both eyes. Surgery is the only treatment (Box 32-5). Signs and symptoms include:

- Cloudy, blurry, or dimmed vision (Fig. 32-3, *A* and *B*).
- Colors seem faded and brownish. Blues and purples are hard to see.
- Sensitivity to light and glares.
- Poor vision at night.
- Halos around lights.
- Double vision in the affected eye.

BOX 32-5	Cataract Surgery—Post-Operative Care

- Have the person wear ordered eyeglasses or eye shield as directed. If ordered, the shield is worn for sleep, including naps.
- Follow measures for visually impaired or blind persons when an eye shield is worn (p. 464). There may be vision loss in the other eye.
- Remind the person not to rub or press the affected eye.
- Do not bump the eye.
- Place the over-bed table and bedside stand on the un-operative side.
- Place the call light and needed items within reach.
- Report eye drainage or complaints of pain at once.
- Remind the person not to bend, stoop, cough, or lift things.

Age-Related Macular Degeneration

Age-related macular degeneration (AMD) blurs central vision. *Central vision* is seen "straight-ahead." AMD causes a blind spot in the center of vision (see Fig. 32-3, *A* and *C*). Central vision is needed for reading, sewing, driving, and seeing faces and fine detail.

Onset is gradual and painless. For advanced AMD, no treatment can prevent vision loss. Laser surgery may stop or slow the disease progress.

Diabetic Retinopathy

In diabetic retinopathy, blood vessels in the retina are damaged. A complication of diabetes, it is a leading cause of blindness. Usually both eyes are affected.

Vision blurs (see Fig. 32-3, *A* and *D*). The person may see spots "floating." Often there are no early warning signs.

The person needs to control diabetes, blood pressure, and cholesterol. Laser surgery may help.

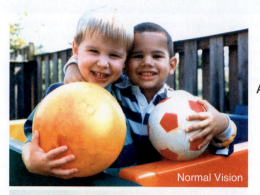

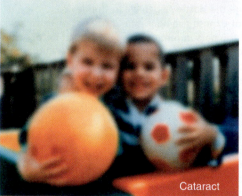

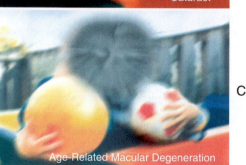

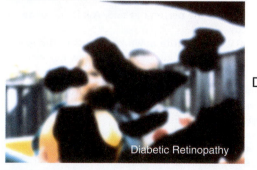

FIGURE 32-3 Vision loss with eye disorders. **A,** Normal vision. **B,** Vision loss from a cataract. **C,** Vision loss from macular degeneration. **D,** Vision loss from diabetic retinopathy. (A and B, Modified from National Eye Institute: *Facts about cataract,* Bethesda, Md, September 2015, National Institutes of Health. C, Modified from National Eye Institute: *Don't lose sight of age-related macular degeneration,* Bethesda, Md, NIH Publication No. 12-3251, revised 2012, National Institutes of Health. D, Modified from National Eye Institute: *Facts about diabetic eye disease,* Bethesda, Md, September 2015, National Institutes of Health.)

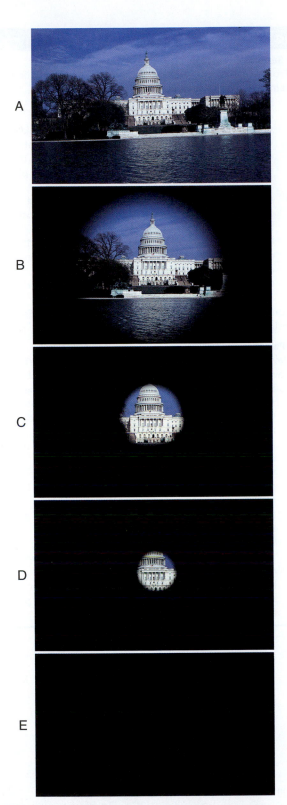

Glaucoma

With glaucoma, fluid builds up in the eye, causing pressure on the optic nerve. The optic nerve is damaged. Vision loss with eventual blindness occurs.

Glaucoma can affect 1 or both eyes. Peripheral vision (side vision) is lost. The person sees through a tunnel (Fig. 32-4), has blurred vision, and sees halos around lights.

Glaucoma has no cure. Prior damage cannot be reversed. Drugs and surgery can control glaucoma and prevent further damage to the optic nerve.

Low Vision

Low vision is vision loss that cannot be corrected with eyeglasses, contact lenses, drugs, or surgery. The vision loss interferes with every-day activities. While wearing eyeglasses or contact lenses, the person has problems:

- Recognizing faces of family and friends
- Doing tasks that require close vision—reading, cooking, sewing, and so on
- Picking out and matching clothing colors
- Reading signs (traffic, stores)
- Doing things because lighting seems dimmer

The person learns to use visual and adaptive (assistive) devices. Examples include:

- Prescription reading glasses
- Large-print reading materials
- Hand-held and video magnifiers
- Audio tapes
- Electronic reading machines
- Computers with large print and speech systems
- Phones, clocks, and watches with large numbers and that talk
- Lighting that can be adjusted

Impaired Vision and Blindness

Some people are totally blind. Others sense some light but have no usable vision. Others have some usable vision but cannot read newsprint. The legally blind person sees at 20 feet what a person with normal vision sees at 200 feet.

Loss of sight is serious. Adjustments can be hard and long. Special education and rehabilitation programs help the person adjust to the vision loss and learn to be independent. The goal is to be as active as possible and have quality of life. The person learns to use visual and adaptive (assistive) devices, braille, long canes, and guide dogs. Follow the practices in Box 32-6 (p. 464) according to the care plan.

FIGURE 32-4 Vision loss from glaucoma. **A,** Normal vision. **B,** Loss of peripheral vision begins. **C, D,** and **E,** Vision loss continues, with eventual blindness.

BOX 32-6   Caring for Blind and Visually Impaired Persons

The Setting

- Report worn or loose carpeting and other flooring. Also report the use of throw rugs or plastic runners.
- Keep furniture, equipment, electrical cords, and other items out of areas where the person will walk.
- Report furniture that has wheels.
- Keep chairs pushed in under the table or desk.
- Keep room doors fully open or fully closed.
- Keep drawers and cabinet, cupboard, and closet doors fully closed.
- Report burnt-out light bulbs.
- Provide preferred lighting. Tell the person when the lights are on or off.
- Adjust window coverings to prevent glares. Sunny days and bright, snowy days cause glares.
- Keep the call light and TV, light, and other controls within reach.
- Turn on night-lights in the person's room and bathroom and in hallways.
- Practice safety measures to prevent falls (Chapter 11).
- Orient the person to the room. Describe the layout. Include the location and purpose of furniture and equipment.
- Let the person touch and find furniture and equipment.
- Do not re-arrange furniture and equipment.
- Use colors and contrast. Solid, bright colors (red, orange, yellow) are best. Avoid pastels, patterns, prints, designs, and stripes. White or yellow against black provides strong contrast. Place light-colored objects against dark backgrounds or dark-colored objects against light backgrounds. For example, use a white plate with a dark placemat or tablecloth.

The Setting—cont'd

- Provide the same meal-time setting. Arrange things in the same way for each meal.
  - Have the person sit in good light.
  - Arrange the place setting.
    - The knife and spoon are to the right of the plate.
    - The fork and napkin are to the left of the plate.
    - The glass or cup is to the right of the plate if the person is right-handed. It is to the left of the plate if left-handed.
  - Arrange main dishes, side dishes, seasonings, and condiments in a straight line or in a semi-circle just beyond the place setting.
  - Explain the location of food and beverages. Use the face of a clock (Chapter 23). Or guide the person's hand to each item on the tray or place setting.
  - Cut meat, open containers, butter bread, and perform other tasks as needed.
- Complete a safety check before leaving the room. (See the inside of the front cover.)

The Person

- Have the person wear comfortable shoes that fit correctly.
- Have the person use hand and stair railings and grab bars.
- Assist with walking as needed. Offer to guide and help the person. Respect the person's answer. If help is accepted:
  - Offer your arm. State which arm is offered. Tap the back of your hand against the person's hand.
  - Have the person hold on to your arm just above the elbow (Fig. 32-5). Do not grab the person's arm.
  - Walk at a normal pace. Walk 1 step ahead of the person. Stand next to the person at the top and bottom of stairs and when crossing streets.
  - Never push, pull, or guide the person in front of you.
  - Pause to change direction, step up, or step down.
  - Warn of stairs, elevators, escalators, doors, turns, furniture, and other obstructions. State if steps are up or down.
  - Have the person hold on to a railing, the wall, or a strong surface if you need to step away. Tell the person that you are leaving and what to hold on to.

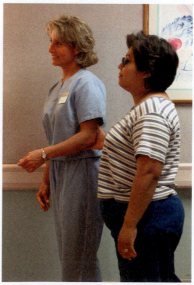

FIGURE 32-5 The blind person walks slightly behind the nursing assistant. She touches the nursing assistant's arm lightly.
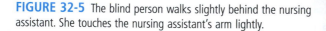

| BOX 32-6 | Caring for Blind and Visually Impaired Persons—cont'd |

The Person—cont'd

- Guide the person to a seat by placing your guiding arm on the seat. The person moves a hand down your arm to the seat.
- Let the person do as much as possible. Do not do things that the person can do. Cutting and seasoning food, getting dressed, and putting on shoes are examples.
- Provide visual and adaptive (assistive) devices. Follow the care plan.

You

- Identify yourself when you enter the room. Give your name, title, and reason for being there. Do not touch the person until he or she is aware of your presence.
- Ask the person how much he or she can see. Do not assume the person is totally blind or has some vision.
- Identify others. Say where each person is and what the person is doing.
- Offer to help. Simply say: "May I help you?" Respect the person's answer.
- Leave the person's belongings where you found them. Do not move or re-arrange things. If you must move things, tell the person what you moved and where.

Communication

- Face the person when speaking. Speak slowly and clearly.
- Use a normal tone of voice. Do not shout or speak loudly.
- Address the person by name. This shows that you are directing a comment or question to him or her.
- Speak directly to the person. Do not talk just to others who are present.
- Feel free to use words such as "see," "look," "read," or "watch TV." You can use "blind" and "visually impaired." You also can use colors, sizes, shapes, patterns, designs, and so on.

Communication—cont'd

- Describe people, places, and things thoroughly. Do not leave out a detail because you do not think it is important.
- Warn of dangers. Give a calm and clear warning. You can say "wait" first. Then describe the danger. For example: "Wait, there is ice on the walk."
- Greet the person by name when he or she enters a room. This alerts the person to your presence. Tell the person who you are. Also identify others in the room.
- Listen to the person. Give verbal cues that you are listening. Say: "yes," "okay," "I see," "tell me more," "I don't understand," and so on.
- Answer questions. Provide specific and descriptive responses.
- Give step-by-step explanations as you give care. Say when the procedure is over.
- Give specific directions.
  - Say: "right behind you," "on your left," or "in front of you." Avoid phrases like "over here" or "over there."
  - Tell the distance. For example: "three steps in front of you" or "at the end of the hallway by the nurses' station."
  - Give landmarks if possible. Sounds and scents can serve as "landmarks." "By the kitchen" is an example.
- Tell the person when you are leaving the room or the area. If appropriate, state where you are going. For example: "I'm going to go into your bathroom now."
- Tell the person when you are ending a conversation. For example: "Thank you for sharing stories about your children."

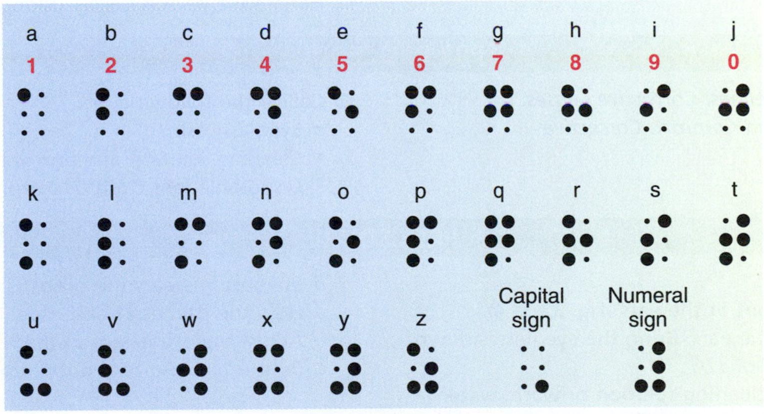

FIGURE 32-6 Braille.

Braille. *Braille is a touch reading and writing system that uses raised dots for each letter of the alphabet* (Fig. 32-6). *The first 10 letters also represent the numbers 0 through 9.* Braille is read by moving the hands from left to right along each line of braille.

Special devices allow computer access—keyboards, displays, and printers. A "braille display" lets the person read the information. Braille printers produce printouts in braille.

Mobility. Blind and visually impaired persons learn to move about using a long cane or a guide dog. Both are used world-wide.

- Long canes are white or silver-gray with red tips. Do not interfere with the arm holding the cane. The person stores the cane when not in use. If you store it, tell the person where.
- The guide dog sees for the person. The dog responds to the master's commands. Commands are disobeyed to avoid danger. For example, the guide dog disobeys a command to cross the street if a car is coming. Do not pet, feed, or distract a guide dog. Such actions can place the person in danger.

Corrective Lenses

Eyeglasses and contact lenses correct many vision problems. Eyeglasses are worn for reading, for seeing at a distance, or for all activities. Contact lenses are usually worn while awake. Some contacts can be worn day and night for up to 30 days.

Eyeglass lenses are hardened glass or plastic. Clean them daily and as needed. Wash glass lenses with warm water. Dry them with a lens cloth or cotton cloth. Plastic lenses scratch easily. Use special cleaning solutions and cloths.

See *Delegation Guidelines: Corrective Lenses.*
See *Promoting Safety and Comfort: Corrective Lenses.*
See procedure: *Caring for Eyeglasses.*

DELEGATION GUIDELINES
Corrective Lenses

Cleaning eyeglasses is a routine care measure. Do not wait until the nurse tells you to clean them. Clean them daily and as needed.

To clean eyeglasses, find out if you need a special cleaning solution. Then follow the manufacturer's instructions.

PROMOTING SAFETY AND COMFORT
Corrective Lenses

Safety
Eyeglasses are costly. Protect them from loss or damage. When not worn, put them in their case. Place the case in the top drawer of the bedside stand.

Some agencies let nursing assistants remove and insert contact lenses. Others do not. Know your agency's policy. If allowed to insert and remove contacts, follow agency procedures.

Caring for Eyeglasses

QUALITY OF LIFE

- Knock before entering the person's room.
- Address the person by name.
- Introduce yourself by name and title.

- Explain the procedure before starting and during the procedure.
- Protect the person's rights during the procedure.
- Handle the person gently during the procedure.

PRE-PROCEDURE

1 Follow *Delegation Guidelines: Corrective Lenses.* See *Promoting Safety and Comfort: Corrective Lenses.*
2 Practice hand hygiene.

3 Collect the following.
  - Eyeglass case
  - Cleaning solution or warm water
  - Disposable lens cloth or cotton cloth

PROCEDURE

4 Remove the eyeglasses.
  a Hold the frames in front of the ears (Fig. 32-7, *A*).
  b Lift the frames from the ears. Bring the eyeglasses down away from the face (Fig. 32-7, *B*).
5 Clean the lenses with a cleaning solution or warm water. Clean in a circular motion. Dry the lenses with the cloth.
6 *If the person will not wear the eyeglasses:*
  a Open the eyeglass case.
  b Fold the glasses. Put them in the case. Do not touch the clean lenses.
  c Place the case in the top drawer of the bedside stand.

7 *If the person wears the eyeglasses:*
  a Hold the frames at each side. Place them over the ears.
  b Adjust the eyeglasses so the nose-piece rests on the nose.
  c Return the case to the top drawer of the bedside stand.

POST-PROCEDURE

8 Provide for comfort. (See the inside of the front cover.)
9 Place the call light and other needed items within reach.
10 Return the cleaning solution to its proper place.
11 Discard the disposable cloth.

12 Complete a safety check of the room. (See the inside of the front cover.)
13 Practice hand hygiene.
14 Report and record your observations.

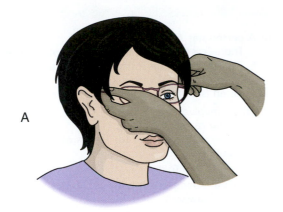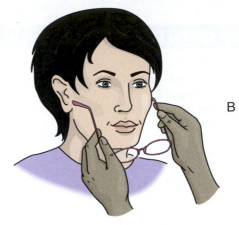

FIGURE 32-7 Removing eyeglasses. **A,** Hold the frames in front of the ears. **B,** Lift the frames from the ears. Bring the glasses down away from the face.

Contact Lenses. Contact lenses fit on the eye. There are hard and soft contacts. Disposable ones are discarded daily, weekly, or monthly. Contacts are cleaned, removed, and stored according to the manufacturer's instructions.

Report and record the following.

- Eye redness or irritation
- Eye drainage
- Complaints of eye pain, blurred or fuzzy vision, or uncomfortable lenses

FOCUS ON P R I D E

The Person, Family, and Yourself

Personal and Professional Responsibility
Hearing aids, contact lenses, and eyeglasses are costly to repair or replace. Protect devices from loss or damage. If a device is lost or damaged, tell the nurse. Take pride in being responsible and honest.

Rights and Respect
Many persons with hearing, speech, and vision problems have overcome great challenges. They take pride in how they have adapted. They deserve to be treated with dignity and respect. Do not pity the person. Treat the person like an adult, not like a child. Focus on the person's abilities, not disabilities.

Always refer to the person first. Then state the disability if needed. For example, a nurse says: "Please take Mrs. Jones a warm blanket. She is blind, so knock and introduce yourself before entering the room. She will place the blanket as she prefers."

Independence and Social Interaction
Adjusting to a hearing, speech, or vision problem is often long and hard. Take time to listen. Be patient, understanding, and sensitive to the person's needs and feelings. Allow the person to be in control to the extent possible. This helps promote independence to improve quality of life.

Delegation and Teamwork
Hearing loss requires changes in communication. Communication measures are part of the care plan. Using gestures, written notes, or an ASL interpreter are examples.

Follow the care plan. A consistent approach is needed. The health team communicates with the person in the same way. Take pride in being part of a caring health team.

Ethics and Laws
The *Americans With Disabilities Act (ADA) of 1990* protects the rights of persons with disabilities. It includes persons with limited hearing, speech, and vision. The ADA covers rights such as employment, access to services and places, and the use of communication devices.

To comply with the ADA, agencies often provide:

- Braille on signs for areas with public access. Lobbies, restrooms, elevators, and cafeterias are examples.
- Communication devices for hearing or speech problems. For example, a device with a keyboard and small screen is connected to a phone line. The device is used instead of a phone.
- ASL interpreters.
- Information in large print and braille.

Know your agency's resources for persons with disabilities. Offer to help. If not sure how to help, ask the nurse. Take pride in helping others.

FOCUS ON PRIDE: *Application*

Hearing, speech, and vision problems do not affect intelligence. Some behaviors insult the person. Treating the person like a child and talking to others but not the person are examples. What are other examples? Identify ways to show dignity and respect.

Circle the BEST answer.

1 Care of the person with Meniere's disease includes
   a Wearing a hearing aid
   b Preventing falls from vertigo
   c Speech therapy
   d Treating infection

2 When talking to a person with hearing loss
   a Shout
   b Change the subject if the person does not seem to understand
   c Avoid using gestures and facial expressions
   d Use short sentences and simple words

3 A hearing aid
   a Corrects a hearing problem
   b Makes sounds louder
   c Makes speech clearer
   d Lowers background noise

4 A hearing aid does not seem to be working. Your *first* action is to
   a See if it is turned on
   b Wash it with soap and water
   c Have it repaired
   d Remove the batteries

5 A person has aphasia. You know that
   a The person cannot hear
   b Mouth and face muscles are affected
   c The person has a language disorder
   d The person cannot speak

6 A person with receptive aphasia has trouble
   a Talking
   b Writing
   c Understanding messages
   d Using gestures

7 A person has a speech disorder. You should
   a Correct the person's speech
   b Discourage the writing of words
   c Leave the TV on while talking
   d Ask the person to repeat as needed

8 A person with a cataract
   a Has cloudy, blurry, or dim vision
   b Loses central vision
   c Has eye pain
   d Is blind

9 A person had cataract surgery. Which would you question?
   a Remind the person not to bend or cough.
   b Let the person rub the eye.
   c Place the over-bed table on the un-operative side.
   d Have the person wear an eye shield during naps.

10 A person has AMD. Which is *true?*
   a There is a blind spot in the center of the eye.
   b Lost vision can be restored with surgery.
   c Peripheral (side) vision is lost.
   d Vision is blurry with spots.

11 Braille involves
   a A long cane for walking
   b Raised dots arranged for letters of the alphabet
   c A guide dog
   d Corrective lenses

12 Which are dangers for blind or visually impaired persons?
   a Closed drawers
   b Doors that are fully open
   c Equipment in hallways
   d Night-lights

13 A person is visually impaired. You should
   a Move furniture to provide variety
   b Avoid words such as "see" and "look"
   c Assume that the person has no sight
   d Provide a consistent meal-time setting

14 A person is blind. To give directions you can say
   a "Over there"
   b "Right here"
   c "Across the room"
   d "On your left"

15 When eyeglasses are not worn they should be
   a Soaked in a cleansing solution
   b Taken to the nurses' station
   c Put in the eyeglass case
   d Placed on the over-bed table

Answers to Chapter 32 questions are on p. 552.

FOCUS ON PRACTICE

Problem Solving

A resident asks for help completing the weekly menu. You are to read each option and mark the choices. Hard of hearing, the resident struggles to hear you. You repeat the meal options many times. What will you do? How can you promote hearing?

Common Health Problems

OBJECTIVES

- Define the key terms and key abbreviations in this chapter.
- Describe cancer and how it is treated.
- Describe musculo-skeletal and nervous system disorders and the care required.
- Describe cardiovascular and respiratory disorders and the care required.

- Describe digestive, urinary, and reproductive disorders and the care required.
- Describe endocrine, immune system, and skin disorders and the care required.
- Explain how to promote PRIDE in the person, the family, and yourself.

KEY TERMS

arthritis Joint (*arthr*) inflammation (*itis*)
arthroplasty The surgical replacement (*plasty*) of a joint (*arthro*)
benign tumor A tumor that does not spread to other body parts
cancer See "malignant tumor"
emesis See "vomitus"
fracture A broken bone
hemiplegia Paralysis (*plegia*) on 1 side (*hemi*) of the body
malignant tumor A tumor that invades and destroys nearby tissues and can spread to other body parts; cancer

metastasis The spread of cancer to other body parts
paralysis Loss of muscle function, sensation, or both
paraplegia Paralysis in the legs, lower trunk, and pelvic organs
pneumonia Inflammation and infection of lung tissue
quadriplegia Paralysis in the arms, legs, trunk, and pelvic organs; tetraplegia
tumor A new growth of abnormal cells that is benign or malignant
vomitus The food and fluids expelled from the stomach through the mouth; emesis

KEY ABBREVIATIONS

AIDS	Acquired immunodeficiency syndrome	**MI**	Myocardial infarction
ALS	Amyotrophic lateral sclerosis	**mm Hg**	Millimeters of mercury
BPH	Benign prostatic hyperplasia	**MS**	Multiple sclerosis
CAD	Coronary artery disease	**O₂**	Oxygen
CO₂	Carbon dioxide	**RA**	Rheumatoid arthritis
COPD	Chronic obstructive pulmonary disease	**ROM**	Range of motion
CVA	Cerebrovascular accident	**STD**	Sexually transmitted disease
HBV	Hepatitis B virus	**TB**	Tuberculosis
HIV	Human immunodeficiency virus	**TIA**	Transient ischemic attack
IBD	Inflammatory bowel disease	**UTI**	Urinary tract infection
IV	Intravenous		

Understanding common health problems gives meaning to the required care. The nurse gives you more information as needed. See Chapter 8 as you study this chapter.

CANCER

Cells reproduce for tissue growth and repair. Cells divide in an orderly way. Sometimes cell division and growth are out of control. A mass or clump of cells develops. This *new growth of abnormal cells is called a **tumor**. Tumors are benign or malignant* (Fig. 33-1).

- *Benign tumors do not spread to other body parts.* They can grow to a large size but rarely threaten life. They usually do not grow back when removed.
- *Malignant tumors (cancer) invade and destroy nearby tissues. They can spread to other body parts.* They may be life-threatening. Sometimes they grow back after removal.

Metastasis is the spread of cancer to other body parts (Fig. 33-2). If not treated and controlled, cancer cells break off the tumor and travel to other body parts. New tumors grow at those sites.

Cancer can occur almost anywhere. Common sites are the skin, lung and bronchus, colon and rectum, breast, prostate, uterus, ovary, urinary bladder, kidney, mouth and pharynx, pancreas, and thyroid gland.

Risk Factors

Cancer is the second leading cause of death in the United States. The National Cancer Institute describes these risk factors.

- *Age.* Advancing age is the most important risk factor. However, cancer can occur at any age.
- *Tobacco.* This includes using tobacco (smoking, snuff, and chewing tobacco) and being around tobacco (second-hand smoke). This risk can be avoided.
- *Radiation.* Sources are sun light, x-rays, and radon gas that forms in the soil and some rocks.
- *Infections.* Certain viruses and bacteria increase the risk of cancers—cervix, penis, vagina, anus, mouth, liver, lymphoma, leukemia, Kaposi's sarcoma (associated with AIDS, p. 490), stomach.
- *Immuno-suppressive drugs.* These drugs lower the body's ability to stop cancer from forming. Such drugs are often used for organ transplant patients to prevent rejection of the transplant.
- *Alcohol.* Alcohol is linked to the increased risk of cancers of the breast, mouth, esophagus, liver, colon, and rectum.
- *Diet.* Fruits and vegetables may protect against cancers of the mouth, esophagus, and stomach. A diet high in fat, protein, calories, and red meat may increase the risk of colon and rectal cancers.
- *Hormones.* The female hormones estrogen and progesterone are known to increase the risk of breast and uterine cancers.
- *Obesity.* Obesity is linked to post-menopausal breast cancer and cancers of the esophagus, pancreas, colon, rectum, kidney, and uterus.
- *Environment.* Air pollution, second-hand smoke, and asbestos are linked to lung cancer. Drinking water with large amounts of arsenic is linked to skin, bladder, and lung cancers.

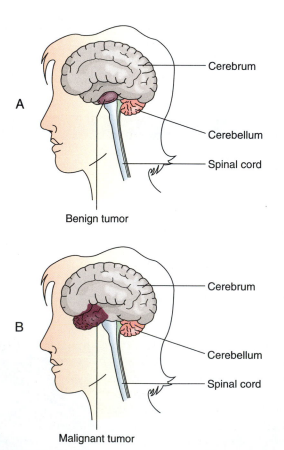

FIGURE 33-1 Tumors. **A,** A benign tumor grows within a local area. **B,** A malignant tumor invades other tissues.

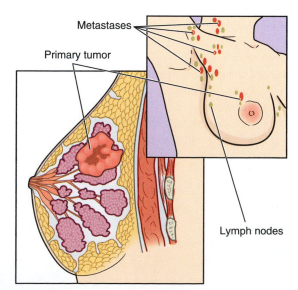

FIGURE 33-2 A tumor in the breast has metastasized to the lymph nodes.

BOX 33-1 Cancer—General Signs and Symptoms

- Unexplained weight loss
- Fever
- Fatigue
- Pain
- Skin changes—darker looking skin, reddened skin, itching, excessive hair growth, *jaundice* (yellowish skin and eyes)
- Change in bowel habits
- Change in bladder function
- Sores that do not heal
- White patches in the mouth
- White spots on the tongue
- Unusual bleeding or discharge
- Thickening or lump in the breast or any other body part
- Indigestion or trouble swallowing
- Change in a wart or mole or new skin change
- Nagging cough or hoarseness

Modified from American Cancer Society: *Signs and symptoms of cancer*, revised August 11, 2014.

Treatment

If detected early, cancer can be treated and controlled (Box 33-1). Treatment depends on the tumor type, its site and size, and if it has spread. The treatment goal may be to:

- Cure the cancer.
- Control the disease.
- Reduce symptoms.

Common treatments are surgery, radiation therapy, and chemotherapy.

- *Surgery* removes tumors.
- *Radiation therapy (radiotherapy)* kills cancer cells. X-ray beams are aimed at the tumor. Sometimes radioactive material is implanted in or near the tumor. Cancer cells and normal cells receive radiation. Both are destroyed. Skin changes occur at the treatment site—dryness, itching, swelling, peeling, redness, blistering. Special skin care measures are ordered. Extra rest is needed for fatigue. Discomfort, nausea, vomiting, diarrhea, and loss of appetite (*anorexia*) are other side effects.
- *Chemotherapy* involves drugs that kill cancer cells. Cancer cells and normal cells are affected. Side effects include hair loss (*alopecia*), poor appetite, nausea, vomiting, diarrhea, and *stomatitis*—inflammation (*itis*) of the mouth (*stomat*). Bleeding and infection are risks from decreased blood cell production.

The Person's Needs

Persons with cancer have many needs. They include:

- Pain relief or control
- Rest and exercise
- Fluids and nutrition
- Preventing skin breakdown
- Preventing constipation or diarrhea
- Dealing with treatment side effects
- Psychological and social needs
- Spiritual needs
- Sexual needs

Anger, fear, and depression are common. Some surgeries are disfiguring. The person may feel unwhole, unattractive, or unclean. The person and family need support.

Spiritual needs are important. A spiritual leader may provide comfort. To many people, spiritual needs are just as important as physical needs.

Persons dying of cancer often receive hospice care (Chapters 1 and 37). Support is given to the person and family.

See *Focus on Communication: The Person's Needs.*

FOCUS ON COMMUNICATION
The Person's Needs

Knowing what to say to a person with cancer can be hard. Do not avoid the person. Talk as you would with any other person. Avoid comments like "I'm sure you will be fine" or "It will be okay."

Often the person needs to talk and have someone listen. Listen and use touch to show you care. Being there when needed is important. You may not have to say anything. Just listen.

MUSCULO-SKELETAL DISORDERS

Musculo-skeletal disorders affect movement. Injury and aging are common causes. Daily living, social activities, and quality of life are affected.

Arthritis

Arthritis means joint (arthr) *inflammation* (itis). Affected joints have swelling, stiffness, and reduced range of motion. The joints are hard to move.

The 2 main types of arthritis are:

- *Osteoarthritis.* Cartilage covering the ends of bones wears away, allowing the bones to rub together. The hands, knees, hips, and spine are often affected (Fig. 33-3, p. 472).
- *Rheumatoid arthritis (RA).* An autoimmune disorder (p. 489), RA attacks the lining of the joint, causing painful swelling. Wrist and finger joints are commonly affected. RA can also affect the neck, shoulders, elbows, hips, knees, ankles, and feet. RA occurs on both sides of the body. For example, both the right and left wrists are affected. RA can cause fever and fatigue. Sometimes other body parts are affected—decreased red blood cell production; dry eyes and mouth; and inflammation of the blood vessels, lungs, and heart.

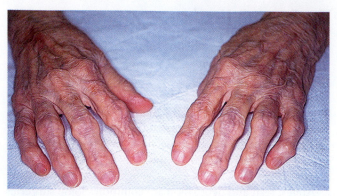

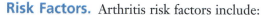

FIGURE 33-3 Bony growths called *Heberden nodes* occur in the finger joints. (From Swartz MH: *Textbook of physical diagnosis,* ed 7, Philadelphia, 2014, Saunders.)

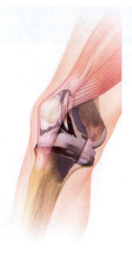

FIGURE 33-4 Knee replacement prosthesis. (Courtesy Zimmer, Inc., A Bristol-Meyers Squibb Company, Warsaw, Ind.)

Risk Factors. Arthritis risk factors include:
- *Aging.* The risk increases with age.
- *Being over-weight.* Stress is placed on the weight-bearing joints—knees, hips, and spine.
- *Gender.* Arthritis is more common in women.
- *Joint injury.* A previous joint injury may develop into osteoarthritis.
- *Family history.* Arthritis tends to run in families.

Treatment. Osteoarthritis and RA have no cure. Treatments are similar.
- *Pain control.* Drugs decrease swelling and inflammation and relieve pain.
- *Heat and cold.* Heat relieves pain, increases blood flow, and reduces stiffness. Sometimes cold is applied after joint use.
- *Exercise.* Exercise helps joint flexibility. It helps with weight control and promotes fitness. The person is taught needed exercises.
- *Rest and joint care.* Good body mechanics, posture, and regular rest protect the joints. Relaxation methods are helpful.
- *Assistive (adaptive) devices.* Canes and walkers provide support. Splints support weak joints and promote alignment. Devices for hands and wrists are useful.
- *Weight control.* Weight loss reduces stress on weight-bearing joints and prevents further joint injury.
- *Healthy life-style.* The focus is on fitness, exercise, rest, managing stress, and good nutrition.
- *Safety.* Falls are prevented. Help is given with activities of daily living (ADL) as needed. Elevated toilet seats are helpful when hips and knees are affected. So are chairs with higher seats and armrests.
- *Joint replacement surgery.* ***Arthroplasty*** *is the surgical replacement* (plasty) *of a joint* (arthro). The damaged joint is removed and replaced with an artificial joint (*prosthesis*). Hip and knee replacements are common (Fig. 33-4). See Box 33-2. Ankle, foot, shoulder, elbow, and finger joints also can be replaced.

BOX 33-2	Care After Joint Replacement—Hip and Knee

- Deep-breathing and coughing exercises to prevent respiratory complications.
- Elastic stockings to prevent *thrombi* (blood clots) in the legs.
- Physical therapy and exercises to strengthen the hip or knee.
- Measures to protect the hip as shown in Figure 33-5.
- Food and fluids for tissue healing and to restore strength.
- Safety measures to prevent falls.
- Measures to prevent infection. Wound, urinary tract, and skin infections must be prevented.
- Measures to prevent pressure injuries.
- Assist devices for moving, turning, re-positioning, and transfers.
- Long-handled devices for reaching things.
- Assistance with walking and a walking aid—cane, walker, or crutches.

Do

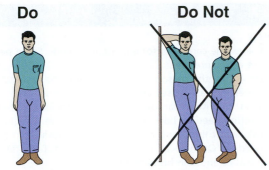

Do not cross your operated leg past the mid-line of the body or turn your kneecap in toward your body.

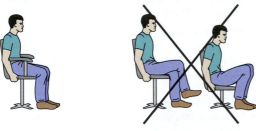

Do not sit in low chairs or cross your legs.

To sit: Use a high chair with arms or add pillows to elevate the seat.

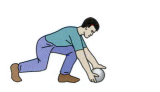

Avoid flexing your hips past 90 degrees.

To bend: Keep the operative leg behind you or as instructed by your therapist.

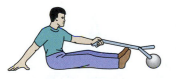
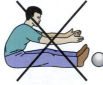

To reach: Use long-handled grabbers or as your therapist advises.

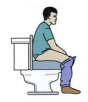

Use an elevated toilet.

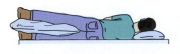
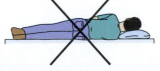

Sleep with a pillow between the legs.

FIGURE 33-5 Measures to protect the hip after hip replacement surgery. (Modified from Monahan FD and others: *Phipps' medical-surgical nursing: health and illness perspectives,* ed 8, St Louis, 2007, Mosby.)

Fractures

A ***fracture is a broken bone.*** Fractures are open or closed (Fig. 33-6).

- *Open fracture (compound fracture)*—the broken bone has come through the skin.
- *Closed fracture (simple fracture)*—the bone is broken but the skin is intact.

Falls, accidents, bone tumors, and osteoporosis (p. 476) are some causes. Signs and symptoms of a fracture are:

- Pain
- Swelling
- Loss of function or movement
- Movement where motion should not occur
- Deformity (abnormal position of the part)
- Bruising and skin color changes at the fracture site
- Bleeding (internal or external)

For healing, bone ends are brought into and held in normal position. This is called *reduction and fixation.*

- Reduction—the bone is moved back into place.
  - Closed reduction—the bone is not exposed.
  - Open reduction—the bone is surgically exposed and moved into alignment.
- Fixation—the bone is held (fixed) in place.
  - External fixation—Pins, screws, or wires are set into the bone outside the skin. The device is removed after healing or when the person is healthy enough for surgery.
  - Internal fixation—Nails, rods, pins, screws, plates, or wires are surgically placed. The device is under the skin.

Casts, traction, splints, and walking boots also are used.

- *Casts.* Casts are made of plaster of Paris, plastic, or fiberglass. Plastic and fiberglass casts dry quickly. A plaster of Paris cast dries in 24 to 48 hours. It is odorless, white, and shiny when dry. When wet, it is gray and cool and has a musty smell. The nurse may ask you to assist with care (Box 33-3, p. 474).
- *Traction.* A steady pull from 2 directions keeps the bone in place. Weights, ropes, and pulleys are used (Fig. 33-9, p. 474). Traction is applied to the neck, arms, legs, or pelvis. To assist with the person's care, see Box 33-4, p. 475.

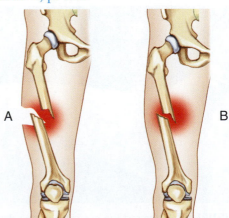

FIGURE 33-6 A, Open fracture. **B,** Closed fracture. (From Patton KT, Thibodeau GA: *The human body in health & disease,* ed 7, St Louis, 2018, Elsevier.)

BOX 33-3   Cast Care

The Cast

- Do not cover the cast with blankets, plastic, or other material. A cast gives off heat as it dries. Covers prevent the escape of heat. Burns can occur if heat cannot escape.
- Promote drying of the cast. Turn the person every 2 hours or as directed. All cast surfaces need exposure to air.
- Maintain the shape of the cast.
  - Do not place a wet cast on a hard surface. It flattens the cast.
  - Use pillows to support the entire length of the cast (Fig. 33-7).
  - Support the wet cast with your palms to turn and position the person (Fig. 33-8). Fingertips can dent the cast, causing pressure areas and skin breakdown.
  - Report rough cast edges. The nurse may cover the cast edges with tape.
  - Keep the cast dry. A wet cast loses its shape. For casts near the perineal area, the nurse may apply a waterproof material after the cast dries.
- Do not remove stockinette or padding around the cast edges.

Positioning

- Position the person as directed.
- Elevate a casted arm or leg on pillows to reduce swelling.
- Have enough help to turn and re-position the person. Plaster casts are heavy and awkward. Balance is lost easily.

Safety

- Follow the care plan for elimination needs. Some persons use a fracture pan.
- Do not let the person insert things into the cast. Itching under the cast causes an intense desire to scratch. Scratching items can open the skin—pencils, coat hangers, knitting needles, back scratchers, and so on. Infection is a risk. Scratching items can wrinkle the stockinette or cotton padding. Or they can be lost into the cast. Both can cause pressure and skin breakdown.
- Do not put powder on the skin under the cast.
- Do not let the person put rings on the fingers or toes.
- Complete a safety check before leaving the room. (See the inside of the front cover.)

Reporting and Recording

- Report these signs and symptoms at once.
  - *Pain*—pressure injury, poor circulation, nerve damage
  - *Swelling and a tight cast*—reduced blood flow to the part
  - *Pale skin*—reduced blood flow to the part
  - *Cyanosis* (bluish skin color)—reduced blood flow to the part
  - *Odor*—infection
  - *Inability to move the fingers or toes*—pressure on a nerve
  - *Numbness*—pressure on a nerve, reduced blood flow to the part
  - *Temperature changes*—cool skin means poor circulation; hot skin means inflammation
  - *Drainage on or under the cast*—infection or bleeding
  - *Chills, fever, nausea, and vomiting*—infection

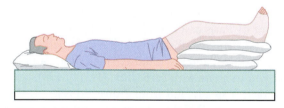

FIGURE 33-7 Pillows support the entire length of the wet cast.

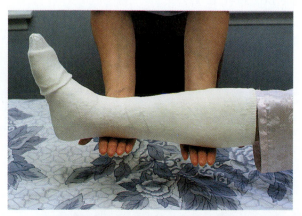

FIGURE 33-8 The cast is supported with the palms.

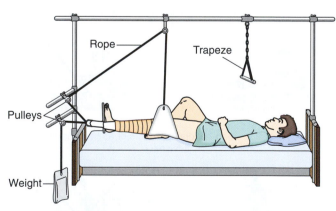

FIGURE 33-9 Traction set-up. Note the weight, pulleys, and rope. A trapeze is used to raise the upper body off the bed. (Modified from Monahan FD and others: *Phipps' medical-surgical nursing: health and illness perspectives,* ed 8, St Louis, 2007, Mosby.)

BOX 33-4   Traction Care

- Keep the person in good alignment.
- Do not remove the traction.
- Keep the weights off the floor. Weights must hang freely from the traction set-up (see Fig. 33-9).
- Do not add or remove weights.
- Check for frayed ropes. Report fraying at once.
- Perform range-of-motion (ROM) exercises for uninvolved joints as directed.
- Position the person as directed. Usually only the supine position is allowed. Slight turning may be allowed.
- Provide the fracture pan for elimination.
- Give skin care as directed.
- Put bottom linens on the bed from the top down. The person uses a trapeze to raise the body off the bed (see Fig. 33-9).
- Check pin, nail, wire, or tong sites for redness, drainage, and odors. Report observations at once.
- Observe for the signs and symptoms listed under cast care (see Box 33-3). Report them at once.
- Complete a safety check before leaving the room. (See the inside of the front cover.)

BOX 33-5   Hip Fracture Care

- Give good skin care. Skin breakdown can be rapid.
- Prevent pressure injuries.
- Prevent wound, skin, and urinary tract infections.
- Encourage deep-breathing and coughing exercises as directed.
- Turn and position the person as directed. Usually the person is not positioned on the operative side.
- Prevent external rotation of the hip. Use trochanter rolls, pillows, or sandbags.
- Keep the leg abducted at all times. Use pillows (Fig. 33-11) or a hip abduction wedge (abductor splint). Do not exercise the affected leg.
- Provide a straight-back chair with armrests. The person needs a high, firm seat.
- Place the chair on the unaffected side.
- Use assist devices to move, turn, re-position, and transfer the person.
- Do not let the person stand on the operated leg unless allowed by the doctor.
- Elevate the leg following the care plan. With an internal fixation device, the leg is not elevated when the person sits in a chair. Elevating the leg puts strain on the device.
- Apply elastic stockings to prevent *thrombi* (blood clots) in the legs.
- Remind the person not to cross his or her legs.
- Assist with walking according to the care plan. The person uses a walker or crutches.
- Follow measures to protect the hip. See Box 33-2 and Figure 33-5.
- Practice safety measures to prevent falls.
- Complete a safety check before leaving the room. (See the inside of the front cover.)

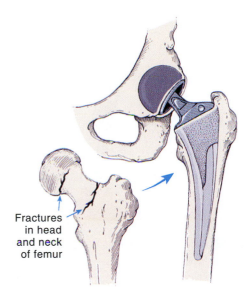

Fractures in head and neck of femur

FIGURE 33-10 Hip fracture repaired with a prosthesis. (Modified from Cooper K, Gosnell K: *Adult health nursing,* ed 7, St Louis, 2015, Mosby.)

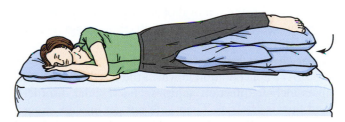

FIGURE 33-11 Pillows are used to keep the hip in abduction. (From Monahan FD and others: *Phipps' medical-surgical nursing: health and illness perspectives,* ed 8, St Louis, 2007, Mosby.)

Hip Fractures. Common in older persons, hip fractures require surgical repair or a hip replacement (Fig. 33-10). Adduction, internal rotation, external rotation, and severe hip flexion are avoided after surgery. Rehabilitation is usually needed.

Post-operative problems present life-threatening risks. They include pneumonia, urinary tract infections, and *thrombi* (blood clots) in the leg veins or lungs. Pressure injuries, constipation, and confusion are other problems. Box 33-5 describes the required care.

Osteoporosis

With osteoporosis, the bone *(osteo)* becomes porous and brittle *(porosis)*. Bones are fragile and break easily. Spine, hip, and wrist fractures are common.

Older people are at risk. For women, the risk increases after menopause from the lack of estrogen. Low levels of dietary calcium and vitamin D cause bone changes.

All ethnic groups are at risk. Other risk factors include a family history of the disease, being thin or having a small frame, eating disorders (Chapter 34), tobacco use, alcoholism, lack of exercise, bedrest, and immobility. Exercise and activity are needed for bone strength. Bone must bear weight to form properly. If not, calcium is lost from the bone. The bone becomes porous and brittle.

Back pain, loss of height, and stooped posture occur. Fractures are a major threat. Even slight activity can cause fractures. They can occur from turning in bed, getting up from a chair, or coughing. Fractures are great risks from falls and accidents.

Prevention is important. Doctors often order calcium and vitamin supplements. Estrogen is ordered for some women. Other preventive measures include:

- Exercising weight-bearing joints—walking, jogging, stair climbing, weight lifting, dancing
- No smoking and limited alcohol
- Back supports or corsets for good posture
- Walking aids
- Safety measures to prevent falls and accidents
- Good body mechanics
- Safe moving, transfer, and turning and positioning procedures

Loss of Limb

An *amputation* is the removal of all or part of an extremity. Severe injuries, tumors, severe infection, gangrene, and vascular disorders are common causes. Diabetes can cause vascular changes leading to amputation.

Gangrene is a condition in which there is death of tissue. Causes include infection, injuries, and vascular disorders. Blood flow is affected. Tissues do not get enough oxygen and nutrients. Tissues become black, cold, shriveled, and die (Fig. 33-12). Surgery is needed to remove dead tissue. Gangrene can cause death.

A *prosthesis* is an artificial replacement for a missing body part (Fig. 33-13). Occupational and physical therapists help the person learn to use the prosthesis.

The person may feel that the limb is still there. Aching, tingling, and itching are common sensations. Or the person complains of pain in the amputated part *(phantom pain)*. This is a normal reaction. It may occur for a short time or for many years.

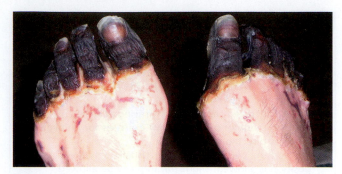

FIGURE 33-12 Gangrene. (From Centers for Disease Control and Prevention/Christina Nelson, MD, MPH, 2012.)

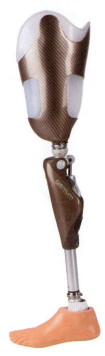

FIGURE 33-13 Above-the-knee prosthesis. (Courtesy Otto Bock Health Care, Minneapolis, Minn.)

NERVOUS SYSTEM DISORDERS

Nervous system disorders can affect mental and physical function. They can affect the ability to speak, understand, feel, see, hear, touch, think, control bowels and bladder, and move.

Stroke

Stroke (*brain attack* or *cerebrovascular accident [CVA]*) occurs when 1 of these happens.

- A blood vessel in the brain bursts and bleeds into the brain (cerebral hemorrhage).
- A blood clot blocks a blood vessel in the brain. Blood flow stops.

Brain cells in the affected area do not get enough oxygen and nutrients. Brain damage occurs. Functions controlled by that part of the brain are lost (Fig. 33-14).

Stroke is a leading cause of death and disability among adults in the United States. See Box 33-6 for warning signs. The person needs emergency care. Blood flow to the brain must be restored as soon as possible.

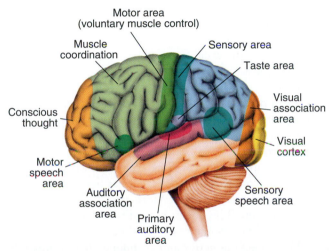

FIGURE 33-14 Functions lost from a stroke depend on the area of brain damage. (Modified from Patton KT, Thibodeau GA: *The human body in health & disease*, ed 7, St Louis, 2018, Elsevier.)

Warning signs may last a few minutes. This is called a *transient ischemic attack (TIA).* (*Transient* means *temporary* or *short term. Ischemic* means *to hold back* [ischein] *blood* [hemic].) The brain's blood supply is interrupted for a short time. A TIA may occur before a stroke.

Unconsciousness, noisy breathing, high blood pressure, slow pulse, redness of the face, and seizures may occur. So can **hemiplegia—*paralysis* (plegia) *on 1 side* (hemi) *of the body.*** The person may lose bowel and bladder control and the ability to speak. (See "Aphasia" in Chapter 32.)

The effects of stroke include:

- Loss of face, hand, arm, leg, or body control
- Hemiplegia
- Changing emotions—crying easily or mood swings sometimes for no reason
- Difficulty swallowing (*dysphagia*)
- Aphasia or slowed or slurred speech
- Changes in sight, touch, movement, and thought
- Impaired memory
- Urinary frequency, urgency, or incontinence
- Loss of bowel control or constipation
- Depression and frustration
- Behavior changes

Rehabilitation starts at once. The person may depend in part or totally on others for care. The goal is to regain the highest possible level of function (Box 33-7).

BOX 33-6 | **Stroke—Warning Signs**

- Sudden numbness or weakness of the face, arm, or leg, especially on 1 side of the body
- Sudden confusion, trouble speaking or understanding speech
- Sudden trouble seeing in 1 or both eyes
- Sudden trouble walking, dizziness, loss of balance or coordination
- Sudden, severe headache with no known cause

From National Institute of Neurological Disorders and Stroke: *Know stroke. Know the signs. Act in time.* NIH Publication Number 13-4872, Bethesda, Md, July 2013, National Institutes of Health.

BOX 33-7 | **Stroke Care Measures**

- Position the person in the lateral (side-lying) position to prevent aspiration.
- Keep the bed in semi-Fowler's position.
- Approach the person from the strong (unaffected) side. The person may have loss of vision on the affected side.
- Turn and re-position the person at least every 2 hours.
- Use assist devices to move, turn, re-position, and transfer the person.
- Encourage deep breathing and coughing.
- Prevent contractures. Assist with ROM exercises.
- Prevent pressure injuries.
- Meet food and fluid needs. A dysphagia diet is common (Chapter 23).
- Apply elastic stockings to prevent *thrombi* (blood clots) in the legs.
- Meet elimination needs. Follow the care plan for:
  - Catheter care or bladder training
  - Bowel training
- Practice safety precautions.
  - Keep the call light and other needed items within reach on the strong (unaffected) side.
  - Check the person often if he or she cannot use the call light. Follow the care plan.
  - Use bed rails according to the care plan.
  - Prevent falls and other injuries.
- Encourage as much self-care as possible. This includes turning, positioning, and transferring. The person uses assistive (adaptive) and walking aids as needed.
- Do not rush the person. Movements are slower after a stroke.
- Follow established communication methods.
- Give support, encouragement, and praise.
- Complete a safety check before leaving the room. (See the inside of the front cover.)

Parkinson's Disease

Parkinson's disease is a progressive disorder affecting movement. Persons over the age of 50 are at risk. One or both sides of the body are affected. Mild at first (Fig. 33-15), signs and symptoms include:

- *Tremors*—often start in the hand. Pill-rolling movements—rubbing the thumb and index finger—may occur. There may be trembling in the hands, arms, legs, jaw, and face.
- *Rigid, stiff muscles*—occur in the arms, legs, neck, and trunk.
- *Stooped posture and impaired balance*—it is hard to walk. The person has a slow, shuffling gait. Falls are a risk.
- *Mask-like expression*—the person cannot blink or smile. A fixed stare is common.

Other signs and symptoms develop over time. They include swallowing and chewing problems, constipation, sleep problems, depression, and emotional changes (fear, insecurity). Memory loss and slow thinking can occur. The person may have slow, monotone, and soft speech.

With no cure, drugs are used to control the disease. Exercise and physical therapy help improve strength, posture, balance, and mobility. Therapy is needed for speech and swallowing problems. The person may need help with eating and self-care. Normal elimination is a goal. Safety measures are needed to prevent falls and injuries.

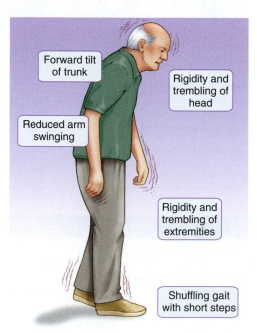

Forward tilt of trunk

Rigidity and trembling of head

Reduced arm swinging

Rigidity and trembling of extremities

Shuffling gait with short steps

FIGURE 33-15 Signs of Parkinson's disease. (From Patton KT, Thibodeau GA: *The human body in health & disease*, ed 7, St Louis, 2018, Elsevier.)

Multiple Sclerosis

Multiple sclerosis (MS) is a central nervous system disease. *Multiple* means *many*. *Sclerosis* means *hardening* or *scarring*. The myelin (which covers nerve fibers) in the brain and spinal cord is destroyed. Nerve impulses are not sent to and from the brain in a normal way. Functions are impaired or lost.

Symptoms usually start between the ages of 15 and 60. Women and whites are at greater risk than other groups. The risk increases if a family member has MS. Signs and symptoms may include:

- Blurred or double vision; blindness in 1 eye
- Muscle weakness in the arms and legs
- Balance and coordination problems
- Tingling, prickling, or numb sensations
- Partial or complete paralysis
- Pain
- Speech problems
- Tremors
- Dizziness
- Concentration, attention, memory, and judgment problems
- Depression
- Bladder problems
- Problems with sexual function
- Hearing loss
- Fatigue
  MS can present in many ways. For example:
- Symptoms appear for a while then seem to go away. The person is in *remission*. Later, symptoms flare up again *(relapse)*.
- More symptoms appear. The condition worsens.
- There are remissions and relapses at first. Eventually symptoms become worse. More symptoms occur with each flare-up. The person's condition declines.

MS has no cure. Some drugs can slow the disease. Persons with MS are kept as active and as independent as possible. The care plan reflects changing needs. Skin care, hygiene, and ROM exercises are important. So are turning, positioning, and deep breathing and coughing. Elimination needs are met. Injuries and complications from bedrest are prevented.

Amyotrophic Lateral Sclerosis

Amyotrophic lateral sclerosis (ALS) attacks the nerve cells that control voluntary muscles. Commonly called *Lou Gehrig's disease*, it is rapidly progressive and fatal. (Lou Gehrig, a New York Yankees baseball player, died of the disease.)

ALS usually strikes persons between 40 and 60 years of age. Most die 2 to 5 years after onset.

Nerve cells in the brain, brainstem, and spinal cord responsible for voluntary muscles are affected. These cells stop sending messages to the muscles. Muscles weaken, waste away *(atrophy)*, and twitch. Over time, the brain cannot start or control voluntary movements. The person cannot move the arms, legs, and body. Muscles for speaking, chewing and swallowing, and breathing also are affected. Eventually respiratory muscles fail.

The disease usually does not affect the mind, intelligence, or memory. Sight, smell, taste, hearing, and touch are not affected. Usually bowel and bladder functions remain intact.

ALS has no cure. Some drugs can slow the disease and improve symptoms. However, damage cannot be reversed. The person is kept active and independent to the extent possible. The care plan reflects changing needs.

Head Injuries

Head injuries result from trauma to the scalp, skull, or brain. Injuries range from a minor bump to a serious, life-threatening brain injury.

Traumatic brain injury (TBI) occurs from violent injury to the brain. Falls, traffic accidents, assaults, and firearms are common causes. So are sports and combat injuries.

Brain tissue is bruised or torn. Bleeding is in the brain or in nearby tissues. Spinal cord injuries are likely.

If the person survives, some permanent damage is likely. Disabilities depend on the severity and site of injury. They include:

- Cognitive problems—thinking, memory, and reasoning
- Sensory problems—sight, hearing, touch, taste, and smell
- Communication problems—expressing or understanding language
- Emotional problems—depression, anxiety, personality changes, aggressive behavior, acting out, socially inappropriate behavior
- Changes in level of consciousness:
  - Coma—the person is unconscious, does not respond, is unaware, and cannot be aroused.
  - Vegetative state—the person is unconscious and unaware of surroundings. He or she has sleep-wake cycles and may open the eyes, make sounds, or move. The person cannot speak or follow commands.
  - Brain death—despite complete loss of brain function, the heart continues to beat. Reflex activity, movement, and spontaneous respirations are absent.

Rehabilitation is required. Nursing care depends on the person's needs and abilities.

Spinal Cord Injury

Spinal cord injuries can seriously damage the nervous system. *Paralysis (loss of muscle function, sensation, or both)* can result. Common causes are traffic accidents, falls, violence (knife and gunshot wounds), sports injuries, alcohol use, cancer, and other diseases.

Problems depend on the amount of damage to the spinal cord and the level of injury. The higher the level of injury, the more functions lost (Fig. 33-16).

- Lumbar injuries—occur in the low back. Sensory and muscle function in the legs is lost. The person has paraplegia. *Paraplegia is paralysis in the legs, lower trunk, and pelvic organs. (Para means beyond; plegia means paralysis).*
- Thoracic injuries—occur in the middle and upper back. Sensory and muscle function below the chest is lost. The person has paraplegia.
- Cervical injuries—occur at the neck. Sensory and muscle function of the arms, legs, and trunk is lost. *Paralysis in the arms, legs, trunk, and pelvic organs is called quadriplegia (tetraplegia). Quad and tetra mean 4. Plegia means paralysis.*

Cervical traction with a special bed may be needed. The spine is kept straight at all times. See Box 33-8 (p. 480) for care measures. Emotional needs are great. Reactions to paralysis and loss of function are often severe. If the person lives, rehabilitation is needed.

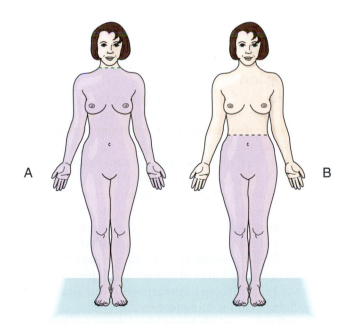

FIGURE 33-16 The *shaded areas* show the area of paralysis. **A,** Quadriplegia (tetraplegia). **B,** Paraplegia.

BOX 33-8	Paralysis—Care Measures

- Practice safety measures to prevent falls. Use bed rails as directed.
- Keep the bed in a low position. Follow the care plan.
- Keep the call light and other needed items within reach. If unable to use the call light, check the person often.
- Prevent burns. Check bath water, heat applications, and food for proper temperature.
- Turn (logroll) and re-position the person at least every 2 hours.
- Prevent pressure injuries. Follow the care plan.
- Use supportive devices for good alignment.
- Follow bowel and bladder training programs.
- Keep intake and output records.
- Maintain muscle function and prevent contractures. Assist with ROM exercises.
- Assist with food and fluid needs. Provide adaptive (assistive) devices as ordered.
- Give emotional and psychological support.
- Follow the rehabilitation plan.
- Complete a safety check of the room. (See the inside of the front cover.)

BOX 33-9	Cardiovascular Disorders—Risk Factors

Factors You *Cannot* Change
- Age—45 years or older for men; 55 years or older for women
- Gender—men are at greater risk than women; risk increases for women after menopause
- Race—African-Americans are at greater risk
- Family history—tends to run in families

Factors You *Can* Change
- Being over-weight
- Stress
- Smoking and tobacco use
- Poor diet—high in fat, salt, sugar, and cholesterol
- Excessive alcohol
- Lack of exercise
- High blood pressure
- Unhealthy blood cholesterol levels
- Diabetes

Modified from MedlinePlus: *How to prevent heart disease*, Bethesda, Md, updated December 18, 2017, U.S. National Library of Medicine.

CARDIOVASCULAR DISORDERS

Cardiovascular disorders are leading causes of death in the United States. Problems occur in the heart or blood vessels.

Hypertension

With *hypertension* (high blood pressure), the systolic pressure is 130 mm Hg (millimeters of mercury) or higher (*hyper*). Or the diastolic pressure is 80 mm Hg or higher. Resting blood pressure is too high. Such measurements must occur several times. See Box 33-9 for risk factors. See Chapter 25 for normal blood pressure ranges.

Narrowed blood vessels are a common cause. The heart pumps with greater force to move blood through narrowed vessels. Kidney disorders, head injuries, some pregnancy problems, and adrenal gland tumors are other causes.

Signs and symptoms develop over time. Headache, blurred vision, dizziness, and nose bleeds occur. Hypertension can lead to stroke, hardening of the arteries, heart attack, heart failure, kidney failure, and blindness.

Life-style changes can lower blood pressure. A diet low in fat and salt, a healthy weight, and regular exercise are needed. No smoking is allowed. Alcohol and caffeine are limited. Managing stress and sleeping well also lower blood pressure. Certain drugs lower blood pressure.

Coronary Artery Disease

The *coronary arteries* supply the heart muscle with blood. In coronary artery disease (CAD) (coronary heart disease, heart disease), the coronary arteries become hardened and narrow. One or all are affected. The heart muscle gets less blood and oxygen (O_2).

The most common cause is atherosclerosis (Fig. 33-17). Plaque—made up of cholesterol, fat, and other substances—collects on artery walls. The narrowed arteries block some or all blood flow. Blood clots can form along the plaque and block blood flow.

Major complications of CAD are angina, myocardial infarction (heart attack), irregular heartbeats, and sudden death. The more risk factors (see Box 33-9), the greater the chance of CAD and its complications.

Treatment goals are to:
- Relieve symptoms (see "Angina")
- Slow or stop atherosclerosis
- Lower the risk of blood clots
- Widen or bypass clogged arteries
- Reduce cardiac events (see "Angina" and "Myocardial Infarction," p. 482)

CAD requires life-style changes (see "Hypertension"). Some drugs decrease the heart's workload and relieve symptoms. Other drugs prevent a heart attack or sudden death. Drugs can delay medical and surgical procedures that open or bypass diseased arteries (Fig. 33-18).

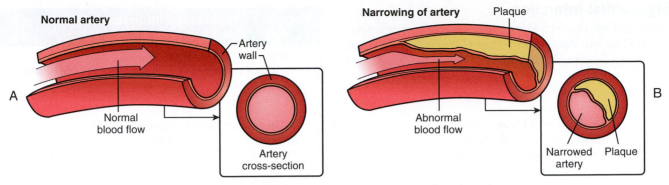

FIGURE 33-17 **A,** Normal artery. **B,** Plaque on the artery wall in atherosclerosis.

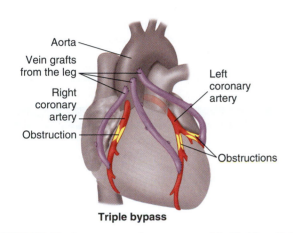

Triple bypass

FIGURE 33-18 Coronary artery bypass surgery. (Modified from Patton KT, Thibodeau GA: *The human body in health & disease,* ed 7, St Louis, 2018, Elsevier.)

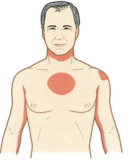

- Mid sternum
- Left shoulder and down both arms
- Neck and arms

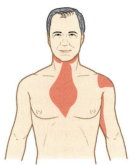

- Substernal radiating to neck and jaw
- Substernal radiating down left arm

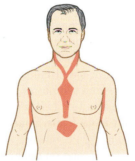

- Epigastric
- Epigastric radiating to neck, jaw, and arms

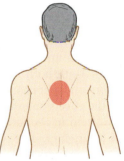

- Intrascapular

FIGURE 33-19 *Shaded areas* show the common locations and patterns of angina. (From Lewis SL and others: *Medical-surgical nursing: assessment and management of clinical problems,* ed 10, St Louis, 2017, Elsevier.)

Angina

Angina is chest pain from reduced blood flow to part of the heart muscle *(myocardium)*. *(Angina* comes from the Latin word *angor* that means *strangling.)* It occurs when the heart needs more O_2. Normally blood flow to the heart increases when O_2 needs increase. Exertion, a heavy meal, stress, and excitement increase the heart's need for O_2. So does smoking and very hot or cold temperatures. In CAD, narrowed vessels prevent increased blood flow.

Chest pain is described as tightness, pressure, squeezing, or burning in the chest. Pain can occur in the shoulders, arms, neck, jaw, or back (Fig. 33-19). Pain in the jaw, neck, and down 1 or both arms is common. The person may be pale, feel faint, and perspire. Dyspnea is common. Nausea, fatigue, and weakness may occur. Some persons complain of "gas" or indigestion. Rest often relieves symptoms in 3 to 15 minutes.

Besides rest, a *nitroglycerin* tablet is taken when angina occurs. Placed under the tongue, the tablet dissolves and is rapidly absorbed into the bloodstream. Kept within reach, the person takes a tablet and then tells the nurse. For some persons, the nurse applies and removes nitroglycerin patches.

Over-exertion, heavy meals and over-eating, emotional stress, cold weather, and hot and humid weather are avoided. Doctor-supervised exercise programs are helpful.

See "Coronary Artery Disease" for the treatment of angina. Increased blood flow to the heart prevents or lowers the risk of heart attack and death. Chest pain lasting longer than a few minutes and not relieved by rest and nitroglycerin may signal a heart attack. Emergency care is needed.

Myocardial Infarction

Myocardial refers to the *heart muscle*. *Infarction* means *tissue death*. With myocardial infarction (MI) part of the heart muscle dies from sudden blockage of blood flow in a coronary artery.

MI also is called:

- Heart attack
- Acute myocardial infarction (AMI)
- Acute coronary syndrome (ACS)

See Box 33-10 for signs and symptoms. MI is an emergency. Efforts are made to:

- Relieve pain.
- Restore blood flow to the heart.
- Stabilize vital signs.
- Give O_2.
- Calm the person.
- Prevent death and life-threatening problems.

The person may need medical or surgical procedures to open or bypass the diseased artery. Cardiac rehabilitation is needed. The goals are to:

- Recover and resume normal activities.
- Prevent another MI.
- Prevent complications such as heart failure or sudden cardiac arrest (sudden cardiac death) (Chapter 36).

Heart Failure

Heart failure or congestive heart failure (CHF) occurs when the weakened heart cannot pump normally. Blood backs up. Tissue congestion occurs.

When the left side of the heart cannot pump normally, blood backs up into the lungs. Respiratory congestion occurs. When the right side of the heart cannot pump normally, blood backs up into the venous system. Swelling occurs *(edema)*. With both left-sided and right-sided failure, the body does not get enough blood. Signs and symptoms occur from the effects on other organs. See Box 33-11. *Pulmonary edema* (fluid in the lungs) can result from heart failure. It is an emergency. The person can die.

Drugs strengthen the heart, decrease strain on the heart, and reduce fluid buildup. A sodium-controlled diet is ordered. Oxygen is given. Semi-Fowler's position is preferred for breathing. Intake and output (I&O), daily weight, elastic stockings, and ROM exercises are part of the care plan.

RESPIRATORY DISORDERS

The respiratory system brings O_2 into the lungs and removes carbon dioxide (CO_2) from the body. Respiratory disorders interfere with this function and threaten life.

Chronic Obstructive Pulmonary Disease

Chronic obstructive pulmonary disease (COPD) involves 2 disorders—chronic bronchitis and emphysema. These disorders interfere with O_2 and CO_2 exchange in the lungs. They obstruct (block) airflow. Lung function is gradually lost.

BOX 33-10	Myocardial Infarction—Signs and Symptoms

- Chest pain
  - Sudden, severe; usually in the center or on the left side
  - Described as pressure, tightness, fullness, squeezing, or aching
  - More severe and lasts longer than angina
  - Not relieved by rest or nitroglycerin
- Pain or numbness in 1 or both arms, the back, neck, jaw, or stomach
- Indigestion or "heartburn"
- *Dyspnea* (difficulty breathing)
- Nausea, vomiting
- Dizziness
- Fainting
- Perspiration and cold, clammy skin
- *Pallor* (pale skin) or *cyanosis* (bluish color)
- Pulse: fast, irregular
- Fear, apprehension, and a feeling of doom

BOX 33-11	Heart Failure—Signs and Symptoms

- Dyspnea (worse with exertion or lying down)
- Sputum: white, pink, blood-tinged, foamy
- Cough
- Lung sounds: gurgling, wheezing
- Confusion
- Dizziness
- Fainting
- Fatigue
- Weakness
- *Pallor* (pale skin)
- *Nocturia* (frequent urination at night)
- Nausea
- Appetite: decreased
- Swelling: feet, ankles, legs, abdomen, neck veins
- Weight gain
- Pulse: rapid, irregular

Cigarette smoking is the greatest risk factor. Pipe, cigar, and other smoking tobaccos are also risk factors. So is exposure to second-hand smoke. Not smoking is the best way to prevent COPD. COPD has no cure.

Chronic Bronchitis. Chronic bronchitis occurs after repeated episodes of bronchitis. *Bronchitis* means *inflammation* (itis) *of the bronchi* (bronch).

Smoker's cough in the morning is often the first symptom. At first the cough is dry. Over time, mucus is coughed up. Mucus may contain pus. The cough becomes more frequent. The person has difficulty breathing and tires easily. Mucus and inflamed breathing passages obstruct airflow. The body cannot get enough O_2.

The person must stop smoking. Oxygen therapy and breathing exercises are common. Respiratory tract infections are prevented. If one occurs, prompt treatment is needed.

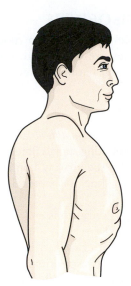

FIGURE 33-20 Barrel chest from emphysema.

Emphysema. In emphysema, the alveoli enlarge and become less elastic. Alveoli do not expand and shrink normally with breathing in and out. As a result, some air is trapped in the alveoli. Trapped air is not exhaled. Over time, more alveoli are involved. O_2 and CO_2 exchange cannot occur in affected alveoli. As more air is trapped in the lungs, the person develops a *barrel chest* (Fig. 33-20).

The person has shortness of breath and a cough. At first, shortness of breath occurs with exertion. Over time, it occurs at rest. Sputum may contain pus. Fatigue is common. The person works hard to breathe in and out. The body does not get enough O_2. Breathing is easier when sitting upright and slightly forward (Chapter 30).

The person must stop smoking. Respiratory therapy, breathing exercises, oxygen, and drug therapy are ordered.

Asthma

With asthma, the airway becomes inflamed and narrow. Extra mucus is produced. Dyspnea results. Wheezing and coughing are common. So are pain and tightness in the chest. Symptoms are mild to severe.

Asthma usually is triggered by allergies. Other triggers include air pollutants and irritants, smoking and second-hand smoke, respiratory infections, exertion, and cold air. Sudden attacks (*asthma attacks*) can occur. There is shortness of breath, wheezing, coughing, rapid pulse, sweating, and cyanosis. The person gasps for air and is very frightened.

Asthma is treated with drugs. Severe attacks may require emergency care.

Influenza

Influenza (*flu*) is a respiratory infection caused by viruses. The flu season is October through March. Older persons are at great risk. Pneumonia is a common complication.

Signs and symptoms of flu include:
- High fever (100°F [Fahrenheit] to 102°F) for 3 to 4 days
- Headache
- General aches and pains
- Fatigue and weakness that can last 2 to 3 weeks
- Chest discomfort
- Cough
- Stuffy nose, sneezing, sore throat

Treatment involves fluids and rest. Drugs are ordered for symptom relief and to shorten the flu episode.

Coughing and sneezing spread flu viruses. Follow Standard Precautions. The flu vaccine is the best prevention. See *Focus on Older Persons: Influenza.*

FOCUS ON OLDER PERSONS

Influenza

Older persons may not have the usual flu signs and symptoms. The following may signal flu in older persons.
- Changes in mental status or behavior
- Worsening of other health problems
- A body temperature below the normal range
- Fatigue
- Decreased appetite and fluid intake

Pneumonia

Pneumonia *means inflammation and infection of lung tissue.* (*Pneumo* means *lungs.*) Affected tissues fill with fluid. O_2 and CO_2 exchange is affected.

Bacteria, viruses, and other microbes are causes. Signs and symptoms include:
- Fever
- Chills
- Painful cough
- Chest pain on breathing
- Rapid pulse and breathing
- Shortness of breath
- Cyanosis
- Thick and white, green, yellow, or rust-colored sputum
- Nausea and vomiting
- Headache
- Tiredness
- Muscle aches

Drugs are ordered for infection and pain. Fluid intake is increased because of fever and to thin secretions. Thin secretions are easier to cough up. Intravenous (IV) therapy and oxygen may be needed. Semi-Fowler's position eases breathing. Rest is important. Standard Precautions are followed. Transmission-Based Precautions depend on the cause. Mouth care is important. Frequent linen changes are needed because of fever.

See *Focus on Older Persons: Pneumonia*, p. 484.

Tuberculosis

Tuberculosis (TB) is a bacterial infection in the lungs. TB is spread by airborne droplets with coughing, sneezing, speaking, singing, or laughing (Chapter 13). Nearby persons can inhale the bacteria. Those with close, frequent contact with an infected person are at risk. TB is more likely to occur in close, crowded areas. Age, poor nutrition, and HIV (human immunodeficiency virus) infection are other risk factors.

TB can be present in the body but not cause signs and symptoms. An active infection may not occur for many years. Only persons with an active infection can spread the disease to others.

Chest x-rays and TB testing can detect the disease. Signs and symptoms are tiredness, loss of appetite, weight loss, fever, chills, and night sweats. Cough and sputum increase over time. Sputum may contain blood. Chest pain occurs.

Drugs for TB are given. Standard Precautions and airborne precautions are needed (Chapter 13). The person must cover the mouth and nose with tissues when sneezing, coughing, or producing sputum. Tissues are discarded in a no-touch waste container. Hand-washing after contact with sputum is essential.

See *Focus on Older Persons: Tuberculosis.*

DIGESTIVE DISORDERS

The digestive system breaks down food for the body to absorb. Solid wastes are eliminated. See Chapter 22 for diarrhea, constipation, flatulence, fecal incontinence, and ostomy care.

Vomiting

Vomitus (emesis) is the food and fluids expelled from the stomach through the mouth. Vomiting signals illness or injury. Aspirated vomitus can obstruct the airway. Vomiting large amounts of blood can lead to shock (Chapter 36). These measures are needed.

- Follow Standard Precautions and the Bloodborne Pathogen Standard.
- Turn the person's head well to 1 side if the person is supine. This prevents aspiration.
- Place a kidney basin under the chin.
- Move vomitus away from the person.
- Provide oral hygiene. This helps remove the bitter taste of vomitus.
- Observe vomitus for blood, color, odor, and undigested food. If it looks like coffee grounds, it contains blood. Report your observations.
- Measure, report, and record the amount of vomitus.
- Save a specimen for laboratory study.
- Dispose of vomitus after the nurse observes it.
- Eliminate odors.
- Provide for comfort. (See the inside of the front cover.)

Diverticular Disease

Small pouches can develop in the colon. The pouches bulge outward through weak spots in the colon wall (Fig. 33-21). A pouch is called a *diverticulum. (Diverticulare* means *to turn inside out). Diverticulosis* is the condition of having these pouches. *(Osis* means *condition of.)* The pouches can become infected or inflamed—*diverticulitis. (Itis* means *inflammation.)*

Many people over 50 years of age have diverticulosis. Aging, obesity, smoking, lack of exercise, low-fiber diet, a diet high in animal fat, and some drugs are risk factors.

When feces enter the pouches, they can become inflamed and infected. The person has abdominal pain and tenderness in the lower left abdomen. Fever, nausea and vomiting, chills, cramping, and constipation or diarrhea are likely.

Diet changes are ordered. Sometimes antibiotics and probiotics are ordered. *Probiotics*—found in dietary supplements and some foods—are live bacteria normally found in the colon. Surgery is done for severe disease, obstruction, and ruptured pouches. The diseased part of the bowel is removed. A colostomy may be needed (Chapter 22).

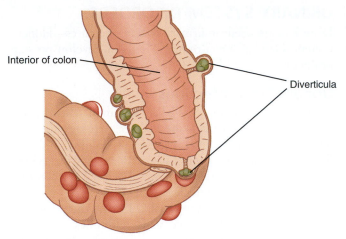

FIGURE 33-21 Diverticulosis. (From Lewis SM and others: *Medical-surgical nursing: assessment and management of clinical problems,* ed 10, St Louis, 2017, Elsevier.)

BOX 33-12	Hepatitis—Signs and Symptoms

- *Jaundice*—yellowish color of the skin or whites of the eyes
- Fatigue
- Pain: abdominal, joint
- Appetite: loss of
- Nausea and vomiting
- Diarrhea
- Bowel movements (BMs): light, clay-colored
- Urine: dark
- Fever
- Headache
- Itching
- Weight loss
- Skin rash

Inflammatory Bowel Disease

Inflammatory bowel disease (IBD) involves chronic inflammation of the digestive tract. Two types of IBD are:

- *Crohn's disease.* The lining of the large intestine, small intestine, or both is inflamed.
- *Ulcerative colitis.* The lining of the large intestine and rectum is inflamed and has ulcers.

Signs and symptoms include:

- Diarrhea
- Abdominal pain and cramping
- Fever
- Bleeding—bright red blood in the toilet, dark blood in the stools, or occult blood (Chapter 26)
- Appetite: loss of
- Weight loss

IBD often occurs before 30 years of age. Risk factors include a family history of IBD, cigarette smoking, some drugs, and a diet high in fat and refined foods.

Complications include bowel obstruction, ulcers in the gastro-intestinal (GI) tract (including the mouth and anus), colon cancer, osteoporosis, and liver disease. Treatment involves diet changes and drug therapy for inflammation, infection, diarrhea, pain, and nutrition. Surgery may be needed to remove damaged parts of the small intestine or colon. A colostomy or ileostomy (Chapter 22) may be necessary.

Hepatitis

Hepatitis is inflammation *(itis)* and infection of the liver *(hepat)* caused by a virus. See Box 33-12 for signs and symptoms. Some people have no symptoms. There are 5 major types of hepatitis.

- *Hepatitis A* is spread by food or water contaminated with feces from an infected person. Hepatitis A is spread by eating or drinking food or water contaminated with feces, eating or drinking from a contaminated vessel, or eating raw shellfish from sewage-polluted water. Having close contact or sex with an infected person can also spread the virus. Handle bedpans, toilets, commodes, incontinence products, and rectal thermometers carefully. The hepatitis A vaccine protects against the disease.
- *Hepatitis B* is caused by the hepatitis B virus (HBV). It is spread through infected blood and body fluids (saliva, semen, vaginal secretions).
  - By sharing blood-contaminated IV needles and syringes
  - By accidental needle-sticks
  - By sex without a condom, especially anal sex
  - During childbirth from mother to baby
- *Hepatitis C* is spread by blood infected with the hepatitis C virus. A person may have no symptoms but can spread the disease. Serious liver disease and damage may appear years later. The virus is spread mainly through sharing blood-contaminated IV needles and syringes and contaminated tools used for tattoos or body piercings.
- *Hepatitis D* occurs only in people infected with hepatitis B. It is spread in the same way as HBV.
- *Hepatitis E* is spread through food or water contaminated by feces from an infected person. This disease is not common in the United States.

See *Promoting Safety and Comfort: Hepatitis,* p. 486.

Cirrhosis

Cirrhosis is a liver condition caused by chronic liver damage. *(Cirrho* means *yellow-orange. Osis* means *condition.)* Scar tissue blocks blood flow through the liver. Normal liver functions are affected.

Chronic alcohol abuse, chronic hepatitis B and C, and extra fat in the liver are common causes. Obesity is becoming a common cause. Signs and symptoms may occur as the disease progresses.

- Weakness and fatigue
- Loss of appetite and weight loss
- Nausea
- *Ascites*—abdominal bloating from fluid buildup in the abdomen (Fig. 33-22)
- *Edema* (swelling) in the feet and legs
- Itching
- Spider-like blood vessels on the skin
- Jaundice

Cirrhosis has many serious complications. Infection, bruising, and bleeding occur. Blood vessels in the esophagus and stomach enlarge and burst. Gallstones may develop. Toxins build up in the brain, causing confusion, personality changes, and memory loss. Diabetes and liver cancer are risks.

Complications are treated. A low-sodium diet is needed for edema and ascites. Diuretic drugs (water pills) are ordered to remove fluid. Antibiotics are ordered for infection. The person must avoid alcohol and may need a liver transplant.

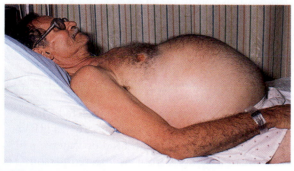

FIGURE 33-22 Fluid in the membrane lining the abdominal cavity *(ascites).* (From Swartz MH: *Textbook of physical diagnosis,* ed 7, Philadelphia, 2014, Saunders.)

URINARY SYSTEM DISORDERS

Disorders can occur in urinary system structures—kidneys, ureters, bladder, and urethra. Men can develop prostate problems.

Urinary Tract Infections

Urinary tract infections (UTIs) are common. Microbes can enter the system through the urethra. Urological exams, intercourse, poor perineal hygiene, immobility, and poor fluid intake are common causes. Persons with urinary catheters are at high risk (Chapter 21). UTI is a common healthcare-associated infection (Chapter 13).

See Box 33-13 for the types of UTIs and their signs and symptoms. UTIs are treated with antibiotics. Fluids are encouraged—usually 2000 mL (milliliters) a day. Normal elimination is promoted. For prevention and treatment, proper perineal care and catheter care are needed.

BOX 33-13   Urinary Tract Infections

Common Signs and Symptoms

- Urinary frequency
- *Oliguria*—scant *(olig)* urine *(uria)*
- Urgency
- *Dysuria*—difficult or painful *(dys)* urination *(uria)*
- Pain or burning on urination
- *Hematuria*—blood *(hemat)* in the urine *(uria)*
- *Pyuria*—pus *(py)* in the urine *(uria)*
- Cloudy urine
- Urine odor
- Pelvic pain—women
- Rectal pain—men

Cystitis—a bladder *(cyst)* infection *(itis)* caused by bacteria

- Additional symptoms
  - Pelvic pressure
  - Lower abdominal discomfort

Pyelonephritis—inflammation *(itis)* of the kidney *(nephr)* pelvis *(pyelo)*

- Additional symptoms
  - Back and side pain
  - High fever
  - Nausea and vomiting
  - Shaking and chills

Prostate Enlargement

The prostate is a walnut-shaped gland in men. It lies in front of the rectum and just below the bladder (Chapter 8). The prostate surrounds the urethra. The prostate grows larger (enlarges) as the man grows older. This is called benign prostatic hyperplasia (BPH). *Benign* means *non-malignant*. *Hyper* means *excessive*. *Plasia* means *formation* or *development*. Benign prostatic hypertrophy is another name for enlarged prostate. (*Trophy* means *growth*.)

BPH is common in older men. The enlarged prostate presses against the urethra, obstructing urine flow (Fig. 33-23). These problems are common.

- Trouble starting a urine stream
- A weak urine stream
- Frequent voidings of small amounts of urine
- Urgency and leaking or dribbling urine
- Frequent voiding at night (*nocturia*)
- Urinary retention (The man is not able to completely empty the bladder.)
- Urinary incontinence
- Pain during urination

For mild BPH, drugs can shrink the prostate or stop its growth. Some microwave and laser treatments destroy excess prostate tissue. Or surgery is done to remove tissue.

Kidney Stones

Kidney stones (*calculi*) are hard deposits in the kidney. Stones vary in shape and size from grains of sand to golf ball–sized (Fig. 33-24). Bedrest, immobility, and poor fluid intake are risk factors. Signs and symptoms include:

- Severe, cramping pain in the back and side just below the ribs
- Pain in the lower abdomen, thigh, and urethra
- Nausea and vomiting
- Fever and chills
- *Dysuria*—difficult or painful (*dys*) urination (*uria*)
- Urinary urgency
- Pain on urination
- *Hematuria*—blood (*hemat*) in the urine (*uria*)
- Cloudy urine
- Foul-smelling urine

Drugs are given for pain relief. The person needs to drink 2000 to 3000 mL (milliliters) a day. Fluids help flush stones out through the urine. All urine is strained (Fig. 33-25). Medical or surgical removal of the stone may be necessary. Diet changes may prevent stones.

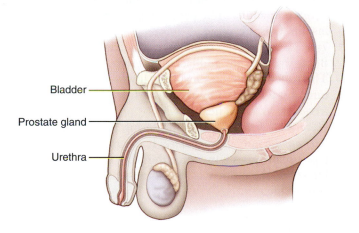

Bladder

Prostate gland

Urethra

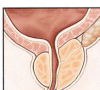

Normal prostate

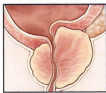

Enlarged prostate

FIGURE 33-23 Enlarged prostate. The prostate presses against the urethra. Urine flow is obstructed.

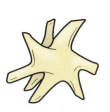

Jagged and yellow

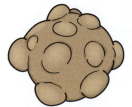

Golf ball–sized and brown

FIGURE 33-24 Kidney stones.

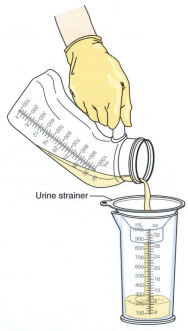

Urine strainer

FIGURE 33-25 Urine is poured through a strainer to collect stones.

BOX 33-14	Kidney Failure—Care Measures

- A diet low in protein, potassium, and sodium
- Fluid restriction
- Measuring blood pressure in the supine, sitting, and standing positions
- Measuring daily weight
- Measuring and recording intake and output
- Turning and re-positioning at least every 2 hours
- Measures to prevent pressure injuries
- ROM exercises
- Measures to prevent itching (bath oils, lotions, creams)
- Measures to prevent injury and bleeding
- Frequent oral hygiene
- Measures to prevent infection
- Deep-breathing and coughing exercises
- Measures to prevent diarrhea or constipation
- Measures to meet emotional needs
- Measures to promote rest

Kidney Failure

In kidney failure (renal failure), the kidneys do not function or are severely impaired. Waste products are not removed from the blood. Fluid is retained. Heart failure and hypertension easily result. The person is very ill.

Kidney failure may be acute or chronic. Treatment involves drugs, restricted fluids, and diet therapy. Chronic kidney disease (CKD; chronic kidney failure) requires dialysis. *Dialysis* is the process of removing waste products from the blood. You assist in the person's care. See Box 33-14.

REPRODUCTIVE DISORDERS

Aging affects the reproductive system (Chapter 9). Injuries, diseases, and surgeries can affect reproductive structures and functions.

Sexually Transmitted Diseases

A sexually transmitted disease (STD) is spread by oral, vaginal, or anal sex. Some people have no signs and symptoms or are not aware of an infection. Others know but are too embarrassed to seek treatment.

STDs often occur in the genital and rectal areas. The ears, mouth, nipples, throat, tongue, eyes, and nose are other sites. Condom use helps prevent the spread of STDs, especially the human immunodeficiency virus (HIV) and acquired immunodeficiency syndrome (AIDS). Some STDs are also spread through skin breaks, by contact with infected body fluids (blood, semen, saliva), or by contaminated blood or needles.

Standard Precautions and the Bloodborne Pathogen Standard are followed.

See *Focus on Older Persons: Sexually Transmitted Diseases.*

FOCUS ON OLDER PERSONS

Sexually Transmitted Diseases

Many older people are sexually active. They get and can spread STDs in the same ways as younger persons. However, many do not think they are at risk. Always practice Standard Precautions and follow the Bloodborne Pathogen Standard. Do not assume that older people are too old to have sex.

ENDOCRINE DISORDERS

The endocrine system is made up of glands. The endocrine glands secrete hormones that affect other organs and glands. Diabetes is the most common endocrine disorder.

Diabetes

In diabetes, the body cannot produce or use insulin properly. Insulin is needed for glucose to move from the blood into the cells. The pancreas secretes insulin. Without enough insulin, sugar builds up in the blood. Blood glucose (sugar) is high. Cells do not have enough sugar for energy and cannot function.

Types of Diabetes. A family history of the disease is a common risk factor for the 3 types of diabetes.

- *Type 1 diabetes*—seen in children and teenagers but can develop in adults. The pancreas produces little or no insulin. Onset is rapid.
- *Type 2 diabetes*—can occur at any age, even in children. Being over-weight and lack of exercise are risk factors. The pancreas secretes insulin. However, the body cannot use it well. Onset is slow. Infections are frequent. Wounds heal slowly.
- *Gestational diabetes*—develops during pregnancy. (*Gestation* comes from *gestare.* It means *to bear.*) This type usually goes away after the baby is born. However, the mother is at risk for type 2 diabetes later in life.

Signs and Symptoms. Signs and symptoms of diabetes are:

- Extreme thirst
- Frequent urination
- Feeling very hungry or tired
- Weight loss without trying
- Sores that heal slowly
- Dry, itchy skin
- Tingling or loss of feeling in the feet
- Blurred vision

Complications. Diabetes must be controlled to prevent complications. Diabetes can damage the heart, blood vessels, eyes, kidneys, and nerves. Heart and blood vessel damage can lead to stroke, heart attack, and slow healing. Foot and leg wounds and ulcers are very serious (Chapter 28). Infection and gangrene can occur. Sometimes amputation is necessary.

Treatment. Type 1 diabetes is treated with daily insulin therapy, healthy eating (Chapter 23), and exercise. Type 2 diabetes is treated with healthy eating, exercise, and weight loss if needed. Type 2 may require oral drugs or insulin. Types 1 and 2 involve controlling blood pressure, cholesterol, and the risk factors for coronary artery disease.

Good foot care is needed. Corns, blisters, calluses, and other foot problems can lead to an infection and amputation. See Chapters 19 and 28.

Blood sugar level can fall too low or go too high. Blood glucose is checked daily or 3 or 4 times a day for:

- *Hypoglycemia* means low *(hypo)* sugar *(glyc)* in the blood *(emia)*.
- *Hyperglycemia* means high *(hyper)* sugar *(glyc)* in the blood *(emia)*.

See Table 33-1 for the causes, signs, and symptoms of hypoglycemia and hyperglycemia. Both can lead to death if not corrected. Call for the nurse at once.

IMMUNE SYSTEM DISORDERS

The immune system protects the body from microbes, cancer cells, and other harmful substances. It defends against threats inside and outside the body. Immune system disorders occur from problems with the immune response. The response may be inappropriate, too strong, or lacking.

Autoimmune Disorders

Autoimmune disorders occur when the immune system attacks the body's own *(auto)* healthy cells, tissues, or organs. Most autoimmune disorders are chronic. Signs and symptoms depend on the disease. Common autoimmune disorders include:

- *Celiac disease.* The person cannot tolerate gluten—a substance in wheat, rye, barley, and some drugs. Abdominal bloating and pain, diarrhea or constipation, weight loss or gain, and fatigue occur when gluten is ingested.
- *Graves' disease.* The thyroid gland produces excess *(hyper)* amounts of the thyroid hormone. The person has anxiety, problems sleeping, rapid heart rate, weight loss, sweating, muscle weakness, shaky hands, and bulging eyes.
- *Hashimoto's disease.* The thyroid gland does not produce enough thyroid hormone. The person has fatigue, weakness, weight gain, sensitivity to cold, muscle aches, stiff joints, facial swelling, and constipation.
- *Lupus.* This disease can damage the joints, skin, kidneys, heart, lungs, and other body parts.
- *Rheumatoid arthritis* (p. 471).
- *Multiple sclerosis* (p. 478).
- *Inflammatory bowel disease* (p. 485).
- *Type 1 diabetes.*

TABLE 33-1	Hypoglycemia and Hyperglycemia		
Hypoglycemia (Low Blood Sugar)		**Hyperglycemia (High Blood Sugar)**	
Causes	**Signs and Symptoms**	**Causes**	**Signs and Symptoms**
Too much insulin or diabetic drugs	Fatigue; weakness	Not enough insulin or diabetic drugs	Weakness
Increased exercise	Dizziness; faintness	Too little exercise	Drowsiness
Omitting or missing a meal	Vision changes	Eating too much food	Vision: blurred
Delayed meal	Hunger	Emotional stress	Hunger; thirst
Eating too little food	Tingling around the mouth	Infection or sickness	Dry mouth (very)
Vomiting	Headache	Undiagnosed diabetes	Headache
Drinking alcohol	Skin: cold and clammy		Skin: dry
	Sweating		Face: flushed
	Respirations: rapid and shallow		Respirations: rapid, deep, and labored
	Pulse: rapid		Pulse: rapid, weak
	Blood pressure: low		Blood pressure: low
	Motions: clumsy and jerky		Breath odor: sweet
	Trembling; shakiness		Leg cramps
	Confusion		Urination: frequent
	Convulsions		Nausea; vomiting
	Unconsciousness		Convulsions
			Coma

BOX 33-15	AIDS—Signs and Symptoms

- Rapid weight loss
- Recurring fever
- Night sweats
- Fatigue: extreme and unexplained
- Swollen lymph glands: underarms, groin, neck
- Diarrhea lasting more than 1 week
- Sore throat
- Sores: mouth, anus, genitals
- Red, brown, pink, or purple blotches: under the skin; inside the mouth, nose, or eyelids
- Memory loss
- Depression
- Loss of coordination
- Paralysis

BOX 33-16	Caring for the Person With AIDS

- Follow Standard Precautions and the Bloodborne Pathogen Standard.
- Provide daily hygiene. Avoid irritating soaps.
- Follow the care plan for oral hygiene. A toothbrush with soft bristles is best.
- Provide oral fluids as ordered.
- Measure and record intake and output.
- Measure weight daily.
- Encourage deep-breathing and coughing exercises as ordered.
- Prevent pressure injuries.
- Assist with ROM exercises and ambulating as ordered.
- Encourage self-care. The person may use assistive (adaptive) devices (walker, commode, eating devices).
- Encourage the person to be as active as possible.
- Change linens and garments when damp or wet.
- Listen and provide emotional support.

HIV/AIDS

Acquired immunodeficiency syndrome (AIDS) is caused by the *human immunodeficiency virus (HIV)*. HIV attacks the immune system. Therefore it destroys the body's ability to fight infections and disease.

HIV is spread through certain body fluids—blood, semen, vaginal fluids, rectal fluids, and breast-milk. HIV is not spread by air, water, insects, casual contact (shaking hands, hugging, dancing, sharing dishes), closed mouth or social kissing, or toilet seats. It is not spread through saliva, tears, or sweat unless these body fluids contain HIV-infected blood.

HIV is transmitted *mainly* by:
- Having sex with someone who has HIV.
  - Anal sex
  - Vaginal sex
  - Multiple sex partners
- Sharing needles, syringes, rinse water, or other equipment used to prepare injection drugs.

If untreated, HIV progresses in stages. AIDS is the most severe stage. Box 33-15 lists the signs and symptoms of AIDS. Some HIV-infected persons are symptom-free for more than 10 years. However, they can spread HIV to others.

Drugs are used to treat or reduce HIV symptoms. They also reduce complications and prolong life. AIDS has no vaccine and no cure at present. It is a life-threatening disease.

You may care for persons who are HIV positive, are HIV carriers, or have AIDS (Box 33-16). You may have contact with the person's blood or body fluids. Protect yourself and others. Follow Standard Precautions and the Bloodborne Pathogen Standard. A person may have the HIV virus but no symptoms. In some persons, HIV or AIDS is not yet diagnosed.

See *Focus on Older Persons: HIV/AIDS.*

SKIN DISORDERS

There are many types of skin disorders. Alopecia, hirsutism, dandruff, lice, and scabies are discussed in Chapter 19. Skin tears and pressure injuries are discussed in Chapters 28 and 29. Burns are discussed in Chapter 36.

Shingles

Shingles (herpes zoster) is caused by the virus that causes chicken pox. The virus lies dormant in nerve tissue. (*Dormant* means *to be inactive.*) The virus can become active years later.

The person has a rash or fluid-filled blisters on 1 side of the body (Fig. 33-26). Burning or tingling pain, numbness, or itching can occur.

Persons who have had chicken pox are at risk. So are persons with weakened immune systems from HIV infections, cancer treatments, transplant surgeries, and stress.

Anti-viral drugs and pain-relief drugs are used. For many healthy people, blisters heal and pain is gone in 3 to 5 weeks. A vaccine is available to prevent shingles.

Shingles lesions are infectious until they crust over. Avoid contact with an infected person if you:
- Have never had chicken pox or the vaccine to prevent chicken pox.
- Are pregnant and have not had chicken pox or the vaccine to prevent chicken pox.
- Have a weakened immune system.

FOCUS ON OLDER PERSONS

HIV/AIDS

Older persons get and spread HIV through sexual contact and IV drug use. Aging and some diseases mask the signs and symptoms of AIDS. Older persons are less likely to be tested for HIV/AIDS. Often the person dies without the disease being diagnosed.

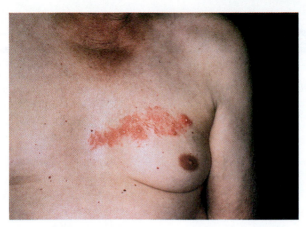

FIGURE 33-26 Shingles. (Courtesy Department of Dermatology, School of Medicine, University of Utah, Salt Lake City, Utah.)

FOCUS ON P R I D E
The Person, Family, and Yourself

Personal and Professional Responsibility

Understanding health problems allows you to safely assist with care. You may want to know more about a health problem that was not covered during your training. Ask the nurse to explain the problem and the care required. Also look up the problem in a medical dictionary or on the Internet. Take pride in learning more.

Rights and Respect

The right to personal choice promotes independence. Some choices are unhealthy. For example, a person with COPD continues to smoke. Or a person with CAD refuses to exercise or make diet changes. The health team teaches the person the risks and encourages healthy changes. The health team cannot force changes. The person needs to understand the risks.

Some persons believe that unhealthy choices improve quality of life. Aware of the risks, they choose not to change. You may not agree with the person's decision, but you must respect the person. Treat the person with dignity and respect.

Independence and Social Interaction

The person and family have many reactions to illness—fear, anger, worry, guilt. Families respond in different ways. A helping and encouraging family provides motivation and support. Family bonds are stronger when the family shares responsibility and relies on each other during stress. The person's health and quality of life also benefit. Some families refuse to help. Or only 1 or 2 members help and support the person. This strains the family and places extra stress on the person.

Promote pride in the family. Compliment their efforts. Encourage the family's help and support.

Delegation and Teamwork

A person's condition can change quickly. A person with angina may have an MI. Hypertension may lead to a stroke. A person may have a severe asthma attack.

Sudden condition changes require the nurse's attention. Assist as directed. You may need to help other patients or residents while the nurse provides care. Always help willingly. The entire nursing team must give "extra effort" during an emergency.

Ethics and Laws

With chronic health problems, staff often care for persons many times. Staff get to know the person. They learn about likes, dislikes, and preferences. Staff learn about the person's family, school or work, hobbies, and so on. Interest in the person adds to quality of care.

However, staff must avoid crossing professional boundaries (Chapter 4). Maintaining these boundaries can be hard when caring for persons you see often and know well. However, you must protect the person's privacy and rights. Watch your behavior closely to avoid crossing boundaries. Tell the nurse if you suspect a person is crossing boundaries.

FOCUS ON PRIDE: *Application*

After a stroke, a person has hemiplegia, aphasia, and dysphagia. Explain how you will modify the care measures listed below. Apply learning from this and other chapters.
- Transferring from the bed to the wheelchair
- Dressing and undressing
- Assisting with food and fluids
- Explaining a procedure
- Performing a safety check of the room

Circle the BEST answer.

1 Which is a general sign of cancer?
   a Painful, swollen joints
   b Feeling very tired
   c A rash with blisters
   d Weight gain

2 Chemotherapy will likely cause
   a Burns
   b Skin breakdown
   c Nausea and vomiting
   d Weight gain

3 A person has arthritis. Care includes
   a Keeping joints abducted
   b Applying traction to affected areas
   c Wearing a cast to prevent movement
   d Rest balanced with exercise

4 A person had hip replacement surgery. Which should you question?
   a Do not cross the legs.
   b Provide a chair with a low seat.
   c Keep a hip abduction wedge between the legs.
   d Provide a long-handled brush for bathing.

5 A person with osteoporosis is at risk for
   a Fractures
   b An amputation
   c Phantom pain
   d Paralysis

6 A cast needs to dry. Which should you question?
   a Turn the person so the cast dries evenly.
   b Cover the cast with blankets and plastic.
   c Elevate the cast on pillows.
   d Support the cast by the palms when lifting.

7 A person is in traction. Care includes
   a Avoiding ROM exercises
   b Keeping the weights on the floor
   c Removing the weights if the person is uncomfortable
   d Using a fracture pan for elimination

8 After hip surgery the operated leg is kept
   a Abducted
   b Adducted
   c Externally rotated
   d Flexed

9 A person had a stroke. Which should you question?
   a Leave the bed in semi-Fowler's position.
   b Perform ROM exercises every 2 hours.
   c Turn and re-position the person every 2 hours.
   d Place needed items on the weak (affected) side.

10 Which statement about Parkinson's disease is *true?*
   a There is a cure.
   b Mental function is affected first.
   c Tremors, slow movements, and a shuffling gait occur.
   d Paralysis occurs but mental function is intact.

11 Which statement about multiple sclerosis is *true?*
   a There is a cure.
   b Only voluntary muscles are affected.
   c Persons older than 65 are at risk.
   d Women are at greater risk than men.

12 A person has quadriplegia from a spinal cord injury. Which should you question?
   a Keep the bed in a low position.
   b Assist with active ROM exercises.
   c Follow the bowel training program.
   d Turn and re-position every hour.

13 In hypertension, the systolic blood pressure is
   a 130 mm Hg or higher
   b 120 mm Hg or higher
   c 90 mm Hg or higher
   d 80 mm Hg or higher

14 A person is being treated for hypertension. Which would you question?
   a No smoking
   b A high-sodium diet
   c Regular exercise
   d A low-fat diet

15 A person has angina. Which is *true?*
   a There is heart muscle damage.
   b Pain is described as crushing or stabbing.
   c Pain is relieved with rest and nitroglycerin.
   d Pain is always on the left side of the chest.

16 A person complains of sudden squeezing chest pain. You should
   a Report the pain if it is not relieved in 15 minutes
   b Report the pain at once
   c Give the person a nitroglycerin tablet
   d Give the person oxygen

17 A person has heart failure. Which should you question?
   a Encourage fluids
   b Measure intake and output
   c Measure weight daily
   d Perform ROM exercises

18 The most common cause of COPD is
   a Smoking
   b Allergies
   c Being over-weight
   d A high-sodium diet

19 A person has emphysema. Which is *true?*
   a The person has an infection.
   b Breathing is usually easier lying down.
   c The person has dyspnea and a cough.
   d There is swelling in an arm or leg.

20 The flu virus is spread by
   a Coughing and sneezing
   b The fecal-oral route
   c Blood
   d Needle sharing

21 Which position eases breathing in the person with pneumonia?
   a Supine
   b Prone
   c Semi-Fowler's
   d Trendelenberg's

22 A person has TB. You had contact with the person's sputum. What should you do?
   a Wash your hands.
   b Put on gloves.
   c Use an alcohol-based hand sanitizer.
   d Tell the nurse.

23 A person is vomiting. You should
 a Position the person supine
 b Leave to get the nurse
 c Do nothing
 d Turn the person's head to the side

24 A person has diverticular disease. How will you assist with care?
 a Giving antibiotics
 b Promoting normal bowel elimination
 c Dietary teaching and planning
 d Assessing risk factors

25 A person has IBD. You may be asked to
 a Collect a sputum specimen for microbes
 b Perform blood glucose testing
 c Collect a stool specimen for occult blood
 d Strain the urine for stones

26 Which is spread by food or water contaminated with feces from an infected person?
 a Hepatitis A
 b Hepatitis B
 c Hepatitis C
 d Hepatitis D

27 Hepatitis requires
 a Sterile gloving
 b Double-bagging
 c Standard Precautions
 d Masks, gowns, and goggles

28 A person has cirrhosis. Which should you question?
 a Measure I&O.
 b Weigh the person daily.
 c Observe vomitus and BMs for blood.
 d Encourage fluids.

29 A person has cystitis. This is a
 a Kidney infection
 b Kidney stone
 c Sexually transmitted disease
 d Bladder infection

30 BPH causes urinary problems because
 a The person has a weak urine stream
 b The person voids frequently at night
 c The enlarged prostate presses against the urethra
 d Voidings are in small amounts

31 Which statement about STDs is *true?*
 a Older persons do not get them.
 b They only affect the genital area.
 c Some persons have no signs or symptoms.
 d STDs require needle use.

32 A person with diabetes is vomiting after a meal. The person is at risk for
 a Hypoglycemia
 b Hyperglycemia
 c Jaundice
 d Bleeding

33 HIV is spread through
 a Body fluids
 b Coughing and sneezing
 c Using public phones and restrooms
 d Hugging or dancing with an infected person

34 HIV can be prevented by
 a Taking immuno-suppressive drugs
 b Getting an HIV vaccine
 c Using probiotics
 d Avoiding risky sexual behaviors

35 A person has shingles. You know that
 a Healing occurs in 3 to 5 days
 b Itching and pain are common
 c Lesions are not infectious
 d Antibiotics are used for treatment

Answers to Chapter 33 questions are on p. 552.

FOCUS ON PRACTICE

Problem Solving

A resident with diabetes is confused, weak, and shaky. What do you do? What might these signs and symptoms indicate? How does understanding the person's health problems help you give better care?

Mental Health Disorders

OBJECTIVES

- Define the key terms and key abbreviations in this chapter.
- Explain the difference between mental health and mental illness.
- List the causes of mental health disorders.
- Describe anxiety disorders and the defense mechanisms used to relieve anxiety.
- Describe schizophrenia.
- Describe bipolar disorder and depression.
- Describe personality disorders.
- Describe substance use disorder and addiction.
- Describe suicide and the persons at risk.
- Describe the care required by persons with mental health disorders.
- Explain how to promote PRIDE in the person, the family, and yourself.

KEY TERMS

addiction A chronic disease involving substance seeking behaviors and use that is compulsive and hard to control despite the harmful effects

anxiety A vague, uneasy feeling in response to stress

compulsion Repeating an act over and over again (a ritual)

defense mechanism An unconscious reaction that blocks unpleasant or threatening feelings

delusion A false belief

delusion of grandeur An exaggerated belief about one's importance, wealth, power, or talents

delusion of persecution A false belief that one is being mistreated, abused, or harassed

detoxification The process of removing a toxic substance from the body

flashback Reliving a trauma in thoughts during the day and in nightmares during sleep

hallucination Seeing, hearing, smelling, or feeling things that are not real

mental Relating to the mind; something that exists in the mind or is done by the mind

mental health The person copes with and adjusts to every-day stresses in ways accepted by society

mental health disorder A disturbance in the ability to cope with or adjust to stress; behavior and function are impaired; mental illness, psychiatric disorder

obsession A frequent, upsetting thought, idea, or image

panic An intense and sudden feeling of fear, anxiety, terror, or dread

phobia An intense fear

psychosis A state of severe mental impairment

stress The response or change in the body caused by any emotional, physical, social, or economic factor

suicide To kill oneself on purpose

suicide contagion Exposure to suicide or suicidal behaviors within one's family, one's peer group, or through media reports of suicide

withdrawal syndrome The physical and mental response after stopping or severely reducing the use of a substance that was used regularly

KEY ABBREVIATIONS

BPD	Borderline personality disorder
OCD	Obsessive-compulsive disorder

PTSD	Post-traumatic stress disorder

The whole person has physical, social, psychological (mental), and spiritual parts. Each part affects the other.

- A physical problem can have social, mental, and spiritual effects.
- A mental health problem can have physical, social, and spiritual effects.
- A social problem can have physical, mental, and spiritual effects.

BASIC CONCEPTS

Mental relates to the mind. It is something that exists in the mind or is done by the mind. Therefore mental health involves the mind. Mental health and mental health disorders involve stress.

- *Stress—the response or change in the body caused by any emotional, physical, social, or economic factor.*
- *Mental health—the person copes with and adjusts to every-day stresses in ways accepted by society.*
- *Mental health disorder—a disturbance in the ability to cope with or adjust to stress. Behavior and function are impaired. Mental illness and psychiatric disorder* are other names.

Causes of mental health disorders include:

- Not being able to cope with or adjust to stress.
- Chemical imbalances.
- Genetics. Many mental health disorders tend to run in families.
- Physical, biological, or psychological factors.
- Substance abuse (p. 499).
- Social and cultural factors.
- Abuse.

ANXIETY DISORDERS

Anxiety is a vague, uneasy feeling in response to stress. The person senses danger or harm—real or imagined. The person acts to relieve the unpleasant feeling. Often anxiety occurs when needs are not met.

Some anxiety is normal. Persons with mental health disorders have higher levels of anxiety. Signs and symptoms depend on the degree of anxiety (Box 34-1).

Coping and defense mechanisms may help relieve anxiety. Unhealthy coping includes over-eating, drinking, smoking, and fighting. Healthy coping includes discussing the problem, exercising, playing music, and wanting to be alone or with others who are helpful.

Defense mechanisms are unconscious reactions that block unpleasant or threatening feelings (Box 34-2). (*Unconscious reactions* are experiences and feelings that cannot be recalled.) Some use of defense mechanisms is normal. In mental health disorders, they are used poorly.

In *generalized anxiety disorder* (GAD), the person has extreme worry and anxiety for little or no reason. The person has extreme anxiety. Getting through the day can be difficult. Worry can prevent the person from normal function.

BOX 34-1 Anxiety—Signs and Symptoms

- Appetite: loss of
- Apprehension
- Attention span: poor
- Blood pressure: increased
- "Butterflies" in the stomach
- Diarrhea
- Directions: difficulty following
- "Lump" in the throat
- Mouth: dry
- Nausea
- Pulse: rapid
- Respirations: rapid
- Sleep: difficulty
- Speech: rapid, voice changes
- Sweating
- Tiredness
- Trembling
- Urinary frequency and urgency
- Weakness

BOX 34-2 Defense Mechanisms

Compensation. *Compensate* means *to make up for, replace, or substitute.* A weakness is replaced with a strength.
EXAMPLE: Not good in sports, a child develops another talent.

Conversion. *Convert* means *to change.* An emotion is changed into a physical symptom.
EXAMPLE: Not wanting to read out loud in school, a child complains of a headache.

Denial. *Deny* means *refusing to accept or believe something that is true.* The person refuses to accept unpleasant or threatening things.
EXAMPLE: After a heart attack, a person continues to smoke.

Displacement. *Displace* means *to move or take the place of.* Behaviors or emotions are moved from 1 person, place, or thing to a safe person, place, or thing.
EXAMPLE: Angry at your boss, you yell at a friend.

Identification. *Identify* means *to relate or recognize.* A person assumes the ideas, behaviors, and traits of another person.
EXAMPLE: A neighbor is a football player. A child practices football in the backyard.

Projection. *Project* means *to blame another.* Another person or object is blamed for unacceptable behaviors, emotions, ideas, or wishes.
EXAMPLE: After over-sleeping, traffic is blamed for being late for work.

Rationalization. *Rational* means *sensible, reasonable, or logical.* An acceptable reason—not the real reason—is given for behaviors or actions.
EXAMPLE: Often late for work, a worker does not get a raise. The worker thinks: "My boss doesn't like me."

Reaction formation. A person acts in a way opposite to how he or she truly feels.
EXAMPLE: A worker does not like the boss. The worker gives the boss a gift.

Regression. *Regress* means *to move back or to retreat.* The person retreats or moves back to an earlier time or condition.
EXAMPLE: A 3-year-old wants a baby bottle when a new baby arrives.

Repression. *Repress* means *to hold down or keep back.* Unpleasant or painful thoughts or experiences are kept from the conscious mind. They cannot be recalled or remembered.
EXAMPLE: A child was sexually abused. Now 33 years old, there is no memory of the event.

Panic Disorder

Panic is an intense and sudden feeling of fear, anxiety, terror, or dread. Onset is sudden, with no real danger. The person cannot function. Signs and symptoms of anxiety are severe (see Box 34-1). The person may also have:

- Chest or stomach pain
- Shortness of breath
- Numbness and tingling in the hands
- Dizziness
- Hot or cold chills
- Feelings of impending doom or loss of control

The person may feel that he or she is having a heart attack or dying. Panic attacks can last for a few minutes or longer. They can occur at any time and during sleep.

Phobias

Phobia means an intense fear. The person has an intense fear of something that has little or no real danger. Common phobias are fear of:

- Being in an open, crowded, or public place (*agoraphobia—agora* means *marketplace*)
- Water (*aquaphobia—aqua* means *water*)
- Being in or trapped in an enclosed or narrow space (*claustrophobia—claustro* means *closing*)
- The slightest uncleanliness (*mysophobia—myso* means *anything that is disgusting*)
- Night or darkness (*nyctophobia—nycto* means *night* or *darkness*)

The person avoids what is feared. When faced with the fear, the person has high anxiety and cannot function.

Obsessive-Compulsive Disorder

The person with obsessive-compulsive disorder (OCD) has obsessions and compulsions. An *obsession is a frequent, upsetting thought, idea, or image.* Microbes, dirt, violent thoughts, and sexual acts are examples. *Compulsion is repeating an act over and over again (a ritual).* The act may not make sense. Anxiety is great if the act is not done.

Common rituals are hand-washing, cleaning, counting to a certain number, or putting things in a certain order. Rituals can take over an hour every day. Hoarding is another OCD behavior. OCD behaviors are distressing and affect daily life.

BOX 34-3	Post-Traumatic Stress Disorder—Signs and Symptoms

- Affection: problems with
- Aggressive and violent behaviors
- Anger: gets mad easily; outbursts
- Avoiding reminders of the harmful event
- Closeness: problems with
- Difficulty around the anniversary of the harmful event
- Emotionally numb: especially to those who were once close
- Flashbacks
- Guilt: intense
- Irritability
- Loss of interest in things once enjoyed
- Physical symptoms:
  - Headache
  - Gastro-intestinal (GI) distress
  - Immune system problems
  - Dizziness
  - Chest pain
  - Discomfort in other body parts
- Sleeping: problems with; bad dreams
- Startles easily
- Trusting people: problems with

Post-Traumatic Stress Disorder

Post-traumatic stress disorder (PTSD) occurs after a terrifying event to self or others. There was physical harm or the threat of physical harm. PTSD can develop at any age. See Box 34-3 for signs and symptoms. PTSD can develop:

- After harm to self or a loved one
- After seeing a harmful event happen to another person

PTSD can result from many traumatic events. They include:

- War, terrorist attack, bombing
- Abuse, mugging, rape, torture
- Kidnapping, being held captive
- Crashes—vehicle, train, plane
- Natural disaster—flood, tornado, hurricane, earthquake

Flashbacks are common. A *flashback is reliving a trauma in thoughts during the day and in nightmares during sleep.* Flashbacks may involve images, sounds, smells, or feelings. Every-day things can trigger them. A door slamming is an example. During a flashback, the trauma seems to be happening all over again.

PTSD can start any time after the event. Treatment can take 6 to 12 weeks or longer. The condition may become chronic.

SCHIZOPHRENIA

Schizophrenia means split (*schizo*) mind (*phrenia*). A severe, chronic, disabling brain disorder, schizophrenia involves:

- *Psychosis—a state of severe mental impairment.* The person does not view the real or unreal correctly.
- *Hallucinations—seeing, hearing, smelling, or feeling things that are not real.* A person may see animals, insects, or people that are not real. Hearing voices is the most common type of hallucination. "Voices" may comment on behavior or order the person to do things, warn of danger, or talk to other voices.
- *Delusions—false beliefs.* For example, the person believes the TV is airing the person's thoughts or that he or she is being harmed. The person may have:
  - *Delusions of grandeur—exaggerated beliefs about one's importance, wealth, power, or talents.* For example, a man believes he is Superman. Or a woman believes she is the Queen of England.
  - *Delusions of persecution—false beliefs that one is being mistreated, abused, or harassed.* For example, a person believes that others are cheating, harassing, poisoning, spying on, or plotting against him or her.
- *Thought disorders.* The person has trouble organizing or logically connecting thoughts. Speech may be garbled and hard to understand. The person may stop speaking in the middle of a thought. Some persons make up words with no meaning.
- *Movement disorders.* These include:
  - Agitated body movements
  - Repeating motions over and over
  - Sitting for hours without moving, speaking, or responding
- *Emotional and behavioral problems.* Normal functions are impaired or absent. The person may:
  - Lose motivation or interest in daily activities.
  - Be unable to plan or do activities.
  - Seem to lack emotions.
  - Neglect personal hygiene.
  - Withdraw socially.
- *Cognitive problems. Cognitive* relates to *understanding, remembering,* and *reasoning.* The person may have trouble paying attention or understanding or remembering information. Symptoms make it hard to perform daily tasks.

Some persons regress. To *regress* means *to retreat or move back to an earlier time or condition.* For example, a 5-year-old wets the bed when there is a new baby. This is normal. Healthy adults do not act like infants or children.

Symptoms usually begin between the ages of 16 and 30. Schizophrenia tends to affect more men than women. In rare cases, it can appear in childhood. People with schizophrenia do not tend to be violent. However, if a person becomes violent, it is often directed at oneself. Some persons with schizophrenia attempt suicide (p. 501).

See *Focus on Communication: Schizophrenia.*

FOCUS ON COMMUNICATION

Schizophrenia

Delusions and hallucinations can frighten a person. Good communication is important.

- Speak slowly and calmly.
- Do not pretend to experience what the person does. Help the person focus on reality.
- Do not try to convince the person that the experience is not real. To the person, it is real.

  For example, a person hears voices. You can say: "I don't hear the voices but I believe you do. Try to listen to my voice and not the other voices."

BIPOLAR DISORDER

Bipolar means 2 (*bi*) poles or ends (*polar*). The person with bipolar disorder has severe extremes in mood, energy, and function. There are emotional highs or "ups" (*mania*) and emotional lows or "downs" (*depression*). Therefore the disorder is also called manic-depressive illness.

The disorder runs in families. It usually develops during the late teens or early adulthood. Life-long management is needed. The person may have problems in school or keeping a job.

Signs and symptoms range from mild to severe (Box 34-4). Mood changes are called "episodes." Some people are suicidal.

BOX 34-4 Bipolar Disorder—Signs and Symptoms

Mania (Manic Episode)
- Increased energy, activity, and restlessness
- Excessively "high," overly happy, "up" mood
- Extreme irritability
- Feeling "jumpy" or "wired"
- Racing thoughts and rapid speech
- Jumping from 1 idea to another
- Easily distracted; problems concentrating
- Sleep problems
- Unrealistic beliefs in one's abilities and powers
- Poor judgment
- Spending sprees
- A lasting period of behavior that is different from usual
- Sex: increased drive; reckless sex
- Drug or alcohol abuse
- Aggressive behavior
- Denial that anything is wrong

Depression (Depressive Episode)
- Sadness; "down" or empty mood
- Hopelessness; lack of joy
- Little energy; decreased activity level
- Worry and anxiety
- Guilt
- Loss of interest in sex or activities once enjoyed
- Feeling tired or "slowed down"
- Problems concentrating, remembering, or making decisions
- Restlessness or irritability
- Sleep problems
- Change in appetite: low or increased
- Chronic pain or other symptoms without a cause
- Thoughts of death or suicide
- Suicide attempts

DEPRESSION

Depression (major depressive disorder; clinical depression) involves the body, mood, and thoughts (see Box 34-4). The person has prolonged feelings of sadness, loss, anger, or frustration that affect daily life. Work, study, sleep, eating, and other activities are affected.

Many factors can cause depression. They include genetics, changes in the brain, and hormones. Thyroid problems, pregnancy, miscarriage, childbirth (post-partum depression), and menopause involve hormonal changes. A stressful event such as illness or death of a partner, parent, or child may cause depression. So can divorce or job loss.

Depression in Older Persons

Not a normal part of aging, depression can occur in older persons. Older persons have many losses—death of family and friends, loss of body functions, loss of independence. See Box 34-5 for the signs and symptoms of depression in older persons.

Some medical conditions and drug side effects can cause symptoms of depression. Depression in older persons is often overlooked or a wrong diagnosis is made. Often the person is thought to have a cognitive disorder (Chapter 35). Therefore depression is often not treated.

BOX 34-5	Depression in Older Persons— Warning Signs

- Changes in mood, energy level, and appetite
- Problems feeling good thoughts; flat feeling
- Sadness; hopelessness
- Concentration: problems with
- Restlessness or feeling on edge
- Worry and stress: increased
- Anger
- Irritability or aggression
- Sleep problems; sleeping too much
- Headaches
- Digestive problems
- Pain
- Alcohol or drugs: need for
- Obsessions or compulsions
- Thinking or behaviors that interfere with daily living or are of concern to others
- Suicidal thoughts
- High-risk activities

Modified from National Institute of Mental Health: *Older adults and mental health*, revised October 2016.

PERSONALITY DISORDERS

Personality disorders involve rigid and maladaptive behaviors. To *adapt* means *to change* or *adjust*. *Mal* means *bad, wrong, or ill*. *Maladaptive* means *to change or adjust in the wrong way*. Because of their behavior, persons with personality disorders cannot function well in society.

Antisocial Personality Disorder

The person has a history of thinking and behaviors that violates the rights of others. The person has no regard for the safety of others. Lacking responsibility, the person has no guilt. The person may display aggressive and violent behaviors. Signs and symptoms include:

- Disregard for right and wrong
- Lying to, charming, or conning others for personal gain or pleasure
- Feeling superior to others
- Engaging in dangerous behavior or criminal acts
- Failing to plan ahead or consider negative consequences
- Being irritable or hostile
- Having poor or abusive relationships
- Failing to fulfill work or financial responsibilities

Borderline Personality Disorder

Borderline personality disorder (BPD) involves a pattern of unstable moods, behaviors, self-image, and functioning. As a result, the person is impulsive and has unstable relationships. Signs and symptoms include:

- Extreme mood swings. Anger, depression, and anxiety may last for a few hours or for days.
- Feelings of emptiness or boredom.
- Intense anger or anger control problems.
- Intense fear of abandonment. Extreme measures are taken to avoid being left, rejected by, or separated from another. The fear may be real or imagined.
- Intense and stormy relationships with loved ones, family, and friends. The person has extremes from love and closeness to dislike and anger.
- Unstable self-image. The person has sudden changes in feelings, opinions, values, and goals.
- Impulsive and dangerous behaviors. Spending sprees, unsafe sex, substance abuse, reckless driving, and binge eating are examples.
- Suicidal behaviors or threats of self-harm. Self-harm behaviors include cutting, burning, and hitting oneself; head banging; and hair pulling.
- Paranoid thoughts. *Paranoia* is a disorder *(para)* of the mind *(noia)*. Paranoid thoughts include delusions and suspicions about a person or situation.
- Dissociative symptoms. *Dissociate* means *to disconnect or separate*. The person feels cut off from oneself, observes oneself from outside the body, or loses touch with reality.

SUBSTANCE USE DISORDER

Substance use disorder (substance abuse) is when the use of alcohol or another substance (a drug) leads to health issues or problems at work, school, or home.

The exact cause is unknown. Influencing factors include genetics, how the substance affects the person, peer pressure, anxiety, depression, and stress. The person with substance use disorder may have other mental health disorders.

Legal substances (such as drugs for pain relief) and illegal substances (such as heroin) are used. Legal drugs are approved for use in the United States. Doctors prescribe them. Illegal drugs are not approved for use. Legal drugs may be bought or obtained illegally. Commonly used substances include:

- *Opiates and other narcotics.* These drugs are strong painkillers that cause drowsiness. Some cause an intense feeling of well-being, happiness, excitement, and joy.
- *Stimulants.* These drugs stimulate the brain and nervous system.
- *Depressants.* These drugs depress the nervous system, causing drowsiness and reduced anxiety. Alcohol is a depressant.
- *Hallucinogens.* These drugs cause sensations and images (hallucinations) that are not real.
- *Marijuana.* This drug affects the brain, causing a "high." Seeing brighter colors and mood changes are common. Legal in some states, medical use includes pain management and nausea from cancer therapy.

Signs and symptoms of substance use disorder are listed in Box 34-6.

See *Focus on Older Persons: Substance Use Disorder.*

FOCUS ON OLDER PERSONS

Substance Use Disorder

Older persons are at risk for substance use disorder. Reasons include:

- Long-term and many prescription drugs
- Not taking drugs properly
- Multiple health problems
- Physical changes from aging
- Using over-the-counter (OTC) drugs and dietary supplements
- Drug interactions

BOX 34-6   Substance Use Disorder—Signs and Symptoms

Behavior Changes

- Missing school or work; decreased school or work performance
- Getting into trouble—fights, violence, accidents, car crashes, illegal activities
- Using a substance in hazardous situations—driving, using a machine
- Secretive or suspicious behaviors; hiding substance use
- Appetite: changes in
- Sleep pattern: changes in
- Personality and attitude: changes in
- Mood swings
- Irritability
- Angry outbursts
- Hyperactivity
- Agitation
- Giddiness
- Motivation: lacking
- Fearful, anxious, or paranoid behaviors for no reason
- Hostile reactions when confronted about the substance use
- Lack of control over use
- Being unable to stop or reduce use
- Making excuses to use the substance
- Confusion
- Needing to use the substance daily or regularly
- Not caring about appearance
- Not taking part in normal activities
- Using the substance when alone

Physical Changes

- Eyes: bloodshot, abnormal pupil size
- Weight: loss or gain
- Appearance: decline in
- Smells: body, breath, clothing
- Tremors
- Speech: slurred
- Coordination: impaired

Social Changes

- Sudden change in friends, hangouts, hobbies
- Legal problems related to substance use
- Unexplained need for money
- Financial problems
- Continued substance use despite harmful effects on health, work, or family

Modified from U.S. Department of Health & Human Services: *Mental health and substance use disorders,* MentalHealth.gov.

Addiction

Addiction is a chronic disease involving substance seeking behaviors and use that is compulsive and hard to control despite the harmful effects. The person must have the substance. Persons addicted to drugs or alcohol cannot stop taking the substance without treatment.

- *Drug addiction*—a strong urge or craving to use the substance. The person cannot stop using the drug. Tolerance develops—needing more of the drug for the same effect.
- *Alcoholism (alcohol dependence)*—a disease that involves:
  - *Craving*—a strong need to drink
  - *Loss of control*—not being able to stop drinking once started
  - *Physical dependence*—withdrawal symptoms
  - *Tolerance*—the need for more alcohol for the same effect

The following signal addiction.

- The substance is taken in larger amounts. Or it is taken longer than intended.
- The person tries to cut down or stop using the substance.
- The person craves or has a strong urge for the substance.
- Much time is spent using the substance or recovering from its effects. Or the person spends much time trying to obtain the substance. This interferes with family, work, school, or interests. Substance use continues despite problems.
- Dangerous activities occur during or after substance use. See Box 34-6.
- The person continues to use the substance even when it causes depression or anxiety or worsens other health problems.
- Substance use causes impaired memory *(blackouts)*.
- The person has tolerance to the substance.
  - The substance has less and less effect on the person.
  - More of the substance is needed for the same effect.
- The person has withdrawal symptoms. *Withdraw means to stop, remove, or take away.* **Withdrawal syndrome is the physical and mental response after stopping or severely reducing the use of a substance that was used regularly.** The body responds with anxiety, restlessness, insomnia, irritability, poor attention, and physical illness.

Treatment

Substance use disorder is not easy to treat. The process is long-term. The person may *relapse*—use the substance again after stopping. Treatment may involve:

- Emergency treatment. An over-dose is life-threatening. Treatment depends on the substance used.
- Detoxification (detox). A *toxin* is a harmful substance that can cause death or serious illness. **Detoxification is the process of removing a toxic substance from the body.**
- Drug therapy. A drug with a similar action on the body is slowly given to reduce withdrawal effects.
- Counseling. See "Care and Treatment" on p. 502.

Complications

Complications can occur from substance abuse. They include:

- Sudden death. This can occur from 1 use of the substance.
- Stroke.
- Lung disease.
- Cancer. Cancers of the mouth and stomach are linked to alcohol abuse.
- Infection. HIV/AIDS and hepatitis B and C are risks from shared needles (Chapter 33).
- Job loss.
- Depression.
- Memory and concentration problems.
- Problems with police and legal issues.
- Relationship problems.
- Unsafe sexual practices. Unwanted pregnancy, sexually transmitted disease, HIV/AIDS, or hepatitis can result.
- Suicide.

EATING DISORDERS

An eating disorder involves extremes in eating patterns. The person has a severe disturbance in eating behavior. Eating disorders can develop during childhood, young adulthood, or later in life. The person may have other mental health disorders.

- *Anorexia nervosa.* Anorexia means no (*a*) appetite (*orexis*). *Nervosa* relates to *nerves* or *emotions*. The person has an intense fear of gaining weight. A fat body image is felt despite being quite thin. Small amounts and only certain foods are eaten. Forced vomiting and intense exercise are common. So is enema and laxative use to rid the body of food. Laxatives are drugs that promote defecation. Diuretic abuse may occur. These drugs cause the kidneys to produce large amounts of urine. Extra fluid is lost. Weight loss results. Serious health problems can result. Death is a risk from cardiac arrest or suicide.
- *Bulimia nervosa.* Binge eating occurs—eating large amounts of food. Then the body is purged (rid) of the food to prevent weight gain. Vomiting, laxatives, enemas, diuretics, fasting, and intense exercise are some methods used.
- *Binge eating disorder.* The person often eats large amounts of food. Eating is out of control. The person does not purge, fast, or exercise after binge eating. Often the person is over-weight or obese. High blood pressure, heart disease, diabetes, and joint pain can occur.

SUICIDE

Suicide means to kill oneself on purpose. Risk factors are listed in Box 34-7. *If a person mentions or talks about suicide, take the person seriously. Call for the nurse at once. Do not leave the person alone.*

Agencies treating persons with mental health disorders must identify persons at risk for suicide. They must:

- Identify specific factors or features that increase or decrease the risk for suicide.
- Meet the person's immediate safety needs.
- Provide the most appropriate setting to treat the person.
- Provide crisis information to the person and family. A crisis "hotline" phone number is an example.
  See *Focus on Communication: Suicide.*
  See *Focus on Older Persons: Suicide.*

BOX 34-7	Suicide Risk Factors

- Depression and other mental health disorders
- Substance use disorder
- Prior suicide attempt
- Family history of a mental health disorder or substance abuse
- Family history of suicide
- Family violence (including physical or sexual abuse)
- Guns or other firearms in the home
- Incarceration (prison or jail)
- Exposure to the suicidal behavior of others (family, friends, media figures)

Modified from National Institute of Mental Health: *Suicide in America: frequently asked questions (2015)*, NIH publication No. TR 14-6389, Bethesda, Md, National Institutes of Health.

FOCUS ON COMMUNICATION

Suicide

A person thinking about suicide may say:

- "I just don't want to live anymore."
- "I wish I was dead."
- "I wish I had never been born."
- "Everyone would be better off without me."

A person may ask you not to tell anyone about the suicidal thoughts. Protecting personal information is important. But the person's safety is the priority. Never promise that you will not tell anyone. *Call for the nurse at once if a person talks about suicide.*

FOCUS ON OLDER PERSONS

Suicide

According to the National Institute of Mental Health, older adults are at risk for suicide. Many older persons suffer from depression (p. 498). Depression often occurs with other serious illnesses. Heart disease, stroke, diabetes, cancer, and Parkinson's disease are examples. The person also may have social and financial problems.

Most older victims did not report depression to their doctors. Or depression was not diagnosed.

Suicide Contagion

Suicide contagion is exposure to suicide or suicidal behaviors within one's family, one's peer group, or through media reports of suicide. The exposure has led to suicides and suicidal behaviors in persons at risk. Adolescents and young adults are at risk for suicide contagion.

Following suicide exposure, those close to the victim need evaluation by a mental health professional. They include family, friends, peers, and co-workers. Persons at risk for suicide need mental health services.

CARE AND TREATMENT

Treatment of mental health disorders involves having the person explore thoughts and feelings. Psychotherapy and behavior, group, occupational, art, and family therapies are used. Often drugs are ordered.

The care plan reflects the needs of the total person. This includes physical, safety and security, and emotional needs.

Communication is important. Be alert to nonverbal communication—the person's and your own. The person may respond to stress with anxiety, panic, anger, or violence. Protect yourself. Once you are safe, the health team can protect the person and others. To protect yourself:

- Call for help. Do not try to handle the situation on your own.
- Keep a safe distance between you and the person.
- Be aware of your setting. Do not let the person block your exit.

See *Focus on Communication: Care and Treatment.*

FOCUS ON COMMUNICATION
Care and Treatment

Nonverbal communication involves eye contact, tone of voice, facial expressions, body movements, and posture. Persons with depression often have little eye contact, poor posture, and speak softly. Some do not say much at all. Facial expressions may not change. Some persons cry.

Persons with anxiety may be restless, unable to sit still, and talk fast. Eye contact may be prolonged and intense. Others have poor eye contact. The eyes may dart about. Be alert to nonverbal cues. Report what you observe.

Your nonverbal communication is important. When interacting with persons with mental health disorders:

- Face the person.
- Maintain eye contact.
- Position yourself near the person but not too close. Do not invade the person's space.
- Crouch, sit, or stand at the person's level if safe to do so.
- Show interest and concern through your posture and facial expressions.
- Speak calmly.

FOCUS ON PRIDE
The Person, Family, and Yourself

Personal and Professional Responsibility
Just as a person does not choose to have a physical illness, a person does not choose a mental health disorder. How you view the illness affects how you treat the person. Treat the person with kindness, respect, and compassion. Provide quality care.

Rights and Respect
Agencies have strict rules to protect the person's rights to privacy and confidentiality (Chapter 2). Do not talk about the person with your family or friends. Never give information to someone not involved in the person's care. This includes the person's family. Direct questions to the nurse. Follow agency policies. Take pride in protecting the person's rights.

Independence and Social Interaction
Social support is important in treating mental health disorders. Interacting with others is a healthy way to manage stress. Family and friends provide a sense of worth and belonging. The care plan includes how they are involved in the person's care.

Supporting a person with a mental health disorder can be demanding. The family needs support. Many communities offer support groups. You can offer encouragement. Tell the family that you value the support they give.

Delegation and Teamwork
Teamwork is important. A person may become hostile, violent, or threaten or attempt suicide. The health team must react quickly to protect the person and others. If someone calls for help, respond at once. Assist as the nurse directs. Take pride in working as a team to ensure safety.

Ethics and Laws
Persons with mental health disorders may say or do things that seem strange or odd to you. Do not laugh at or insult the person. Do not joke with others about the person.

Ethics deals with right and wrong conduct. Be professional. Treat the person with dignity and respect. Take pride in the way you treat others.

FOCUS ON PRIDE: *Application*

Why are persons with mental health disorders at risk for violations of their rights? How must the health team protect the person's rights?

REVIEW QUESTIONS

Circle the BEST answer.

1 Stress is
 a A way to cope with or adjust to every-day living
 b A response or change in the body caused by some factor
 c A mental health disorder
 d An unwanted thought or idea

2 These statements are about defense mechanisms. Which is *true*?
 a Using them signals a mental health disorder.
 b They relieve anxiety.
 c They prevent mental health disorders.
 d Persons with mental health disorders use them well.

3 A phobia is
 a The event that causes stress
 b A false belief
 c An intense fear of something
 d A ritual

4 A person cleans and cleans. This behavior is
 a A delusion
 b A hallucination
 c A compulsion
 d An obsession

5 A person has nightmares about a trauma. The person is having
 a Flashbacks
 b Phobias
 c Panic attacks
 d Anxiety

6 Schizophrenia
 a Involves obsessions and compulsions
 b Can be cured with drugs and therapy
 c Usually begins in late adulthood
 d Is a disabling brain disorder

7 Bipolar disorder means that the person
 a Is very suspicious
 b Has anxiety
 c Is very unhappy and feels unwanted
 d Has severe extremes in mood

8 In bipolar disorder, an "emotional high" is called
 a Depression
 b A hallucination
 c Mania
 d An obsession

9 Which is a sign of depression in older persons?
 a Hallucinations
 b Appetite changes
 c Increased activity
 d Garbled speech

10 In antisocial personality disorder, the person
 a Lacks regard for the rights and safety of others
 b Has a sad, anxious, or empty mood
 c Withdraws from people and interests
 d Is paranoid and avoids social situations

11 Which statement about substance use disorder is *true*?
 a Legal substances cannot cause addiction.
 b Substance abuse causes problems at work, home, or school.
 c Complications of substance abuse are minor.
 d There is no treatment for substance abuse.

12 A person has withdrawal syndrome. This means that
 a The person has a physical and mental response when the drug is not taken
 b The person needs higher doses of the drug
 c The effect is reduced with the same amount of drug
 d The person has a relapse after treatment

13 Binge eating followed by purging occurs in
 a Anorexia nervosa
 b Binge eating disorder
 c Bulimia nervosa
 d Borderline personality disorder

14 A person talks about suicide. What should you do?
 a Call for the nurse.
 b Identify factors that increase the risk of suicide.
 c Ask what method the person plans to use.
 d Restrain the person.

15 A patient's family member asks what to say when the person talks about suicide. You should
 a Give advice
 b Direct the question to the nurse
 c Suggest a local support group
 d Call a crisis hotline

Answers to Chapter 34 questions are on p. 552.

FOCUS ON PRACTICE

Problem Solving

A patient is being treated for bipolar disorder. The patient is pacing, appears restless, and is talking very fast about work that needs to be done at home. The patient says: "I don't need to be here. I'm leaving and you can't stop me!" What will you do? How will you protect yourself if the patient becomes violent?

OBJECTIVES

- Define the key terms and key abbreviations in this chapter.
- Describe confusion and its causes.
- List the measures that help confused persons.
- Explain the difference between delirium and dementia.
- Describe the signs, symptoms, and behaviors of Alzheimer's disease (AD).
- Explain the care required by persons with AD and other dementias.
- Describe the effects of AD on the family.
- Explain validation therapy.
- Explain how to promote PRIDE in the person, the family, and yourself.

KEY TERMS

cognitive function Involves memory, thinking, reasoning, ability to understand, judgment, and behavior

confusion A state of being disoriented to person, time, place, situation, or identity

delirium A state of sudden, severe confusion and rapid changes in brain function

delusion A false belief

dementia The loss of cognitive function that interferes with routine personal, social, and occupational activities

elopement When a patient or resident leaves the agency without staff knowledge

hallucination Seeing, hearing, smelling, or feeling something that is not real

paranoia A disorder *(para)* of the mind *(noia);* false beliefs (delusions) and suspicion about a person or situation

sundowning Signs, symptoms, and behaviors of AD increase during hours of darkness

KEY ABBREVIATIONS

AD Alzheimer's disease
ADL Activities of daily living

NIA National Institute on Aging

Changes in the brain and nervous system occur with aging and certain diseases (Box 35-1). Cognitive function may be affected. *(Cognitive* relates to *knowledge.)* Quality of life is affected. *Cognitive function involves memory, thinking, reasoning, ability to understand, judgment, and behavior.*

BOX 35-1	Nervous System Changes From Aging

- Nerve cells are lost.
- Nerve conduction slows.
- Reflexes, responses, and reaction times are slower.
- Vision, hearing, taste, smell, and touch decrease.
- Sensitivity to pain decreases.
- Blood flow to the brain is reduced.
- Sleep patterns change.
- Memory is shorter; forgetfulness occurs.
- Dizziness can occur.

CONFUSION

Confusion is a state of being disoriented to person, time, place, situation, or identity. *Disoriented* means *to be apart from* (dis) *one's awareness* (oriented). Disease, brain injury, infections, hearing and vision loss, and drug side effects are some causes. Reduced blood flow to the brain with aging can cause personality and mental changes.

Memory and the ability to make good judgments are lost. A person may not know people, the time, or the place. Daily activities may be affected. Behavior changes are common—anger, restlessness, depression, irritability.

Treatment is aimed at the cause. Confusion may be temporary or permanent. Some measures help improve function (Box 35-2). You must meet the person's basic needs.

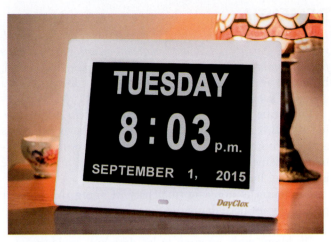

FIGURE 35-1 A large clock can help persons who are confused. (Photo courtesy of DayCloxUSA.com.)

BOX 35-2	Confusion—Care Measures

- Follow the care plan.
- Provide for safety.
- Face the person. Speak clearly.
- Call the person by name each time you have contact.
- State your name. Show your name tag.
- Give the date and time each morning. Repeat as needed during the day or evening.
- Explain what you are going to do and why.
- Give clear, simple directions and answers to questions.
- Break tasks into small steps.
- Ask clear and simple questions. Allow time to respond.
- Make sure the person can see a calendar and clock (Fig. 35-1). Remind the person of holidays, birthdays, and other events.
- Have the person wear needed eyeglasses and hearing aids.
- Use touch to communicate (Chapter 7).
- Place familiar objects and photos within view.
- Provide newspapers, magazines, TV, radio, phone, and other electronic device. Read to the person if appropriate.
- Discuss current events.
- Maintain the day-night cycle.
  - Open window coverings during the day. Close them at night.
  - Use night-lights in rooms, bathrooms, hallways, and other areas at night.
  - Have the person wear day-time clothes during the day.
- Provide a calm, relaxed, and peaceful setting. Prevent loud noises, rushing, and crowded hallways and dining rooms.
- Follow the person's routine. Meals, bathing, exercise, TV, bedtime, and other activities have a schedule. This promotes a sense of order and what to expect.
- Do not re-arrange furniture or the person's belongings.
- Encourage the person to take part in self-care.

Delirium

Delirium is a state of sudden, severe confusion and rapid changes in brain function. Usually temporary and reversible, it occurs with physical or mental illness. Other causes include surgery, drug or alcohol abuse, drug side effects, and infections. Delirium often lasts about 1 week. However, it may take several weeks for normal mental function to return.

Delirium signals illness. It is an emergency. The cause must be found and treated. See Box 35-3 for signs and symptoms.

BOX 35-3	Delirium—Signs and Symptoms

- Alertness: changes in (usually more alert in the morning and less alert at night)
- Sensation: changes in
- Awareness: changes in
- Movement: very active or slow moving
- Drowsiness
- Confusion about time or place
- Memory: decreased short-term memory and recall (cannot remember events since the delirium began)
- Thinking: changes in
- Concentration: problems with
- Speech: does not make sense
- Incontinence
- Emotional changes:
  - Agitation
  - Anger
  - Depression
  - Euphoria
  - Irritability

Modified from MedlinePlus, *Delirium*, Bethesda, Md, updated December 5, 2017, U.S. National Library of Medicine, National Institutes of Health.

DEMENTIA

Dementia is the loss of cognitive function that interferes with routine personal, social, and occupational activities. (De means from. Mentia means mind.) Changes in personality, mood, behavior, and communication are common. Dementia is a group of symptoms, not a specific disease.

Dementia is caused by damage to brain cells. Causes are listed in Box 35-4. Some dementias can be reversed. Signs and symptoms improve when the cause is removed. Permanent dementias result from changes in the brain. There is no cure. Function declines over time.

Dementia is not a normal part of aging. Most older people do not have dementia. Early warning signs include:
- Memory loss (losing things, forgetting names)
- Problems with common tasks (dressing, cooking, driving)
- Problems with language and communication; forgetting simple words
- Getting lost in familiar places
- Misplacing things and putting things in odd places (for example, putting a watch in the oven)
- Personality, mood, and behavior changes
- Poor or decreased judgment (for example, going out in the snow without shoes)

See *Focus on Older Persons: Dementia.*

BOX 35-4	Dementia—Causes

Treatable Causes of Dementia
- Drug and alcohol abuse
- Drug side effects
- Head injuries; bleeding in the brain
- Heart, lung, and blood vessel problems
- Hypoglycemia
- Hypoxia
- Infections
- Nutritional problems
- Poisoning
- Thyroid problems
- Tumors

Causes of Permanent Dementia
- AIDS-related dementia
- Alcohol-related dementia
- Alzheimer's disease
- Brain tumors
- Huntington's disease—a genetic brain disorder
- Multi-infarct dementia (MID)—many (multi) strokes leave areas of damage (infarct)
- Multiple sclerosis
- Parkinson's disease
- Stroke
- Syphilis
- Traumatic brain injury

FOCUS ON OLDER PERSONS

Dementia

Depression is the most common mental health disorder in older persons. It is often overlooked or mistaken for dementia. Dementia, depression, aging, and some drug side effects have similar signs and symptoms. See "Depression in Older Persons" in Chapter 34.

ALZHEIMER'S DISEASE

Alzheimer's disease (AD) is the most common type of permanent dementia. Many brain cells are destroyed and die. Over time, the brain shrinks from nerve cell death and tissue loss (Fig. 35-2). Two abnormal structures are thought to cause damage.
- Plaques—protein pieces that build up in the spaces between nerve cells.
- Tangles—twisted protein fibers that build up inside cells.

With aging, most people develop some plaques and tangles. In AD, plaque and tangle development is severe. Memory areas of the brain are often affected before other areas.

AD onset is gradual. Usually symptoms appear after age 60. Persons with AD can live for 3 to 10 years or longer. More persons with AD are women because women live longer than men.

The greatest risk factor is increasing age. The risk increases after age 65. About one-third ($\frac{1}{3}$) of people age 85 and older have AD. A family history of AD increases the person's risk.

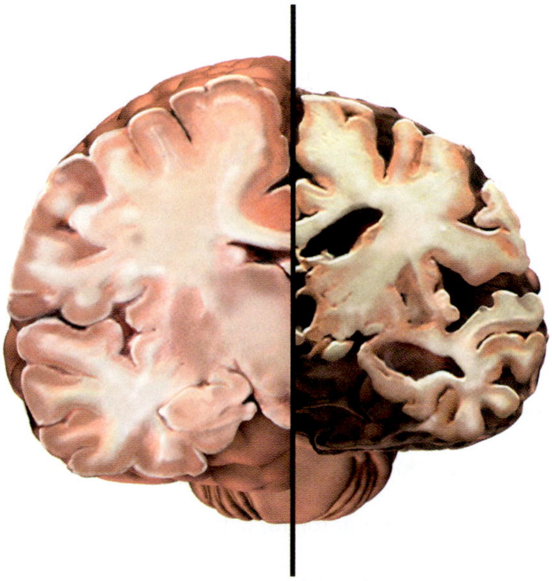

FIGURE 35-2 Nerve cell death and tissue loss shrink the brain in the person with AD. (From Alzheimer's Association: *Brain tour,* 2011.)

BOX 35-5 Alzheimer's Disease—Signs

Warning Signs
- Asks the same question over and over.
- Repeats the same story—word for word, again and again.
- Forgets activities once done regularly and with ease—cooking, repairs, playing cards, and so on.
- Loses the ability to pay bills or balance a checkbook.
- Gets lost in familiar places.
- Misplaces household items.
- Neglects hygiene. Wears the same clothes over and over.
- Relies on someone for decisions or answers that he or she would have handled.

Other Signs
- Forgets recent events, conversations, and appointments.
- Forgets simple directions.
- Forgets names of family members and every-day things (clock, TV, and so on).
- Forgets words, cannot find the right word, loses train of thought.
- Substitutes unusual words and names for what is forgotten.
- Speaks in a native language.
- Curses or swears.
- Forgets important dates and events.
- Takes longer to do things.
- Gives away large amounts of money.
- Does not recognize or understand numbers.
- Has problems following conversations.
- Has problems reading and writing.
- Has problems driving to familiar places.
- Forgets where he or she is.
- Forgets how he or she got to a certain place.
- Does not know how to get back home.
- Wanders from home.
- Cannot tell or understand time or dates.
- Cannot solve every-day problems (iron is left on, stove burners left on, food burning on the stove, and so on).
- Distrusts others.
- Is stubborn.
- Does not want to do things and withdraws socially.
- Is restless.
- Becomes suspicious and fearful.
- Sleeps more than usual.

Warning signs modified from Eric Pfeiffer, MD, *The seven warning signs of Alzheimer's disease,* University of South Florida Suncoast Alzheimer's and Gerontology Center. Reprinted with permission.

BOX 35-6 Alzheimer's Disease and Normal Aging

Signs of AD	Normal Age-Related Changes
Poor judgment and decision making.	Makes a bad decision once in a while.
Cannot manage a budget.	Misses a monthly payment.
Loses track of the date or season.	Forgets which day it is but remembers later.
Problems having a conversation.	Sometimes forgets which word to use.
Misplaces things. Cannot retrace steps to find them.	Loses things from time to time.

Modified from Alzheimer's Association, *10 early signs and symptoms of Alzheimer's,* 2017.

Signs of AD

According to the Alzheimer's Association, the most common early symptom of AD is difficulty remembering newly learned information. *The classic sign is a gradual loss of short-term memory.* At first, the only symptom may be forgetfulness.

With AD there is a slow, steady decline in mental functions.
- Memory
- Thinking
- Reasoning
- Judgment
- Language
- Behavior
- Mood
- Personality

The person has problems with work and every-day functions. Problems with family and social relationships occur.

Box 35-5 lists the warning and other signs of AD. See Box 35-6 for the differences between AD and normal age-related changes.

Stages of AD

Signs and symptoms become more severe as AD progresses. The disease ends in death. AD is described in 3 stages (Box 35-7; Fig. 35-3, p. 508).

BOX 35-7 Alzheimer's Disease—3 Stages

Mild AD
- Memory problems
- Wandering and getting lost
- Problems handling money and paying bills
- Repeating questions
- Taking longer to complete daily tasks
- Losing things or misplacing them in odd places
- Personality and behavior changes

Moderate AD
- Increased memory loss and confusion
- Problems recognizing family and friends
- Cannot learn new things
- Problems with tasks having multiple steps—getting dressed is an example
- Problems coping with new situations
- Hallucinations, delusions, and paranoia (pp. 508 and 510)
- Impulsive behavior

Severe AD
- Depends on others for care
- Cannot communicate
- Weight loss
- Seizures
- Skin infections
- Difficulty swallowing
- Groaning, moaning, or grunting
- Increased sleeping
- In bed most or all of the time
- Loss of bowel and bladder control

Modified from National Institute on Aging: *What are the signs of Alzheimer's disease?*, National Institutes of Health, content reviewed May 16, 2017.

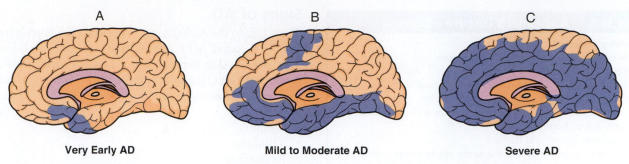

FIGURE 35-3 A, Very early AD. **B,** Mild to moderate AD. **C,** Severe AD. (NOTE: Blue shading shows the areas of the brain affected.) (Redrawn from National Institute on Aging: *Alzheimer's disease: Unraveling the mystery*, Bethesda, Md, September 2008, National Institutes of Health.)

Behavior and Function Changes

AD changes how a person behaves and acts. Besides the signs and symptoms in Boxes 35-5 and 35-7, these behaviors and changes are common.

- Sundowning
- Hallucinations
- Delusions
- Catastrophic reactions
- Wandering and getting lost
- Agitation and aggression
- Paranoia (p. 510)
- Repetitive behaviors (p. 510)
- Rummaging and hiding things (p. 510)
- Changes in intimacy and sexuality (p. 510)
- Communication changes (p. 511)
- Screaming (p. 511)

Besides brain changes, the following can affect behavior.

- Health problems—illness, pain, infection, drugs, lack of sleep, constipation, hunger, thirst, poor vision or hearing, alcohol abuse, too much caffeine
- Emotions—sadness, fear, feeling overwhelmed, stress, anxiety
- Changes in routine
- Problems in the person's setting:
  - A strange setting. The person does not know the setting well.
  - Too much noise (TV, music, people talking at once) can cause confusion and frustration.
  - Not understanding signs. The person may think that a WET FLOOR sign means to urinate on the floor.
  - Mirrors. The person may think that a mirror image is another person in the room.

See *Promoting Safety and Comfort: Behavior and Function Changes.*

Sundowning. With *sundowning, signs, symptoms, and behaviors of AD increase during hours of darkness.* As daylight ends and darkness starts, confusion and restlessness increase. So do anxiety, agitation, and other symptoms. Behavior is worse after sundown. It may continue during the night.

Sundowning may relate to being tired or hungry. Poor light and shadows may cause the person to see things that are not there. The person may be afraid of the dark.

Hallucinations and Delusions. A *hallucination is seeing, hearing, smelling, or feeling something that is not real.* Senses are dulled. Affected persons see animals, insects, or people that are not present. Some hear voices. They may feel bugs crawling or feel that they are being touched.

Poor vision or hearing may be a cause. The person should wear needed eyeglasses and hearing aids. Other causes include infection, pain, and drugs.

Delusions are false beliefs. To the person, the beliefs are real. People with AD think they are another person. Some believe they are in jail, are being killed, or are being attacked. A person may believe the caregiver is someone else. Many other false beliefs can occur.

Catastrophic Reactions. These are extreme responses to normal events or things. The person reacts as if there is a disaster or tragedy. The person may scream, cry, or be agitated or combative (ready to fight). These reactions are common from too many stimuli. Eating, music or TV playing, and being asked questions all at once can overwhelm the person.

Wandering and Getting Lost. Persons with AD are not oriented to person, time, and place. They may wander off and not find their way back. Wandering is by foot, car, bike, or other means. They may be with you one moment and gone the next.

Judgment is poor. They cannot tell what is safe or dangerous. Life-threatening accidents are great risks. They can walk into traffic or a nearby river, lake, ocean, or forest. If not properly dressed, heat or cold exposure is a risk.

Wandering may have no cause. Or the person is looking for something or someone—the bathroom, the bedroom, a child, or a partner. Pain, drug side effects, stress, restlessness, too much stimulation, and anxiety are other causes. A wandering pattern may reflect a life-long routine—leaving work, getting children from school, and so on. Sometimes finding the cause prevents wandering.

See *Promoting Safety and Comfort: Wandering and Getting Lost.*

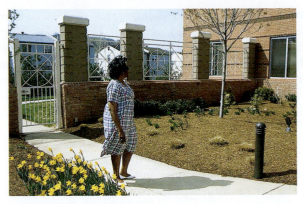

FIGURE 35-4 An enclosed garden allows persons with AD to wander in a safe setting.

> ### PROMOTING SAFETY AND COMFORT
> #### *Wandering and Getting Lost*
>
> **Safety**
> Patients and residents may try to wander to another nursing unit or out of the agency. *Leaving the agency without staff knowledge is called elopement.* Serious injury and death have resulted. State and federal guidelines to prevent elopement are followed.
>
> All staff must be alert to persons who wander. Wandering is allowed in safe areas (Fig. 35-4). Unsafe areas include kitchens, shower rooms, and utility rooms.
>
> Tell other staff that a person wanders. You cannot be with the person all the time. All staff can help monitor the person. Help other staff in the same way. If you see a person wandering into an unsafe area, gently guide the person to a safe place (Fig. 35-5). Tell the nurse.

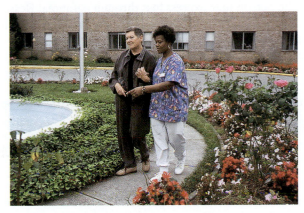

FIGURE 35-5 Guide the person who wanders to a safe area.

MedicAlert® + Alzheimer's Association Safe Return®. *MedicAlert® + Alzheimer's Association Safe Return®* is a nationwide 24-hour emergency service for persons who wander or have a medical emergency. The purpose is to find and safely return persons who wander and become lost. A small fee is charged.

A family member provides required information and a photo. The person receives an ID (wallet card and bracelet or necklace). If reported missing, the person's information is sent to the police. When the person is found, someone calls the toll-free number on the ID. *MedicAlert® + Alzheimer's Association Safe Return®* then calls the family member or caregiver. The person is returned home.

Agitation and Aggression. When agitated, the person is restless or worried and cannot settle down. The person may pace, move about, or not sleep. Agitation may lead to aggression. The person may yell, scream, swear, hit, pinch, grab, or try to hurt someone. Common causes are:
- Pain or discomfort.
- Anxiety, depression, or stress.
- Drug interactions.
- Fatigue.
- Too many or too few stimuli.
- Hunger or thirst.
- Elimination needs, constipation, and incontinence.
- Feeling lost or abandoned.
- Care measures (bathing, dressing) that upset or frighten the person.
- Change in routine, caregiver, or setting.
- Caregivers. A caregiver may rush the person or be impatient. Or mixed verbal and nonverbal messages are sent. For example, a caregiver talks too fast or too loud. Consider how your behaviors affect the person.

Paranoia. *Paranoia is a disorder (para) of the mind (noia). The person has false beliefs (delusions) and suspicion about a person or situation.* Paranoia is a type of delusion. The person believes others are mean, lying, not fair, or "out to get" him or her. The person may be suspicious, fearful, or jealous.

Paranoia may worsen as memory loss gets worse. The National Institute on Aging (NIA) uses these examples.

- The person forgets where he or she put something. The person thinks the item was stolen.
- The person forgets you are a caregiver. The person thinks you are a stranger and does not trust you.
- The person forgets people whom he or she has met. The person believes strangers are harmful.
- The person forgets the directions you give. The person thinks you are trying to trick him or her.

The person may express loss through paranoia. Reasons for the loss do not make sense. Therefore the person blames or accuses others.

See *Promoting Safety and Comfort: Paranoia.*

PROMOTING SAFETY AND COMFORT
Paranoia

Safety

Behaviors may not mean paranoia. Fears of harm, strangers, stealing, mistreatment, and so on may be real. Some people abuse vulnerable adults (Chapter 4). This includes sexual and financial abuse.

Abuse may be by phone, mail, e-mail, or in person. The abuser may be a friend or family member. Financial abuse occurs when money or belongings are stolen. Financial abuse can include:

- Forging checks or cashing checks without permission
- Taking retirement and Social Security benefits
- Using the person's credit cards or bank accounts
- Changing names on wills, bank accounts, insurance policies, or titles to homes or cars
- "Scams" such as identity theft, phone prizes, and threats
- Borrowing money and not paying it back
- Giving away or selling the person's property without permission
- Forcing the person to sign over property
Protect the person from harm, abuse, and mistreatment. Report the following at once.
- What the person is saying
- The person seems afraid or worried about money
- Some of the person's items are missing
- The person's behaviors
- Signs and symptoms of problems
- Visitors or family members acting strangely

Repetitive Behaviors. *Repetitive* means *to do over and over.* The person repeats the same motions, words, or questions over and over. For example, the same napkin is folded over and over. Or the person says the same words or asks the same question over and over. Such behaviors are not harmful. However, they can annoy caregivers and the family.

Rummaging and Hiding Things. To *rummage* means *to search for things by moving things around, turning things over, or looking through something such as a drawer or closet.* The behavior may have no meaning. Or the person is looking for a certain item but cannot tell you what or why.

The person may hide things, throw things away, or lose things. Eyeglasses, hearing aids, and dentures must stay with the person. Always make sure these items are safe. Money, jewelry, and other important items usually are sent home with the family.

Changes in Intimacy and Sexuality. *Intimacy* is a special bond between people who love and respect each other. It includes the way people talk and act toward each other. *Sexuality* involves the way partners physically express their feelings for each other. The person with AD may:

- Depend on and cling to a partner.
- Not remember life with a partner.
- Not remember feelings for a partner.
- Fall in love with another person.
- Have side effects from drugs that affect sexual interest.
- Have memory loss, brain changes, or depression that affects sexual interest.
- Have abnormal sexual behaviors.

Sexual behaviors are labeled abnormal because of how and when they occur. Sexual behaviors may involve the wrong person, the wrong place, or the wrong time. Persons with AD cannot control behavior.

Healthy persons do not undress or expose themselves in front of others. They do not masturbate or engage in sexual acts in public. They know their sexual partners. Persons with AD often mistake someone else for a sexual partner. The person kisses and hugs the other person.

Being overly *(hyper)* interested in sex is called *hypersexuality.* The person may try to seduce others. Or the person may masturbate often. These behaviors are symptoms of AD. They may not mean that the person wants to have sex. If masturbating in public, lead the person to his or her room. Provide for privacy and safety.

The nurse encourages the partner to show affection. Their normal practices are encouraged. Examples include hand holding, hugging, kissing, touching, and dancing.

Some behaviors are not sexual. Touching, scratching, and rubbing the genitals can signal infection, pain, or discomfort in the urinary or reproductive systems. Poor hygiene and incontinence are other causes. Good hygiene prevents itching. Clean the person promptly and thoroughly after elimination. Do not let the person stay wet or soiled. The nurse assesses the person for urinary or reproductive system problems.

Communication Changes. Communication skills gradually decline. The person has trouble expressing thoughts and emotions. Communication changes include:

- Struggling to find the right word
- Forgetting what he or she wants to say
- Repeating familiar words
- Relying on gestures more than words
- Problems understanding the meaning of words
- Attention problems during conversations
- Losing one's train of thought when talking
- Problems blocking background noises—radio, TV, music, phones, and so on
- Frustration with communication problems
- Being sensitive to touch, tone, and voice volume

In time, the person cannot understand others and communicate verbally.

See *Caring About Culture: Communication Changes.*
See *Focus on Communication: Communication Changes.*

CARING ABOUT CULTURE

Communication Changes

For some, English is a second language. For example, the first language learned is Spanish, Italian, French, Russian, Chinese, or Japanese. With AD, the person may forget or no longer understand English. He or she uses and understands only the first language learned.

Screaming. At first, persons with AD have problems finding the right words. As AD progresses, they speak in short sentences or just words. Often speech is not understandable.

Screaming to communicate is common in persons who are very confused and have poor communication skills. They may scream a word or a name. Or they just make screaming sounds.

Possible causes include hearing and vision problems, pain or discomfort, fear, and fatigue. Too much or not enough stimulation is another cause. A person may react to a caregiver or family member by screaming. See Box 35-8.

FOCUS ON COMMUNICATION

Communication Changes

To promote communication with the person with AD, see Box 35-8. Avoid:

- *Giving orders.* For example: "Sit down and eat" is bossy. It does not show respect. Instead say: "Let me help you sit down."
- *Wanting the truth.* For example, do not say: "Don't you remember?" or "What day is it?" Instead say: "Today is Friday."
- *Correcting errors.* For example, do not say: "I just told you it's time to get dressed. You already had breakfast." Instead say: "Let me help you get dressed."
- *Pointing out errors.* Instead of saying: "You missed a button," say: "Let's try it this way."
- *Giving many choices.* For example: "What would you like for dinner?" involves many choices. Instead, limit choices. Say: "Do you want potatoes or rice?"
- *Asking open-ended questions.* For example, do not say: "How did you sleep last night?" Instead, ask "yes" or "no" questions. Say: "Did you sleep okay last night?"

BOX 35-8	**Communication—Persons With AD or Other Dementias**

- Treat the person with dignity and respect.
- Approach the person in a calm, quiet manner.
- Approach the person from the front—not from the side or the back. This avoids startling the person.
- Make eye contact to get the person's attention. Maintain eye contact.
- Have the person's attention before you start speaking.
- Identify yourself and other people by name.
- Call the person by name.
- Avoid pronouns (he, she, them, it, and so on). For example, instead of saying: "She is here," say: "Mary is here."
- Follow the rules and measures to promote communication (Chapter 7).
- Control distractions and noise. TV, radio, and music are examples.
- Speak in a calm, gentle voice.
- Be aware of your body language. Smile and avoid frowning, grimacing, or other negative actions.
- Use gestures or cues. Point to objects.
- Comfort the person with touch. Hold the person's hand while you talk.
- Speak slowly. Use simple words and short sentences.
- Ask or say 1 thing at a time. Present 1 idea, statement, or question at a time.
- Give simple, step-by-step instructions.

- Explain all procedures and activities.
- Repeat instructions as needed. Allow time to respond or react.
- Ask simple questions with simple answers. Do not ask complex questions.
- Do not "baby talk" or use a "baby voice."
- Let the person speak. Do not interrupt or rush the person.
- Give the person time to respond.
- Try other words if the person does not seem to understand.
- Provide the word the person is looking for if he or she is struggling to communicate a thought.
- Do not criticize, correct, interrupt, argue, or try to reason with the person.
- Give consistent responses.
- Practice the measures in Chapter 32.
  - To promote hearing
  - To communicate with speech-impaired persons
  - For blind and visually impaired persons
- Try these measures for the screaming person.
  - Provide a calm, quiet setting.
  - Play soft music.
  - Have the person wear hearing aids and eyeglasses.
  - Have a family member or favorite caregiver comfort and calm the person.
  - Use touch to calm the person.

CARE OF PERSONS WITH AD AND OTHER DEMENTIAS

The person may be cared for at home until symptoms become severe. Adult day care may help. Often assisted living or nursing center care is required. Other illnesses may require hospital care. You may care for persons with AD or other dementias in such settings. The person and family need your support and understanding.

People with AD do not choose the behaviors, signs, and symptoms of the disease. They cannot control what is happening to them. *The disease is responsible, not the person.*

Currently AD has no cure. Symptoms worsen over many years. Over time, the person depends on others for care. Safety, hygiene, food and fluids, elimination, and activity needs must be met. So must comfort and sleep needs. Good skin care and alignment prevent skin breakdown and contractures. The person's care plan and the agency's safety plan will include many of the measures listed in Box 35-9.

The person can have other health problems and injuries. However, the person may not be aware of pain, fever, constipation, incontinence, or other signs and symptoms. Carefully observe the person. Report any change in usual behavior.

Infection is a risk. The person cannot fully tend to self-care. Infection can occur from poor hygiene. This includes poor skin care, oral hygiene, and perineal care after elimination. Inactivity and immobility can cause pneumonia and pressure injuries.

The person needs to feel useful, worthwhile, and active. This promotes self-esteem. Therapies and activities focus on strengths and past successes. For example:

- A person who used to cook helps clean fruit.
- Once a good dancer, activities are planned so the person can dance.
- A person likes to clean. The person helps with dusting.

Supervised activities meet the person's needs and cognitive abilities. Activities are based on what the person enjoys and can do. Some people like crafts, exercise, gardening, and listening and moving to music. Others like sing-alongs, board games, and reminiscing. (*Reminiscence* or *to reminisce* is *to talk about or recall past events.*) Some like to string beads, fold towels, or roll dough.

Massage, soothing touch, music, and aromatherapy are comforting and relaxing. The person may need hospice care as death nears (Chapter 37).

You must treat these persons with dignity and respect. They have the same rights as everyone else. Speak in a calm voice. Always explain what you are going to do.

See *Focus on Older Persons: Care of Persons With AD and Other Dementias.*

See *Focus on Surveys: Care of Persons With AD and Other Dementias.*

Text continued on p. 516.

FOCUS ON OLDER PERSONS

Care of Persons With AD and Other Dementias

Many nursing centers have secure Alzheimer's units. Entrances and exits are locked. Residents cannot wander away. They have a safe setting to move about. Some persons have aggressive behaviors that disrupt or threaten others. They need a secured unit.

According to the *Omnibus Budget Reconciliation Act of 1987 (OBRA)*, secured units are physical restraints. The center must follow OBRA rules and use the least restrictive approach. A dementia diagnosis and a doctor's order are needed to be on a secured unit. At least every 90 days, the health team reviews the person's need for a secured unit. The person's rights are always protected.

At some point, the secured unit is no longer needed. For example, a person's condition progresses to severe AD (see Box 35-7). The person cannot sit or walk. Wandering is not a concern. The person is transferred to another unit.

FOCUS ON SURVEYS

Care of Persons With AD and Other Dementias

To ensure quality of life, surveyors look at all aspects of dementia care. For example:

- Are bathing, dressing, and grooming needs met?
- Is independence promoted? For example, does the staff give cues so the person can dress himself or herself?
- Is the person reminded to use the toilet at regular times?
- Is the person in a calm, quiet setting for meals?
- Are enough fluids offered to prevent dehydration?
- Does the staff respond to the person in a dignified manner?
- Is a safe setting provided?
- Does the staff provide supervision for safe behaviors?

Federal laws require that nursing assistant education and training include dementia management and preventing abuse. Annual in-service training also is required. Surveyors will review employee records to make sure requirements are met.

| BOX 35-9 | Care of Persons With AD and Other Dementias |

Environment
- Follow set routines.
- Avoid changing rooms or roommates.
- Place picture signs by room doors, bathrooms, dining rooms, and other areas (Fig. 35-6).
- Keep personal items where the person can see and reach them.
- Stay within the person's sight to the extent possible.
- Place memory aids (large clocks and calendars) where the person can see them.
- Keep noise levels low.
- Play music and show movies from the person's past.
- Select tasks and activities that fit the person's abilities and interests.

Safety
- Reassure the person that you are there to help.
- Remove harmful, sharp, and breakable items from the area. This includes knives, scissors, glasses, dishes, razors, and tools.
- Provide plastic eating and drinking utensils. They help prevent breakage and cuts.
- Place safety plugs in electrical outlets. Or cover outlets with safety plates.
- Keep cords and electrical items out of reach.
- Remove electric appliances from the bathroom. Hair dryers, curling irons, make-up mirrors, and electric shavers are examples.
- Provide safe storage for:
  - Personal care items (Chapter 18)
  - Cleaners and drugs
  - Dangerous equipment and tools
  - Cigarettes, cigars, pipes, matches, and other smoking materials
  - Car keys

Safety—cont'd
- Keep childproof caps on drug containers and cleaners.
- Remove knobs from stoves or place safety covers on the knobs (Fig. 35-7).
- Remove dangerous appliances, power tools, and firearms and weapons from the home.
- Supervise the person who smokes.
- Practice safety measures to prevent:
  - Falls (Chapter 11)
  - Fires (Chapter 10)
  - Burns (Chapter 10)
  - Poisoning (Chapter 10)
- Lock doors to kitchens, utility rooms, and housekeeping closets. Keep them locked.

Wandering
- Follow agency policy for locking doors and windows. Locks are often at the top and bottom of doors (Fig. 35-8). The person is not likely to look for a lock in such places.
- Keep door alarms and electronic doors turned on. Respond to alarms at once.
- Follow agency policy for fire exits. Everyone must be able to leave the building for a fire.
- Have the person wear an ID bracelet or *MedicAlert*® + *Alzheimer's Association Safe Return*® ID at all times.
- Know when the person is more likely to wander.
- Follow the care plan for daily routine, activities, and exercise. Meet food, fluid, and elimination needs.
- Involve the person in activities—folding napkins, dusting a table, sorting socks, rolling yarn, sweeping, sanding blocks of wood, or watering plants.
- Do not use restraints. Restraints require a doctor's order. They also tend to increase confusion and disorientation.

Continued

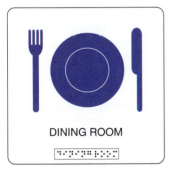
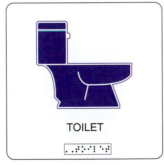

FIGURE 35-6 Signs give cues to persons with dementia.

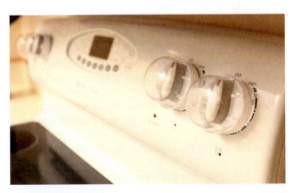

FIGURE 35-7 Safety covers are on stove knobs.

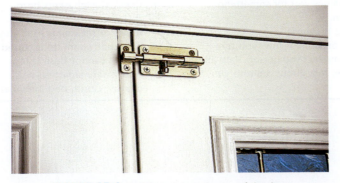

FIGURE 35-8 A slide lock is at the top of the door.

BOX 35-9　Care of Persons With AD and Other Dementias—cont'd

Wandering—cont'd

- Do not argue with the person who wants to leave. The person will not understand.
- Go with the person who insists on going outside. Provide proper clothing. Guide the person inside after a few minutes.
- Allow wandering in enclosed areas. The agency may have enclosed and safe areas for wandering.

Sundowning

- Complete treatments and activities early in the day.
- Encourage exercise and activity early in the day.
- Keep the person on a schedule. Waking up, meal times, and bedtime should involve a set routine.
- Avoid caffeine (coffee, tea, colas, chocolate), sweets, and alcohol late in the day. Provide a calm, quiet setting late in the day.
- Do not restrain the person.
- Meet nutrition and elimination needs. Unmet needs can increase restlessness.
- Use night-lights at night.
- Do not try to reason with the person. He or she will not understand.
- Do not ask the person to explain the problem. Communication changes impair understanding and speech.

Hallucinations and Delusions

- Have the person wear eyeglasses and hearing aids as needed.
- Do not argue with the person. He or she will not understand.
- Reassure the person. Say that you will keep the person safe.
- Distract the person with an item or activity. Or take the person to another room. Taking the person for a walk may be helpful.
- Turn off TV or movies when violent and disturbing programs are on. The person may believe the story is real.
- Comfort the person if he or she seems afraid. Use touch to calm and reassure the person (Fig. 35-9).
- Eliminate noises that can be misinterpreted. TV, radio, music, furnaces, air conditioners, and other things could affect the person.
- Check lighting. Eliminate glares, shadows, or reflections.
- Cover or remove mirrors. The person could misinterpret his or her reflection.
- Remove anything that could be used to hurt the self or others.
- Report behavior changes. They may signal a physical illness.

Paranoia

- Do not react if the person blames you for something.
- Do not argue with the person.
- Tell the person that he or she is safe.
- Use touch or gently hug the person to show you care.
- Search for missing things to distract the person. Talk about what you found. For example, talk about a photo you found.

Catastrophic Reactions

- Approach the person from the front. Do not startle from behind or the side.
- Be calm. Do not appear rushed. Give the person time to calm down.
- Use touch correctly. Know how the person responds to touch. Touch can comfort some people. Others do not like being touched.
- Explain in simple terms what you want the person to do. For example: "It's time for bed. I'll help you into bed."
- Do not argue with the person.
- Follow the person's daily routine, including naps and bedtime.
- Distract the person with an item or activity.

Agitation and Aggression

- Look at how your behaviors affect the person.
- Provide a calm, quiet setting.
- Follow the care plan and a set routine for ADL (activities of daily living). Meet basic needs.
- Observe for early signs of agitation and aggression. Try to remove the cause before behaviors worsen.
- Do not ignore the problem. Try to find the cause.
- Allow personal choice. Let the person decide things to the extent possible.
- Try to distract the person. A snack, safe object, or activity may help.
- Reassure the person.
  - Speak calmly.
  - Listen to concerns.
  - Try to show that you understand the person's anger or fears.
- Keep personal items within the person's sight. Photos and treasures are examples.
- Reduce glares, noise, and clutter.
- Limit the number of people in the room.
- Use gentle touch.
- Provide soothing music.
- Read to the person with a gentle voice.
- Provide quiet times.
- Limit the amount of caffeine (coffee, tea, colas, chocolate) and sweets.
- See Chapter 7 for dealing with the angry person.
- See Chapter 10 for workplace violence.

Rummaging and Hiding Things

- Keep harmful items and products out of sight and reach.
- Remove spoiled items from refrigerators and cabinets. The person may look for food and snacks. He or she may not know or be able to taste spoiled food.
- Guide the person away from other patient or resident rooms.
- Keep wastebaskets covered or out of sight. The person may rummage through a wastebasket or throw things away.
- Check wastebaskets before you empty them. Look for items thrown away or hidden. Do the same before discarding linens or returning food trays.
- Keep bathroom doors closed and toilet seats down. The person cannot flush things down the toilet.
- Allow rummaging in a safe place. The agency may have a drawer, closet, bag, box, basket, or chest with safe items.

BOX 35-9   Care of Persons With AD and Other Dementias—cont'd

Repetitive Behaviors

- Allow harmless acts. Holding a purse, folding napkins, and petting a stuffed animal are examples.
- Distract the person. Music, picture books, exercise, and movies may provide distraction.
- Take the person for a walk.
- Know when repetitive behaviors are likely. For example, a person constantly calls for a nurse at bedtime.
- Use a calm voice and gentle touch.
- Do not argue with the person.
- Answer questions. You may have to answer the same question many times.
- Follow the care plan for memory aids. Clocks, calendars, and photos are examples.

Sleep

- Develop a regular bedtime. Bedtime should be the same each evening.
- Provide a quiet, peaceful mood in the evening—dim lights, low noise level, and soft music.
- Follow bedtime rituals.
- Use night-lights in rooms, hallways, bathrooms, and other areas. They help the person see and prevent accidents and disorientation.
- Limit caffeine.
- Limit naps during the day.
- Follow the person's exercise plan. Play music to the exercise.
- Reduce noises.

Personal Hygiene and Grooming

- Allow the person to do as much as possible.
- Provide good skin care. Keep the skin free of urine and feces.
- Promote personal hygiene.
  - Use the person's preferred bathing method (tub bath, shower).
  - Make sure the bathroom is warm and well-lit.
  - Do not force the person into a shower or tub. Do not argue with the person. People with AD are often afraid of bathing. Try bathing when the person is calm.
  - Provide privacy and keep the person warm.
  - Check for a comfortable water temperature.
  - Place a towel over the shoulders or lap. The person feels less exposed.
  - Do not rush the person.
  - Tell the person what you will do step-by-step.
  - Give the person a washcloth to hold.

Personal Hygiene and Grooming—cont'd

- Provide oral hygiene.
  - Explain what to do 1 step at a time. For example: "Pick up the toothpaste. Take off the cap. Squeeze the toothpaste on the toothbrush. Put the toothbrush in your mouth. Brush."
- Assist with dressing and undressing.
  - Choose clothing that is comfortable and simple to put on. Front-opening garments are easy to put on. Pullover tops are harder. And the person may become frightened when the head is inside a garment.
  - Select clothing that closes with Velcro. Such items are easy to put on and take off. Buttons, zippers, snaps, and other closures can frustrate the person.
  - Offer simple clothing choices (Fig. 35-10). Let the person choose between 2 shirts or 2 blouses, 2 pants or 2 slacks, and so on.
  - Lay clothing out in the order it will be put on. Hand the person 1 item at a time. Tell or show the person what to do. Do not rush.

Other Basic Needs

- Follow a daily routine. This helps the person know when certain things will happen.
- Meet food and fluid needs. Provide finger foods. Cut food and pour liquids as needed. Watch for signs of dysphagia. See Chapter 23.
- Promote urinary and bowel elimination and prevent incontinence.
- Provide incontinence care as needed.
- Promote exercise and activity during the day. This helps reduce wandering and sundowning behaviors. The person may also sleep better.
- Reduce coffee, tea, and cola intake. These contain caffeine—a stimulant. It can increase restlessness, confusion, and agitation.
- Provide a quiet, restful setting. Soft music is better than loud TV programs.
- Play music during care activities such as bathing and during meals.
- Have equipment ready for any procedure. This lessens the time for care measures.
- Observe for signs and symptoms of health problems (Chapters 6 and 33).
- Prevent infection.

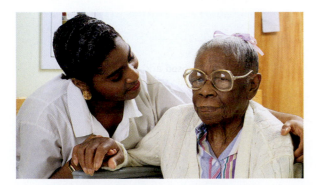

FIGURE 35-9 Use touch to calm the person.

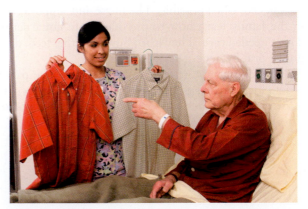

FIGURE 35-10 The person is offered simple clothing choices.

The Family

The person may live at home or with a partner, children, or other family members. Or someone stays with the person. Home care may help for a while. Adult day care and assisted living are options (Chapter 1). Nursing center care is needed when:

- The family cannot meet the person's needs.
- The person no longer knows the caregiver.
- Family members have health problems.
- Money problems occur.
- The person's behavior presents dangers to self and others.

Doctor's visits, drugs, home care, and assisted living are costly. So is nursing center care. The person's medical care can drain finances.

Home care and nursing center care are stressful. The family has physical, emotional, social, and financial stresses. Adult children are in the *sandwich generation*. Their own children need attention while an ill parent needs care. Caring for 2 families is stressful. Often adult children have jobs too.

Caregivers can suffer from anger, anxiety, guilt, depression, and sleep problems. Some cannot concentrate or are irritable. Health problems can develop. They need to focus on their own health. They need a healthy diet, exercise, and plenty of rest. Asking family and friends for help is hard for some people.

Caregivers need support and encouragement. The NIA suggests how family members can take care of themselves. See Box 35-10. AD support groups are sponsored by hospitals, nursing centers, and the Alzheimer's Association. The Alzheimer's Association has chapters across the country. Support groups offer encouragement and advice. Members share feelings, anger, frustration, guilt, and other emotions. They also share coping and caregiving ideas.

The family often feels hopeless. No matter what is done, the person gets worse. Much time, money, energy, and emotion are needed to care for the person. Anger and resentment may result. Guilt feelings are common. The family knows that the person did not choose the disease and its signs, symptoms, and behaviors. Sometimes behaviors are embarrassing. The family may be upset and angry that the loved one cannot show love or affection.

The family is an important part of the health team. They help plan care when possible. The nurse and support group help the family learn how to provide a safe home setting and give needed care. They learn how to bathe, feed, dress, and give oral hygiene.

In nursing centers, some family members take part in unit activities. For many persons, family members provide comfort. They also need support and understanding from the health team.

BOX 35-10   Family Caregivers—Taking Care of Yourself

- Ask for help when you need it. Asking for something specific may be useful. For example:
  - "Can you make Mom's dinner Sunday night?"
  - "Can you stay with Dad from 2 to 4 Monday afternoon?"
  - "Can Mom stay at your house Saturday afternoon?"
- Join a support group.
- Take breaks every day.
- Spend time with friends.
- Maintain hobbies and interests.
- Eat healthy foods and exercise often.
- See a doctor regularly.
- Keep health, legal, and financial information current.
- Remember that these feelings are normal—being sad, lonely, frustrated, confused, angry. Say to yourself:
  - "I'm doing the best I can."
  - "What I'm doing would be hard for anyone."
  - "I'm not perfect and that's okay."
  - "I can't control some things."
  - "I need to do what works for right now."
  - "Even when I do everything I can, there will still be problem behaviors. They are caused by the illness, not what I do."
  - "I will enjoy our peaceful times together."
  - "I will get counseling if caregiving becomes too much."
- Meet spiritual needs—attending religious services, believing that larger forces or a higher power is at work.
- Understand that you may feel powerless and hopeless about what is happening.
- Understand that you may feel a sense of loss and sadness.
- Understand why you are caring for a person with AD. Was the choice made out of love, loyalty, duty, religious obligation, money concerns, fear, habit, or self-punishment?
- Let yourself feel "uplifts." Examples include good feelings about the person, support from caring people, and time for your interests.

Modified from National Institute on Aging: *Alzheimer's caregiving: caring for yourself*, Bethesda, Md, content reviewed May 17, 2017, National Institutes of Health.

Validation Therapy

Validation therapy is a way to communicate with persons with dementia. *Validate* means *to show that a person's feelings and needs are fair and have meaning.* Behaviors signal the need to express feelings and needs—safety, security, comfort, love and belonging, feeling useful, and so on. Caregivers help the person express feelings and needs verbally or nonverbally. With validation, the person's reality (what the person thinks is real and true) is accepted. The person is treated with dignity and self-worth.

Validation therapy is based on these principles.

* All behavior has meaning.
* A person may have unresolved issues and emotions from the past.
* A person's mind may return to the past to resolve issues and emotions.
* Caregivers need to listen and provide empathy.

* Attempts are not made to correct thoughts or bring the person back to reality (reality orientation). For example:
  * A person talks about waiting for the bus to go to work. The caregiver does not say: "You don't work anymore." Instead, the caregiver says: "Tell me about your work."
  * A resident says she is at the train station waiting for her husband. Killed in a war, her husband never came home. The caregiver does not remind the resident of what happened. Instead, the caregiver asks the resident about her husband.
  * A patient was 3 years old when his father died. He holds a ball constantly. He calls for his father and repeats "play ball, play ball." The caregiver does not remind the patient that his father is not alive. Instead, the caregiver says: "Tell me about playing ball."

Validation therapy is useful for some persons. If used in your agency, you will be trained to use validation therapy correctly.

FOCUS ON PRIDE

The Person, Family, and Yourself

Personal and Professional Responsibility

Everyone has different talents, abilities, and interests. Persons with dementia are no different. Understanding the person's past and his or her hobbies, talents, family, and work helps you give better care.

Learn about the person. Engage the person in activities once enjoyed. Treat each person as unique with a history, interests, strengths, and needs.

Rights and Respect

The person has the right to privacy and confidentiality. Protect the person from exposure. Only those involved in the person's care are present during care. The person is allowed to visit in private. Do not share information about the person with others.

The person has the right to keep and use personal items. A pillow, blanket, afghan, or sweater may have meaning. The person may not know why or recognize the item. Still, it is important and provides comfort. Keep personal items safe. Protect property from loss or damage.

Independence and Social Interaction

Persons with dementia have problems with ADL. Eating, bathing, dressing, and elimination are examples. Maintaining routines can help the person remain independent longer. For example, a person uses the bathroom, washes hands, brushes teeth, brushes hair, and dresses in the morning. The person is more independent when ADL are done in this order. Changing the order causes confusion.

Break down tasks into simple steps. Kindly tell the person each step. Repeat directions as needed. Allow extra time for each task. Resist the urge to take over. Let the person do what is safely possible.

Delegation and Teamwork

Persons with dementia may respond better to certain staff or caregivers. This can vary by day or time of day. Do not be offended if someone else provides care. The team works together to meet the person's needs.

Sometimes the person resists care from everyone. Convincing the person to allow care is often useless. Use a calm and caring approach. Try giving care at a different time. Never use force.

Ethics and Laws

Persons with AD often have changes in mood, behavior, and personality. The person may become easily agitated or angry. The person cannot control words and actions. Some behaviors are hard to deal with.

You must control your reactions to stress. Be professional. Tell the nurse if you feel frustrated, angry, or impatient. You may need an assignment change. Never take out your anger on the person. The person must be protected from physical and verbal abuse and mistreatment.

FOCUS ON PRIDE: Application

Caregivers affect the person's quality of life. Describe care that values the person. What qualities must the caregiver have? How must the caregiver treat the person?

REVIEW QUESTIONS

Circle the BEST answer.

1 A person is confused. Which should you question?
   a Restrain in bed at night.
   b Give clear, simple directions.
   c Use touch to communicate.
   d Open drapes during the day.

2 A person has AD. Which is *true*?
   a AD is a normal part of aging.
   b Diet and drugs can cure the disease.
   c AD and delirium are the same.
   d AD ends in death.

3 During the final stage of AD, the person is likely to
   a Wander and become lost
   b Follow simple commands
   c Need total assistance with ADL
   d Repeat questions over and over

4 A person has AD. To communicate, you should
   a Give orders
   b Limit choices
   c Correct mistakes
   d Ask open-ended questions

5 A person with AD is screaming. You know that this is
   a A way to communicate
   b An agitated reaction
   c Caused by a delusion
   d A repetitive behavior

6 Which statement about sundowning is *true*?
   a AD behaviors improve at night.
   b Encouraging activity late in the day can help.
   c Being tired or hungry can increase restlessness.
   d Dim lighting or darkness is calming.

7 A person with AD has delusions. Which should you question?
   a Distract the person with an activity.
   b Tell the person you will provide protection.
   c Tell the person the beliefs are not real.
   d Use touch to calm the person.

8 Which can cause delusions in persons with AD?
   a Mirrors
   b Eyeglasses
   c Hearing aids
   d Night-lights

9 A person with AD keeps telling you that someone is stealing things. What should you do?
   a Nothing. The person has paranoia.
   b Tell the nurse. Someone could be abusing the person.
   c Replace missing items.
   d Send other items home with the family.

10 A person with AD is at risk for elopement. Which should you question?
   a Make sure door alarms are turned on.
   b Make sure an ID bracelet is worn.
   c Assist with exercise as ordered.
   d Remind the person not to wander.

11 Which can help with rummaging?
   a Keep the person's room locked.
   b Provide safe places to rummage.
   c Ask the person to explain the behavior.
   d Hide items the person looks for.

12 Which is *unsafe* for persons with AD?
   a Safety plugs are placed in electrical outlets.
   b Cleaners and drugs are locked up.
   c The person keeps smoking materials.
   d Sharp objects are removed from the setting.

13 A person with AD is upset. Which is a *correct* response?
   a Try to reason with the person.
   b Ask what is bothering the person.
   c Ignore the problem.
   d Provide reassurance and try to find the cause.

14 You are caring for a person with AD. You should avoid
   a Trying to bring the person back to reality
   b Offering support to the family
   c Following a set routine
   d Providing a quiet setting

15 Validation therapy involves
   a Support groups and counseling for persons with severe AD
   b Drugs to treat AD
   c Helping the person with AD express needs and feelings
   d Orienting the person with AD to reality

Answers to Chapter 35 questions are on p. 552.

Answers to Chapter 35 questions are on p. 552.

FOCUS ON PRACTICE

Problem Solving

A person has moderate AD. While preparing for a bath, the person becomes upset and repeats: "Go away" over and over. How will you respond? How might you meet hygiene needs?

Emergency Care

OBJECTIVES

- Define the key terms and key abbreviations in this chapter.
- Describe the rules of emergency care.
- Identify the signs of cardiac arrest and the emergency care required.
- Describe the emergency care for heart attack.
- Describe the emergency care for poisoning.
- Describe the emergency care for hemorrhage, fainting, and shock.

- Describe the emergency care for stroke.
- Explain how to care for a person during a seizure.
- Describe the emergency care for concussions.
- Describe the emergency care for burns.
- Perform the procedures described in this chapter.
- Explain how to promote PRIDE in the person, the family, and yourself.

KEY TERMS

anaphylaxis A life-threatening sensitivity to an antigen
cardiac arrest See "sudden cardiac arrest"
convulsion See "seizure"
fainting The sudden loss of consciousness from an inadequate blood supply to the brain
first aid The emergency care given to an ill or injured person before medical help arrives
hemorrhage The excessive loss of blood in a short time
respiratory arrest Breathing stops but heart action continues for several minutes

resuscitate To revive from apparent death or unconsciousness using emergency measures
seizure Violent and sudden contractions or tremors of muscle groups caused by abnormal electrical activity in the brain; convulsion
shock Results when tissues and organs do not get enough blood
sudden cardiac arrest (SCA) The heart stops suddenly and without warning; cardiac arrest

KEY ABBREVIATIONS

AED	Automated external defibrillator	**EMS**	Emergency Medical Services
AHA	American Heart Association	**RRT**	Rapid Response Team
BLS	Basic Life Support	**SCA**	Sudden cardiac arrest
CPR	Cardiopulmonary resuscitation	**VF; V-fib**	Ventricular fibrillation

Emergencies can occur anywhere. Sometimes you can save a life if you know what to do. First aid and Basic Life Support (BLS) courses prepare you to give emergency care.

The BLS procedures in this chapter are given as basic information. They do not replace certification training. You need a BLS course for health care providers.

BLS guidelines are updated as new information becomes available. You are responsible for following current guidelines. Updates can be found on-line at the American Heart Association's website.

EMERGENCY CARE

First aid is the emergency care given to an ill or injured person before medical help arrives. The goals of first aid are to:

- Prevent death.
- Prevent injuries from becoming worse.

In an emergency, the Emergency Medical Services (EMS) system is activated. Emergency personnel (paramedics, emergency medical technicians) rush to the scene. They treat, stabilize, and transport persons with life-threatening problems. They have guidelines for care and communicate with doctors in hospital emergency rooms. The doctors can direct their care. Their ambulances have emergency drugs, equipment, and supplies. To activate the EMS system, do 1 of the following.

- Dial 911.
- Call the local fire or police department.
- Call the phone operator.

Each emergency is different. The rules in Box 36-1 apply to any emergency. Hospitals and other agencies have procedures for emergencies. In hospitals, Rapid Response Teams (RRTs) are called when a person shows signs of a life-threatening condition. An RRT may include a doctor, a nurse, and a respiratory therapist. The RRT's goal is to prevent death.

See *Focus on Communication: Emergency Care.*
See *Promoting Safety and Comfort: Emergency Care.*

FOCUS ON COMMUNICATION

Emergency Care

Some illnesses and injuries are life-threatening. To find out what happened and the person's condition, you can say:

- "Are you okay?"
- "Tell me what's wrong."
- "Where does it hurt?"
- "If you can, please point to where it hurts."
- "Can you move your arms and legs?"

PROMOTING SAFETY AND COMFORT

Emergency Care

Safety

Contact with blood, body fluids, secretions, and excretions is likely. Follow Standard Precautions and the Bloodborne Pathogen Standard to the extent possible.

For an emergency in an agency, call for the nurse at once. You may need to activate the EMS system or the RRT. Assist as the nurse instructs.

In nursing centers, a nurse decides when to activate the EMS system. The nurse tells you how to help. If a person has stopped breathing or is in sudden cardiac arrest, the nurse may start cardiopulmonary resuscitation (CPR). Some centers allow nursing assistants to start CPR. Others do not. Know your center's policy about CPR.

Comfort

Mental comfort is important. Help the person feel safe and secure. Give reassurance. Explain the care you provide. Use a calm approach.

BOX 36-1	Emergency Care Rules

- Call for help. Or have someone activate the EMS system. *Do not hang up until the operator has hung up.* Give the following information.
  - Your location—street address and city, cross streets or roads, and landmarks
  - Phone number you are calling from
  - What seems to have happened (for example: heart attack, crash, fire)—police, fire equipment, and ambulances may be needed
  - How many people need help
  - Conditions of victims, obvious injuries, and life-threatening situations
  - What aid is being given
- Wait for help if the scene is not safe enough to approach.
- Know your limits. Do not do more than you are able. Do not perform an unfamiliar procedure. Do what you can under the circumstances.
- Stay calm. This helps the person feel more secure.
- Know where to find emergency supplies.
- Follow Standard Precautions and the Bloodborne Pathogen Standard to the extent possible.
- Check for life-threatening problems. Check for breathing, a pulse, and bleeding.
- Keep the person lying down or as you found him or her. Moving the person could make an injury worse.
- Move the person only if the setting is unsafe. Examples include:
  - A burning car or building
  - A building that might collapse
  - Stormy conditions with lightning
  - In water
  - Near electrical wires
- Perform necessary emergency measures.
- Do not remove clothes unless you have to. To remove clothing, tear or cut garments along the seams. (For CPR, remove clothing or move it out of the way.)
- Keep the person warm. Cover the person with a blanket, coats, or sweaters.
- Reassure the person. Explain what is happening and that help was called.
- Do not give the person fluids.
- Keep on-lookers away. They invade privacy and tend to stare, give advice, and comment about the person's condition. The person may think the situation is worse than it is.

BLS FOR ADULTS

When the heart and breathing stop, the person is clinically dead. Blood is not circulated (moved) through the body. Heart, brain, and other organ damage occurs within minutes. The American Heart Association's (AHA's) BLS procedures support circulation and breathing.

Sudden Cardiac Arrest

Sudden cardiac arrest (SCA) or cardiac arrest is when the heart stops suddenly and without warning. Within seconds, breathing stops too. Permanent brain and other organ damage occurs unless circulation and breathing are restored.

There are 3 major signs of SCA.

- *No response.*
- *No breathing or no normal breathing.* The person may have *agonal gasps (agonal respirations)* early during SCA. (*Agonal* means *to struggle.* Agonal is used in relation to death and dying.) Agonal gasps do not bring enough oxygen into the lungs. Agonal gasps are not normal breathing.
- *No pulse.*

The skin is cool, pale, and gray. The person is not coughing or moving.

SCA is a sudden, unexpected, and dramatic event. It can occur anywhere and at any time—while driving, shoveling snow, playing golf or tennis, watching TV, eating, or sleeping. Common causes include cardiovascular disorders (Chapter 33) and dysrhythmias (arrhythmias). Electrical shock, chest trauma, and substance use (Chapter 34) are other causes. The person is at risk for an abnormal heart rhythm called ventricular fibrillation (p. 524). The heart cannot pump blood. A normal rhythm must be restored or the person will die.

Chains of Survival. The AHA's BLS courses teach *Chains of Survival.* The Chains of Survival identify pathways of care for out-of-hospital and in-hospital cardiac arrests (Box 36-2). Care is provided as soon as possible. Any delay reduces the person's chance of survival.

See *Focus on Communication: Chains of Survival.*

BOX 36-2	Chains of Survival

Out-of-Hospital Chain of Survival
1. Recognizing cardiac arrest and activating the EMS system.
2. Immediate high-quality CPR.
3. Rapid defibrillation. See p. 524.
4. Basic and advanced EMS. Care is given by EMS staff, doctors, nurses, and respiratory therapists. They give drugs and perform life-saving measures.
5. Advanced life support and post-arrest care.

In-Hospital Chain of Survival
1. Surveillance and prevention.
2. Recognizing cardiac arrest and activating the RRT.
3. Immediate high-quality CPR.
4. Rapid defibrillation.
5. Advanced life support and post-arrest care.

Modified from American Heart Association: *Highlights of the 2015 American Heart Association guidelines update for CPR and ECC,* copyright 2015.

FOCUS ON COMMUNICATION

Chains of Survival

Getting help is a critical step. If alone, activate the EMS system with your phone while continuing to give care. If alone with no phone, leave the adult to activate the EMS system and get an AED (if available) before giving care. (AED stands for automated external defibrillator. See p. 524.)

If you are not alone, have someone activate the EMS system and have someone get an AED. You may not know names. Point to each person. Make eye contact. Say: "Call 911. Get an AED." Begin care. Follow up soon. Make sure the person called for help and that an AED is on the way.

Respiratory Arrest

Respiratory arrest is when breathing stops but heart action continues for several minutes. If breathing is not restored, cardiac arrest occurs. Respiratory arrest can occur from:

- Problems affecting nerves, muscles, or areas of the brain that control breathing—amyotrophic lateral sclerosis (ALS), spinal cord injuries, stroke (Chapter 33); drug or alcohol over-dose; drug side-effects
- Lung disorders and problems—pneumonia, chronic obstructive pulmonary disease (Chapter 33), pulmonary embolism (Chapter 28), chest injuries
- Blocked airflow—choking (Chapter 10 and p. 527), drowning, suffocation
- Inhaling harmful substances—smoke, chemicals, fumes

Rescue Breathing. Rescue breaths are given when there is a pulse but no breathing or only agonal gasping. To give rescue breaths:

- Open the airway (p. 523).
- Give 1 breath every 5 to 6 seconds for adults.
- Give each breath over 1 second. The chest should rise when breaths are given.
- Check the pulse every 2 minutes. If no pulse, begin CPR.

Adult CPR

Cardiopulmonary resuscitation (CPR) supports circulation and breathing. *To resuscitate means to revive from apparent death or unconsciousness using emergency measures.* CPR provides blood and oxygen to the heart, brain, and other organs until advanced emergency care is given. CPR involves:

- Chest compressions, p. 522
- Airway, p. 523
- Breathing, p. 523
- Defibrillation, p. 524

CPR must be started at once when a person has SCA. CPR procedures require speed, skill, and efficiency.

See *Promoting Safety and Comfort: Adult CPR, p. 522.*

Chest Compressions. In cardiac arrest, the heart has stopped beating. Blood must be pumped through the body another way. Chest compressions force blood through the circulatory system.

Before starting chest compressions, check for a pulse. Use the carotid artery on the side near you. To find the carotid pulse, place 2 or 3 fingertips on the trachea (windpipe). Then slide your fingers down off the trachea to the groove of the neck (Fig. 36-1). Check for a pulse for at least 5 seconds but no more than 10 seconds. While checking for a pulse, look for signs of circulation. See if the person is breathing or is coughing or moving.

The heart lies between the sternum (breastbone) and the spinal column. When pressure is applied to the sternum, the sternum is depressed (moved down). This compresses the heart between the sternum and spinal column (Fig. 36-2). For effective chest compressions, the person must be supine on a hard, flat surface—floor or back-board. You are at the person's side.

Hand position is important (Fig. 36-3). Use the heels of your hands—1 on top of the other. For proper placement:
- Expose the chest. Remove clothing or move it out of the way. You need to see bare skin for proper hand position.
- Place the heel of 1 hand (usually your dominant hand) in the center of the bare chest. The heel of this hand is between the nipples on the lower half of the sternum.
- Place the heel of your other hand on top of the heel of the first hand.

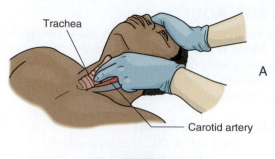

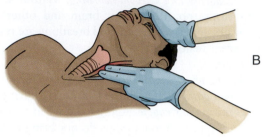

FIGURE 36-1 Locating the carotid pulse. **A,** Two fingers are placed on the trachea. **B,** The fingertips are moved down into the groove of the neck to the carotid artery.

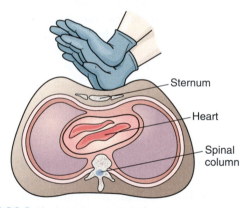

FIGURE 36-2 The heart lies between the sternum and the spinal column. The heart is compressed when pressure is applied to the sternum.

FIGURE 36-3 Hand position for CPR. **A,** The heel of the dominant hand is in the center of the chest. It is between the nipples and on the lower half of the sternum. **B,** The heel of the non-dominant hand is on top of the dominant hand.

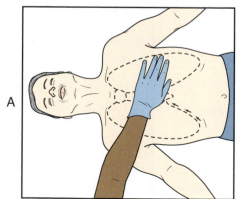

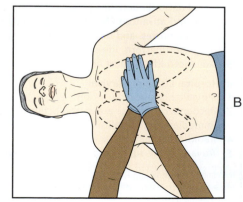

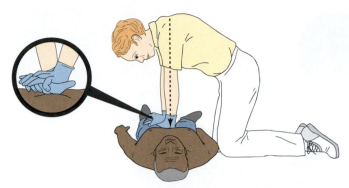

FIGURE 36-4 Giving chest compressions. The arms are straight. The shoulders are over the hands. The fingers are interlocked.

To give chest compressions, your arms are straight. Your shoulders are directly over your hands. And your fingers are interlocked (Fig. 36-4). Press down at least 2 inches. Then release pressure without removing your hands. Releasing pressure allows the chest to recoil—to return to its normal position. Recoil lets the heart fill with blood. Avoid leaning on the chest between compressions.

The AHA recommends that you:

* Give compressions at a rate of 100 to 120 per minute.
* Interrupt chest compressions only when necessary. Interruptions should be less than 10 seconds. Without chest compressions, blood does not flow to the heart, brain, and other organs.

Airway. The respiratory passages (airway) must be open to restore breathing. The airway is often obstructed (blocked) during SCA. The person's tongue falls toward the back of the throat and blocks the airway. The head tilt–chin lift method opens the airway (Fig. 36-5).

* Place the palm of 1 hand on the forehead.
* Tilt the head back by pushing down on the forehead with your palm.
* Place the fingers of your other hand under the lower jaw near the chin. Use your index and middle fingers. Do not use your thumb.
* Lift the jaw. This brings the chin forward.
* Do not close the mouth. The mouth should be slightly open.

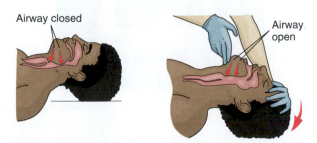

Airway closed   Airway open

FIGURE 36-5 The head tilt–chin lift method opens the airway. One hand is on the forehead. Pressure is applied to tilt the head back. The chin is lifted with the fingers of the other hand.

Breathing. Air is not inhaled when breathing stops. To get oxygen, the person is given *breaths*. That is, a rescuer inflates the person's lungs.

Each breath should take 1 second. *You should see the chest rise with each breath.* Two breaths are given after every 30 chest compressions.

Mouth-to-Mouth Breathing. Mouth-to-mouth breathing (Fig. 36-6) is 1 way to give breaths. You place your mouth over the person's mouth. Contact with the person's blood, body fluids, secretions, or excretions is likely. To give mouth-to-mouth breathing:

1 Keep the airway open with the head tilt–chin lift method.
2 Pinch the nostrils shut. Use your thumb and index finger on the hand on the forehead. Shutting the nostrils keeps air from coming out the nose.
3 Take a breath. A regular breath is needed, not a deep breath.
4 Place your mouth tightly over the person's mouth. Seal the mouth with your lips.
5 Blow air into the person's mouth. You should see the chest rise as the lungs fill with air.
6 Repeat the head tilt–chin lift method if the chest did not rise.
7 Remove your mouth from the person's mouth. Then take in a quick breath.
8 Give another breath. You should see the chest rise.

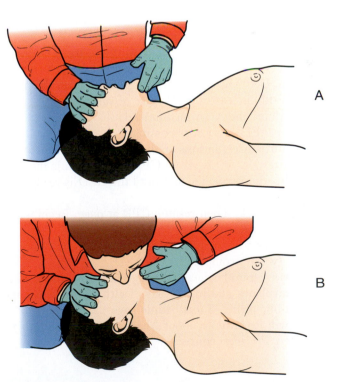

A

B

FIGURE 36-6 Mouth-to-mouth breathing. **A,** The airway is opened. The nostrils are pinched shut. **B,** The person's mouth is sealed by the rescuer's mouth.

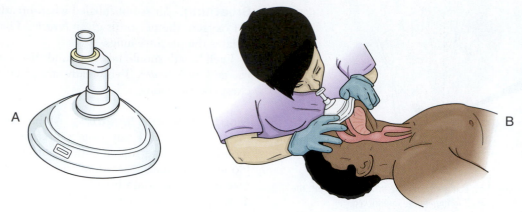

FIGURE 36-7 **A,** Mask for giving breaths. **B,** The mask is in place.

Barrier Device Breathing. A barrier device is used for giving breaths when possible. The device prevents contact with the person's mouth and blood, body fluids, secretions, or excretions. A face mask is an example of a barrier device (Fig. 36-7, *A*). The mask is placed over the person's mouth and nose and sealed against the face (Fig. 36-7, *B*). The seal must be tight. Then open the airway with the head tilt–chin lift method.

Defibrillation. *Ventricular fibrillation (VF, V-fib)* is an abnormal heart rhythm (Fig. 36-8). It causes sudden cardiac arrest. Rather than beating in a regular rhythm, the heart shakes and quivers like a bowl of Jell-O. The heart does not pump blood. The heart, brain, and other organs do not receive blood and oxygen.

A *defibrillator* delivers a shock to the heart. The shock stops the VF (V-fib). This allows a regular heart rhythm to return. Defibrillation as soon as possible after the onset of VF (V-fib) increases the chance of survival.

For adults, the AHA recommends that rescuers:
- Use an AED as soon as possible.
- Minimize interruptions in chest compressions before and after a shock is given. CPR is given while the AED pads are applied and until the AED is ready to check the rhythm.
- Give 1 shock. Then resume CPR at once. Begin with chest compressions.
- Check for a heart rhythm after about 2 minutes of CPR (when prompted by the AED).

AEDs are found in health care agencies (Fig. 36-9). They are on airplanes and in airports, health clubs, malls, and other public places. Some people have them at home.

You will learn more about AEDs in the AHA's *BLS for Healthcare Providers* course.

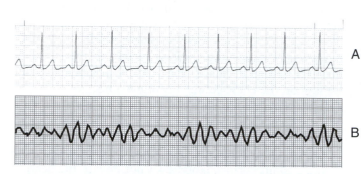

FIGURE 36-8 **A,** Normal rhythm. **B,** Ventricular fibrillation. (From Ignatavicius DD, Workman ML: *Medical-surgical nursing: patient-centered collaborative care,* ed 8, St Louis, 2016, Elsevier.)

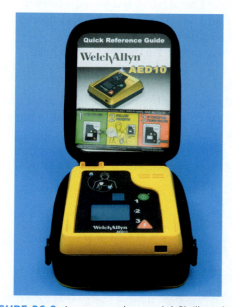

FIGURE 36-9 An automated external defibrillator (AED).

Performing Adult CPR. CPR is done only for cardiac arrest. You must determine if cardiac arrest or fainting (p. 528) has occurred. *CPR is done if the person does not respond, is not breathing or only gasping (has no normal breathing), and has no pulse.*

CPR is done alone or by 2 people. When done alone, 1 rescuer gives chest compressions and breaths. With 2 rescuers, 1 person gives chest compressions and 1 gives breaths (Fig. 36-10). Rescuers switch tasks about every 2 minutes to avoid fatigue and inadequate compressions. The second rescuer uses the AED if available.

See *Focus on Communication: Performing Adult CPR.*
See *Promoting Safety and Comfort: Performing Adult CPR.*
See procedure: *Adult CPR—1 Rescuer.*
See procedure: *Adult CPR With AED—2 Rescuers, p. 526.*

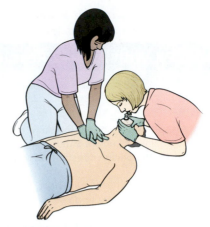

FIGURE 36-10 Two people perform CPR.

FOCUS ON COMMUNICATION
Performing Adult CPR

Good communication is needed for 2-rescuer CPR. The rescuer giving compressions counts out loud so the other rescuer is ready to give breaths. Clear communication prevents delays and lessens interruptions in chest compressions.

PROMOTING SAFETY AND COMFORT
Performing Adult CPR

Safety
Never practice CPR on another person. Serious damage can occur. Mannequins are used to learn and practice CPR.

A safe setting is needed. Move the person only if the scene is unsafe (see Box 36-1). Do not approach the person if it is unsafe for you.

The person must be on a hard, flat surface for CPR. Logroll the person so there is no twisting of the spine. Place the arms alongside the body. For the person in bed, place a board under the person. Or move the person to the floor.

Follow Standard Precautions and the Bloodborne Pathogen Standard to the extent possible. This includes the use of gloves and a barrier device.

Basic Life Support guidelines are updated as new information becomes available. You are responsible for following current guidelines. Updates can be found on-line at the American Heart Association's website.

Adult CPR—1 Rescuer

PROCEDURE

1 Make sure the scene is safe.
2 Check for a response. Tap or gently shake the person. Call the person by name, if known. Shout: "Are you okay?"
3 Shout for help if the person does not respond.
4 Activate the EMS system or the agency's RRT.
　a *If alone with a phone,* use it while continuing to give care.
　b *If alone without a phone,* leave the person to activate the EMS system before starting CPR.
　c *If help arrives,* send him or her to activate the EMS system.
5 Get an AED.
　a *If alone,* get the AED before starting CPR.
　b *If help arrives,* ask him or her to get the AED.
6 Check for breathing and a carotid pulse at the same time. Look for no breathing or only gasping. Start CPR for no breathing (or only gasping) and no definite pulse within 10 seconds.
7 Position the person for CPR if not already done. The person is supine on a hard, flat surface.

8 Expose the chest.
9 Give CPR.
　a Place 2 hands on the lower half of the sternum. Give 30 chest compressions at a rate of 100 to 120 per minute. Establish a regular rhythm. Count out loud. Allow the chest to recoil between compressions.
　b Open the airway. Use the head tilt–chin lift method.
　c Give 2 breaths. Use a barrier device if one is available. Each breath should take only 1 second. The chest should rise. If the first breath does not make the chest rise:
　　1 Open the airway. Use the head tilt–chin lift method.
　　2 Give another breath.
10 Continue CPR with 30 chest compressions followed by 2 breaths. Limit compression interruptions to less than 10 seconds. Use the AED when available. See procedure: *Adult CPR With AED—2 Rescuers, p. 526.*
11 Continue CPR until help takes over or the person begins to move. If movement occurs, place the person in the recovery position (p. 527).

Basic Life Support guidelines are updated as new information becomes available. You are responsible for following current guidelines. Updates can be found on-line at the American Heart Association's website.

Adult CPR With AED—2 Rescuers

PROCEDURE

1 Make sure the scene is safe.
2 *Rescuer 1:*
  a Check for a response. Tap or gently shake the person. Call the person by name, if known. Shout: "Are you okay?"
  b Shout for help if the person does not respond.
3 *Rescuer 2:*
  a Activate the EMS system or the agency's RRT using a phone (if available) or leave to do so.
  b Get an AED.
4 *Rescuer 1:* Follow steps 6 through 10 in procedure: *Adult CPR—1 Rescuer.*
5 *Rescuer 2:*
  a Open the AED case.
  b Turn on the AED (Fig. 36-11, *A*).
  c Apply adult electrode pads to the chest (Fig. 36-11, *B*). Follow the AED's instructions and diagram.
  d Attach the connecting cables to the AED (Fig. 36-11, *C*).
  e Clear away from the person. Make sure no one is touching the person (Fig. 36-11, *D*).
  f Let the AED check the heart rhythm.
  g Make sure everyone is clear of the person if the AED advises a "shock" (see Fig. 36-11, *D*). Loudly tell others not to touch the person. Say: "Everyone, clear!" Look to make sure no one is touching the person.
  h Press the SHOCK button if the AED advises a "shock" (Fig. 36-11, *E*).

6 *Rescuers 1 and 2—perform 2-rescuer CPR.*
  a Begin with compressions. One rescuer gives 30 chest compressions. The rescuer pauses for the other rescuer to give 2 breaths.
  b The other rescuer gives 2 breaths after every 30 chest compressions.
7 Pause for a rhythm check when prompted by the AED (after about 2 minutes of CPR). Repeat steps 5, e–h. Change positions and continue CPR. Begin with compressions.
8 Continue CPR and use of the AED until help takes over or the person begins to move. If movement occurs, place the person in the recovery position.

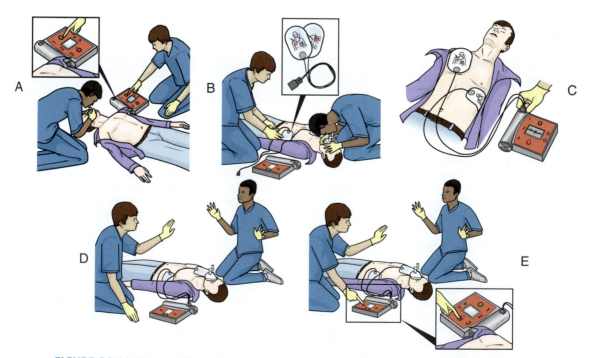

FIGURE 36-11 Using an AED. **A,** The rescuer turns on the AED. **B,** Electrode pads are placed on the chest. **C,** The cables are connected to the AED. **D,** The rescuers "clear" the person. The rescuer makes sure no one is touching the person. **E,** The SHOCK button is pressed to deliver a shock.

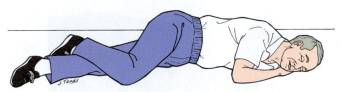

FIGURE 36-12 Recovery position.

Hands-Only CPR. With cardiac arrest, survival depends on others nearby. In public, trained BLS providers are often not available. Bystanders may worry that they will not do CPR correctly or may cause injury.

"Hands-Only CPR" (compression-only CPR) can be done by others in the out-of-hospital setting. In "Hands-Only CPR," CPR for an adult or adolescent involves 2 steps.

1 Call 911.

2 Push hard and fast in the center of the chest.

"Hands-Only CPR" is for persons *not* trained in BLS. As a health care provider, use the CPR method learned in a BLS course.

Recovery Position

The recovery position is used when the person is breathing and has a pulse but is not responding (Fig. 36-12). The position helps keep the airway open and prevents aspiration.

Logroll the person into the recovery position. Keep the head, neck, and spine straight. A hand supports the head. *Do not use this position if the person might have neck injuries or other trauma.*

CHOKING

Foreign bodies can obstruct (block) the airway. This is called *choking* or *foreign-body airway obstruction (FBAO)*. Air cannot pass into the lungs. The body does not get enough oxygen. It can lead to cardiac arrest.

Airway obstruction can be mild or severe. With severe airway obstruction, air does not move in and out of the lungs. If the obstruction is not removed, the person will die. Abdominal thrusts are used to relieve severe airway obstruction. See Chapter 10 for emergency care of the choking person.

HEART ATTACK

Heart attack (myocardial infarction) occurs when part of the heart muscle dies from the sudden blockage of blood flow in a coronary artery (Chapter 33). Signs and symptoms include:

- Chest pain (not relieved by rest)
- Pain or discomfort in 1 or both arms, the back, neck, jaw, or stomach
- Shortness of breath
- Perspiration and cold, clammy skin
- Feeling light-headed
- Nausea and vomiting

If you suspect a heart attack, have the person sit and rest. Loosen tight clothing. Activate the EMS system at once. Prompt treatment can reduce the amount of heart muscle damage. Follow the rules in Box 36-1. Start CPR for cardiac arrest.

POISONING

A poison is any substance harmful to the body when ingested, inhaled, injected, or absorbed through the skin. See Chapter 10 for measures to prevent poisoning.

Some common signs and symptoms of poisoning are:

- Burns or redness around the mouth and lips
- A chemical odor to the breath
- Burns, stains, or odors on the person, on clothing, or around the person
- Empty drug bottles or spilled drugs
- Vomiting
- Dyspnea
- Drowsiness
- Confusion

For contact with a poison, call the Poison Control Center (1-800-222-1222). Also follow these emergency measures.

- *Poison in the eyes*—rinse the eyes with running water.
- *Poison on the skin*—remove clothing in contact with the poison. Rinse the skin with running water.
- *Inhaled poison*—leave the area. Get the person to fresh air at once.
- *Swallowed poison*—do not have the person try to vomit or give the person anything to cause vomiting. Do not give the person anything to eat or drink unless told to do so by the Poison Control Center.
- Activate the EMS system if the person stops breathing, collapses, or has a seizure (p. 529). Provide BLS if the person is not responding or breathing. See p. 529 for emergency care for seizures.
- Follow the rules in Box 36-1. Also follow the directions from the Poison Control Center.

HEMORRHAGE

Life and body functions need an adequate blood supply. If a blood vessel is cut or torn, bleeding occurs. The larger the blood vessel, the greater the bleeding and blood loss. *Hemorrhage is the excessive loss of blood in a short time.* If bleeding is not stopped, the person will die.

Hemorrhage is internal or external. You cannot see internal hemorrhage. The bleeding is inside body tissues and body cavities. Pain, shock, vomiting blood, coughing up blood, cold and moist skin, and loss of consciousness signal internal hemorrhage. There is little you can do for internal bleeding.

- Follow the rules in Box 36-1. This includes activating the EMS system.
- Keep the person warm, flat, and quiet until help arrives.
- Do not give fluids.

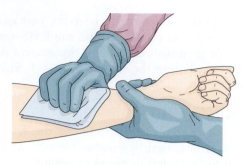

FIGURE 36-13 Direct pressure is applied to the wound to stop bleeding.

If not hidden by clothing, external bleeding is usually seen. Bleeding from an artery occurs in spurts. There is a steady flow of blood from a vein. To control bleeding:
- Follow the rules in Box 36-1. This includes activating the EMS system.
- Do not remove any objects that have pierced or stabbed the person.
- Place a sterile dressing directly over the wound. Or use any clean material (handkerchief, towel, cloth, or sanitary napkin).
- Apply firm pressure directly over the bleeding site (Fig. 36-13). Do not release pressure until the bleeding stops. If needed, wrap an elastic bandage firmly over the dressing or material.
- Do not remove the dressing or material. If bleeding continues, apply more dressings on top and apply more pressure.
- Bind the wound when bleeding stops. Tape or tie the dressing in place. You can tie the dressing with such things as clothing, a scarf, or a necktie.
  See *Promoting Safety and Comfort: Hemorrhage.*

PROMOTING SAFETY AND COMFORT
Hemorrhage
Safety
Contact with blood is likely with hemorrhage. Follow Standard Precautions and the Bloodborne Pathogen Standard to the extent possible. Wear gloves if possible. Practice hand hygiene as soon as you can.

FAINTING

Fainting is the sudden loss of consciousness from an inadequate blood supply to the brain. Hunger, fatigue, fear, and pain are common causes. Some people faint at the sight of blood or injury. Standing in 1 position too long and being in a warm, crowded room are other causes. Hemorrhage and other serious problems can cause fainting.

Dizziness, perspiration (sweating), and blackness before the eyes are warning signals. The person looks pale. The pulse is weak. Respirations are shallow if consciousness is lost.

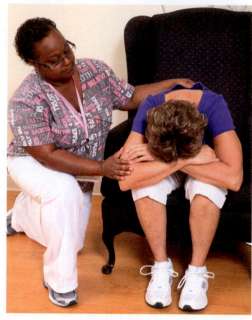

FIGURE 36-14 The person bends forward and lowers her head to prevent fainting.

Emergency care includes the following.
- Have the person sit or lie down to prevent fainting.
  - If sitting, the person bends forward and places the head between the knees (Fig. 36-14).
  - If lying down, raise the person's legs.
- Loosen tight clothing (belts, ties, scarves, collars, and so on).
- Keep the person lying down if fainting has occurred. Raise the legs about 12 inches.
- Do not let the person get up quickly.
- Help the person to a sitting position after recovery from fainting. Observe for fainting.
- Provide BLS if there is no response or breathing.

SHOCK

Shock results when tissues and organs do not get enough blood. Blood loss, allergic reaction, poisoning, heart attack (myocardial infarction), burns, and severe infection are causes. Signs and symptoms include:
- Low or falling blood pressure
- Rapid and weak pulse
- Rapid respirations
- Cold, moist, and pale skin
- Thirst
- Nausea and vomiting
- Restlessness
- Confusion and loss of consciousness as shock worsens
  Shock is possible in any acutely ill or severely injured person. Follow the rules in Box 36-1. Keep the person lying down. If no injuries from trauma, raise the legs about 6 to 12 inches. Lower the feet if the position causes pain. Maintain an open airway and control bleeding. Begin CPR for cardiac arrest.

Anaphylactic Shock

Some people are allergic or sensitive to foods, insects, chemicals, and drugs. For example, allergies to *penicillin* are common. An *antigen* is a substance that the body reacts to. The body releases chemicals to fight or attack the antigen. The person may react with an area of redness, swelling, or itching. Or the reaction may involve the entire body.

Anaphylaxis is a life-threatening sensitivity to an antigen. (*Ana* means *without. Phylaxis* means *protection.*) The reaction can occur within seconds. Signs and symptoms include:

- An itchy rash
- Swelling of the face, eyes, or lips
- Flushed or pale skin
- Feeling warm
- Dyspnea or wheezing from airway narrowing or a swollen tongue or throat
- Feeling that there is a "lump" in the throat
- A fast and weak pulse
- Nausea, vomiting, or diarrhea
- A feeling of dread or doom
- Dizziness or fainting
- Signs and symptoms of shock

Anaphylactic shock is an emergency. The EMS system must be activated. Drugs are needed to reverse the allergic reaction. Keep the person lying down and the airway open. Start CPR for cardiac arrest.

Some persons carry *epinephrine*—a drug used to treat life-threatening allergic reactions. The person injects the drug into the outer thigh. One dose is given for anaphylaxis. The person may give a second dose if:

- There is no response to the first dose.
- EMS arrival will take longer than 5 to 10 minutes.

STROKE

Stroke (cerebrovascular accident) occurs when the brain is suddenly deprived of its blood supply (Chapter 33). Usually only part of the brain is affected. A stroke may be caused by a thrombus, an embolus, or hemorrhage if a blood vessel in the brain ruptures.

Signs of stroke vary (Chapter 33). They depend on the size and location of brain injury. The National Institute of Neurological Disorders and Stroke lists these major signs.

- Sudden numbness or weakness of the face, arm, or leg, especially on 1 side of the body
- Sudden confusion or trouble speaking or understanding speech
- Sudden trouble seeing in 1 or both eyes
- Sudden trouble walking, dizziness, or loss of balance or coordination
- Sudden, severe headache with no known cause

If you suspect a stroke, activate the EMS system at once. The most effective stroke treatments must be given within 3 hours of symptom onset. Find out when symptoms began. Tell the EMS staff the time. Follow the rules in Box 36-1. Keep the person comfortable, warm, and quiet. Provide BLS and emergency care for seizures if necessary.

SEIZURES

Seizures (convulsions) are violent and sudden contractions or tremors of muscle groups caused by abnormal electrical activity in the brain. Movements are uncontrolled. The person may lose consciousness. Causes include head injury during birth or from trauma, high fever, brain tumors, poisoning, and nervous system disorders or infections. Lack of blood flow to the brain can also cause seizures.

The major types of seizures are:

- *Partial seizure.* Only 1 part of the brain is involved. A body part may jerk. Or the person has a hearing or vision problem or stomach discomfort. The person does not lose consciousness.
- *Generalized tonic-clonic (grand mal) seizure.* This type has 2 phases. In the *tonic* phase, the person loses consciousness. If standing or sitting, the person falls to the floor. The body is rigid because all muscles contract at once. The *clonic* phase follows. Muscle groups contract and relax. This causes jerking and twitching movements. Incontinence may occur. A deep sleep is common after the seizure. Confusion and headache may occur on awakening.
- *Generalized absence (petit mal) seizure.* This type usually lasts a few seconds. There is loss of consciousness, twitching of the eyelids, and staring. No first aid is necessary. However, guide the person away from dangers—stairs, streets, a hot stove, fireplaces, and so on.

Emergency Care for Seizures

You cannot stop a seizure. However, you can protect the person from injury.

- Follow the rules in Box 36-1. This includes activating the EMS system.
- Do not leave the person alone.
- Lower the person to the floor. This protects the person from falling.
- Note the time the seizure started.
- Place something soft under the head (Fig. 36-15, p. 530). It prevents the head from striking the floor. You can use a pillow, a cushion, or a folded blanket, towel, or jacket. Or cradle the person's head in your lap.
- Remove eyeglasses and loosen tight jewelry and clothing around the neck. Ties, scarves, collars, and necklaces are examples.
- Turn the person onto the side. Make sure the head is turned to the side. See Figure 36-15.
- Do not put any object or your fingers between the teeth. The person can bite down on your fingers or injure his or her teeth or jaw.
- Do not try to stop the seizure or control movements.
- Move furniture, equipment, and sharp objects out of the way. The person may strike these objects during the seizure.
- Note the time the seizure ends.
- Make sure the mouth is clear of food, fluids, and saliva after the seizure.
- Provide BLS if the person is not breathing after the seizure.

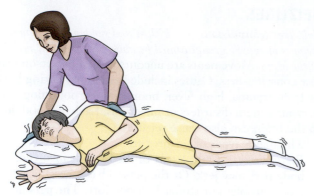

FIGURE 36-15 A pillow protects the person's head during a seizure.

CONCUSSIONS

Head injuries can be minor or serious and life-threatening. Concussion is the most common brain injury. A concussion results from a bump or blow to the head or jolt to the head or body. The head and brain move quickly back and forth.

The following danger signs in adults signal the need for emergency care.

- Headache—gets worse or does not go away
- Stiff neck
- Weakness, numbness, or decreased coordination
- Nausea or vomiting more than once
- Slurred speech
- Very sleepy; drowsy; cannot be awakened
- One eye pupil is larger than the other
- Convulsions or seizures
- Cannot recognize people, places, or things
- Increased confusion, restlessness, or agitation
- Unusual behavior
- Loss of consciousness

Emergency care for a concussion includes the following.

- Follow the rules in Box 36-1. This includes activating the EMS system.
- Provide BLS if the person is not responding or breathing.
- Place your hands on both sides of the head to keep the head aligned with the spine. Prevent movement.
- Apply firm pressure with a clean cloth to a bleeding area. See "Hemorrhage" on p. 527. Be careful not to move the person's head.
- Do not apply direct pressure to the skull if the skull may be fractured. Cover the wound with sterile gauze dressing.
- Do not remove any object from a wound.
- Logroll the person as a unit onto the side if vomiting occurs.
- Apply ice packs to swollen areas.

BURNS

Burns can severely disable a person. They can also cause death. Most burns occur in the home. Infants, children, and older persons are at risk. Common causes of burns and fires are:

- Scalds from hot liquids
- Playing with matches and lighters
- Electrical injuries
- Cooking accidents (barbecues, microwave ovens, stoves, ovens)
- Falling asleep while smoking
- Fireplaces
- Space heaters
- No smoke alarms or non-functioning smoke alarms
- Sunburn
- Chemicals

Some burns are severe (Fig. 36-16). Severity depends on burn size and depth, the body part involved, and age. Burns to the face, hands, feet, groin, buttocks, or over a joint are more serious than burns to an arm or leg. Infants, young children, and older persons are at high risk for death.

Emergency care for severe burns includes the following.

- Follow the rules in Box 36-1. This includes activating the EMS system.
- Do not touch the person if he or she is in contact with an electrical source. Have the power source turned off. Do not approach the person or try to remove the electrical source with any object until the power source is turned off.
- Remove the person from the fire or burn source.
- Stop the burning process. Put out flames with water or roll the person in a blanket. Or smother flames with a coat, sheet, or towel.
- Apply cold or cool water for 10 to 15 minutes. Water temperature is between 59°F and 77°F (Fahrenheit) (15°C and 25°C [centigrade]). Do not put ice directly on the burn.
- Remove hot clothing that is not sticking to the skin. If you cannot remove hot clothing, cool the clothing with water.
- Remove jewelry and any tight clothing that is not sticking to the skin.
- Provide rescue breathing and CPR as needed.
- Cover burns with sterile, dry dressings. Or use a sheet or any other clean cloth.
- Do not put oil, butter, salve, or ointments on the burns.
- Keep blisters intact. Do not break blisters.
- Elevate the burned area above heart level if possible.
- Cover the person with a blanket or coat to prevent heat loss.

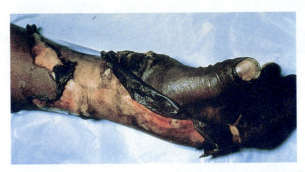

FIGURE 36-16 A severe burn. (From Ignatavicius DD, Workman ML: *Medical-surgical nursing: patient-centered collaborative care,* ed 8, St Louis, 2016, Elsevier.)

FOCUS ON P R I D E
The Person, Family, and Yourself

Personal and Professional Responsibility

Understanding emergency care allows you to safely assist in an emergency. This chapter includes basic information. BLS courses for health care providers offer further training. You also practice emergency procedures. CPR and use of an AED are examples.

Most agencies require nursing assistants to be certified in BLS. You must pass a written and skills test for certification. In the skills test, you show how to provide BLS. Take the course seriously. What you learn can save a life.

Rights and Respect

Protect the right to privacy. Do not expose the person unnecessarily. The person may be in a lounge, dining area, or public place. Do what you can to provide privacy. As always, treat the person with dignity and respect.

Independence and Social Interaction

Quality of life and independence are important. In an emergency, choices may be few. However, they are given when possible. For example, the person has the right to choose a hospital.

The EMS staff has guidelines if a person refuses care. For example, the person must be competent and able to legally make medical decisions. The person must also be informed of the risks, benefits, and alternatives to recommended care.

Delegation and Teamwork

On-lookers can threaten privacy and confidentiality. Your main concern is the person's illness or injuries. You cannot give care and manage on-lookers. Ask someone else to deal with on-lookers. If someone else is giving care, keep on-lookers away from the person. Work together to protect the person's privacy.

Ethics and Laws

People are curious. They want to know what happened, the extent of injuries or illness, and if the person will be okay. Do not discuss the situation. Do not offer ideas of what is wrong. Information about care, treatment, and condition is confidential. Keep the person's information private. It is the right thing to do.

FOCUS ON PRIDE: *Application*

Emergencies are stressful. A calm, professional approach helps the person and family feel more secure. Describe professional conduct in an emergency. Explain how you will prepare yourself to respond.

Circle the BEST answer.

1 When giving first aid, you should
  a Know your own limits
  b Move the person
  c Give the person fluids
  d Keep the person cool

2 The signs of sudden cardiac arrest are
  a Restlessness, rapid breathing, and a weak pulse
  b Confusion, hemiplegia, and slurred speech
  c No response, no normal breathing, and no pulse
  d Dizziness, pale skin, and slow breathing

3 Rescue breathing for an adult involves
  a Giving each breath over 2 seconds
  b Watching the abdomen rise with each breath
  c Giving a breath every 3 to 5 seconds
  d Giving a breath every 5 to 6 seconds

4 Which hand placement is correct for adult chest compressions?
  a 1 hand in the center of the chest
  b 2 hands below the sternum
  c 2 hands on the lower half of the sternum
  d 2 fingers on the lower half of the sternum

5 To check for breathing,
  a Use the head tilt–chin lift method to open the airway
  b Look for no breathing or agonal gasping
  c Look, listen, and feel for air moving in and out of the lungs
  d Take 10 to 15 seconds to listen for breathing

6 Which pulse is used during adult CPR?
  a The carotid pulse
  b The apical pulse
  c The brachial pulse
  d The femoral pulse

7 Which compression rate is used for CPR?
  a 30 compressions per minute
  b 100 to 120 compressions per minute
  c 15 compressions per minute
  d 60 to 100 compressions per minute

8 For adult CPR,
  a Give 2 breaths after every 15 compressions
  b Give 2 breaths after every 30 compressions
  c Give 1 breath after every 5 compressions
  d Give 2 breaths when you are tired from giving compressions

9 Two rescuers are giving adult CPR. When should the AED be used?
  a After 5 cycles of CPR
  b After 2 minutes of CPR
  c As soon as the AED arrives
  d When EMS staff arrives

10 A person swallowed a chemical. You should
  a Have the person drink a glass of water
  b Have the person try to vomit
  c Call the Poison Control Center
  d Contact the chemical's manufacturer

11 A person is hemorrhaging from the forearm. Your *first* action is to
  a Lower the arm
  b Apply pressure to the brachial artery
  c Tape a dressing in place
  d Apply direct pressure to the wound

12 A person is about to faint. What should you do?
  a Have the person sit or lie down.
  b Take the person outside for fresh air.
  c Have the person stand very still.
  d Raise the head if the person is lying down.

13 Which is a sign of shock?
  a High blood pressure
  b Slow pulse
  c Slow and deep respirations
  d Cold, moist, and pale skin

14 Which statement about heart attack is *true?*
  a It is the same as cardiac arrest.
  b It can cause cardiac arrest.
  c Symptoms resolve with rest.
  d It is a severe response to an antigen.

15 Emergency care for stroke involves
  a Asking when the person's symptoms began
  b Giving the person sips of water
  c Controlling bleeding
  d Positioning the person bent forward with the head lowered

16 A person is having a tonic-clonic (grand mal) seizure. You should
  a Place an object between the person's teeth
  b Loosen tight jewelry and clothing around the neck
  c Try to stop the person's movements
  d Place the person's head on a firm surface

17 After falling down stairs, a person is confused and has a headache. You should
  a Place the person in the recovery position
  b Give the person a pain-relief drug
  c Prevent movement of the head and neck
  d Help the person to bed to lie down

18 While waiting for help to arrive, cover a severe burn with
  a A sterile, dry dressing or clean cloth
  b Butter or oil
  c Salve or an ointment
  d Nothing

Answers to Chapter 36 questions are on p. 552.

FOCUS ON PRACTICE

Problem Solving

A resident has a seizure during an activity. What emergency care will you provide? After the seizure, the person is only gasping. Explain what you would do step-by-step. How will you and the nursing team provide for the person's privacy?

End-of-Life Care

OBJECTIVES

- Define the key terms and key abbreviations in this chapter.
- Describe palliative care and hospice care.
- Describe the factors affecting attitudes about death.
- Describe the 5 stages of dying.
- Explain how to meet the needs of the dying person and family.
- Explain the purposes of the *Patient Self-Determination Act.*

- Describe 3 advance directives.
- Identify the signs of approaching death and the signs of death.
- Explain how to assist with post-mortem care.
- Perform the procedure in this chapter.
- Explain how to promote PRIDE in the person, the family, and yourself.

KEY TERMS

advance directive A document stating a person's wishes about health care when that person cannot make his or her own decisions
autopsy The examination of the body after death
end-of-life care The support and care given during the time surrounding death
palliative care Care that involves relieving or reducing the intensity of uncomfortable symptoms without producing a cure

post-mortem care Care of the body after *(post)* death *(mortem)*
reincarnation The belief that the spirit or soul is reborn in another human body or in another form of life
rigor mortis The stiffness or rigidity *(rigor)* of skeletal muscles that occurs after death *(mortis)*
terminal illness An illness or injury from which the person will not likely recover

KEY ABBREVIATIONS

DNR	Do Not Resuscitate
ID	Identification

OBRA	Omnibus Budget Reconciliation Act of 1987

End-of-life care describes the support and care given during the time surrounding death. Sometimes death is sudden. Often it is expected. Some people gradually fail. End-of-life care may involve days, weeks, or months.

Your feelings about death affect the care you give. You will help meet the dying person's physical, psychological, social, and spiritual needs. Therefore you must understand the dying process. Then you can approach the dying person with caring, kindness, and respect.

TERMINAL ILLNESS

Many illnesses and diseases have no cure. The body cannot function after some injuries. Recovery is not expected. The disease or injury ends in death. *An illness or injury from which the person will not likely recover is a* **terminal illness**.

Types of Care

Terminally ill persons can choose palliative care or hospice care. The person may opt for palliative care and then change to hospice care.

- *Palliative care. Palliate* means *to soothe or relieve.* **Palliative care** *involves relieving or reducing the intensity of uncomfortable symptoms without producing a cure.* The focus is on comfort. The intent is to improve quality of life and provide family support. Palliative care can be given along with disease treatment.
- *Hospice care.* The focus is on the physical, emotional, social, and spiritual needs of dying persons and their families (Chapter 1). Often the person has less than 6 months to live. Cure or life-saving measures are not concerns. Pain relief and comfort are stressed. The goal is to improve quality of life. Follow-up care and support groups for survivors are hospice services. Hospice also supports the health team in dealing with a person's death.

ATTITUDES ABOUT DEATH

Experiences, culture, religion, and age influence attitudes about death. Many people fear death. Others do not believe they will die. Some look forward to and accept death. Attitudes about death often change as a person grows older and with changing needs.

Cultural and Spiritual Needs

Practices and attitudes about death differ among cultures. See *Caring About Culture: Death Rites.* In some cultures, dying people are cared for at home by the family. Some families prepare the body for burial.

Spiritual needs relate to the human spirit and to religion and religious beliefs. Many people strengthen religious beliefs when dying. Religion can comfort the dying person and the family.

Attitudes about death are often closely related to religion. Some believe life after death is free of suffering and hardship. They also believe in reunion with loved ones. Many believe sins and misdeeds are punished in the afterlife. Others do not believe in the afterlife. To them, death is the end of life.

There are also religious beliefs about the body's form after death. Some believe the body keeps its physical form. Others believe that only the spirit or soul is present in the afterlife. *Reincarnation is the belief that the spirit or soul is reborn in another human body or in another form of life.*

Many religions have rites and rituals during the dying process and at the time of death and after. Prayers, blessings, scripture readings, and religious music are common sources of comfort. So are visits from a cleric.

See *Focus on Communication: Cultural and Spiritual Needs.*

CARING ABOUT CULTURE

Death Rites

In *Vietnam,* dying persons may be helped to recall past good deeds and to achieve a fitting mental state. Death at home may be preferred. In some areas, a coin or jewels (a wealthy family) or rice (a poor family) is put in the dead person's mouth. The belief is that they will help the soul go through encounters with gods and devils and the soul will be born rich in the next life.

In *India,* Hindu persons are often accepting of God's will. The person's desire to be clear-headed as death nears must be assessed in planning treatment. The family and person need a time and place for prayer. The Hindu priest reads from Holy Sanskrit books. Some priests tie strings (meaning a blessing) around the waist. Cremation is usually preferred.

(NOTE: *Each person is unique. A person may not follow all of the beliefs and practices of his or her culture. Follow the care plan.*)

Modified from D'Avanzo CE: *Pocket guide to cultural health assessment,* ed 4, St Louis, 2008, Mosby.

FOCUS ON COMMUNICATION

Cultural and Spiritual Needs

Your cultural or religious practices and beliefs may differ from those of patients and residents. Do not judge the person by your standards. Do not make negative comments or insult the person's beliefs. Respect the person as a whole. This includes his or her beliefs and customs.

Age

Adults fear pain and suffering, dying alone, and the invasion of privacy. They also fear loneliness and separation from loved ones. They worry about the care and support of those left behind. Adults often resent death because it affects plans, hopes, dreams, and ambitions.

Infants and toddlers do not understand death. They know or sense that something has changed. They sense a caregiver's absence or a different caregiver. They also sense changes in when and how their needs are met. They may feel a sense of loss.

Between 2 and 6 years old, children think death is temporary. It can be reversed. The dead person continues to live and function and can come back to life. Such ideas come from fairy tales, cartoons, movies, video games, and TV. Children this age often blame themselves when someone or something dies. To them, death is punishment for being bad. They know when family members or pets die. They notice dead birds or bugs. Answers to questions about death often cause fear and confusion. Children who are told "He is sleeping" may be afraid to go to sleep.

Between 6 and 11 years, children learn that death is final. They do not think they will die. Death happens to others, especially adults. It can be avoided. Children relate death to punishment and body mutilation. It also involves witches, ghosts, goblins, and monsters. Understanding increases as children grow older and have more experiences with death.

Older persons know death will occur. Many have lost family and friends. Some welcome death as freedom from pain, suffering, and disability. Like younger adults, many fear dying alone.

THE STAGES OF DYING

Dr. Elisabeth Kübler-Ross described 5 stages of dying. They also are called the "stages of grief." *Grief* is the person's response to loss.

- *Stage 1: Denial.* The person refuses to believe that he or she is dying. "No, not me" is a common response. The person believes a mistake was made.
- *Stage 2: Anger.* The person thinks "Why me?" There is anger and rage. Dying persons envy and resent those with life and health. Family, friends, and the health team are often targets of anger.
- *Stage 3: Bargaining.* Anger has passed. The person now says: "Yes, me but…" The person may bargain with God or a higher power for more time. Promises are made in exchange for more time. Bargaining is usually private and spiritual.
- *Stage 4: Depression.* The person thinks "Yes, me" and is very sad. The person mourns lost things and the future loss of life. The person may cry or say little. Sometimes the person talks about people and things that will be left behind.
- *Stage 5: Acceptance.* The person is calm, at peace, and accepts death. The person has said what needs to be said. Unfinished business is complete. This stage may last for many months or years. Reaching the acceptance stage does not mean death is near.

Dying persons do not always pass through each stage. A person may stay in one stage. Some move back and forth between stages. For example, a person moves from acceptance back to bargaining and then moves forward to acceptance.

COMFORT NEEDS

End-of-life care involves physical, mental and emotional, and spiritual comfort. See "Cultural and Spiritual Needs." Comfort goals are to:

- Prevent or relieve suffering to the extent possible.
- Respect and follow end-of-life wishes.

Dying persons may want family and friends present. They may want to talk about fears, worries, and anxieties. Some want to be alone. Often they need to talk during the night. Things are quiet, distractions are few, and there is more time to think. You need to listen and use touch.

- *Listening.* The person needs to talk and share worries and concerns. Let the person express feelings and emotions. Do not worry about saying the wrong thing or finding comforting words. You do not need to say anything. Being there is what counts.
- *Touch.* Touch shows care and concern when words cannot. Sometimes the person does not want to talk but needs you nearby. Do not feel that you must talk. Silence, along with touch, is a powerful and meaningful way to communicate.

Some people want to see a spiritual leader. Or they want to take part in religious practices. Provide privacy during prayer and spiritual times. Be courteous to the spiritual leader. The person has the right to have religious items nearby—medals, pictures, statues, writings, and so on. Handle them with care and respect.

See *Focus on Communication: Comfort Needs.*
See *Focus on Older Persons: Comfort Needs.*

FOCUS ON COMMUNICATION

Comfort Needs

Knowing what to say to the dying person is hard for many health team members. Unless you have been near death yourself, do not say: "I understand what you are going through." The statement is a communication barrier. Instead, you can say:

- "Would you like to talk? I have time to listen."
- "You seem sad. Can I help?"
- "Is it okay if I quietly sit with you for a while?"

FOCUS ON OLDER PERSONS

Comfort Needs

Persons with Alzheimer's disease (AD) become more and more disabled. Those with advanced AD cannot share their concerns, discomforts, or problems. It is hard to provide emotional and spiritual comfort.

Focus on the person's senses—hearing, touch, sight—to promote comfort. Comforting touch or massage can be soothing. So can soft music or sounds from nature—birds chirping, gentle breezes, ocean waves, and so on.

Physical Needs

Dying may take a few minutes, hours, days, or weeks. Body processes slow. The person is weak. Levels of consciousness change. The person is independent to the extent possible. As the person weakens, basic needs are met by others. Every effort is made to promote physical and psychological comfort. The person is allowed to die in peace and with dignity.

Pain. Pain can range from none to severe. Report signs and symptoms of pain at once (Chapters 17 and 25). Some persons cannot tell you about pain. Watch for signs of pain or discomfort.

- Restlessness, agitation
- Frowning, grimacing
- Sighing
- Moaning
- Whimpering, crying
- Tense muscles
- Rapid pulse

Skin care, personal and oral hygiene, back massages, and good alignment promote comfort. So do frequent position changes and supportive devices. Turn the person slowly and gently. Follow the care plan to prevent and control pain. The nurse can give pain-relief drugs.

Breathing Problems. Shortness of breath and difficulty breathing *(dyspnea)* are common end-of-life problems. Semi-Fowler's position and oxygen (Chapter 30) are helpful. An open window for fresh air may be helpful. So might a fan circulating air.

Noisy breathing—the *death rattle*—is common as death nears. This is from mucus collecting in the airway. These measures may help.

- The side-lying position
- Suctioning by the nurse
- Drugs to reduce the amount of mucus

Vision, Hearing, and Speech. Vision blurs and gradually fails. The person turns toward light. A darkened room may frighten the person. The eyes may be half-open. Secretions may collect in the eye corners.

Because of failing vision, explain who you are and what you are doing to the person or in the room. The room should be well lit. Avoid bright lights and glares.

Good eye care is needed (Chapter 18). If the eyes stay open, a nurse may apply a protective ointment. Then the eyes are covered with moist pads to prevent injury.

Hearing is one of the last functions lost. Many people hear until the moment of death. Even unconscious persons may hear. Always assume that the person can hear. Speak in a normal voice. Give reassurance and explain care. Offer words of comfort. Avoid upsetting topics. Do not talk about the person.

Speech becomes harder. It may be hard to understand the person. Sometimes the person cannot speak. Anticipate the person's needs. Do not ask questions with long answers. Ask a few "yes" or "no" questions. Despite speech problems, you must talk to the person.

Mouth, Nose, and Skin. Oral hygiene promotes comfort. Give routine mouth care if the person can eat and drink. Give frequent oral hygiene as death nears and when taking oral fluids is difficult. Oral hygiene is needed if mucus collects in the mouth and the person cannot swallow. A lip balm may be used for dry lips.

Crusting and irritation of the nostrils can occur. Nasal secretions, an oxygen cannula, and a naso-gastric tube are common causes. Carefully clean the nose. Apply lubricant as directed by the nurse and the care plan.

Circulation fails. Body temperature rises as death nears although the skin is cool, pale, and mottled (blotchy). Sweating increases. Skin care, bathing, and preventing pressure injuries are necessary. Linens and gowns are changed as needed. Although the skin feels cool, only light bed coverings are needed. Blankets may cause warmth and restlessness. However, observe for signs of cold—shivering, hunching shoulders, and pulling covers. Prevent drafts and provide more blankets.

Nutrition. Nausea, vomiting, and loss of appetite are common at the end of life. Drugs for nausea and vomiting are ordered.

You may need to feed the person. Favorite foods may help loss of appetite. So may small, frequent meals.

As death nears, loss of appetite is common. The person may choose not to eat or drink. Do not force the person to eat or drink. Tell the nurse.

Elimination. Urinary and fecal incontinence may occur. Use incontinence products or waterproof under-pads as directed. Give perineal care as needed. Constipation and urinary retention are common. Enemas and catheters may be needed. Follow the care plan for catheter care.

The Person's Room. Provide a comfortable and pleasant room. It should be well lit and well ventilated. Remove unnecessary equipment. Some equipment is upsetting to see (suction machines, drainage containers). If possible, keep such items out of the person's sight.

Mementos, pictures, cards, flowers, and religious items provide comfort. The person and family arrange the room as they wish. This helps meet love, belonging, and esteem needs. The room should reflect the person's choices.

Mental and Emotional Needs

Mental and emotional needs are very personal. Some persons are calm and at peace. Others are anxious or depressed or have specific fears and concerns. Examples include:

- Severe pain
- When and how death will occur
- What will happen to loved ones
- Dying alone

Simple measures may be soothing—touch, holding hands, back massage, soft lighting, music at a low volume.

THE FAMILY

This is a hard time for the family. It may be hard to find comforting words. To show you care, use touch and be available, courteous, and considerate.

Sometimes the family keeps a *vigil*. That is, someone is always with the person even at night. They watch over or pray for the person. Provide for the family's comfort.

Respect the right to privacy. The person and family need time together. However, do not neglect care because the family is present. Most agencies let family members help give care. Or you can suggest that they take a beverage or meal break.

The family may be very tired, sad, and tearful. Watching a loved one die is very painful. So is dealing with the eventual loss of that person. The family goes through stages like the dying person. They need support, understanding, courtesy, and respect. A spiritual leader may provide comfort. Communicate this request to the nurse at once.

LEGAL ISSUES

Much attention is given to the right to die. Some people make end-of-life wishes known.

Advance Directives

The *Patient Self-Determination Act* and the *Omnibus Budget Reconciliation Act of 1987 (OBRA)* give persons the right to accept or refuse treatment. They also give the right to make advance directives. An **advance directive** is a document stating *a person's wishes about health care when that person cannot make his or her own decisions.* Advance directives usually forbid certain care if there is no hope of recovery. Quality of care cannot be less because of the person's advance directives.

See *Focus on Surveys: Advance Directives.*

FOCUS ON SURVEYS

Advance Directives

Federal and state laws require that agencies educate staff about policies and procedures for advance directives. A surveyor may ask you about advance directives. For example:

- Did you receive information from the agency about advance directives?
- When did you receive such information?
- What do advance directives mean to you?
- What care do you give when a person has an advance directive?

Living Wills. A living will is about measures that support or maintain life when death is likely. Tube feedings, ventilators, and resuscitation are examples. A living will may instruct doctors:

- Not to start measures that prolong dying
- To remove measures that prolong dying

Durable Power of Attorney for Health Care. This advance directive gives the power to make health care decisions to another person. That person is often called a *health care proxy*. Usually this is a family member, friend, or lawyer. When a person cannot make health care decisions, the health care proxy can do so. This advance directive does not cover property or financial matters.

"Do Not Resuscitate" Orders. "Do Not Resuscitate" (DNR) or "No Code" orders mean that the person will not be resuscitated (Chapter 36). The person is allowed to die with peace and dignity. The orders are written after consulting with the person and family. The family and doctor make the decision if the person is not mentally able to do so.

SIGNS OF DEATH

As death nears, these signs may occur fast or slowly.

- Movement, muscle tone, and sensation are lost. This usually starts in the feet and legs. Mouth muscles relax, the jaw drops. The mouth may stay open. The facial expression is often peaceful.
- Gastro-intestinal functions slow down. Abdominal distention, fecal incontinence, nausea, and vomiting are common.
- Body temperature rises. The person feels cool or cold, looks pale, and perspires heavily.
- Circulation fails. The pulse is fast or slow, weak, and irregular. Blood pressure starts to fall.
- The respiratory system fails. Slow or rapid and shallow respirations are observed. Mucus collects in the airway. Breathing sounds are noisy and gurgling *(death rattle)*.
- Pain decreases as the person loses consciousness. However, some people are conscious until the moment of death.

The signs of death include *no pulse, no respirations,* and *no blood pressure.* The pupils are fixed and dilated. A doctor determines that death has occurred. He or she pronounces the person dead. If a doctor is not present in a nursing center, a nurse calls the doctor to report the signs of death. The time and place are noted for the death certificate.

CARE OF THE BODY AFTER DEATH

Care of the body after (post) *death* (mortem) *is called **post-mortem care***. You may be asked to assist the nurse. Post-mortem care begins when the person is pronounced dead.

Post-mortem care is done to maintain a good appearance of the body. Discoloration and skin damage are prevented. Valuables and personal items are gathered for the family.

Within 2 to 4 hours after death, rigor mortis develops. ***Rigor mortis** is the stiffness or rigidity* (rigor) *of skeletal muscles that occurs after death* (mortis). The body is positioned in normal alignment before rigor mortis sets in. The family may want to see the body. The body should appear in a comfortable and natural position.

In some agencies, the body is prepared only for viewing by the family. The funeral director completes post-mortem care.

Sometimes an autopsy is done. An ***autopsy** is the examination of the body after death.* (*Autos* means *self. Opsis* means *view.*) It is done to determine the cause of death. Post-mortem care is not done. Doing so could remove or destroy evidence.

Post-mortem care involves moving the body. For example, soiled areas are bathed and the body is placed in good alignment. Moving the body can cause air in the lungs, stomach, and intestines to be expelled. When air is expelled, sounds are produced. Do not let those sounds alarm or frighten you. They are normal and expected.

See *Delegation Guidelines: Care of the Body After Death.*

See *Promoting Safety and Comfort: Care of the Body After Death.*

See procedure: *Assisting With Post-Mortem Care.*

DELEGATION GUIDELINES
Care of the Body After Death

To assist with post-mortem care, you need this information from the nurse.
- If dentures are inserted or placed in a denture cup
- If tubes and dressings are removed or left in place
- If rings are removed or left in place
- If the family wants to view the body
- Special agency policies and procedures

PROMOTING SAFETY AND COMFORT
Care of the Body After Death

Safety
Standard Precautions and the Bloodborne Pathogen Standard are followed. You may have contact with blood, body fluids, secretions, and excretions.

Assisting With Post-Mortem Care

PRE-PROCEDURE

1 Follow *Delegation Guidelines: Care of the Body After Death.* See *Promoting Safety and Comfort: Care of the Body After Death.*
2 Practice hand hygiene.
3 Collect the following.
   - Post-mortem kit (shroud or body bag, gown, ID [identification] tags, gauze squares, safety pins)
   - Disposable bed protectors
   - Wash basin
   - Bath towel and washcloths
   - Denture cup
   - Items for shaving facial hair (Chapter 19)
   - Tape
   - Dressings
   - Gloves
   - Cotton balls
   - Valuables envelope
4 Provide for privacy.
5 Raise the bed for body mechanics.
6 Make sure the bed is flat.

Assisting With Post-Mortem Care—cont'd

PROCEDURE

7 Put on the gloves.
8 Position the body supine. Arms and legs are straight. A pillow is under the head and shoulders. Or raise the head of the bed 15 to 20 degrees if this is agency policy.
9 Close the eyes. Gently pull the eyelids over the eyes. Apply moist cotton balls gently over the eyelids if the eyes do not stay closed.
10 Insert dentures or put them in a labeled denture cup. Follow agency policy.
11 Close the mouth. If necessary, place a rolled towel under the chin to keep the mouth closed.
12 Remove all jewelry, except for wedding rings if this is agency policy. List the jewelry that you removed. Place the jewelry and the list in a valuables envelope.
13 Place a cotton ball over the rings. Tape them in place as the nurse directs.
14 Remove drainage containers.
15 Remove tubes and catheters with gauze squares as the nurse directs.
16 Shave facial hair if agency policy or if desired by the family.
17 Bathe soiled areas with plain water. Dry thoroughly.
18 Place a disposable bed protector under the buttocks.
19 Remove soiled dressings. Replace them with clean ones.
20 Put a clean gown on the body. Position the body as in step 8.

21 Brush and comb the hair if necessary.
22 Cover the body to the shoulders with a sheet if the family will view the body.
23 Gather belongings. Put them in a bag labeled with the person's name. Be sure to include eyeglasses, hearing aids, and other valuables.
24 Remove supplies, equipment, and linens. Straighten the room. Provide soft lighting.
25 Remove and discard the gloves. Practice hand hygiene.
26 Let the family view the body. Provide for privacy. Return to the room after they leave.
27 Practice hand hygiene. Put on gloves.
28 Fill out the ID tags. Tie 1 to the ankle or to the right big toe.
29 Place the body in the body bag or cover it with a sheet. Or apply a shroud (Fig. 37-1).
   a Position the shroud under the body.
   b Bring the top down over the head.
   c Fold the bottom up over the feet.
   d Fold the sides over the body.
   e Pin or tape the shroud in place.
30 Attach the second ID tag to the shroud, sheet, or body bag.
31 Leave the denture cup with the body.
32 Pull the privacy curtain around the bed. Or close the door.

POST-PROCEDURE

33 Remove and discard the gloves. Practice hand hygiene.
34 Clean the unit after the body has been removed. Wear gloves for this step.
35 Remove and discard the gloves. Practice hand hygiene.

36 Report the following.
   • The time the body was taken by the funeral director
   • What was done with jewelry, other valuables, and personal items
   • What was done with dentures

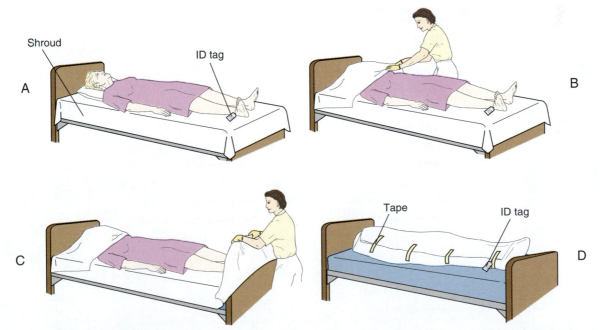

FIGURE 37-1 Applying a shroud. **A,** Position the shroud under the body. **B,** Bring the top down over the head. **C,** Fold the bottom up over the feet. **D,** Fold the sides over the body. Tape or pin the sides together. Attach the ID tag.

Personal and Professional Responsibility

To give quality care to the dying person:

- Promote comfort. Report complaints or signs of pain at once. Follow the comfort measures in the care plan.
- Protect the person's privacy.
- Provide support to the person and family. Be kind. Show compassion and respect.
- Offer the family time alone with the person.

Take pride in supporting the person and family during a difficult time. The family has many emotions during the dying process and after a loved one's death (Fig. 37-2).

Rights and Respect

Understanding the person's needs and desires allows you to give better care. Respect the person's right to die in peace and with dignity. The right to privacy and the right to be treated with dignity and respect apply after death.

Independence and Social Interaction

The person is encouraged to take part in care to the extent possible. Some days the person can do more than other days. Follow the nurse's directions and the care plan. Do not force the person to do more than he or she can physically or mentally do.

Delegation and Teamwork

Over time, the health team often bonds with the person. This is common in hospice and long-term care. The person's death is difficult for the staff. Sadness and grief may occur.

Tell the nurse if you have trouble coping with a person's death. Support others who need help. A kind word, a hug, or taking time to listen show concern. Take pride in being a part of a caring and supportive team.

Ethics and Laws

The dying person has rights under OBRA.

- *The right to privacy before and after death.* The person has the right not to have his or her body seen by others. Proper draping and screening are important.
- *The right to visit others in private.* Moving the dying person to a private room provides privacy. The family can also stay as long as they like.
- *The right to confidentiality before and after death.* The final moments and cause of death are confidential. So are statements, conversations, and family reactions.
- *The right to be free from abuse, mistreatment, and neglect.* The person has the right to kind and respectful care before and after death. Report signs of abuse, mistreatment, or neglect at once.
- *Freedom from restraint.* Restraints are used only if ordered by the doctor. Dying persons are often too weak to be dangerous to themselves or others.
- *The right to personal possessions.* The person may want photos and religious items nearby. Protect the person's property from loss or damage before and after death. They may be family treasures or mementos.
- *The right to a safe and home-like setting.* Everyone must keep the setting safe and home-like. Try to keep equipment and supplies out of view. The room should be free from unpleasant odors and noises.
- *The right to personal choice.* The dying person may refuse treatment. Advance directives are common. Respect the person's choices to refuse treatment or not prolong life.

Genuine concern for the dying person is shown in the care you give. How can you show respect at the end of life and with post-mortem care? How can you show care and concern for the grieving family?

ROGER'S BELL

Mom neared the end of her travail,
she suffered much...so thin, so frail.
I worried a lot; "What if she fell?"
Then I remembered "Roger's Bell!"
I put the bell beside her bed.
"Just ring it anytime," I said,
"and I'll be there to help you stand,
or rub your back, or hold your hand."
I'd tell Mom most every night
to ring that bell if things weren't right.
And once or twice she rang the bell,
she did it for me, I could tell.
The final weeks were Carol's hell...
yet she ignored the nightstand bell.

The bell was quiet the day she died,
when friends she barely knew had cried.
I went to the nightstand...said a prayer,
picked up the bell...Do I dare?
"Why have it there beside your bed,
when now I need your help instead?"
She answered, "If you're sad and lonely too,
ring the bell and I'll be there with you!"
– Now Mom doesn't need my steady hand,
– she marches on...leading the band.
Her ordeal is over, her task complete,
and she watches over me, till again we meet.

–Bob Pinkerton

FIGURE 37-2 When he was dying of cancer, Linda Pinkerton Davis gave her husband, Roger, a nightstand bell. Several years later, Linda gave "Roger's bell" to her mom, Carol. Carol's husband wrote the poem after her death. (Printed with permission from Robert Pinkerton, July 2017.)

REVIEW QUESTIONS

Circle the BEST answer.

1 Which is *true*?
   a Death from terminal illness is sudden.
   b Doctors know when death will occur.
   c An illness is terminal when recovery is not likely.
   d All severe injuries end in death.

2 Reincarnation is the belief that
   a There is no afterlife
   b The spirit or soul is reborn into another human body or form of life
   c The body keeps its physical form in the afterlife
   d Only the spirit or soul is present in the afterlife

3 Adults and older persons usually fear
   a Reincarnation
   b The 5 stages of dying
   c Advance directives
   d Dying alone

4 Persons in the stage of denial
   a Are angry
   b Are calm and at peace
   c Refuse to believe they are dying
   d Are sad and quiet

5 A person tries to gain more time during the stage of
   a Anger
   b Bargaining
   c Depression
   d Acceptance

6 When caring for the dying person, you should
   a Use touch and listen
   b Do most of the talking
   c Ask questions with long answers
   d Speak in a loud voice

7 As death nears, the last sense lost is
   a Sight
   b Taste
   c Smell
   d Hearing

8 The dying person's care includes the following. Which should you question?
   a Eye care
   b Mouth care
   c Active range-of-motion exercises
   d Position changes

9 The dying person is positioned in
   a The supine position
   b The Fowler's position
   c Good body alignment
   d The dorsal recumbent position

10 A "DNR" order means that
   a CPR will not be done
   b The person has a living will
   c Life-prolonging measures will be carried out
   d The person is kept alive as long as possible

11 The signs of death are
   a Convulsions and incontinence
   b No pulse, respirations, or blood pressure
   c Loss of consciousness and convulsions
   d The eyes stay open, no muscle movements, and the body is rigid

12 Post-mortem care is done
   a After rigor mortis sets in
   b When the funeral director arrives for the body
   c After the family has viewed the body
   d After the doctor pronounces the person dead

Answers to Chapter 37 questions are on p. 552.

FOCUS ON PRACTICE

Problem Solving

A person is nearing the end of life. You want to provide mouth care. The family arrives. Is this a good time to give care? What will you say to the family?

OBJECTIVES

- Define the key terms and key abbreviations in this chapter.
- Identify the sources for jobs and places to work.
- Describe what employers look for when hiring staff.
- Describe how to prove completion of a nursing assistant training and competency evaluation program (NATCEP).
- Explain how to complete a job application.
- Describe in-person, phone, and video interviews.
- Explain how to prepare and dress for an interview.

- Identify common interview questions.
- Explain how to conduct yourself during an interview.
- Describe the questions you cannot be asked during an interview or on a job application.
- Explain what to do after an interview.
- Explain how to accept or decline a job offer.
- Explain how to promote PRIDE in the person, the family, and yourself.

KEY TERMS

discrimination Unjust treatment based on age, race, sex, and other personal qualities
job application An agency's official form listing questions that require factual answers from the person seeking employment

job interview When an employer asks a job applicant questions about his or her education and career
reasonable accommodation To assist or change a position or workplace to allow an employee to do his or her job despite having a disability

KEY ABBREVIATIONS

EEOC Equal Employment Opportunity Commission
NATCEP Nursing assistant training and competency evaluation program

OBRA Omnibus Budget Reconciliation Act of 1987

Successfully completing a nursing assistant training and competency evaluation program (NATCEP) is a step toward employment. During your NATCEP or after, you will likely focus on getting a job. This chapter will help you do so in a professional and efficient manner.

SOURCES OF JOBS

There are easy ways to learn about jobs and places to work.
- Newspaper ads
- Local and state employment services
- Agencies you would like to work at
- Phone book yellow pages
- People you know—instructor, family, and friends
- The Internet
- Your school's or college's job placement counselors
- Job fairs
- Your clinical experience site

Your clinical experience site is an important source. The staff observe students as future employees. They look for good work ethics. They watch how students treat patients, residents, and co-workers. If your clinical agency is not hiring, the staff may suggest other places to apply.

WHAT EMPLOYERS LOOK FOR

If you owned a business, who would you hire? Your answer helps you better understand the agency's point of view. Agencies want staff who:

- Are dependable
- Are well-groomed
- Have needed job skills and training
- Have values and attitudes that fit with the agency

To function well, you need good work ethics. Review Chapter 5 and the *Focus on PRIDE* boxes at the end of each chapter to develop positive attitudes and work practices.

You must be at work on time and when scheduled. Undependable people cause everyone problems. Other staff have extra work. Fewer staff give care. Quality of care suffers. You want co-workers to work when scheduled. Otherwise, you have extra work. You have less time to spend with patients and residents. Likewise, co-workers expect you to work when scheduled.

Job Skills and Training

The agency checks the nursing assistant registry and requests proof of successful NATCEP completion. To prove NATCEP completion, an agency will accept 1 or more of the following.

- A certificate of course completion
- A high school, college, or technical school transcript
- An official grade report (report card)

Give the agency a *copy* of your certificate, transcript, or grade report. Never give the original to anyone. Keep originals in a safe place for future use. Some agencies want a transcript sent directly from the school or college.

See *Promoting Safety and Comfort: Job Skills and Training.*

PROMOTING SAFETY AND COMFORT

Job Skills and Training

Safety

To work in long-term care, you must complete a state-approved NATCEP. This is a requirement of the *Omnibus Budget Reconciliation Act of 1987 (OBRA)*. The agency requests proof of training. The nursing assistant registry is checked. Nursing centers cannot hire persons convicted of abuse, neglect, or mistreatment. This also is an OBRA requirement.

JOB APPLICATIONS

A *job application is an agency's official form listing questions that require factual answers from the person seeking employment* (Fig. 38-1, pp. 544-545). Personal information (legal name, address, phone number), work history, education, qualifications, and references are examples.

You get a job application from the *personnel office (human resources office)* or on-line. For a paper application, use a black pen to complete the form. You can complete the application at the agency. Or you can take it home for return by mail or in person. You must be well-groomed and behave pleasantly when seeking or returning a job application. It may be your first chance to make a good impression.

On-line job applications require a computer. Follow the agency's instructions for completing an on-line application.

Completing a Job Application

To complete a job application, see Box 38-1, p. 546. The application may be your first chance to impress the agency. A neat, readable, and complete application gives a good image. A sloppy or incomplete one does not.

A job application is easier to complete with a file of your education and work history. The file should contain:

- A copy of your high school diploma or general equivalency diploma (GED).
- A copy of any grade reports, degrees, certificates, or military training.
- A copy of your NATCEP certificate of completion.
- Nursing assistant registry information for each state in which you are certified (licensed, registered).
- Copies of communications with your state's nursing assistant registry agency.
- Copies of court records for criminal convictions.
- A copy of your Social Security card.
- Names, addresses, and phone numbers of references.
- Names, addresses, and phone numbers of current and past employers. Include:
  - Your job title
  - Dates employment started and ended
  - Your supervisor's name
  - Hourly salary
- Proof of in-services attended and continuing education units (CEUs).

When requesting a job application, also ask for the agency's nursing assistant job description (Chapter 3).

Text continued on p. 546.

EMPLOYMENT APPLICATION

APPLICANT INSTRUCTIONS

If you need help filling out this application form or for any phase of the employment process, please notify the person that gave you this form and every effort will be made to accommodate your needs in a reasonable amount of time.

1. Please read "APPLICANT NOTE" below.
2. Complete both sides of this page.
3. If more space is needed to complete any question, use comments section at the bottom of this page.
4. Print clearly: incomplete or illegible applications will not be processed. PLEASE NOTE "NOT APPLICABLE" IF NOT ANSWERING A QUESTION.
5. Provide only requested information. Failure to do so may result in disqualification of your application.
6. Some packets may include an AFFIRMATIVE ACTION QUESTIONNAIRE. This information is being gathered for affirmative action under Section 503 of the Rehabilitation Act of 1973. The information is voluntary and will be kept confidential. An applicant will not be subject to any adverse treatment for refusing to complete the questionnaire.
7. DO NOT FILL OUT ANY OTHER ATTACHED FORMS OR PAGES UNTIL INSTRUCTED.

TODAY'S DATE: _____

NAME: _____
LAST   FIRST   MI

SOCIAL SECURITY NUMBER: _____

HOME PHONE: _____ WORK PHONE: _____

CURRENT ADDRESS: _____
STREET

CITY   STATE   ZIP

PRIOR ADDRESS: _____
STREET

CITY   STATE   ZIP

APPLICANT NOTE

This application form is intended for use in evaluating your qualifications for employment. This is not an employment contract. Please answer all appropriate questions completely and accurately. False or misleading statements during the interview and on this form are grounds for terminating the application process or, if discovered after employment, terminating employment. All qualified applicants will receive consideration without discrimination based on sex, marital status, race, color, age, creed, national origin, sexual orientation, military reserve membership, ancestry, religion, height, weight, use of a guide or support animal because of blindness, deafness or physical handicap, or the presence of disabilities. A conviction will not necessarily bar an applicant from employment. Additional testing of job-related skills and for the presence of drugs in your body may be required prior to employment. After an offer of employment, and prior to reporting to work, you may be required to submit to a medical review. Depending on company policy and the needs of the job, you will be required to complete a medical history form and may be required to be examined by a medical professional designated by the company.

AVAILABILITY

For which position are you applying? _____

What date can you start?_____ What category would you prefer? ❑ Full time   ❑ Part time   ❑ Temporary   ❑ Labor pool

For which schedules are you available?* ❑ Weekdays   ❑ Weekends   ❑ Evenings   ❑ Nights   ❑ Overtime   ❑ Shift   ❑ Other_____

*reasonable efforts will be made to accommodate sincerely held moral and ethical beliefs, (WI) religious beliefs and practices (All other States)

JOB-RELATED SKILLS

NOTE: Do not fill out any part of this section you believe to be non-job related.

❑ Yes   ❑ No   If the job requires, do you have the appropriate valid drivers license?
Name on license _____ DL#_____ Type _____ State of Issue_____

❑ Yes   ❑ No   Have you had any moving violations within the last seven years? Please describe._____
Please list any other skills, licenses or certificates that may be job-related or that you feel would be of value to this job or company. _____

❑ Yes   ❑ No   Have you been given a job description or had the essential functions of the job explained to you?

❑ Yes   ❑ No   Do you understand these essential functions?

❑ Yes   ❑ No   Can you perform the essential functions of this job with or without reasonable accommodation?

SECURITY

List states and counties of residence for the past seven years: _____

❑ Yes   ❑ No   Have you used any names or Social Security Numbers other than given above? If so, please list in comments, below.

❑ Yes   ❑ No   Have you been convicted of a crime in the past seven years? If so, please describe in the boxes below. (Conviction will not necessarily be a bar to employment. In accordance with company policy and applicable state and federal laws, factors such as age at time of the offense, remoteness of the offense, time since last conviction, nature of the job sought and rehabilitation effort will be reviewed.)

INCIDENT	CITY/STATE	CHARGE
1.		
2.		

COMMENTS   (ASK FOR AN ADDITIONAL PAGE IF NECESSARY)

_____
_____
_____
_____

FIGURE 38-1 A sample job application. (Courtesy ADP Screening and Selection Services, Ft. Collins, Colo.)

PREVIOUS EMPLOYERS

PLEASE NOTE: Your application will <u>not be</u> considered unless every question in this section is answered. Since we will make every effort to contact previous employers, the **correct telephone numbers of past employers are critical.** Ask for a phone book or call information if necessary. FOR EMPLOYERS OUTSIDE THE U.S., A CURRENT FAX NUMBER IS MANDATORY.

MOST RECENT EMPLOYER   ☐ Yes   ☐ No   Are you currently working for this employer?
☐ Yes   ☐ No   If yes, may we contact?

PHONE (   )
FAX   (   )

COMPANY NAME _____   CITY _____   STATE _____

FROM _____ TO _____
DATES EMPLOYED   JOB TITLE _____   SUPERVISOR NAME _____

DUTIES _____

PER
SALARY _____ (HOUR, WEEK, MONTH)   REASON FOR LEAVING _____

SECOND MOST RECENT EMPLOYER

PHONE (   )
FAX   (   )

COMPANY NAME _____   CITY _____   STATE _____

FROM _____ TO _____
DATES EMPLOYED   JOB TITLE _____   SUPERVISOR NAME _____

DUTIES _____

PER
SALARY _____ (HOUR, WEEK, MONTH)   REASON FOR LEAVING _____

THIRD MOST RECENT EMPLOYER

PHONE (   )
FAX   (   )

COMPANY NAME _____   CITY _____   STATE _____

FROM _____ TO _____
DATES EMPLOYED   JOB TITLE _____   SUPERVISOR NAME _____

DUTIES _____

PER
SALARY _____ (HOUR, WEEK, MONTH)   REASON FOR LEAVING _____

REFERENCES
Include only individuals familiar with your work ability. Do not include relatives.

NAME	ADDRESS/PHONE	YEARS KNOWN/RELATIONSHIP
1.		
2.		

EDUCATION
NOTE: Do not fill out any part of this section you believe to be non-job related.
Please circle highest grade completed.   7   8   9   10   11   12   13   14   15   16   16+

If your school records are under a different name than listed on page 1, please enter that name _____

NAME	CITY/STATE	GRADUATED	DEGREE?
HIGH SCHOOL			
COLLEGE			
OTHER			

CERTIFICATION AND RELEASE
I certify that I have read and understand the applicant note on page one of this form and that the answers given by me to the foregoing questions and the statements made by me are complete and true to the best of my knowledge and belief. I understand that any false information, omissions or misrepresentations of facts called for in this application, whether on this document or not, may result in rejection of my application or discharge at any time during my employment. I authorize the company and/or its agents, including consumer reporting bureaus, to verify any of this information. I authorize all former employers, persons, schools, companies and law enforcement authorities from any liability for any damage whatsoever for issuing this information. I also understand that the use of illegal drugs is prohibited during employment. If company policy requires, I am willing to submit to drug testing to detect the use of illegal drugs prior to and during employment.

SIGNATURE _____   DATE _____

© ADP SCREENING & SELECTION SERVICES 2002

FIGURE 38-1, cont'd

BOX 38-1	Guidelines for Completing a Job Application

- Read and follow the directions. They may ask you to print using black ink. Following directions on the job application gives insight about your ability to follow directions on the job.
- Write neatly. Writing must be readable. A messy application gives a bad image. Readable writing gives the correct information. The agency cannot contact you if unable to read your phone number. You may miss getting the job.
- Complete the entire form. If an item does not apply to you, write "N/A" for non-applicable. Or draw a line through the space. This shows that you read the section. It also shows that you did not skip the item on purpose.
- Report any felony convictions as directed. Write "no" or "none" as appropriate. Criminal background and fingerprint checks are common requirements (Chapter 3).
- Give information about employment gaps. If you did not work for a time, the agency wonders why. Providing this information shows you are honest. Some reasons are an illness, school, raising children, or caring for a family member.
- Tell why you left a job, if asked. Be brief but honest. People leave jobs for one that pays better. Some leave for career advancement. Others leave for reasons given for employment gaps. If fired from a job, give an honest but positive answer. Do not talk badly about the agency.
- Give references. List the names, titles, addresses, and phone numbers of at least 4 non-family references. Have this information written down before completing an application. (Always ask references if an agency can contact them.) You may get the job faster if the agency can check references quickly. The agency should not have to wait for missing or incomplete information. This wastes your time and the agency's time. Also, the agency wonders if you are hiding something with incomplete reference information.
- Be prepared to provide the following.
  - Social Security number
  - Proof of the legal right to work in the United States
  - Proof of successful NATCEP completion
  - Identification—driver's license or government-issued ID card
- Give honest answers. Lying on an application is fraud. It is grounds for being fired.

THE JOB INTERVIEW

A *job interview* is when an employer asks a job applicant questions about his or her education and career. The agency gets to know and evaluate you. You learn about the agency.

The interview may be when you complete the job application. Some agencies review applications before scheduling interviews. An interview may be conducted by 1 person or 2 or more people.

When an interview is scheduled, write down the interviewer's name and the interview date and time. If you need directions to the agency, ask for them when the interview is scheduled.

When expecting a call from the agency, answer your phone. Do not let your phone go to an answering machine or voice mail. If the caller has to leave a message, you need an appropriate and professional greeting.

Types of Interviews

Interviews may be in-person, by phone, or by video. You need good communication skills. (See Chapters 6 and 7.)
- *In-person interview.* You and the interviewer meet in the same room face-to-face. Appropriate dress and body language are needed.
- *Phone interview.* A phone interview may be used to decide if an in-person interview will follow. If distance is a factor, a phone interview may be sufficient for the agency and you.
- *Video interview.* You use a computer at home or another site. Appropriate dress and body language are needed.

For phone and video interviews:
- Use a quiet room. Turn off phones, music, TV, and other electronic devices. Do not use a room where phones ring, people are talking, or pets are present.
- Be ready to answer the phone or turn on the computer at the scheduled time.
- Have your wireless phone or computer charged. Consider plugging into a power source to prevent your computer from turning off.
- Speak clearly and slowly. Do not shout.
- Listen carefully. Let the interviewer finish speaking before you answer.
- Smile. Smile even for a phone interview. Attitude and facial expression affect your voice tone.

Preparing for the Interview

Box 38-2 lists common interview questions. Prepare your answers ahead of time. Also prepare a list of your skills for the interviewer.

You must present a good image. You need to be neat, clean, and well-groomed. How you dress is important. Follow the guidelines in Box 38-3.

Show that you are dependable. No matter the type of interview, be on time. For an in-person interview, do a practice run (dry run). Go to the agency some day before the interview. Note how long it takes to get there and where to park. Also find the personnel office. A practice run gives an idea of the time needed from your home to the personnel office.

When you arrive at the agency, turn off your phone and other devices. Tell the receptionist your name, why you are there, and the interviewer's name. Then sit quietly in the waiting area. Do not smoke, chew gum, or use your phone or other devices for calls, e-mails, text messages, or other reasons. While waiting, review your answers to the common interview questions. Waiting may be part of the interview. The interviewer may ask staff about how you acted while waiting. Smile and be polite and friendly.

BOX 38-2	Common Interview Questions

What the Interviewer May Ask

- Tell me about yourself.
- Tell me about your career goals.
- What are you doing to reach these goals?
- Describe what *professional* behavior means to you.
- Tell me about your last job. Why did you leave?
- What did you like the most about your last job? The least?
- What would your supervisor and co-workers tell me about you? Your dependability? Your skills? Your flexibility?
- Which functions are hard for you? How do you handle this difficulty?
- How do you set priorities?
- How have your experiences prepared you for this job?
- What would you like to change about your last job?
- How do you handle problems with patients, residents, families, and co-workers?
- Why do you want to work here?
- Why should this agency hire you?

What to Ask the Interviewer

- Which job functions are the most important?
- What employee qualities and traits are important to you?
- What nursing care pattern is used here (Chapter 1)?
- Who will I work with?
- When are performance evaluations done? Who does them? How are they done?
- What performance factors are evaluated?
- How does the supervisor handle problems?
- What are the most common reasons that nursing assistants lose their jobs here? What are common reasons for resigning? (To *resign* means *to leave a job.*)
- How do you see this job in the next year? In the next 5 years?
- What is the greatest reward from this job? The greatest challenge?
- What do you like the most about nursing assistants who work here? The least?
- Why should I work here rather than in another agency?
- How much will I make an hour?
- What hours will I work?
- What uniforms are required?
- What benefits do you offer?
  - Health and dental insurance?
  - Continuing education?
  - Vacation time?
- Do you have a new employee orientation program? How long is it?
- May I have a tour of the agency and the unit I will work on? Can I meet the nurse manager and unit staff?
- Can I have a few minutes to talk to the nurse manager?

BOX 38-3	Grooming and Dressing for an Interview

- Bathe and brush your teeth. Wash your hair. Men should shave facial hair or groom beards and mustaches.
- Use deodorant or antiperspirant.
- Make sure your hands and fingernails are clean.
- Apply make-up in a simple, attractive manner.
- Style your hair in a neat and attractive way.
- Do not wear jeans, shorts, tank tops, halter tops, or other casual clothing.
- Iron clothing. Sew on loose buttons and mend garments.
- Wear clothing that covers tattoos (body art).
- Wear a simple dress, skirt or slacks and blouse, or suit (women). Wear a suit or slacks and a shirt (men). A jacket or tie is optional. A long-sleeved white or light blue shirt is best. See Figure 38-2.
- Wear socks (men and women) or hose (women). Hose should be free of runs and snags.
- Make sure shoes are clean and in good repair.
- Avoid heavy perfumes, colognes, and after-shave lotions. A light fragrance is okay.
- Wear only simple jewelry that complements your clothes. Avoid adornments in body piercings. For multiple ear piercings, wear only 1 set of earrings.
- Stop in the restroom when you arrive at the agency. Check your hair, make-up, clothes, and hands.

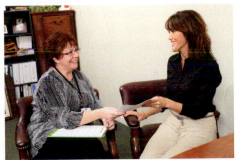
A

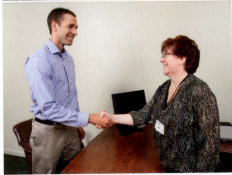
B

FIGURE 38-2 Dress for an interview. **A,** This woman wears a simple blouse and slacks. **B,** This young man wears a simple shirt and slacks.

During the Interview

Politely greet and address the interviewer as Miss, Mrs., Ms., Mr., or Doctor. For an in-person interview, a firm hand-shake is correct for men and women. Stand until asked to sit. Sit with good posture and in a professional way. If offered a beverage, you may accept. Be sure to thank the person.

Good eye contact is needed for in-person and video interviews. Look directly at the interviewer to answer or ask questions. Poor eye contact sends negative information—shy, insecure, dishonest, or lacking interest.

Watch your body language (Chapter 7)—facial expressions, gestures, posture, and body movements. What you say is important. However, your body tells a great deal. Avoid distracting habits—slumping; biting nails; playing with jewelry, clothing, or your hair; crossing your arms; and crossing and swinging legs back and forth. Focus on the interview. Do not touch or read things on the person's desk.

Give complete and honest answers. Speak clearly and with confidence. Avoid short and long answers. "Yes" and "no" answers give little information. Briefly explain "yes" and "no" responses (Chapter 7).

The interviewer will ask about your skills. Share your skills list. An agency-required skill may not be on your list. Explain that you are willing to learn if your state allows nursing assistants to perform the skill.

Review the job description with the interviewer. Ask questions. Advise the interviewer of functions you cannot perform because of training, legal, ethical, or religious reasons. Honesty now prevents problems later.

Find the right job for you. An employer wants to hire staff who will be happy in the job and the agency. Box 38-2 lists some questions for you to ask at the end of the interview. The interviewer's answers will help you decide if the job is right for you.

The interview lasts 15 to 20 minutes. You may be offered a job at this time. Or you are told when to expect a call or letter. Follow-up is acceptable. Ask when you can check on your application. Always thank the interviewer. Say that you look forward to hearing from him or her. Shake the person's hand after an in-person interview.

Questions You Cannot Be Asked

The U.S. Equal Employment Opportunity Commission (EEOC) is a government agency. To guard against discrimination in hiring, the EEOC has guidelines for questions that cannot be asked during an interview or on a job application. *Discrimination* *involves unjust treatment based on age, race, sex, and other personal qualities.* See Box 38-4.

See *Focus on Communication: Questions You Cannot Be Asked.*

BOX 38-4	Interview Questions Not Allowed by the EEOC

- *Age.* Generally, you cannot be asked your age, your birth date, or any question that refers to your age. However, under OBRA, you must be at least 16 years old. Some states have limits on the tasks allowed for persons under 18 years of age.
- *Color, race, gender, or national origin.* This includes questions related to your place of birth or that of your parents; language spoken; or how you learned to read, write, or speak a language.
- *Religion or spiritual beliefs.* You cannot be asked about your religion, religious practices, church, priest or pastor, or religious holidays observed.
- *Sex.* No questions are allowed about sex or your sexuality.
- *Disabilities.* You cannot be asked if you have disabilities or what they are. This includes treatment for alcoholism. However, you can be asked if you can perform the job with reasonable accommodation. *Reasonable accommodation means to assist or change a position or workplace to allow an employee to do his or her job despite having a disability.*
- *Pregnancy or plans for pregnancy.* You cannot be asked if you are pregnant, planning to get pregnant, or about your pregnancy history.
- *Marital status.* You cannot be asked if you are married, single, divorced, separated, engaged, or widowed.
- *Children.* You cannot be asked if you have children, how many children or their ages, or who will care for children while you are at work.
- *Arrest record.* You cannot be asked about arrests. However, you can be asked about criminal convictions.
- *Finances.* You cannot be asked about credit cards or bank accounts or if you own your home or car.
- *Number of sick days used in the last year.* You cannot be asked about your medical history. However, you may have to take a medical exam or have some tests done after a job offer is made.
- *Citizenship.* You cannot be asked if you are a United States citizen. You cannot be asked to provide proof of citizenship. However, if hired, you can be asked to provide proof of the legal right to work in the United States.

FOCUS ON COMMUNICATION

Questions You Cannot Be Asked

If asked a question listed in Box 38-4, you have the right to decline to answer. Decline politely. You can say: "I'm sorry, but the EEOC does not allow you to ask that question. What else can I answer for you?"

After the Interview

A thank-you letter or note is advised within 24 hours after the interview (Fig. 38-3). Write neatly and clearly. Use a computer or typewriter if your writing is hard to read. The thank-you note should include:

- The date
- The interviewer's formal name with Miss, Ms., Mrs., Mr., or Dr.
- A statement thanking the person for the interview
- Comments about the interview, the agency, and your eagerness to hear about the job
- Your signature, using your first and last names

December 12

Dear [Interviewer's name],

Thank you for the interview yesterday. I enjoyed meeting you and learning more about the nursing center. I was impressed by the friendliness of the staff and would enjoy working in that environment.

Again, thank you. I look forward to hearing from you soon.

Sincerely,
[Your full name]

FIGURE 38-3 Sample thank-you note written after a job interview.

ACCEPTING OR DECLINING A JOB OFFER

When you accept a job, agree on a starting date, pay rate, and work hours. Ask where to report on your first day. Ask for all information in writing. That way you and the agency have the same understanding of the job offer. Use the written offer later if questions arise. Also ask for the employee handbook and other agency information. Read everything before you start working.

Accept the best job for you. To decline a job offer, thank the person for offering you a job. If asked why you are refusing, give a positive response. For example: "Thank you for offering me a job. I'm going to accept a job closer to my home."

Sometimes a job is not offered. You may not hear from the agency. Or the agency calls, writes, or e-mails saying that you will not be offered the job. If this happens, thank the person for letting you know. Ask that the agency keep your application active. For example: "Thank you for letting me know. I'm disappointed but please keep me in mind for other openings."

DRUG TESTING

State laws vary about drug testing. Drug testing may be part of the application process. If so, review the job application before signing it. The application usually states 1 of the following (see Fig. 38-1).

- Drug testing is part of the application screening process for new staff.
- A job offer depends on passing a drug test.

FOCUS ON PRIDE
The Person, Family, and Yourself

Personal and Professional Responsibility
Agencies invest much time and money in new staff. Changing jobs often can reflect poorly on you. Before applying, find out about the agency. This helps you decide if the agency is a good fit for you. Also, your interest in the agency can make a good impression during an interview.

Rights and Respect
You have the right to protection from discrimination. Application and interview questions must relate to your ability to do the job. See Box 38-4 for questions that are not allowed.
Job-related questions are allowed if asked to all applicants, regardless of age or gender. These questions are allowed.
- What languages do you read, write, and speak fluently?
- Can you perform the duties of this job? Do you need any special accommodations to perform the job?
- Have you ever been convicted of a crime?
Know your rights. Plan how to respond if you suspect a question violates your rights.

Independence and Social Interaction
Some agencies perform social media background checks. State laws vary about what information can be accessed—public or private. Age, sex, disability, color, race, gender, national origin, or religion must not be considered in hiring decisions. Employers must focus only on information related to the job.
Show good judgment when using social media (Chapter 5). Facebook, Twitter, Instagram, and LinkedIn are examples. Be professional. Agencies may view them.

Delegation and Teamwork
Non–health care work experiences, education, and training are important. They give employers information about your dependability, teamwork, and work quality. Draw from your experiences. Give examples of your positive work ethics.

Ethics and Laws
Patient and resident safety is of great importance. Employers watch for safe and ethical conduct. They must act when conduct is unsafe or unethical. Background checks, drug testing, and interview questions help agencies decide if an applicant will meet safety and ethical standards.
Poor conduct outside of work can affect your job. Take pride in making good choices inside and outside the workplace.

FOCUS ON PRIDE: Application
Being prepared for an interview is helpful. You may be nervous about what questions will be asked, how you will answer, and if you will make a good impression. Describe how you will prepare yourself for a job interview. How will you respond to a question not allowed by the EEOC?

Circle the BEST answer.

1 When should you ask questions about your job description?
a After completing the job application
b Before completing the job application
c When your interview is scheduled
d During the interview

2 Lying on a job application is
a Negligence
b Fraud
c Libel
d Defamation

3 When completing a job application
a Use pencil
b Leave spaces blank that do not apply to you
c Give information about employment gaps
d List family members as references

4 Which do employers look for the *most*?
a Cooperation
b Courtesy
c Empathy
d Dependability

5 What should you wear to a job interview?
a A uniform
b Party clothes
c Slacks and a shirt or blouse
d What is most comfortable

6 For a phone interview you should
a Shout answers so they are heard
b Take another call during the interview
c Have the interviewer leave a message
d Use a quiet room

7 Which is poor behavior during a job interview?
a Crossing your arms and legs
b Good eye contact with the interviewer
c Shaking hands with the interviewer
d Asking the interviewer questions

8 Which is the *best* response to an interview question?
a Brief explanations
b "Yes" or "no"
c Long answers
d A written response

9 An interviewer asks the following. Which should you decline to answer?
a Tell me about yourself.
b Are you married?
c Have you ever been convicted of a crime?
d What are your career goals?

10 After an interview
a Ask if the agency plans to hire you
b Ask to be paid for your time at the interview
c Write a thank-you note
d Do not apply to any other agencies

11 When accepting a job offer, avoid discussing
a Starting date
b Personal finances
c Pay rate
d Work hours

12 Drug testing may be required before an agency hires you.
a True
b False

Answers to Chapter 38 questions are on p. 552.

FOCUS ON PRACTICE

Problem Solving

You are asked the following questions at a job interview. How will you respond to each?
- Why did you decide to become a nursing assistant?
- What are your strengths and weaknesses?
- Describe a problem in your clinical training. How did you resolve it?
- Give an example of when you had to prioritize. How did you decide what to do first, second, and so on?

Review Question Answers

CHAPTER 1
1. d
2. a
3. c
4. b
5. b
6. a
7. d
8. a
9. b
10. a
11. a
12. c
13. c
14. b
15. d

CHAPTER 2
1. T
2. T
3. F
4. T
5. F
6. T
7. F
8. T
9. F
10. F
11. a
12. b
13. c
14. d
15. b
16. a
17. a
18. d
19. c
20. d
21. a
22. c
23. b
24. b

CHAPTER 3
1. T
2. F
3. T
4. F
5. F
6. d
7. c
8. b
9. a
10. c
11. b
12. c
13. d
14. d
15. a

CHAPTER 4
1. c
2. d
3. a
4. b
5. a
6. c
7. b
8. a
9. d
10. c
11. b
12. a
13. b
14. d
15. c
16. b
17. a
18. b
19. c
20. a

CHAPTER 5
1. T
2. T
3. F
4. T
5. T
6. F
7. T
8. F
9. b
10. d
11. c
12. a
13. b
14. a
15. d
16. a
17. c
18. a
19. b
20. a
21. c
22. d

CHAPTER 6
1. F
2. T
3. F
4. F
5. F
6. d
7. c
8. b
9. c
10. a
11. b
12. c
13. b

14. d
15. a
16. a
17. c
18. b
19. c
20. d
21. b
22. a

CHAPTER 7
1. c
2. d
3. b
4. c
5. d
6. d
7. b
8. a
9. b
10. d
11. c
12. d
13. b
14. b
15. c
16. a

CHAPTER 8
1. a
2. b
3. a
4. c
5. c
6. a
7. b
8. c
9. d
10. d
11. c
12. b
13. a
14. b
15. b
16. b
17. c
18. d
19. a
20. d
21. a
22. b

CHAPTER 9
1. b
2. a
3. b
4. d
5. c
6. c
7. a

8. d
9. b
10. d
11. b
12. a
13. a
14. a
15. c
16. d

CHAPTER 10
1. d
2. c
3. c
4. d
5. b
6. d
7. b
8. a
9. c
10. b
11. c
12. b
13. a
14. d
15. b
16. c
17. a
18. c
19. b
20. d

CHAPTER 11
1. a
2. c
3. c
4. a
5. b
6. c
7. d
8. b
9. c
10. b
11. a
12. c
13. c
14. b
15. d

CHAPTER 12
1. F
2. T
3. T
4. F
5. F
6. T
7. T
8. T
9. F
10. F

11. T
12. F
13. F
14. T
15. F
16. d
17. c
18. b
19. c
20. a
21. b
22. a
23. c
24. d

CHAPTER 13
1. F
2. T
3. T
4. F
5. F
6. T
7. F
8. F
9. b
10. b
11. a
12. a
13. b
14. d
15. c
16. c
17. a
18. d
19. c
20. d
21. c
22. b
23. a
24. a
25. c

CHAPTER 14
1. a
2. b
3. c
4. a
5. a
6. c
7. b
8. a
9. d
10. c
11. b
12. b
13. c
14. a

CHAPTER 15
1. c
2. b
3. a
4. b
5. a
6. a
7. b
8. c
9. d
10. b
11. a
12. d
13. d
14. c

CHAPTER 16
1. b
2. d
3. c
4. b
5. b
6. c
7. a
8. d
9. d
10. c
11. b
12. c

CHAPTER 17
1. F
2. T
3. F
4. T
5. F
6. T
7. T
8. T
9. F
10. b
11. d
12. c
13. b
14. a
15. c
16. b
17. a
18. b
19. a
20. c
21. d
22. a
23. b
24. b
25. a

CHAPTER 18
1 T
2 F
3 F
4 F
5 F
6 F
7 T
8 T
9 F
10 F
11 T
12 a
13 c
14 d
15 c
16 b
17 d
18 c
19 a
20 d
21 b
22 b

CHAPTER 19
1 F
2 F
3 T
4 F
5 F
6 d
7 b
8 c
9 a
10 d
11 c
12 b
13 d
14 a
15 c

CHAPTER 20
1 c
2 d
3 a
4 a
5 b
6 b
7 a
8 d
9 c
10 c
11 d
12 a

CHAPTER 21
1 c
2 d
3 a
4 a
5 c
6 b
7 d
8 c
9 a
10 d

CHAPTER 22
1 b
2 a
3 b
4 c
5 c
6 a
7 c
8 d
9 b
10 d
11 c
12 d

CHAPTER 23
1 b
2 b
3 d
4 c
5 d
6 a
7 a
8 c
9 a
10 d
11 b
12 c
13 c
14 d
15 a
16 a
17 c
18 d

CHAPTER 24
1 c
2 b
3 d
4 a
5 d
6 b
7 c
8 d
9 b
10 a
11 b
12 c
13 b
14 a

CHAPTER 25
1 b
2 a
3 c
4 a
5 d
6 c
7 d
8 c
9 c
10 a
11 c
12 d
13 b
14 c
15 d
16 a
17 c
18 c

CHAPTER 26
1 c
2 d
3 b
4 a
5 c
6 d
7 a
8 b

CHAPTER 27
1 T
2 F
3 T
4 F
5 F
6 T
7 T
8 T
9 F
10 F
11 c
12 a
13 a
14 c
15 a
16 d
17 a
18 b

CHAPTER 28
1 c
2 b
3 a
4 d
5 b
6 d
7 a
8 a
9 c
10 b
11 c
12 b
13 a
14 c
15 b
16 a

CHAPTER 29
1 T
2 T
3 T
4 T
5 F
6 T
7 F
8 F
9 b
10 d
11 a
12 c
13 b
14 b
15 d
16 a
17 c
18 a
19 c
20 d
21 c
22 b

CHAPTER 30
1 c
2 c
3 b
4 b
5 d
6 c
7 d
8 a
9 b
10 a
11 c
12 d
13 a
14 c

CHAPTER 31
1 T
2 F
3 T
4 T
5 F
6 T
7 T
8 T
9 c
10 b
11 a
12 d
13 c
14 c

CHAPTER 32
1 b
2 d
3 b
4 a
5 c
6 c
7 d
8 a
9 b
10 a
11 b
12 c
13 d
14 d
15 c

CHAPTER 33
1 b
2 c
3 d
4 b
5 a
6 b
7 d
8 a
9 d
10 c
11 d
12 b
13 a
14 b
15 c
16 b
17 a
18 a
19 c
20 a
21 c
22 a
23 d
24 b
25 c
26 a
27 c
28 d
29 d
30 c
31 c
32 a
33 a
34 d
35 b

CHAPTER 34
1 b
2 b
3 c
4 c
5 a
6 d
7 d
8 c
9 b
10 a
11 b
12 a
13 c
14 a
15 b

CHAPTER 35
1 a
2 d
3 c
4 b
5 a
6 c
7 c
8 a
9 b
10 d
11 b
12 c
13 d
14 a
15 c

CHAPTER 36
1 a
2 c
3 d
4 c
5 b
6 a
7 b
8 b
9 c
10 c
11 d
12 a
13 d
14 b
15 a
16 b
17 c
18 a

CHAPTER 37
1 c
2 b
3 d
4 c
5 b
6 a
7 d
8 c
9 c
10 a
11 b
12 d

CHAPTER 38
1 d
2 b
3 c
4 d
5 c
6 d
7 a
8 a
9 b
10 c
11 b
12 a

The Patient Care Partnership—Understanding Expectations, Rights, and Responsibilities (A Summary)

High-Quality Care
- The hospital provides needed care with skill, compassion, and respect.
- The patient has the right to know the identities of those involved in care.
  - Doctors, nurses, and other staff
  - Students and other trainees

Clean and Safe Setting
- The hospital has policies and procedures to:
  - Avoid mistakes.
  - Prevent abuse or neglect.
- The patient is told of unexpected or significant events.
  - What happened
  - Needed changes in care

Involvement in Care
- The patient has the right to make informed decisions about treatment choices.
  - What are the benefits and risks of each treatment?
  - Is the treatment experimental or part of a research study?
  - What can be expected from treatment?
  - How might long-term effects of treatment affect quality of life?
  - What will the patient and family need to do after hospital discharge?
  - What are the costs of using uncovered services or providers?
- The patient has the right to consent to or refuse treatment. The patient is told of the effects of refusing recommended treatment.
- The patient is expected to give information about:
  - Past illnesses, surgeries, or hospital stays
  - Allergic reactions
  - Drugs or dietary supplements that are taken
  - Any health plan admission requirements
- The health team is expected to respect the patient's health care goals, values, and spiritual beliefs. The patient is responsible for sharing his or her wishes with the doctor, family, and care team.

Involvement in Care—cont'd
- The patient is expected to communicate about who makes decisions when the patient is unable.
- The patient shares *power of attorney*, *living will*, or *advance directive* documents with the doctor, family, and health team (Chapter 37).
- The hospital provides help with making difficult decisions. Counselors or chaplains are available.

Protection of Privacy
- The hospital protects the confidentiality of:
  - The patient's relationships with the doctor and health team
  - Information about the patient's health and care
- The hospital provides a "Notice of Privacy Practices" describing:
  - How patient information is used, disclosed, and protected
  - How to obtain a copy of the hospital's records about patient care

Preparing to Leave the Hospital
- The hospital helps identify sources for follow-up care. The hospital's financial interest in any referrals is disclosed.
- The hospital coordinates hospital activities with community caregivers. The hospital requests permission to share information about care.
- The hospital provides information and training about self-care in the home setting.

Help With Bills and Insurance Claims
- The hospital files insurance, Medicare, or Medicaid claims.
- Patients can contact the business office for questions about insurance coverage.
- The hospital tries to help patients find financial help or make other arrangements if the person is without health coverage. The patient provides needed information to obtain coverage or assistance.

Modified from American Hospital Association: *The patient care partnership: understanding expectations, rights, and responsibilities.*

Appendix B

National Nurse Aide Assessment Program (NNAAP®) Written Examination Content Outline

The NNAAP® written examination is comprised of 70 multiple-choice items; 10 of these items are pretest (non-scored) items on which statistical information will be collected.

I   Physical Care Skills

- **A** Activities of Daily Living   14% of exam
  - 1 Hygiene
  - 2 Dressing and Grooming
  - 3 Nutrition and Hydration
  - 4 Elimination
  - 5 Rest/Sleep/Comfort
- **B** Basic Nursing Skills   39% of exam
  - 1 Infection Control
  - 2 Safety/Emergency
  - 3 Therapeutic and Technical Procedures
  - 4 Data Collection and Reporting
- **C** Restorative Skills   8% of exam
  - 1 Prevention
  - 2 Self Care/Independence

II Psychosocial Care Skills

- **A** Emotional and Mental Health Needs   11% of exam
- **B** Spiritual and Cultural Needs   2% of exam

III Role of the Nurse Aide

- **A** Communication   8% of exam
- **B** Client Rights   7% of exam
- **C** Legal and Ethical Behavior   3% of exam
- **D** Member of the Health Care Team   8% of exam

National Nurse Aide Assessment Program (NNAAP®) Skills Evaluation

List of Skills

1 Hand hygiene (hand washing)
2 Applies one knee-high elastic stocking
3 Assists to ambulate using transfer belt
4 Assists with use of bedpan
5 Cleans upper or lower denture
6 Counts and records radial pulse
7 Counts and records respirations
8 Donning and removing PPE (gown and gloves)
9 Dresses client with affected (weak) right arm
10 Feeds client who cannot feed self
11 Gives modified bed bath (face and one arm, hand and underarm)
12 Measures and records blood pressure
13 Measures and records urinary output
14 Measures and records weight of ambulatory client
15 Performs modified passive range of motion (PROM) for one knee and one ankle
16 Performs modified passive range of motion (PROM) for one shoulder
17 Positions on side
18 Provides catheter care for female
19 Provides foot care on one foot
20 Provides mouth care
21 Provides perineal care (peri-care) for female
22 Transfers from bed to wheelchair using transfer belt

Minimum Data Set: Selected Pages
Sample Pages from Functional Status Form

Resident _____   Identifier _____   Date _____

Section G	Functional Status

G0110. Activities of Daily Living (ADL) Assistance
Refer to the ADL flow chart in the RAI manual to facilitate accurate coding

Instructions for Rule of 3
- When an activity occurs three times at any one given level, code that level.
- When an activity occurs three times at multiple levels, code the most dependent, exceptions are total dependence (4), activity must require full assist every time, and activity did not occur (8), activity must not have occurred at all. Example, three times extensive assistance (3) and three times limited assistance (2), code extensive assistance (3).
- When an activity occurs at various levels, but not three times at any given level, apply the following:
  - When there is a combination of full staff performance, and extensive assistance, code extensive assistance.
  - When there is a combination of full staff performance, weight bearing assistance and/or non-weight bearing assistance code limited assistance (2).

If none of the above are met, code supervision.

1. ADL Self-Performance
Code for **resident's performance** over all shifts - not including setup. If the ADL activity occurred 3 or more times at various levels of assistance, code the most dependent - except for total dependence, which requires full staff performance every time

Coding:

Activity Occurred 3 or More Times

0. **Independent** - no help or staff oversight at any time
1. **Supervision** - oversight, encouragement or cueing
2. **Limited assistance** - resident highly involved in activity; staff provide guided maneuvering of limbs or other non-weight-bearing assistance
3. **Extensive assistance** - resident involved in activity, staff provide weight-bearing support
4. **Total dependence** - full staff performance every time during entire 7-day period

Activity Occurred 2 or Fewer Times

7. **Activity occurred only once or twice** - activity did occur but only once or twice
8. **Activity did not occur** - activity did not occur or family and/or non-facility staff provided care 100% of the time for that activity over the entire 7-day period

2. ADL Support Provided
Code for **most support provided** over all shifts; code regardless of resident's self-performance classification

Coding:

0. **No** setup or physical help from staff
1. **Setup** help only
2. **One** person physical assist
3. **Two+** persons physical assist
8. ADL activity itself **did not occur** or family and/or non-facility staff provided care 100% of the time for that activity over the entire 7-day period

	1. Self-Performance	2. Support
	↓ Enter Codes in Boxes ↓	
A. Bed mobility - how resident moves to and from lying position, turns side to side, and positions body while in bed or alternate sleep furniture	☐	☐
B. Transfer - how resident moves between surfaces including to or from: bed, chair, wheelchair, standing position (**excludes** to/from bath/toilet)	☐	☐
C. Walk in room - how resident walks between locations in his/her room	☐	☐
D. Walk in corridor - how resident walks in corridor on unit	☐	☐
E. Locomotion on unit - how resident moves between locations in his/her room and adjacent corridor on same floor. If in wheelchair, self-sufficiency once in chair	☐	☐
F. Locomotion off unit - how resident moves to and returns from off-unit locations (e.g., areas set aside for dining, activities or treatments). **If facility has only one floor**, how resident moves to and from distant areas on the floor. If in wheelchair, self-sufficiency once in chair	☐	☐
G. Dressing - how resident puts on, fastens and takes off all items of clothing, including donning/removing a prosthesis or TED hose. Dressing includes putting on and changing pajamas and housedresses	☐	☐
H. Eating - how resident eats and drinks, regardless of skill. Do not include eating/drinking during medication pass. Includes intake of nourishment by other means (e.g., tube feeding, total parenteral nutrition, IV fluids administered for nutrition or hydration)	☐	☐
I. Toilet use - how resident uses the toilet room, commode, bedpan, or urinal; transfers on/off toilet; cleanses self after elimination; changes pad; manages ostomy or catheter; and adjusts clothes. Do not include emptying of bedpan, urinal, bedside commode, catheter bag or ostomy bag	☐	☐
J. Personal hygiene - how resident maintains personal hygiene, including combing hair, brushing teeth, shaving, applying makeup, washing/drying face and hands (**excludes** baths and showers)	☐	☐

Resident _____   Identifier _____   Date _____

Section G	**Functional Status**

G0120. Bathing

How resident takes full-body bath/shower, sponge bath, and transfers in/out of tub/shower (**excludes** washing of back and hair). Code for **most dependent** in self-performance and support

Enter Code ☐

A. Self-performance
   0. **Independent** - no help provided
   1. **Supervision** - oversight help only
   2. **Physical help limited to transfer only**
   3. **Physical help in part of bathing activity**
   4. **Total dependence**
   8. **Activity itself did not occur** or family and/or non-facility staff provided care 100% of the time for that activity over the entire 7-day period

Enter Code ☐

B. Support provided
   (Bathing support codes are as defined in item **G0110 column 2, ADL Support Provided**, above)

G0300. Balance During Transitions and Walking

After observing the resident, **code the following walking and transition items for most dependent**

Coding:
   0. **Steady at all times**
   1. **Not steady, but <u>able</u> to stabilize without staff assistance**
   2. **Not steady, <u>only able</u> to stabilize with staff assistance**
   8. **Activity did not occur**

↓ **Enter Codes in Boxes**

☐	**A. Moving from seated to standing position**
☐	**B. Walking** (with assistive device if used)
☐	**C. Turning around** and facing the opposite direction while walking
☐	**D. Moving on and off toilet**
☐	**E. Surface-to-surface transfer** (transfer between bed and chair or wheelchair)

G0400. Functional Limitation in Range of Motion

Code for limitation that interfered with daily functions or placed resident at risk of injury

Coding:
   0. **No impairment**
   1. **Impairment on one side**
   2. **Impairment on both sides**

↓ **Enter Codes in Boxes**

☐	**A. Upper extremity** (shoulder, elbow, wrist, hand)
☐	**B. Lower extremity** (hip, knee, ankle, foot)

G0600. Mobility Devices

↓ **Check all that were normally used**

☐	**A. Cane/crutch**
☐	**B. Walker**
☐	**C. Wheelchair** (manual or electric)
☐	**D. Limb prosthesis**
☐	**Z. None of the above** were used

G0900. Functional Rehabilitation Potential
Complete only if A0310A = 01

Enter Code ☐

A. Resident believes he or she is capable of increased independence in at least some ADLs
   0. **No**
   1. **Yes**
   9. **Unable to determine**

Enter Code ☐

B. Direct care staff believe resident is capable of increased independence in at least some ADLs
   0. **No**
   1. **Yes**

From Centers for Medicare & Medicaid Services: MDS 3.0, http://www.cms.gov/Medicare/Quality-Initiatives-Patient-Assessment-Instruments/NursingHomeQualityInits/MDS30RAIManual.html.

Glossary

A

abduction Moving a body part away from the mid-line of the body

abuse The willful infliction of injury, unreasonable confinement, intimidation, or punishment that results in physical harm, pain, or mental anguish; depriving the person (or the person's caregiver) of the goods or services needed to attain or maintain well-being

acetone See "ketone"

activities of daily living (ADL) The activities usually done during a normal day in a person's life

acute illness A sudden illness from which the person is expected to recover

addiction A chronic disease involving substance seeking behaviors and use that is compulsive and hard to control despite the harmful effects

adduction Moving a body part toward the mid-line of the body

admission The official entry of a person into a health care setting

advance directive A document stating a person's wishes about health care when that person cannot make his or her own decisions

alopecia Hair loss

ambulation The act of walking

anaphylaxis A life-threatening sensitivity to an antigen

anorexia The loss of appetite

antibiotic A drug that kills certain microbes that cause infection

antisepsis The processes, procedures, and chemical treatments that kill microbes or prevent them from causing an infection; *anti* means *against* and *sepsis* means *infection*

anxiety A vague, uneasy feeling in response to stress

aphasia The total or partial loss (*a*) of the ability to use or understand language (*phasia*)

apnea The lack or absence (*a*) of breathing (*pnea*)

arthritis Joint (*arthr*) inflammation (*itis*)

arthroplasty The surgical replacement (*plasty*) of a joint (*arthro*)

artery A blood vessel that carries blood away from the heart

asepsis The absence (*a*) of disease-producing microbes (*sepsis* means *infection*)

aspiration Breathing fluid, food, vomitus, or an object into the lungs

assault Intentionally attempting or threatening to touch a person's body without the person's consent

assisted living residence (ALR) Provides housing, personal care, support services, health care, and social activities in a home-like setting to persons needing help with daily activities

atrophy The decrease in size or wasting away of tissue

autopsy The examination of the body after death

B

base of support The area on which an object rests

battery Touching a person's body without his or her consent

bed mobility How a person moves to and from a lying position, turns from side to side, and re-positions in a bed or other furniture

bed rail A device that serves as a guard or barrier along the side of the bed; side rail

benign tumor A tumor that does not spread to other body parts

biohazardous waste Items contaminated with blood, body fluids, secretions, or excretions; *bio* means *life* and *hazardous* means *dangerous or harmful*

blindness The absence of sight

blood pressure (BP) The amount of force exerted against the walls of an artery by the blood

body alignment The way the head, trunk, arms, and legs are aligned with one another; posture

body language Messages sent through facial expressions, gestures, posture, hand and body movements, gait, eye contact, and appearance

body mechanics Using the body in an efficient and careful way

body temperature The amount of heat in the body that is a balance between the amount of heat produced and the amount lost by the body

bony prominence An area where the bone sticks out or projects from the flat surface of the body; pressure point

boundary crossing A brief act or behavior of being over-involved with the person; the intent of the act or behavior is to meet the person's needs

boundary sign Acts, behaviors, or thoughts that warn of a boundary crossing or boundary violation

boundary violation An act or behavior that meets your needs, not the person's

bradypnea Slow (*brady*) breathing (*pnea*); respirations are fewer than 12 per minute

braille A touch reading and writing system that uses raised dots for each letter of the alphabet; the first 10 letters also represent the numbers 0 through 9

bullying Repeated attacks or threats of fear, distress, or harm by a bully toward a victim

C

calorie The fuel or energy value of food

cancer See "malignant tumor"

capillary A very tiny blood vessel; food, oxygen, and other substances pass from capillaries into the cells

cardiac arrest See "sudden cardiac arrest"

carrier A human or animal that is a reservoir for microbes but does not develop the infection

catheter A tube used to drain or inject fluid through a body opening

catheterization The process of inserting a catheter

cell The basic unit of body structure

certification Official recognition by a state that standards or requirements have been met

chart See "medical record"

chemical restraint Any drug used for discipline or convenience and not required to treat medical symptoms

Cheyne-Stokes respirations Respirations gradually increase in rate and depth and then become shallow and slow; breathing may stop (apnea) for 10 to 20 seconds

child abuse and neglect The intentional harm or mistreatment of a child under 18 years old; it involves any recent act or failure to act on the part of a parent or caregiver; it results in death, serious physical or emotional harm, sexual abuse, or exploitation; and it presents a likely or immediate risk for harm

chronic illness An on-going illness that is slow or gradual in onset; it has no known cure; it can be controlled and complications prevented with proper treatment

circumcised The fold of skin (foreskin) covering the glans of the penis was surgically removed

civil law Laws concerned with relationships between people

clean technique See "medical asepsis"

cognitive function Involves memory, thinking, reasoning, ability to understand, judgment, and behavior

colostomy A surgically created opening (stomy) between the colon (colo) and the body's surface

coma A state of being unaware of one's setting and being unable to react or respond to people, places, or things

comatose Being unable to respond to stimuli

communicable disease A disease caused by pathogens that spread easily; contagious disease

communication The exchange of information—a message sent is received and correctly interpreted by the intended person

compulsion Repeating an act over and over again (a ritual)

condom catheter A soft sheath that slides over the penis and is used to drain urine

confidentiality Trusting others with personal and private information

confusion A state of being disoriented to person, time, place, situation, or identity

constipation The passage of a hard, dry stool

constrict To narrow

contagious disease See "communicable disease"

contamination The process of becoming unclean

contracture The lack of joint mobility caused by abnormal shortening of a muscle

convulsion See "seizure"

crime An act that violates a criminal law

criminal law Laws concerned with offenses against the public and society in general

cross-contamination Passing microbes from 1 person to another by contaminated hands, equipment, or supplies

culture The characteristics of a group of people—language, values, beliefs, habits, likes, dislikes, and customs—passed from 1 generation to the next

cyanosis Bluish color (cyano) to the skin, lips, mucous membranes, and nail beds

D

dandruff Excessive amounts of dry, white flakes from the scalp

deafness Hearing loss in which it is impossible for the person to understand speech through hearing alone

defamation Injuring a person's name and reputation by making false statements to a third person

defecation The process of excreting feces from the rectum through the anus; a bowel movement

defense mechanism An unconscious reaction that blocks unpleasant or threatening feelings

dehydration A decrease in the amount of water in body tissues

delegate To authorize another person to perform a nursing task in a certain situation

delirium A state of sudden, severe confusion and rapid changes in brain function

delusion A false belief

delusion of grandeur An exaggerated belief about one's importance, wealth, power, or talents

delusion of persecution A false belief that one is being mistreated, abused, or harassed

dementia The loss of cognitive and social function caused by changes in the brain; the loss of cognitive function that interferes with routine personal, social, and occupational activities

denture An artificial tooth or a set of artificial teeth

detoxification The process of removing a toxic substance from the body

development Changes in mental, emotional, and social function

developmental task A skill that must be completed during a stage of development

diarrhea The frequent passage of liquid stools

diastolic pressure The pressure in the arteries when the heart is at rest

digestion The process that breaks down food physically and chemically so it can be absorbed for use by the cells

dilate To expand or open wider

disability Any lost, absent, or impaired physical or mental function

disaster A sudden, catastrophic event in which people are injured and killed and property is destroyed

discomfort See "pain"

discrimination Unjust treatment based on age, race, sex, and other personal qualities

disinfection The process of killing pathogens

dorsal recumbent position The back-lying or supine position

dorsiflexion Bending the toes and foot up at the ankle

dysphagia Difficulty (*dys*) swallowing (*phagia*)

dyspnea Difficult, labored, or painful (*dys*) breathing (*pnea*)

dysuria Painful or difficult (*dys*) urination (*uria*); burning on urination

E

edema The swelling of body tissues with water

elder abuse Any knowing, intentional, or negligent act by a caregiver or any other person to an older adult; the act causes harm or serious risk of harm

electronic health record (EHR) An electronic version of a person's medical record; electronic medical record

electronic medical record (EMR) See "electronic health record"

elopement When a patient or resident leaves the agency without staff knowledge

emesis See "vomitus"

enabler A device that limits freedom of movement but is used to promote independence, comfort, or safety

end-of-life care The support and care given during the time surrounding death

end-of-shift report A report that the nurse gives at the end of the shift to the on-coming shift; change-of-shift report

endorsement A state recognizes the certificate, license, or registration issued by another state; reciprocity or equivalency

enema The introduction of fluid into the rectum and lower colon

enteral nutrition Giving nutrients into the gastro-intestinal (GI) tract (*enteral*) through a feeding tube

entrapment Getting caught, trapped, or entangled in spaces created by the bed rails, the mattress, the bed frame, the head-board, or the foot-board

equivalency See "endorsement"

ergonomics The science of designing the job to fit the worker; *ergo* means *work*, *nomos* means *law*

eschar Thick, leathery dead tissue that may be loose or adhered to the skin; it is often black or brown

ethics Knowledge of what is right conduct and wrong conduct

extension Straightening a body part

external rotation Turning the joint outward

F

fainting The sudden loss of consciousness from an inadequate blood supply to the brain

false imprisonment Unlawful restraint or restriction of a person's freedom of movement

fecal impaction The prolonged retention and buildup of feces in the rectum

fecal incontinence The inability to control the passage of feces and gas through the anus

feces The semi-solid mass of waste products in the colon that is expelled through the anus; stool or stools

fever Elevated body temperature

first aid The emergency care given to an ill or injured person before medical help arrives

flashback Reliving a trauma in thoughts during the day and in nightmares during sleep

flatulence The excessive formation of gas or air in the stomach and intestines

flatus Gas or air passed through the anus

flexion Bending a body part

flow rate The number of drops per minute (gtt/min) or milliliters per hour (mL/hr)

footdrop The foot falls down at the ankle; permanent plantar flexion

Fowler's position A semi-sitting position; the head of the bed is raised between 45 and 60 degrees

fracture A broken bone

fraud Saying or doing something to trick, fool, or deceive a person

freedom of movement Any change in place or position of the body or any part of the body that the person is able to control

friction The rubbing of 1 surface against another

full visual privacy Having the means to be completely free from public view while in bed

functional incontinence The person has bladder control but cannot use the toilet in time

G

gait belt See "transfer belt"

gavage The process of giving a tube feeding

geriatrics The care of aging people

gerontology The study of the aging process

glucosuria Sugar (*glucose*) in the urine (*uria*)

gossip To spread rumors or talk about the private matters of others

graduate A measuring container for fluid

growth The physical changes that are measured and that occur in a steady, orderly manner

H

hallucination Seeing, hearing, smelling, or feeling something that is not real

harassment To trouble, torment, offend, or worry a person by one's behavior or comments

hazardous chemical Any chemical that is a physical hazard or a health hazard

health team The many health care workers whose skills and knowledge focus on the person's total care; interdisciplinary health care team

healthcare-associated infection (HAI) An infection that develops in a person cared for in any setting where health care is given; the infection is related to receiving health care

hearing loss Not being able to hear the range of sounds associated with normal hearing

hematuria Blood (*hemat*) in the urine (*uria*)

hemiplegia Paralysis (*plegia*) on 1 side (*hemi*) of the body

hemoglobin The substance in red blood cells that carries oxygen and gives blood its red color

hemoptysis Bloody (*hemo*) sputum (*ptysis* means *to spit*)

hemorrhage The excessive loss of blood in a short time

high-Fowler's position A semi-sitting position; the head of the bed is raised 60 to 90 degrees

hirsutism Excessive body hair

holism A concept that considers the whole person; the whole person has physical, social, psychological, and spiritual parts that are woven together and cannot be separated

hormone A chemical substance secreted by the endocrine glands into the bloodstream

hospice A health care agency or program for persons who are dying

hydration Having an adequate amount of water in body tissues

hyperextension Excessive straightening of a body part

hypertension When the systolic pressure is 130 mm Hg or higher (*hyper*) or the diastolic pressure is 80 mm Hg or higher

hyperventilation Breathing (*ventilation*) is rapid (*hyper*) and deeper than normal

hypotension When the systolic pressure is below (*hypo*) 90 mm Hg or the diastolic pressure is below 60 mm Hg

hypoventilation Breathing (*ventilation*) is slow (*hypo*), shallow, and sometimes irregular

hypoxia Cells do not have enough (*hypo*) oxygen (*oxia*)

I

ileostomy A surgically created opening (*stomy*) between the ileum (small intestine [*ileo*]) and the body's surface

immunity Protection against a disease or condition; the person will not get or be affected by the disease

indwelling catheter A catheter left in the bladder so urine drains constantly into a drainage bag; retention or Foley catheter

infection A disease state resulting from the invasion and growth of microbes in the body

infection control Practices and procedures that prevent the spread of infection

informed consent The process by which a person receives and understands information about a treatment or procedure and is able to decide if he or she will receive it

insomnia A chronic condition in which the person cannot sleep or stay asleep all night

intact skin Normal skin and skin layers without damage or breaks

intake The amount of fluid taken in; input

internal rotation Turning the joint inward

intimate partner violence (IPV) Physical, sexual, or psychological harm by a current or former partner or spouse

intravenous (IV) therapy Giving fluids through a needle or catheter inserted into a vein; IV and IV infusion

invasion of privacy Violating a person's right not to have his or her name, photo, or private affairs exposed or made public without giving consent

involuntary seclusion Separating the person from others against his or her will, keeping the person to a certain area, or keeping the person away from his or her room without consent

J

job application An agency's official form listing questions that require factual answers from the person seeking employment

job description A document that describes what the agency expects you to do

job interview When an employer asks a job applicant questions about his or her education and career

joint The point at which 2 or more bones meet to allow movement

K

ketone A substance appearing in urine from the rapid breakdown of fat for energy; acetone, ketone body

ketone body See "ketone"

Kussmaul respirations Very deep and rapid respirations

L

lateral position The person lies on 1 side or the other; side-lying position

law A rule of conduct made by a government body

libel Making false statements in print, in writing (including e-mail and text messages), through pictures or drawings, through broadcast (radio, TV, or video), posted on-line on websites, or through video sites and social media sites

lice See "pediculosis"

licensed practical nurse (LPN) A nurse who has completed a practical nursing program and has passed a licensing test; called licensed vocational nurse (LVN) in California and Texas

licensed vocational nurse (LVN) See "licensed practical nurse (LPN)"

logrolling Turning the person as a unit, in alignment, with 1 motion

low vision Vision loss that cannot be corrected with eyeglasses, contact lenses, drugs, or surgery; vision loss interferes with every-day activities

M

malignant tumor A tumor that invades and destroys nearby tissues and can spread to other body parts; cancer

malpractice Negligence by a professional person

medical asepsis Practices used to reduce the number of microbes and prevent their spread from 1 person or place to another person or place; clean technique

medical record The legal account of a person's condition and response to treatment and care; chart

medical symptom An indication or characteristic of a physical or psychological condition

menopause When menstruation stops and menstrual cycles end; there has been at least 1 year without a menstrual period

menstruation The process in which the lining of the uterus (endometrium) breaks up and is discharged from the body through the vagina

mental Relating to the mind; something that exists in the mind or is done by the mind

mental health The person copes with and adjusts to every-day stresses in ways accepted by society

mental health disorder A disturbance in the ability to cope with or adjust to stress; behavior and function are impaired; mental illness, psychiatric disorder

metabolism The burning of food for heat and energy by the cells

metastasis The spread of cancer to other body parts

microbe See "microorganism"

microorganism A small (*micro*) living thing (*organism*) seen only with a microscope; microbe

mixed incontinence The combination of stress incontinence and urge incontinence

musculo-skeletal disorders Injuries and disorders of the muscles, tendons, ligaments, joints, and cartilage

N

need Something necessary or desired for maintaining life and mental well-being

neglect The failure of responsible persons to provide food and water, shelter, health care, or protection for a vulnerable person

negligence An unintentional wrong in which a person did not act in a reasonable and careful manner and a person or the person's property was harmed

nocturia Frequent urination (*uria*) at night (*noc*)

non-pathogen A microbe that does not usually cause an infection

nonverbal communication Communication that does not use words

nursing assistant A person who has passed a nursing assistant training and competency evaluation program (NATCEP); performs delegated nursing tasks under the supervision of a licensed nurse

nursing care plan A written guide about the person's nursing care; care plan

nursing diagnosis A health problem that can be treated by nursing measures

nursing process The method nurses use to plan and deliver nursing care; its 5 steps are assessment, nursing diagnosis, planning, implementation, and evaluation

nursing task Nursing care or a nursing function, procedure, activity, or work that can be delegated to nursing assistants when it does not require a nurse's professional knowledge or judgment

nursing team Those who provide nursing care—RNs, LPNs/LVNs, and nursing assistants

nutrient A substance that is ingested, digested, absorbed, and used by the body

nutrition The processes involved in the ingestion, digestion, absorption, and use of food and fluids by the body

O

objective data Information that is seen, heard, felt, or smelled by an observer; signs

observation Using the senses of sight, hearing, touch, and smell to collect information

obsession A frequent, upsetting thought, idea, or image

oliguria Scant amount (*olig*) of urine (*uria*); less than 500 mL in 24 hours

ombudsman Someone who supports or promotes the needs and interests of another person

opposition Touching an opposite finger with the thumb

oral hygiene Mouth care

organ Groups of tissue with the same function

orthopnea Breathing (*pnea*) deeply and comfortably only when sitting (*ortho*)

orthopneic position Sitting up (*ortho*) and leaning over a table to breathe (*pneic*)

orthostatic hypotension Abnormally low (*hypo*) blood pressure when the person suddenly stands up (*ortho* and *static*); postural hypotension

orthotic device A device used to support a muscle, promote a certain motion, or correct a deformity; *ortho* means *to straighten*

ostomy A surgically created opening that connects an internal organ to the body's surface; see "colostomy" and "ileostomy"

output The amount of fluid lost

over-flow incontinence Small amounts of urine leak from a full bladder

oxygen concentration The amount (percent) of hemoglobin containing oxygen

P

pain To ache, hurt, or be sore; discomfort

palliative care Care that involves relieving or reducing the intensity of uncomfortable symptoms without producing a cure

panic An intense and sudden feeling of fear, anxiety, terror, or dread

paralysis Loss of muscle function, sensation, or both

paranoia A disorder (*para*) of the mind (*noia*); false beliefs (delusions) and suspicion about a person or situation

paraplegia Paralysis in the legs, lower trunk, and pelvic organs

pathogen A microbe that is harmful and can cause an infection

pediculosis Infestation with wingless insects that feed on blood; lice

perineal care Cleaning the genital and anal areas; pericare

peristalsis Involuntary muscle contractions in the digestive system that move food down the esophagus through the alimentary canal

phobia An intense fear

physical restraint Any manual method or physical or mechanical device, material, or equipment attached to or near the person's body that he or she cannot remove easily and that restricts freedom of movement or normal access to one's body

pivot To turn one's body from a set standing position

planning Setting priorities and goals

plantar flexion The foot (*plantar*) is bent (*flexion*); bending the foot down at the ankle

pneumonia Inflammation and infection of lung tissue

poison Any substance harmful to the body when ingested, inhaled, injected, or absorbed through the skin

polyuria Abnormally large amounts (*poly*) of urine (*uria*)

post-mortem care Care of the body after (*post*) death (*mortem*)

postural hypotension See "orthostatic hypotension"

posture See "body alignment"

pressure injury Localized damage to the skin and underlying soft tissue; the injury is usually over a bony prominence or related to a medical or other device and results from pressure or pressure in combination with shear

pressure point See "bony prominence"

priority The most important thing at the time

professional boundary That which separates helpful behaviors from behaviors that are not helpful

professional sexual misconduct An act, behavior, or comment that is sexual in nature

professionalism Following laws, being ethical, having good work ethics, and having the skills to do your work

pronation Turning the joint downward

prone position Lying on the abdomen with the head turned to 1 side

prosthesis An artificial replacement for a missing body part

protected health information Identifying information and information about the person's health care that is maintained or sent in any form (paper, electronic, oral)

psychosis A state of severe mental impairment

pulse The beat of the heart felt at an artery as a wave of blood passes through the artery

pulse oximetry Measures (*metry*) the oxygen (*oxi*) concentration in arterial blood

pulse rate The number of heartbeats or pulses in 1 minute

Q

quadriplegia Paralysis in the arms, legs, trunk, and pelvic organs; tetraplegia

R

range of motion (ROM) The movement of a joint to the extent possible without causing pain

reasonable accommodation To assist or change a position or workplace to allow an employee to do his or her job despite having a disability

reciprocity See "endorsement"

recording The written account of care and observations; charting

reflex incontinence Urine is lost at predictable intervals when a specific amount of urine is in the bladder

registered nurse (RN) A nurse who has completed a 2-, 3-, or 4-year nursing program and has passed a licensing test

regurgitation The backward flow of stomach contents into the mouth

rehabilitation The process of restoring the person to his or her highest possible level of physical, psychological, social, and economic function

reincarnation The belief that the spirit or soul is reborn in another human body or in another form of life

religion Spiritual beliefs, needs, and practices

remove easily The manual method, device, material, or equipment used to restrain the person that can be removed intentionally by the person in the same manner it was applied by the staff

reporting The oral account of care and observations

representative A person with the legal right to act on the patient's or resident's behalf when he or she cannot do so for himself or herself

respiration The process of supplying the cells with oxygen and removing carbon dioxide from them; breathing air into (inhalation) and out of (exhalation) the lungs

respiratory arrest Breathing stops but heart action continues for several minutes

restorative aide A nursing assistant with special training in restorative nursing and rehabilitation skills

restorative nursing care Care that helps persons regain health, strength, and independence

resuscitate To revive from apparent death or unconsciousness using emergency measures

reverse Trendelenburg's position The head of the bed is raised and the foot of the bed is lowered

rigor mortis The stiffness or rigidity (*rigor*) of skeletal muscles that occurs after death (*mortis*)

rotation Turning the joint

S

scabies A skin disorder caused by a female mite

seizure Violent and sudden contractions or tremors of muscle groups caused by abnormal electrical activity in the brain; convulsion

self-neglect A person's behaviors and way of living that threaten his or her health, safety, and well-being

semi-Fowler's position The head of the bed is raised 30 degrees; or the head of the bed is raised 30 degrees and the knee portion is raised 15 degrees

semi-prone side position See "Sims' position"

sexuality The physical, emotional, social, cultural, and spiritual factors that affect a person's feelings and attitudes about his or her sex

shear When layers of the skin rub against each other; when the skin remains in place and underlying tissues move and stretch, tearing underlying capillaries and blood vessels and causing tissue damage

shearing When the skin sticks to a surface while muscles slide in the direction the body is moving

shock Results when tissues and organs do not get enough blood

side-lying position See "lateral position"

signs See "objective data"

Sims' position A left side-lying position in which the upper leg (right leg) is sharply flexed so it is not on the lower leg (left leg) and the lower arm (left arm) is behind the person; semi-prone side position

skin tear A break or rip in the outer layers of the skin; the epidermis (top skin layer) separates from the underlying tissues

slander Making false statements through the spoken word, sounds, sign language, or gestures

sleep deprivation The amount and quality of sleep are decreased

sleepwalking The sleeping person leaves the bed and walks about

slough Dead tissue that is shed from the skin; it is usually light colored, soft, and moist; may be stringy at times

sputum Mucus from the respiratory system that is expectorated (expelled) through the mouth

sterile The absence of *all* microbes

sterilization The process of destroying *all* microbes

stoma A surgically created opening seen on the body's surface; see "colostomy" and "ileostomy"

stool Excreted feces

stethoscope An instrument used to listen to the sounds produced by the heart, lungs, and other body organs

straight catheter A catheter that drains the bladder and then is removed

stress The response or change in the body caused by any emotional, physical, social, or economic factor

stress incontinence When urine leaks during exercise and certain movements that cause pressure on the bladder

subjective data Things a person tells you about that you cannot observe through your senses; symptoms

sudden cardiac arrest (SCA) The heart stops suddenly and without warning; cardiac arrest

suffocation When breathing stops from the lack of oxygen

suicide To kill oneself on purpose

suicide contagion Exposure to suicide or suicidal behaviors within one's family, one's peer group, or through media reports of suicide

sundowning Signs, symptoms, and behaviors of Alzheimer's disease (AD) increase during hours of darkness

supination Turning the joint upward

supine position The back-lying or dorsal recumbent position

suppository A cone-shaped, solid drug that is inserted into a body opening; it melts at body temperature

surveyor A person who collects information by observing and asking questions

symptoms See "subjective data"

system Formed by organs that work together to perform special functions

systolic pressure The pressure in the arteries when the heart contracts

T

tachypnea Rapid (*tachy*) breathing (*pnea*); respirations are more than 20 per minute

teamwork Staff members work together as a group; each person does his or her part to give safe and effective care

terminal illness An illness or injury from which the person will not likely recover

thermometer A device used to measure (*meter*) temperature (*thermo*)

tinnitus A ringing, roaring, hissing, or buzzing sound in the ears or head

tissue A group of cells with similar functions

transfer How a person moves to and from surfaces

transfer belt A device applied around the waist and used to support a person who is unsteady or disabled; gait belt

transient incontinence Temporary or occasional incontinence that is reversed when the cause is treated

treatment The care provided to maintain or restore health, improve function, or relieve symptoms

Trendelenburg's position The head of the bed is lowered and the foot of the bed is raised

tumor A new growth of abnormal cells that is benign or malignant

U

ulcer A shallow or deep crater-like sore of the skin or mucous membrane

uncircumcised The male has foreskin covering the head of the penis

urge incontinence The loss of urine in response to a sudden, urgent need to void; the person cannot get to a toilet in time; over-active bladder

urinary frequency Voiding at frequent intervals

urinary incontinence The involuntary loss or leakage of urine

urinary retention Not being able to completely empty the bladder

urinary urgency The need to void at once

urination The process of emptying urine from the bladder; voiding

V

vein A blood vessel that returns blood to the heart

verbal communication Communication that uses written or spoken words

vertigo Dizziness

vital signs Temperature, pulse, respirations, and blood pressure; and pain in some agencies

voiding See "urination"

vomitus The food and fluids expelled from the stomach through the mouth; emesis

vulnerable adult A person 18 years old or older who has a disability or condition that makes him or her at risk to be wounded, attacked, or damaged

W

withdrawal syndrome The physical and mental response after stopping or severely reducing the use of a substance that was used regularly

work ethics Behavior in the workplace

workplace violence Violent acts (including assault or threat of assault) directed toward persons at work or while on duty

wound A break in the skin or mucous membrane

Key Abbreviations

AD	Alzheimer's disease		**Hg**	Mercury
ADL	Activities of daily living		**HIPAA**	Health Insurance Portability and Accountability Act of 1996
AE	Anti-embolism; anti-embolic		**HIV**	Human immunodeficiency virus
AED	Automated external defibrillator			
AHA	American Heart Association		**IBD**	Inflammatory bowel disease
AIDS	Acquired immunodeficiency syndrome		**ID**	Identification
ALR	Assisted living residence		**I&O**	Intake and output
ALS	Amyotrophic lateral sclerosis		**IPV**	Intimate partner violence
AMD	Age-related macular degeneration		**IV**	Intravenous
ASL	American Sign Language			
			L/min	Liters per minute
BLS	Basic Life Support		**LPN**	Licensed practical nurse
BM; BMs	Bowel movement; bowel movements		**LVN**	Licensed vocational nurse
BP	Blood pressure			
BPD	Borderline personality disorder		**MDRO**	Multidrug-resistant organism
BPH	Benign prostatic hyperplasia		**MDS**	Minimum Data Set
			mg	Milligram
C	Centigrade		**MI**	Myocardial infarction
CAD	Coronary artery disease		**mL**	Milliliter
CDC	Centers for Disease Control and Prevention		**mL/hr**	Milliliters per hour
C. diff	*Clostridium difficile*		**mm**	Millimeter
CMS	Centers for Medicare & Medicaid Services		**mm Hg**	Millimeters of mercury
			MRSA	Methicillin-resistant *Staphylococcus aureus*
CNS	Central nervous system		**MS**	Multiple sclerosis
CO₂	Carbon dioxide		**MSD**	Musculo-skeletal disorder
COPD	Chronic obstructive pulmonary disease			
CPR	Cardiopulmonary resuscitation		**NATCEP**	Nursing assistant training and competency evaluation program
CVA	Cerebrovascular accident		**NCSBN**	National Council of State Boards of Nursing
DNR	Do Not Resuscitate		**NG**	Naso-gastric
DON	Director of nursing		**NIA**	National Institute on Aging
			NPO	Nothing per mouth; nothing by mouth
E. coli	*Escherichia coli*		**NPUAP**	National Pressure Ulcer Advisory Panel
EEOC	Equal Employment Opportunity Commission			
EHR	Electronic health record		**O₂**	Oxygen
EMR	Electronic medical record		**OBRA**	Omnibus Budget Reconciliation Act of 1987
EMS	Emergency Medical Services		**OCD**	Obsessive-compulsive disorder
EPHI; ePHI	Electronic protected health information		**OPIM**	Other potentially infectious materials
			OSHA	Occupational Safety and Health Administration
F	Fahrenheit		**oz**	Ounce
FBAO	Foreign-body airway obstruction			
FDA	Food and Drug Administration		**PASS**	*Pull* the safety pin, *aim* low, *squeeze* the lever, *sweep* back and forth
GI	Gastro-intestinal		**PHI**	Protected health information
gtt	Drops		**PPE**	Personal protective equipment
gtt/min	Drops per minute		**PROM**	Passive range of motion
			PTSD	Post-traumatic stress disorder
HAI	Healthcare-associated infection			
HBV	Hepatitis B virus			

RA	Rheumatoid arthritis
RACE	Rescue, alarm, confine, extinguish
RBC	Red blood cell
RN	Registered nurse
ROM	Range of motion; range-of-motion
RRT	Rapid Response Team
SCA	Sudden cardiac arrest
SDS	Safety data sheet
SNF	Skilled nursing facility
SpO₂	Saturation of peripheral oxygen (oxygen concentration)
STD	Sexually transmitted disease
TB	Tuberculosis
TIA	Transient ischemic attack
TJC	The Joint Commission
TPR	Temperature, pulse, and respirations

U/A	Urinalysis
USDA	United States Department of Agriculture
UTI	Urinary tract infection
VF; V-fib	Ventricular fibrillation
VRE	Vancomycin-resistant *Enterococci*
WBC	White blood cell

Index

Page numbers followed by "*f*" indicate figures, "*t*" indicate tables, and "*b*" indicate boxes.

567